# PLANNING HEALTH PROMOTION PROGRAMS

## AN INTERVENTION MAPPING APPROACH

### Fourth Edition

L. Kay Bartholomew Eldredge
Christine M. Markham
Robert A.C. Ruiter
María E. Fernández
Gerjo Kok
Guy S. Parcel

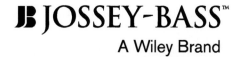

**JB** JOSSEY-BASS™

A Wiley Brand

Published by Jossey-Bass

A Wiley Brand

One Montgomery Street, Suite 1000, San Francisco, CA 94104-4594—www.josseybass.com

Jossey-Bass books and products are available through most bookstores. To contact Jossey-Bass directly call our Customer Care Department within the U.S. at 800-956-7739, outside the U.S. at 317-572-3986, or fax 317-572-4002.

Wiley publishes in a variety of print and electronic formats and by print-on-demand. Some material included with standard print versions of this book may not be included in e-books or in print-on-demand. If this book refers to media such as a CD or DVD that is not included in the version you purchased, you may download this material at http://booksupport.wiley.com. For more information about Wiley products, visit www.wiley.com.

**Library of Congress Cataloging-in-Publication Data**

Bartholomew Eldredge, L. Kay, author.
  Planning health promotion programs : an intervention mapping approach / L. Kay Bartholomew Eldredge,
Christine M. Markham, Robert A.C. Ruiter, Maria E. Fernandez, Gerjo Kok, Guy S. Parcel.
– Fourth edition.
      p. ; cm.
  Preceded by Planning health promotion programs / L. Kay Bartholomew ... [et al.]. 3rd ed. c2011.
  Includes bibliographical references and index.
  ISBN 978-1-119-03549-7 (cloth) ISBN 978-1-119-03556-5 (epdf)
  ISBN 978-1-119-03539-8 (epub)
  I. Title.
  [DNLM: 1. Health Promotion. 2. Evidence-Based Medicine. 3. Health Education. 4. Planning Techniques. 5. Program Development--methods. WA 590]
   RA427.8
   362.1–dc23                                            2015027299

Cover design: Wiley
Cover image: © Valenty/Shutterstock

Printed and bound by CPI Group (UK) Ltd, Croydon, CR0 4YY

FOURTH EDITION

*HB Printing* C9781119035497_141124

# CONTENTS

Figures and Tables . . . . . . . . . . . . . . . . . . . . . . . vii
Acknowledgments . . . . . . . . . . . . . . . . . . . . . . . xiii
About the Authors . . . . . . . . . . . . . . . . . . . . . . . xvii

**Part One:   Foundations                                          1**

**Chapter 1   Overview of Intervention Mapping** . . . . . . . . . . .3
Competency . . . . . . . . . . . . . . . . . . . . . . . . . . . 3
Perspectives . . . . . . . . . . . . . . . . . . . . . . . . . . 7
Intervention Mapping Steps . . . . . . . . . . . . . . . . . 12
Core Processes for Using Theory and Evidence . . . . . . . . 20
The Role of Culture in Intervention Planning . . . . . . . . . 28
Navigating the Book . . . . . . . . . . . . . . . . . . . . . 30
Important Repeating Concepts in the Book . . . . . . . . . . 31
Summary . . . . . . . . . . . . . . . . . . . . . . . . . . . 32
Discussion Questions and Learning Activities . . . . . . . . 38
References . . . . . . . . . . . . . . . . . . . . . . . . . . 39

**Chapter 2   Behavior-Oriented Theories Used in Health Promotion** . 57
Competency . . . . . . . . . . . . . . . . . . . . . . . . . . 57
Perspectives . . . . . . . . . . . . . . . . . . . . . . . . . . 58
Overview of Theories . . . . . . . . . . . . . . . . . . . . . 65
Learning Theories . . . . . . . . . . . . . . . . . . . . . . . 66
Theories of Information Processing . . . . . . . . . . . . . . 70
Theories of Health Behavior . . . . . . . . . . . . . . . . . 74
Theories of Reasoned Action . . . . . . . . . . . . . . . . . 78
Theories of Goal-Directed Behavior . . . . . . . . . . . . . 84
Theories of Automatic Behavior, Impulsive Behavior, and Habits . 89
Stage Theories . . . . . . . . . . . . . . . . . . . . . . . . 95
Attribution Theory and Relapse Prevention . . . . . . . . . . 99
Theories of Persuasive Communication . . . . . . . . . . . 101
Theories of Self-Regulation . . . . . . . . . . . . . . . . . 105
Social Cognitive Theory . . . . . . . . . . . . . . . . . . . 109
Theories of Stigma and Discrimination . . . . . . . . . . . . 113

Diffusion of Innovations Theory . . . . . . . . . . . . . . 116
Summary . . . . . . . . . . . . . . . . . . . . . . . . . 120
Discussion Questions and Learning Activities . . . . . . . . 120
References . . . . . . . . . . . . . . . . . . . . . . . 121

**Chapter 3   Environment-Oriented Theories** . . . . . . . . . . **145**
Competency . . . . . . . . . . . . . . . . . . . . . . . . 145
Perspectives . . . . . . . . . . . . . . . . . . . . . . . 146
General Environmental-Oriented Theories . . . . . . . . . . 149
Interpersonal-Level Theories . . . . . . . . . . . . . . . 155
Organizational-Level Theories . . . . . . . . . . . . . . . 160
Community-Level Theories . . . . . . . . . . . . . . . . . 167
Societal and Governmental Theories . . . . . . . . . . . . 184
Summary . . . . . . . . . . . . . . . . . . . . . . . . . 192
Discussion Questions and Learning Activities . . . . . . . . 192
References . . . . . . . . . . . . . . . . . . . . . . . 193

**Part Two:   Intervention Mapping Steps**                    **209**

**Chapter 4   Intervention Mapping Step 1: Logic Model
            of the Problem** . . . . . . . . . . . . . . . . **211**
Competency . . . . . . . . . . . . . . . . . . . . . . . . 211
Perspectives . . . . . . . . . . . . . . . . . . . . . . . 212
Tasks for Step 1 . . . . . . . . . . . . . . . . . . . . . 214
Summary . . . . . . . . . . . . . . . . . . . . . . . . . 261
Discussion Questions and Learning Activities . . . . . . . . 262
References . . . . . . . . . . . . . . . . . . . . . . . 263

**Chapter 5   Intervention Mapping Step 2: Program Outcomes
            and Objectives—Logic Model of Change** . . . . . . **283**
Competency . . . . . . . . . . . . . . . . . . . . . . . . 283
Perspectives . . . . . . . . . . . . . . . . . . . . . . . 284
Tasks for Step 2 . . . . . . . . . . . . . . . . . . . . . 286
Summary . . . . . . . . . . . . . . . . . . . . . . . . . 330
Discussion Questions and Learning Activities . . . . . . . . 331
References . . . . . . . . . . . . . . . . . . . . . . . 332

**Chapter 6   Intervention Mapping Step 3: Program Design** . . . . **345**
Competency . . . . . . . . . . . . . . . . . . . . . . . . 345
Deciding How to Start . . . . . . . . . . . . . . . . . . . 345
Perspectives . . . . . . . . . . . . . . . . . . . . . . . 350
Tasks for Step 3 . . . . . . . . . . . . . . . . . . . . . 355

Summary . . . . . . . . . . . . . . . . . . . . . 416

Discussion Questions and Learning Activities . . . . . . . . . 417

References . . . . . . . . . . . . . . . . . . . . 418

**Chapter 7   Intervention Mapping Step 4: Program Production . . 435**

Competency . . . . . . . . . . . . . . . . . . . . 435

Perspectives . . . . . . . . . . . . . . . . . . . . 436

Tasks for Step 4 . . . . . . . . . . . . . . . . . . 437

Summary . . . . . . . . . . . . . . . . . . . . . 475

Discussion Questions and Learning Activities . . . . . . . . . 475

References . . . . . . . . . . . . . . . . . . . . 476

**Chapter 8   Intervention Mapping Step 5: Program**
**              Implementation Plan . . . . . . . . . . . . . . 483**

Competency . . . . . . . . . . . . . . . . . . . . 483

Perspectives . . . . . . . . . . . . . . . . . . . . 484

Tasks for Step 5 . . . . . . . . . . . . . . . . . . 494

Summary . . . . . . . . . . . . . . . . . . . . . 528

Discussion Questions and Learning Activities . . . . . . . . . 529

References . . . . . . . . . . . . . . . . . . . . 530

**Chapter 9   Intervention Mapping Step 6: Evaluation Plan**
              with Patricia Dolan Mullen · · · · · · · · · · · · **541**

Competency . . . . . . . . . . . . . . . . . . . . 541

Perspectives . . . . . . . . . . . . . . . . . . . . 541

Tasks for Step 6 . . . . . . . . . . . . . . . . . . 546

Summary . . . . . . . . . . . . . . . . . . . . . 584

Discussion Questions and Learning Activities . . . . . . . . . 585

References . . . . . . . . . . . . . . . . . . . . 585

**Chapter 10  Using Intervention Mapping to Adapt**
**              Evidence-Based Interventions**
              with Linda Highfield, Marieke A. Hartman, Patricia Dolan
              Mullen, and Joanne N. Leerlooijer · · · · · · · · · · · **597**

Competency . . . . . . . . . . . . . . . . . . . . 597

Perspectives . . . . . . . . . . . . . . . . . . . . 598

Intervention Mapping for Adaptation . . . . . . . . . . . 603

Summary . . . . . . . . . . . . . . . . . . . . . 642

Discussion Questions and Learning Activities . . . . . . . . . 643

References . . . . . . . . . . . . . . . . . . . . 643

**Index                                                    651**

# FIGURES AND TABLES

## Figures

| | | |
|---|---|---|
| 1.1 | Intervention Mapping Steps | 13 |
| 1.2 | Logic Model of the Problem | 15 |
| 1.3 | Logic Model of Change | 16 |
| 2.1 | Logic Model for Methods, Determinants, Behaviors, Environmental Conditions, and Health | 62 |
| 4.1 | Logic Model of the Problem | 227 |
| 4.2 | Epilepsy PRECEDE Model | 234 |
| 4.3 | Integrating Qualitative and Quantitative Methods | 244 |
| 4.4 | It's Your Game PRECEDE Logic Model | 259 |
| 5.1 | Logic Model of Change | 285 |
| 5.2 | IYG Logic Model of Change | 320 |
| 6.1 | Intervention Logic Model | 348 |
| 6.2 | Schematic Representation of Shift in Environmental Levels | 349 |
| 6.3 | Cultivando La Salud | 358 |
| 6.4 | Developing Tailored Feedback | 366 |
| 7.1 | MINDSET Top Level Flow Diagram Depicting Data Input to Produce a Tailored Action Plan | 444 |
| 7.2 | Example Draft Screen Map Mock-Ups for MINDSET | 445 |
| 7.3 | Flowchart and Screen Maps Outlining the Data Input Process for MINDSET | 446 |
| 7.4 | Screen Maps Outlining the Generation of Tailored Decision Support Recommendations for MINDSET | 447 |
| 7.5 | Tasks for Producing a Print Piece | 461 |
| 7.6 | Tasks for Producing a Video | 462 |
| 7.7 | Activity Sequence for an It's Your Game Computer Lesson: Healthy Dating Relationships | 470 |
| 7.8 | Example of an It's Your Game Computer Lesson Tailored by Sexual Experience | 471 |
| 7.9 | Design Document for a *Reel World* Series | 472 |
| 7.10 | Example Role Play Activity From It's Your Game | 473 |
| 7.11 | It's Your Game Parent Newsletter (Sample Pages) | 474 |

7.12 Screen Captures Depicting Change Methods and Practical Applications From It's Your Game . . . Keep It Real Computer Activities  474

8.1 The EBI and Implementation Intervention Targets and Outcomes  487

9.1 Intervention Logic Model  547

9.2 Illustration of the PRECIS Criteria to Characterize Research Studies  572

9.3 IYG Intervention Logic Model for Evaluation  581

10.1 Adapting an Evidence-based Health Promotion Intervention  605

10.2 Logic Model of the Problem With Guiding Questions  606

10.3 Logic Model of Change With Guiding Questions  607

10.4 Parts of a Program  616

10.5 Case Study Logic Model of the Problem  632

10.6 Case Study Logic Model of Change  633

## Tables

1.1 Provisional List of Answers Regarding Condom Use Among Adolescents  22

1.2 Examples of Theories for Intervention Mapping Steps and Questions  25

1.3 Programs Developed Using Intervention Mapping  34

2.1 Examples of When to Use Theory in Intervention Planning  58

2.2 Theories Arrayed by Level  61

2.3 The Precaution-Adoption Process Model  97

3.1 A Comparison of Empowering Processes and Empowered Outcomes Across Levels of Analysis  154

3.2 Principles Underlying Effective Tactics  181

4.1 Questions to Guide Recruitment of Stakeholders  216

4.2 Group Facilitation Processes  219

4.3 Examples of Secondary Data Sources for Health, Behavior, Environment, and Quality-of-Life Description  247

4.4 Community Asset Assessment  252

5.1 Performance Objectives for Consistently and Correctly Using Condoms During Sexual Intercourse  296

5.2 Environmental Performance Objectives for the ToyBox-Study  299

5.3 Environmental Performance Objectives for T.L.L. Temple Foundation Stroke Project  300

5.4   Performance Objectives to Reduce Stigma and Promote
      HIV Testing                                              301
5.5   Performance Objectives for Condom Use Among HIV+
      Men Who Have Sex With Men (MSM) Using a Self-
      Regulatory Approach                                      303
5.6   Judging Importance of Determinants of Performance
      Objectives                                               307
5.7   Sample Matrix for Children in the Toy-Box Study          310
5.8   Sample of Rows From Matrices for Interpersonal and
      Organizational Environmental Change in the ToyBox-
      Study                                                    311
5.9   Examples of Cells From a Behavior Matrix: Consistently
      and Correctly Using Condoms During Sexual Intercourse    315
5.10  List of Action Words for Writing Change Objectives:
      Organized by Levels of Complexity of Learning Tasks      317
5.11  Examples of Cells From a Simulated Matrix to Address a
      Habitual Behavior                                        319
5.12  Behavioral Outcomes, Environmental Outcomes, and
      Performance Objectives for It's Your Game . . . Keep It
      Real                                                     323
5.13  Work on Determinants of Middle School Students'
      Choosing Not to Have Sex                                 324
5.14  Work on Determinants of Parents' Communication With
      Child                                                    325
5.15  Matrix for Behavioral Outcome: Student Chooses Not to
      Have Sex                                                 325
5.16  Matrix for Behavioral Outcome: Student has Healthy Rela-
      tionships With Friends, Girlfriends, or Boyfriends       327
5.17  Sample Cells for Matrix for Interpersonal Environmen-
      tal Outcome: Parent Communicates With Child About
      Dating and Sexual Health Topics                          328
6.1   Scope and Sequence of the T.L.L. Temple Foundation
      Stroke Project                                           359
6.2   Communication Channels and Vehicles                      361
6.3   Examples of Objectives and Methods for Changing Aware-
      ness and Risk Perception                                 371
6.4   Examples of Objectives and Methods at Various Levels     373
6.5   Basic Methods at the Individual Level                    376
6.6   Methods to Increase Knowledge                            381
6.7   Methods to Change Awareness and Risk Perception          382
6.8   Methods to Change Habitual, Automatic, and Impulsive
      Behaviors                                                383

6.9   Methods to Change Attitudes, Beliefs, and Outcome
      Expectations                                                    385
6.10  Methods to Change Social Influence                              387
6.11  Methods to Change Skills, Capability, and Self-Efficacy
      and to Overcome Barriers                                        388
6.12  Methods to Reduce Public Stigma                                 391
6.13  Basic Methods for Change of Environmental Conditions            392
6.14  Methods to Change Social Norms                                  393
6.15  Methods to Change Social Support and Social Networks            394
6.16  Methods to Change Organizations                                 395
6.17  Methods to Change Communities                                   396
6.18  Methods to Change Policy                                        398
6.19  Methods and Applications for Emergency Department
      Matrices in the T.L.L. Temple Foundation Stroke Project         408
6.20  Scope and Sequence for It's Your Game . . . Keep It Real        411
6.21  Sample of Methods and Applications for Students From
      It's Your Game . . . Keep It Real                               414
6.22  Sample of Methods and Applications for Parents From It's
      Your Game . . . Keep It Real                                    415
7.1   Design Document Highlights From the T.L.L. Temple
      Foundation Stroke Project—Community Component
      Materials                                                       442
7.2   Additional Design Document Details for the Stroke Project       443
7.3   Suitability Assessment of Materials Rationale                   450
7.4   Pretesting and Pilot-Testing Purposes and Methods              466
8.1   Examples of Change Objectives From the Peace of Mind
      Program                                                         515
8.2   Peace of Mind Program Implementation Intervention Plan          517
8.3   It's Your Game . . . Keep It Real: Matrices of Change
      Objectives for Implementation                                   520
8.4   It's Your Game . . . Keep It Real: Methods, Practical Appli-
      cations, and Program Materials to Enhance Program
      Implementation                                                  527
9.1   Evaluation Stakeholders                                         544
9.2   Evaluation of a School HIV Prevention Program                   551
9.3   Process Evaluation Questions for a Program to Increase
      Colorectal Cancer Screening (CRCS) Among
      U.S. Veterans                                                   554
9.4   Diabetes Program Performance Standards                          555
9.5   Hypothetical Process Evaluation of Diabetes Counseling
      Program                                                         556
9.6   Comparison of Domains of Asthma Knowledge                       563

9.7   Evaluation Plan Summary: School AIDS Prevention
      Program                                                          578
9.8   Partial Evaluation Plan for It's Your Game . . . Keep It Real
      (IYG)                                                            582
10.1  Terms for Thinking About Evidence                               610
10.2  Websites for Full EBIs and General Intervention Strategies      612
10.3  Adaptation "To-Do List" for Telephone-Counseling
      Program                                                          619
10.4  Examples From the Design Document Template for the
      Telephone-Counseling Program                                    622

# ACKNOWLEDGMENTS

Our thanks to colleagues who contributed to chapters and provided case studies in the fourth edition.

Rik Crutzen, PhD, is assistant professor at the Department of Health Promotion, Maastricht University, the Netherlands. He also serves as an honorary principal research fellow in behavior change at the Centre for Technology Enabled Health Research (CTEHR), Coventry University, United Kingdom. The overarching theme of his research is how technological innovations can be used in the field of public health to optimize the impact of these innovations. He contributed to Chapters 6 and 7.

Nell H. Gottlieb, PhD, is emeritus professor of health education in the Department of Kinesiology and Health Education at the University of Texas at Austin and formerly was professor of behavioral sciences at the School of Public Health, University of Texas Health Science Center at Houston. Dr. Gottlieb received her PhD degree in medical sociology from Boston University. Her interests are in multilevel health promotion intervention development and evaluation. Dr. Gottlieb is pursuing a second career as an artist; however, her work on this Intervention Mapping text over the years is apparent in all chapters.

Marieke A. Hartman, PhD, is a postdoctoral research fellow (sponsored by the U.S. National Cancer Institute) in health promotion and behavioral sciences at the University of Texas Health Science Center at Houston (UTHealth) School of Public Health. Her research interests are in bridging public health/health promotion research and practice through community-based dissemination and implementation research. She has used Intervention Mapping to adapt and evaluate theory- and evidence-based interventions for culturally diverse populations. She contributed to Chapters 9 and 10.

Linda Highfield, PhD, is assistant professor of management, policy, and community health at the UTHealth School of Public Health. Dr. Highfield holds a PhD in epidemiology from Texas A&M University and spent five years as the director of research for the Episcopal Health Charities prior to joining the faculty at UTHealth. Dr. Highfield's research interests include geospatial analysis methods and translation of evidence-based interventions to real-world settings. Her current work focuses on improving access to mammography screening for underserved women. She contributed to Chapters 4, 8, and 10.

Joanne N. Leerlooijer, PhD, received her PhD from Maastricht University and is now with the Division of Human Nutrition, Wageningen University, the Netherlands. She has supported organizations in various countries in Africa and Asia in health promotion planning using Intervention Mapping. She has developed training, tools, and guidelines to make Intervention Mapping a practical framework for nonacademic organizations that promote sexual and reproductive health and rights of young people. She contributed to Chapter 10.

Patricia Dolan Mullen, DrPH, MLS, is a distinguished teaching professor and president's scholar for teaching, health promotion, and behavioral sciences, UTHealth School of Public Health. She designed and taught the School's program evaluation and systematic review courses. She has served on many expert panels, including the U.S. Community Preventive Services Task Force. Her current research interests include promoting the use of evidence-based programs and policy, especially cancer prevention and preconception counseling. She has developed programs to help practitioners identify, select, and adapt evidence-based programs. She contributed to Chapters 9 and 10.

Melissa Peskin, PhD, associate professor of health promotion and behavioral sciences and epidemiology at the UTHealth School of Public Health, is an expert in the development, implementation, and evaluation of adolescent sexual health promotion interventions. She is lead author for the iCHAMPSS case study.

Serena Rodriguez, MA, MPH, is a PhD candidate in health promotion and behavioral sciences at the UTHealth School of Public Health, and has taught Intervention Mapping. She contributed to Chapter 10 and to referencing and editing the entire book.

Diane Santa Maria, DrPH, MSN, RN, assistant professor at the UTHealth School of Nursing, contributed examples of the application of Intervention Mapping in clinical settings for each of the Intervention Mapping step chapters.

Herman Schaalma, PhD (1960–2009), was associate professor of social psychology at Maastricht University, the Netherlands. He held the Dutch AIDS Fund–endowed chair for AIDS prevention and health promotion with a special focus on the development of culturally sensitive prevention programs. He received his doctorate in health sciences from Maastricht University. His research applied psychology to understanding and predicting behavior, carefully specifying health promotion goals and objectives, developing innovative health promotion interventions, and promoting the adoption and implementation of health promotion programs.

Dr. Schaalma's contributions to Intervention Mapping over the years continue to be apparent in all chapters of the book.

Ross Shegog, PhD, associate professor, health promotion and behavioral sciences, UTHealth School of Public Health, is an expert in the development of technology-based health promotion interventions for chronic disease management and adolescent health. He is lead author on the MINDSET case study and contributed examples from MINDSET to Chapters 4 and 7. He also contributed a section on eHealth applications in Chapter 6.

Andrew Springer, DrPH, assistant professor, health promotion and behavioral sciences, UTHealth School of Public Health (Austin Regional Campus), has expertise in community-based participatory research methods to develop, implement, and evaluate interventions to enhance physical activity and nutrition among children. He contributed to Chapter 4.

Maartje M. van Stralen, PhD, assistant professor, prevention and public health, Faculty of Earth and Life Sciences, Vrije University Amsterdam, the Netherlands, is an expert in the development, implementation, and evaluation of interventions promoting exercise and other energy balance–related behaviors associated with overweight and obesity. She is the lead author of the Active *plus* case study.

Susan Tortolero Emery, PhD, Professor, health promotion and behavioral sciences and epidemiology at the UTHealth School of Public Health, is a codeveloper with Christine Markham, Ross Shegog, and Melissa Peskin of It's Your Game . . . Keep It Real, which is presented as a case study example in each of the Intervention Mapping step chapters.

Melissa Valerio, PhD, MPH, is associate professor and regional dean of the San Antonio Regional Campus at the UTHealth School of Public Health. Dr. Valerio coteaches Intervention Mapping to master's and doctoral students and has applied the methods to multiple studies to address chronic disease in vulnerable populations in Detroit, Michigan, and the Central and South Texas region. Her research focuses on addressing health literacy in her interventions, with a specific focus on cognitive understanding and processing of self-management regimens and patient/provider communication. She contributed to Chapter 7.

An instructor's supplement, which includes case studies, Power-Point lecture slides, and student assessments, is available at http://www.wiley.com/go/bartholomew4e. Please follow the URL and select the link for "Companion Site" in the "For Instructors" box. You will be instructed to sign-up and then a Wiley representative will contact you and provide you with access to the site. Additional materials, such as videos, podcasts, and readings, can be found at www.josseybasspublichealth.com. Comments about this book are invited and can be sent to publichealth@wiley.com.

**L. Kay Bartholomew Eldredge**, EdD, MPH, is professor and distinguished teaching professor, health promotion and behavioral sciences, and associate dean for academic affairs at the UTHealth School of Public Health. Dr. Bartholomew has worked in the field of health education and health promotion since her graduation from Austin College in 1974, first at a city-county health department and later at Texas Children's Hospital and Baylor College of Medicine. She teaches courses in health promotion intervention development and conducts research in chronic disease self-management. Dr. Bartholomew received her MPH degree from the UTHealth School of Public Health and an EdD degree in educational psychology from the University of Houston College of Education.

**Christine M. Markham** is associate professor and associate department chair of health promotion and behavioral sciences, and associate director, Center for Health Promotion and Prevention Research, at the UTHealth School of Public Health. Her research focuses on child and adolescent health, with an emphasis on sexual and reproductive health, dating violence prevention, and chronic disease management. She received her master's degree in anthropology from the University of Pennsylvania and her PhD in behavioral sciences from the UTHealth School of Public Health. She has been instrumental in demonstrating the use of Intervention Mapping as an effective approach for adapting existing programs to meet the needs of a new population and has taught Intervention Mapping in the United States and the Netherlands.

**Robert A. C. Ruiter**, PhD, is professor of applied psychology with a special interest in the application of neuroscience in applied social psychology (endowed chair) and head of the Department of Work and Social Psychology at the Faculty of Psychology and Neuroscience, Maastricht University, the Netherlands. He obtained his MPH degree in 1995 with specializations in health education and health policy and management and his PhD in psychology, both at Maastricht University. Dr. Ruiter combines laboratory-based research in the working mechanisms of persuasion with applied research in the development of behavior change interventions using Intervention Mapping in the domains of public health and traffic safety. Topics include vaccination, HIV/AIDS, maternal health, and risky decision making in adolescents in both national and international research collaborations.

**María E. Fernández**, PhD, is professor, health promotion and behavioral sciences, at the UTHealth School of Public Health. She is associate director for the Center for Health Promotion and Prevention Research, where she leads cancer control and chronic disease research and health promotion efforts. Her research focus is the reduction of health disparities, the development and evaluation of cancer control interventions for low-income and minority populations, the use of technology for health promotion, and implementation and dissemination science. Since the mid-1990s Dr. Fernández has contributed to the refinement of Intervention Mapping through her teaching and use of the framework.

**Gerjo Kok**, PhD, is former dean and professor of applied psychology, Faculty of Psychology and Neuroscience, Maastricht University, the Netherlands. A social psychologist, he received his doctorate in social sciences from the University of Groningen, the Netherlands. From 1984 to 1998 he was professor of health education at Maastricht University. He held the Dutch AIDS Fund–endowed professorship for AIDS prevention and health promotion from 1992 to 2004. His main interest is in the application of social psychological theory to health promotion behavior, energy conservation, traffic safety, and the prevention of stigmatization.

**Guy S. Parcel**, PhD, is dean emeritus and former professor, health promotion and behavioral sciences, at the UTHealth School of Public Health. Dr. Parcel has authored or coauthored over 200 scientific papers and book chapters over the past 40 years. He has directed research projects funded by the National Institutes of Health and the Centers for Disease Control and Prevention to develop and evaluate programs to address sexual risk behavior in adolescents, diet and physical activity in children, smoking prevention in adolescents, and self-management of childhood chronic diseases, including asthma and cystic fibrosis. Dr. Parcel received his BS and MS degrees in health education at Indiana University and his PhD at Pennsylvania State University with a major in health education and a minor in child development and family relations.

# PART ONE

# FOUNDATIONS

# CHAPTER 1

# OVERVIEW OF INTERVENTION MAPPING

## Competency

• Choose and use a systematic approach to planning health promotion programs.

In this chapter we present the perspectives underlying Intervention Mapping and a preview of the program-planning framework. The purpose of Intervention Mapping is to provide health promotion program planners with a framework for effective decision making at each step in intervention planning, implementation, and evaluation. Health promotion has been defined as combinations of educational, political, regulatory, and organizational supports for behavior and environmental changes that are conducive to health (Green & Kreuter, 2005), and health education is a subset of health promotion applications that are primarily based on education. This book uses the terms *health educator, health promoter,* and *program planner* interchangeably to mean someone who is planning an intervention meant to produce health outcomes. One difficulty which planners may encounter is that of knowing exactly how to create health promotion or education programs that are based on theory, empirical findings from the literature, and data collected from a population. Existing literature, appropriate theories, and additional research data are basic tools for any health educator, but often it is unclear how and where these tools should be used in program planning. In Intervention Mapping, these tools are systematically applied in each step of program development.

**LEARNING OBJECTIVES AND TASKS**

• Explain the rationale for a systematic approach to intervention development

• Describe ecological and systems approaches to intervention development

• Explain the causal logic of public health problems and solutions

• List the steps, tasks, and processes of Intervention Mapping

• Explain how to use theory and evidence in intervention development

## BOX 1.1. MAYOR'S PROJECT

Imagine a health promoter in a city health department. The city's mayor, who has recently received strong criticism for inattention to a number of critical health issues, has now announced that a local foundation has agreed to work with the city to provide funding to address health issues. Youth violence, childhood obesity, adolescent smoking, and other substance abuse as well as the high incidence of HIV/AIDS are among the many issues competing for the mayor's attention. Not only does the allocated sum of money represent a gross underestimation of what is needed to address these issues, but also the city council is strongly divided on which health issue should receive priority. Council members do agree, however, that to dilute effort among the different issues would be a questionable decision, likely resulting in little or no impact on any single issue. As a response to increasing pressures, the mayor makes a bold political move and invites stakeholders who have advocated for these health issues and others to work with the health department to decide on the issue that should be chosen and to build and implement an intervention. The mayor agrees to help secure yearly funds, contingent on the project's effectiveness in producing significant, measurable improvements in the chosen issue at the end of each fiscal year.

The health promoter is to be the project lead from the city health department. Although she is apprehensive about the professional challenge as well as the complications inherent in facilitating a highly visible, political project, the health promoter feels encouraged by the prospect of working with community and public health leaders and is energized by the possibilities in the new project.

The first step the health promoter takes is to put together the planning group for the project. She considers the stakeholders concerned with health in the city. These are individuals, groups, or other entities that can affect or be affected by whatever project is chosen. She develops a list of community, health services, and public health leaders and invites these individuals to an initial meeting where they will discuss the project and make plans to expand this core group. She uses a "snowball" approach whereby each attendee suggests other community members who may be interested in this project. The superintendent of schools begins the process by suggesting interested parents, teachers, and administrators. After the first meeting, the health educator has a list of 25 people to invite to join the planning group.

Twenty-five people is a lot for one group, and the project lead knows that this multifaceted group will have to develop a common vocabulary and understanding, work toward consensus to make decisions, maintain respect during conflicts, and involve additional people through-out the community in the process. Members must be engaged, create working groups, believe that the effort is a partnership and not an involuntary mandate, and work toward sustainability of the project (Becker, Israel, & Allen, 2005; Cavanaugh & Cheney, 2002; Economos & Irish-Hauser, 2007; Faridi, Grunbaum, Gray, Franks, & Simoes, 2007).

The composition of the city's planning group is diverse, and group members are spurred by the mayor's challenge and enthusiastic to contribute their expertise. With this early momentum, the group devotes several weeks to a needs assessment, guided by the PRECEDE model (Green

& Kreuter, 1999). The members consider the various quality-of-life issues relevant to each of the health problems, the segments of the population affected by each issue, associated environmental and behavioral risk factors for each health problem, and determinants of the risk factors.

Planning group members recognize the importance of all of the health issues discussed by the group, and they want to work with community members to ascertain what problem might be most relevant to the community and most feasible to address. Even though the planning group comprises many segments of the city's leadership, health sector, and neighborhoods, the members realize that they do not have a deep enough understanding of what health problems might be of most relevance in their community. A subgroup takes on the role of community liaison to meet with members of various communities within the city to discuss health problems. The community liaison group wants to understand community members' perceptions of their needs, but it is equally concerned with understanding the strengths of the communities and their unique potential contributions to a partnership to tackle a health problem. The subgroup invites members of each interested neighborhood to join the planning group. Jointly, the planning group, the communities, and the funders agree to select a problem as the focus of an intervention. The health promoter knows that with a group this large she will have to strategize about using smaller work groups for different tasks. However, knowing the history of the city and the feeling of some stakeholder groups that they are often excluded from initiatives, she welcomes all interested participants.

The group's initial work on the needs assessment identifies childhood obesity as an important problem, one that the community members could agree to work on, and one that disproportionately affects lower-income and minority children. This initial work facilitates group cohesion and cultivates even greater enthusiasm about generating a solution for the health problem; however, despite the considerable needs assessment work that remains to be done (see Mayor's Project, Chapter 4), several members of the group even begin to imagine the victory that would be had if the group were to produce a change in half the allotted time because so much of the needed background information has already been gathered. The project lead knows that there remains a lot of work to be done but is comfortable with the group's enthusiasm as well as their pace and productivity. Once the group decides which issue to address, it faces the challenge of moving to the program-planning phase. In her previous work the health promoter used Intervention Mapping to develop programs and felt fairly confident about scheduling the first planning meeting devoted specifically to intervention.

What the health promoter hasn't anticipated is that in the course of conducting the initial part of the needs assessment, each group member independently began to conceive of the next step in the planning process as well as to visualize the kind of intervention that would be most suitable to address the problem. The day of the meeting arrives, and on the agenda is a discussion of how the group should begin program planning. What follows is a snapshot of dialogue from the planning group that illustrates several differing perspectives.

*School Board Member:* As we see from the work of our community liaison group, parents are concerned about obesity in children. According to community development techniques, we have to start where the people are. I think we should begin by conducting a series of focus groups with parents and have them tell us what to do.

*City Council Representative:* But we also heard a lot about the barriers to eating good food and exercising. Some of these barriers are environmental. I think we ought to develop a program for the Department of Parks and Recreation.

*Community Member Parent:* Well, I think a school-based program is most important. Our children need to learn what to eat.

*Community Member/Teacher:* Yes, children do have a role. Helping children make nutritious choices is important, but what about the quality of food they are served at home and in the schools?

*Community Agency Participant:* I think the program should focus on excess television watching and sedentary behavior. All community members just need to get up and move!

*Parks and Recreation Representative:* We are talking about one dimension of the problem at a time. This is a very big, very complicated problem. How will we ever address everything? Maybe it is just too big. Maybe we need to take on a simpler problem.

*Religious Leader:* Well, it is big. Maybe we will need an agency coordinator. I say we find a nonprofit group to serve as a community coordinating center from which various interventions and services can be implemented. That way, programs are sustainable and a variety of activities can be offered.

*Youth Club Board Member:* One of the national obesity programs has great brochures and videos—in three languages. We have numerous testimonials from kids, teachers, and parents about how motivated they were by these interventions. This approach is quick and easy; it's low cost; and I've already made sure we can get the materials. Plus, if the materials come from a national center, they must be effective.

*Community Member:* But, are those materials really powerful enough? It seems like a problem as complex as obesity would have to be addressed in many different ways. For example, what about the food service providers in schools? I think we have to think more carefully about how to address the many factors that may be causing this problem and making it hard to solve.

*Health Care Provider:* We know it takes more than learning information to change behavior. We have to address factors such as attitudes and self-efficacy. But how do we measure a change in attitudes? I think we should measure behavior directly.

*Educator:* Well, clearly we have to begin by designing a curriculum. What are our learning objectives?

The health promoter is worried but undeterred by the cacophony of comments about program development. She is prepared to lead group members through a series of systematic steps to construct the intervention and realizes that the group could work through their differences in the process. She is pleased to have a group with so much cumulative experience. The planning group decides to complete the needs assessment by organizing the information about obesity using an effective model that has been applied to many health issues (Green & Kreuter, 2005). (See Intervention Mapping [IM] Step 1, Chapter 4.) The members agree to take an ecological perspective, that is, the belief that most health problems are multidetermined and that one must intervene at individual, organizational, community, and societal levels to resolve a problem (Kok, Gottlieb, Commers, & Smerecnik, 2008). But, as the group dialogue indicates, each group member brought a different set of experiences and training to the meeting. This is a common experience in group activities. Each member makes an important and relevant contribution worthy of consideration in the creation of the intervention. To help the group move to solutions to the problem that they describe in the needs assessment, they will specify behavior and environmental conditions that should change and also the determinants of the desired change (IM Step 2, Chapter 5); design an intervention, including theory- and evidence-based change methods and applications (IM Step 3, Chapter 6); produce a deliverable program (IM Step 4, Chapter 7) and specify how it will be implemented (IM Step 5, Chapter 8); and make plans for program evaluation (IM Step 6, Chapter 9).

## Perspectives

Intervention Mapping is a planning approach that is based on using theory and evidence as foundations for taking an ecological approach to assessing and intervening in health problems and engendering community participation.

## Theory and Evidence

We agree with Kurt Lewin's adage that nothing is as useful as a good theory (Hochbaum, Sorenson, & Lorig, 1992). The use of theory is necessary in evidence-informed health promotion to ensure that we can describe and address the factors that cause health problems and the methods to achieve change. Teachers of health promotion and education suggest that the field would be well served with better guidance in how to use theory to understand health and social problems (DiClemente, Salazar, & Crosby, 2011; Glanz & Bishop, 2010; Glanz, Rimer, & Viswanath, 2015; Jones &

Donovan, 2004). In the text, we address this need by providing guidance on the how-to of theory selection and use (Brug, Oenema, & Ferreira, 2005).

In Intervention Mapping we use theory from a problem-driven perspective. Program planners, even those who are primarily researchers, often approach theory in a way that is fundamentally different from either theory generation or single theory-testing. A person who wants to find a solution to a public health problem has a different task from one who wants to create or test a theory. In practice, problem-driven, applied behavioral or social science may use one theory or multiple theories, empirical evidence, and new research to assess a problem and to solve or prevent a problem. In this approach, the main focus is on problem solving, and the criteria for success are formulated as outcomes related to the problem. Contributions to theory development may be quite useful, but they are peripheral to the problem-solving process.

Choices have to be made when developing an intervention, and theories are one tool to enable planners to make better choices. Health promotion planners are likely to bring multiple theoretical and experiential perspectives to a problem rather than to define a practice or research agenda around a specific theoretical approach. To understand a problem, the planning team begins with a question about a specific health or social problem (Buunk & Van Vugt, 2013; Ruiter, Massar, Van Vugt, & Kok, 2012). The team then accesses social and behavioral science theories and research evidence of causation of the health problem and its behavioral and environmental contributors. Causal theories help describe the health problem and its causes. Change theories suggest approaches to problem solutions. The planner then proceeds to gather evidence for the factors theory suggests. By the term *evidence,* we mean not only data from research studies as represented in the scientific literature but also the opinion and experience of community members and planners. In this way, theoretical and empirical evidence is brought to bear on meeting a health or social need. Intervention Mapping provides a detailed framework for this process.

## Ecological Models and Systems Thinking

The social ecological model, an underpinning for Intervention Mapping, has been used extensively in health promotion and is consonant with and encompassed by systems thinking (Kok et al., 2008; *American Journal of Community Psychology,* 2007; McLeroy, 2006; National Cancer Institute, 2007; Trochim, Cabrera, Milstein, Gallagher, & Leischow, 2006). In the social ecological model, health is a function of individuals and of the environments in which individuals live, including family, social networks, organizations, communities, and societies (Berkman, Kawachi, & Glymour, 2014; Crosby, Salazar, & DiClemente, 2011; Marmot, 2000; Richard, Gauvin, & Raine, 2011; Stokols, 1996).

A system is activities, actors, and settings that are affected by or affect a certain problem situation (Foster-Fishman, Nowell, & Yang, 2007). Using a systems perspective to assess the needs and strengths of the population; to understand a health problem and its causes; to form a group of stakeholders to plan, conduct, and disseminate an intervention; and to select the most effective leverage points to address a health-related problem can increase the effectiveness of planning. In particular, planners should understand that interventions are events in systems and that other factors within a system can reinforce or dampen the influence of an intervention on the specific behavior or environmental change being targeted (Hawe, Shiell, & Riley, 2009). See Chapter 3.

The social ecological paradigm focuses on the interrelationships between individuals (biological, psychological, and behavioral characteristics) and their environments. These environments include physical, social, and cultural aspects that exist across the individual's life domains and social settings. A nested structure of environments allows for multiple influences both within levels and across levels. Throughout the book, we have adopted the approach of D. G. Simons-Morton, B. G. Simons-Morton, Parcel, and Bunker (1988) of looking at agents (decision makers or role actors) at each ecological level: interpersonal (e.g., parents), organizational (e.g., managers of school food services), community (e.g., newspaper editors), or societal (e.g., legislators). Interventions at the various levels focus on agents (individuals or groups, such as boards or committees) in positions to exercise control over aspects of the environment. For example, adolescent uptake of smoking might be influenced by peers and parents at the interpersonal level of environment and by regulations and access at the social and community levels of environment. The picture that emerges is a complex web or system of causation as well as a rich context for intervention.

We present, as a beginning point, a template for simple, linear logic models focusing on the presumed cause-effect pathways related to health problems and their solutions articulated from theory and empirical research (Bartholomew & Mullen, 2011). See Chapter 4. However, we encourage the reader to adapt the logic model template to the complexity of the problem being analyzed, and we assume that the intervention, the system activity being targeted, and the proposed outcome are part of a complex multilevel system. An intervention at one environmental level can influence causal factors at multiple levels. For example, a program to conduct health-related lobbying may influence a legislative behavior (passing laws) that may influence individual health behavior. In illustration, one of our colleagues worked with a coalition in a large metropolitan area to use media and social advocacy to influence the police department and the U.S. Department of Labor to crack down on the use of young Hispanic children as dancers in bars and nightclubs (an activity that can lead to such health risk behaviors as substance abuse and prostitution). Once policy-level change occurred, parents expressed more resolve to manage their children.

## Participation in Health Promotion Planning

All health promotion program development, implementation, and evaluation should be based on broad participation of community members (Israel et al., 2008; Krieger et al., 2002; Minkler, 2004, 2005; Minkler, Thompson, Bell, Rose, & Redman, 2002; Wallerstein & Duran, 2006; Yoo et al., 2004). Inclusive community participation helps ensure that program focus reflects concerns for the local community. Broad participation can bring a greater breadth of skills, knowledge, and expertise to a project and can improve external validity of interventions and evaluation by recognition of the local knowledge of community members and practitioners (Israel, Schulz, Parker, & Becker, 1998; Israel et al., 2008). Green and Mercer (2001) also suggested that evidence-based health promotion interventions may be more acceptable to communities and potential participants when the research that has produced the evidence does not originate under special circumstances in distant places. In a discussion of environmental health promotion, Kreuter, De Rosa, Howze, and Baldwin (2004) described community participation as particularly important for

> "wicked problems" wherein stakeholders may have conflicting interpretations of the problem and the science behind it, as well as different values, goals and life experiences. Accordingly, policy makers, public health professionals, and other stakeholders who grapple with these problems cannot expect to effectively resolve them by relying solely on expert-driven approaches to problem solving. (p. 441)

Planners can benefit greatly by applying principles for facilitating participatory action and partnerships suggested by Israel and colleagues (1998, 2008) and used by others to evaluate community-based participatory program efforts (Belansky, Cutforth, Chavez, Waters, & Bartlett-Horch, 2011; Horn, McCracken, Dino, & Brayboy, 2008; Israel et al., 2005 (see Chapter 4). Their principles are to:

- Recognize a partner community as a unit of identity
- Build upon community strengths and resources
- Facilitate collaborative, equitable decision making in which partners negotiate desired roles in all project phases and attend to social inequalities
- Foster colearning among partners
- Balance knowledge generation with community benefit

- Focus on ecological perspectives, local problems, and multiple determinants of health
- Develop systems using an iterative process
- Disseminate information, results, and benefits to all partners
- Develop a commitment and long-term process

## Ethical Practice of Health Promotion

A systematic, thoughtful planning process can provide part of the road map required to establish ethical health promotion practice. Kass (2001) has presented a framework for evaluation of public health programs against standards of ethical integrity as have the American Association of Public Health (Thomas, Sage, Dillenberg, & Guillory, 2002) and the World Health Organization (World Health Organization, 2011). The Society for Public Health Education (SOPHE) has developed specific ethical and professional guidelines for public health educators (Society for Public Health Education, n.d.). Combined, these sources suggest the following guidelines for intervention:

- Program goals should always be related to the health of the public. Furthermore, health educators should be proactive in confronting issues that can adversely affect health of persons and communities and should provide services equitably. Intervention Mapping supports this principle by directing planners to focus on health issues and to begin planning with a full appraisal of the health problem and its causes.

- Interventions should be based on thorough evidence to increase the chance of effectiveness. Intervention Mapping supports this principle by basing programs on clear evidence of effectiveness. The Intervention Mapping steps help planners systematically consider the following types of evidence: importance, causes (including behavior and environment), and consequences of the health problem; effective approaches to behavioral and environmental change; and useful approaches to implementation. Kass (2001) suggested that when our programs are based only on the most intuitively "obvious" assumptions, we are at the most risk of developing programs that do not work.

- Development of interventions should include diverse participation. As the SOPHE suggested, Intervention Mapping directs planners to involve communities in program development and implementation, consider and accommodate diverse perspectives and values in program development, encourage informed decision making among individuals, and be transparent in disclosure of all program aspects, including benefits, other outcomes, unexpected consequences, and burdens.

- Intervention planners should consider the rights of persons and take action to protect them. Furthermore, public health practitioners are expected to support the worth, dignity, and uniqueness of all people and ground their practice in the ethical principles of respect for autonomy, promotion of social justice, promotion of good, and avoidance of harm. They must address the known and potential burdens of the program, including risks to privacy and confidentiality, liberty, self-determination, and justice.

Intervention Mapping suggests that planners consider burdens to participants and minimize them by adopting alternate approaches.

The emphasis on participation helps ensure that communities have input into judgments about tolerable levels of intervention and evaluation burden as well as an acceptable balance of burden-to-risk based on community values. Members of communities will not necessarily agree on risks and benefits, and a participatory planning process enables disclosure, discussion, consensus, and plans for moving forward through disagreement. Another way that the Intervention Mapping approach helps protect against inequitable burden is the focus on an ecological approach to both problem analysis and intervention. Most problems have contributions from the at-risk group or persons with the problem and from factors and agents in the environment. All significant contributors to the problem should comprise the focus for interventions, and planners should avoid the temptation to blame the victim by burdening the persons with the problem with full responsibility for its solution.

## Intervention Mapping Steps

Each step of Intervention Mapping comprises several tasks (Figure 1.1). The completion of the tasks included in a step creates a product that is the guide for the subsequent step. Completion of all steps creates a blueprint for designing, implementing, and evaluating an intervention based on a foundation of theoretical, empirical, and practical information. Even though Intervention Mapping describes six steps, the process is iterative rather than completely linear. Program developers move back and forth between tasks and steps as they gain new information and perspective. However, the process is also cumulative; planners base each step on the previous steps, and inattention to a step can jeopardize the potential effectiveness of the intervention by compromising the validity of the foundation on which later steps are conducted. Sometimes planners can get carried away by momentum in the process of the planning group and forget a step, or they may perform a step with less-than-optimal rigor. Fortunately, most of the time planners can backtrack and include, repeat, or elaborate on a neglected step.

| STEP | TASKS |
|---|---|

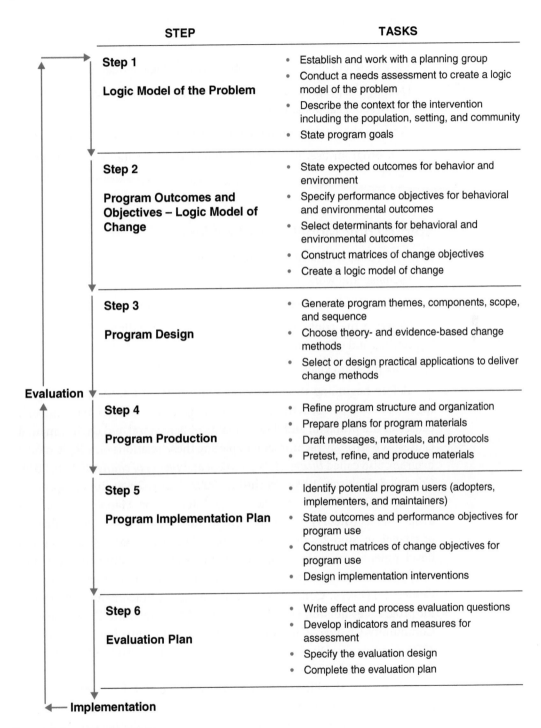

**Step 1**

**Logic Model of the Problem**

- Establish and work with a planning group
- Conduct a needs assessment to create a logic model of the problem
- Describe the context for the intervention including the population, setting, and community
- State program goals

**Step 2**

**Program Outcomes and Objectives – Logic Model of Change**

- State expected outcomes for behavior and environment
- Specify performance objectives for behavioral and environmental outcomes
- Select determinants for behavioral and environmental outcomes
- Construct matrices of change objectives
- Create a logic model of change

**Step 3**

**Program Design**

- Generate program themes, components, scope, and sequence
- Choose theory- and evidence-based change methods
- Select or design practical applications to deliver change methods

**Step 4**

**Program Production**

- Refine program structure and organization
- Prepare plans for program materials
- Draft messages, materials, and protocols
- Pretest, refine, and produce materials

**Step 5**

**Program Implementation Plan**

- Identify potential program users (adopters, implementers, and maintainers)
- State outcomes and performance objectives for program use
- Construct matrices of change objectives for program use
- Design implementation interventions

**Step 6**

**Evaluation Plan**

- Write effect and process evaluation questions
- Develop indicators and measures for assessment
- Specify the evaluation design
- Complete the evaluation plan

Evaluation

Implementation

**Figure 1.1** Intervention Mapping Steps

The six steps of the Intervention Mapping process are the following:

1. Develop a logic model of the problem based on a needs assessment

2. State program outcomes and objectives—a logic model for change

3. Develop the program plan, including scope, sequence, change methods, and practical applications

4. Produce the intervention, including program materials and messages

5. Plan program use, including adoption, implementation, and maintenance

6. Develop an evaluation plan

## Step 1: Logic Model of the Problem

In Step 1 (Chapter 4), the planning team will:

1. Establish and work with a planning group

2. Conduct a needs assessment to create a logic model of the problem

3. Describe the context for the intervention, including the population, setting, and community

4. State program goals

Before beginning to actually plan an intervention, the planner puts together a team to assess the health problem, behavioral and environmental causes of the problem, and determinants of behavioral and environmental causes. We strongly recommend depicting these relations on a logic model diagram, also called *theory of the problem* and *theory of change* (Chen, 2014; Connell & Kubisch, 1996; Frechtling, 2007; Kirby, 2004; Rossi, Lipsey, & Freeman, 2004; Weiss & Coyne, 1997). Intervention Mapping introduces a logic model (theory) of the problem in Step 1 and a logic model (theory) of change in Step 2. Logic models are indispensable guides for program development and evaluation, are an increasingly common requirement in applications to funding agencies, and are taught and supported by the Centers for Disease Control and Prevention as the fundamental framework for program evaluation (ActKnowledge & Aspen Institute Roundtable on Community Change, 2003; Centers for Disease Control and Prevention, 1999; Centers for Disease Control and Prevention, 2011; W. K. Kellogg Foundation, 2006, 2010).

We suggest the PRECEDE model as a framework for creating a logic model (theory) of the problem—graphic representations of the causal relations between health problems and their causes (whether demonstrated or hypothesized) (Glanz et al., 2015; Green & Kreuter, 2005). See Figure 1.2. To develop this model beginning with a health problem, the planning team addresses the questions of What is the problem and who has it? How many people have it or will get it? Moving to the right, in the model, the

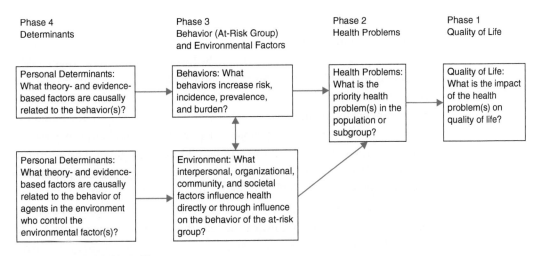

Phase 4
Determinants

Phase 3
Behavior (At-Risk Group)
and Environmental Factors

Phase 2
Health Problems

Phase 1
Quality of Life

Personal Determinants:
What theory- and evidence-
based factors are causally
related to the behavior(s)?

Behaviors: What
behaviors increase risk,
incidence, prevalence,
and burden?

Health Problems:
What is the
priority health
problem(s) in the
population or
subgroup?

Quality of Life:
What is the impact
of the health
problem(s) on
quality of life?

Personal Determinants:
What theory- and evidence-
based factors are causally
related to the behavior of
agents in the environment
who control the
environmental factor(s)?

Environment: What
interpersonal, organizational,
community, and societal
factors influence health
directly or through influence
on the behavior of the at-risk
group?

**Figure 1.2**  Logic Model of the Problem

planner addresses what quality-of-life effects occur because of this health problem. Moving to the left of the health problem, the questions are about causes. What behaviors among the priority population may cause the health problem or make it worse? What environmental factors contribute to the health problem either directly or through behavior? Finally, we address the *why* questions. Why do people in the priority population do the behavior (risk behavior)? Why do people in the environment create the conditions that contribute to the health problem directly or through behavior of the priority population?

In addition to developing the logic model of the problem, an equally important continuous effort is to understand the character of the community, its members, its strengths, and its knowledge of the health problem and potential solutions. Finally in this step, the planning team sets goals for intervention, including behavioral and environmental change, as well as health and quality-of-life outcomes.

## Step 2: Program Outcomes and Objectives and Logic Model of Change

In Step 2, the planner completes the following tasks:

1. State expected outcomes for behavior and environment

2. Specify performance objectives for behavioral and environmental outcomes

3. Select determinants for behavioral and environmental outcomes

4. Construct matrices of change objectives

5. Create a logic model of change

Step 2 (Chapter 5) specifies who and what will change because of the intervention. A logic model (theory) of change shows what change is needed to prevent, reduce, or manage the health problem, and it depicts the proposed mechanisms of change. It depicts the proposed causal relations between theory- and evidence-based change methods, the determinants they are expected to influence, and behavioral and environmental outcomes that will address the health problem (Figure 1.3). The planner begins this step using the logic model of the problem (Step 1) as a guide. The questions to ask are: What needs to change in the behavior of the priority population (behavioral outcome) or in the environment (environmental outcome)? Then, moving to the right: What impact will these changes have on the health problem? Moving toward the left, the *why* questions become: Why would the priority population make these changes? Why would agents in the environment make these changes? In Step 2, the tasks focus on what needs to change by specifying the program outcomes and objectives. In Step 3, the logic model of change is completed with the *how* of change by identifying the theoretical methods for change and the practical applications of selected change methods.

Once the planning team has identified the health-promoting behaviors, environmental conditions, and their determinants, the next task in Step 2 is to develop matrices of change objectives. Performance objectives are the description of the specific behaviors that the at-risk group or the environmental agents have to perform to achieve the desired change. The change objectives combine determinants and performance objectives and are the basis for choosing theory- and evidence-based change methods and other

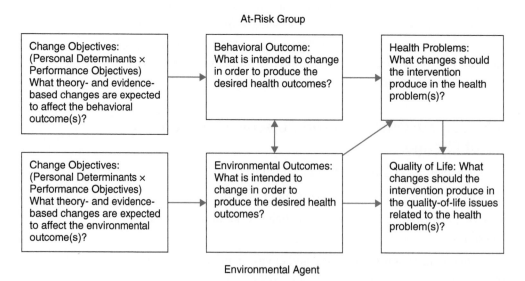

**Figure 1.3** Logic Model of Change

program content. The matrices represent detailed change at relevant ecological levels (individual, interpersonal, organizational, community, or societal) and are the most immediate target of an intervention. When Step 2 is completed, planners can think explicitly about the intervention in Step 3.

To develop performance objectives for environmental outcomes, planners identify roles of environmental agents at each relevant ecological level. For example, superintendents, principals, and teachers may have roles for school environmental change. Statements of what must change at each ecological level and who must make the change are more specific intervention foci than are traditional program goals and objectives. For example, in a program to increase fruit and vegetable consumption by children in elementary school, matrices would be created for both the child and the food service personnel. The food service matrix might contain more than one role: for example, the manager's purchasing practices; the dietitian's menu development, and the cooks' food preparation.

## Step 3: Program Design

In Step 3 (Chapter 6), the planner completes the following tasks:

1. Generate program themes, components, scope, and sequence

2. Choose theory- and evidence-based change methods

3. Select or design practical applications to deliver change methods

In this step, the planning team works from the logic model of change and matrices (Step 2) to design a coherent, deliverable intervention. Designing the intervention means first matching theory- and evidence-based methods to the change objectives they are meant to influence and selecting or devising practical applications to deliver the methods to the various priority populations. An intervention change method is a defined process by which theories postulate and empirical research provides evidence for how change may occur. Whereas a method is a theory-based technique to influence determinants, an application is a way of organizing, operationalizing, and delivering the intervention methods. Examples include a meeting with community members (application) to encourage community participation (change method), role model stories (application) for modeling (change method), and signing a public pledge (application) for commitment (change method). The planning team will strategize practical applications that will reach the priority population and that the population will find acceptable. For example, a planning group might want an intervention that influences parents' outcome expectations regarding human papillomavirus (HPV) vaccination so that they get the vaccination for their children. Change methods might include cultural similarity, modeling, verbal persuasion, and anticipated regret. One application for all of these methods

18

could be a videotaped testimonial by parents who have made the decision to have their children vaccinated for HPV and can model positive aspects of their decision.

Once the planning group has a basic plan of methods and applications, it will be able to describe intervention themes, components, scope, and sequence. All of these tasks are done with the full planning group, but perhaps it is particularly important to listen carefully to practical program ideas from community members who may implement the intervention or participate in it. Also, throughout these tasks reference to the matrices is important to ensure that the final applications will address the change objectives adequately.

## Step 4: Program Production

In Step 4 (Chapter 7), the planner completes the following tasks:

1. Refine program structure and organization
2. Prepare plans for program materials
3. Draft messages, materials, and protocols
4. Pretest, refine, and produce materials

The products in this step are all of the support materials needed in an intervention. This step gives specific guidance for designing communications that convey the intent and form of the intervention as planned in Step 3. It also describes pretesting and pilot testing of applications, activities, materials, and messages before they are finally produced. The most common scenario for producing a new intervention is that most of the needed materials will have to be developed de novo. Nevertheless some materials may be available and can be adapted to address change objectives, methods, and applications. Only after completing Intervention Mapping Steps 1–4 can a planner adequately evaluate whether existing materials fit the program objectives.

## Step 5: Program Implementation Plan

In Step 5 (Chapter 8), the planner completes the following tasks:

1. Identify potential program users (adopters, implementers, and maintainers)
2. State outcomes and performance objectives for program use
3. Construct matrices of change objectives for program use
4. Design implementation interventions

The purpose of this step is to design a plan to promote program implementation (beginning with adoption and extending through maintenance).

Consideration of program implementation actually begins in Step 1 (needs assessment) and continues in this step. To devise an implementation intervention, the planning team will develop new matrices, using the process from Step 2, with these matrices addressing performance objectives and determinants of program adoption, implementation, and maintenance. Linking of each performance objective with a determinant produces a change objective to promote program use. The team then matches change methods and applications to these objectives to develop theory-informed plans for program adoption, implementation, and maintenance.

In this step, the planning team would ask, "Where can the intervention reach the relevant populations?" "In the chosen venues, who would be in charge of adoption? Implementation? Maintenance?" "What specific performance would be necessary at each stage?" and "What would motivate performance?"

The tasks for this step require the planner to identify potential implementers. Sometimes the program adopters, for example, health department administrators, are different from those who will do the day-to-day implementation. Further, those who are in roles to ensure program maintenance may be a different group. This process will be greatly helped by making sure that the right people are at the table in the planning group. It is never too late to be more inclusive by adding new members. For example, to adopt a program to change school lunch nutritional content, a school principal might order the program for review, ask food service managers for opinions about the program, and form a task force for food service change. To implement the program, the focus may change from the principal to the food service staff, who can make changes in menus, orders, and preparation. For maintenance of the program, the performance objectives might switch back to administrators, who can integrate the new procedures into the routine practices of the school. The planner then uses theory and evidence to hypothesize determinants of the adoption, implementation, and maintenance performance objectives. The product for Step 5 is a detailed plan for accomplishing program use by influencing behavior of individuals or groups who will make decisions about adopting and using the program.

## Step 6: Evaluation Plan

In Step 6 (Chapter 9), the planner completes the following tasks:

1. Write effect and process evaluation questions

2. Develop indicators and measures for assessment

3. Specify the evaluation design

4. Complete the evaluation plan

An evaluation plan is actually begun in the needs assessment and is developed throughout each step. In the process of Intervention Mapping, planners make decisions about goals to change behavior, environment, health and quality of life, change objectives, change methods, applications, and implementation. The decisions, although informed by theory and evidence from research, still may not be optimal or may even be completely wrong. Through effect and process evaluation, planners can determine the impact of the intervention and can begin to understand the influence of decisions that were made at each planning step (Grant, Treweek, Dreischulte, Foy, & Guthrie, 2013; Patton, 2008, 2012; Rossi et al., 2004; Steckler & Linnan, 2002; Windsor, Clark, Boyd, & Goodman, 2003).

To evaluate the effect of an intervention, researchers analyze the change in health and quality-of-life problems, behavior and environment, and their determinants. Optimally, planners have defined these factors in a measurable way during the preceding steps. Effect evaluation may show positive, negative, or mixed effects or show no effect at all. Planners want to understand the reasons behind the effects that were achieved, regardless of what those effects were. They need to know more about the process and the changes in intermediate variables. They ask such questions as the following: "Were the behaviors and determinants well specified?" "Were change methods well matched to influence determinants?" "Were practical applications appropriate to deliver the change methods and did they reach the populations?" "Was the implementation complete and appropriate?"

## Core Processes for Using Theory and Evidence

Processes for understanding a problem or answering a question with empirical data and theory can be complex and time-consuming; sometimes planners do not persevere through the difficulties. Consequently, the understanding of a health problem often is incomplete, and attempts to solve the problem are faulty. Therefore, we provide detail about how to undertake these core processes and give examples in the Intervention Mapping steps where they are used (Steps 1, 2, 3, and 5). The core processes include the following:

1. Posing questions

2. Brainstorming to figure out what the planning team already knows about potential answers to the question

3. Reviewing findings from the empirical literature for both theory- and evidence-based answers to the question

4. Reviewing theories for additional constructs

5. Assessing and addressing needs for new data

6. Developing a working list of answers, then moving on to the next question (Buunk & Van Vugt, 2013; Ruiter et al., 2012)

## Posing Questions

The first task for the core processes is to pose a question. The first questions asked are often to analyze causes of the health problem, and later questions concern determinants of behavior and environmental conditions, interventions, and program implementation (Buunk & Van Vugt, 2013; Ruiter et al., 2012). This example illustrates the process of posing questions. A work group in one of our health education methods classes began work on a project to prevent pregnancy and the transmission of HIV and other sexually transmitted infections (STIs) among urban adolescents. Over the course of the project, they asked a number of questions, including the following:

- *Health problem.* What are the health problems related to HIV, STIs, and pregnancy in adolescents (ages 13–18) in the United States?

- *Behaviors.* What are important risk behaviors for the transmission of HIV and STIs, and for pregnancy among adolescents? How do these risk behaviors vary for different groups, such as boys and girls?

- *Determinants.* After defining the health problems and the behavioral risks, the group asked a question concerning determinants of the risk behavior of not using condoms: Why do adolescents have sexual intercourse without using condoms? Why don't adolescent males use condoms when having vaginal sex with steady girlfriends? Why do girls have sex with boys who do not use condoms? The group then asked questions about determinants of the health-promoting behavior: Why would girls carry condoms? Why would adolescents discuss condom use with their partners?

- *Change methods.* Then the focus of the questions shifted to potential solutions or theory- and evidence-based change methods: How can we help specific subgroups of adolescents use condoms? Which change methods can be translated into appropriate practical applications?

## Brainstorming Answers

The second core process is "brainstorming" or "free association." In response to the question, planning group members propose (unedited) possible answers. In this way, the group members can ascertain their current knowledge and practice wisdom and can make a list of provisional answers. Making a provisional list of answers to a question is a creative process that primarily involves free association with the aim of generating as many explanations as possible in response to a question (Buunk & Van Vugt, 2013; Ruiter et al., 2012). The planners can later drop explanations that are poorly supported in the literature. Planners should avoid getting stuck on a single explanation too soon. In formulating these provisional explanations, health educators, as applied behavioral scientists, typically use theoretical and empirical knowledge, whether consciously or not. Doing so is unavoidable at this stage, but the brainstorming should be as open as possible and should not be limited to data- or theory-informed items.

As the students worked to discover determinants for condom use, they generated many answers to the question: Why do adolescents have sexual intercourse without using condoms? (See example in Table 1.1.) The students brainstormed determinants based on what they knew from many sources about condom use. They stimulated creativity by asking related questions, by taking the sexually active adolescent's perspective, and by narrowing the question to particular populations and situations. At this stage their answers included a combination of personal beliefs, local knowledge, practice wisdom, and evidence-informed answers.

**Table 1.1**    Provisional List of Answers Regarding Condom Use Among Adolescents

| Original Provisional List | Additions From Empirical Literature | Theoretical Additions (Some From Empirical Literature) | Additions From New Research |
|---|---|---|---|
| Lack of knowledge of HIV transmission | Do not perceive condoms as pregnancy prevention | Intention to use condoms | Disconfirmed lack of knowledge about HIV or STIs |
| Lack of knowledge of STIs | Perceive condoms as embarrassing | Subjective norms | Argument that condoms don't work is an excuse, not a belief |
| Peers don't use condoms | Did not express personal responsibility for having condoms | Perceived norms | Experience with condoms associated with embarrassment |
| Perception that condoms don't work | Lower family connectedness | Self-efficacy for negotiating and discussing condom use with their partner | Teens wanted to be more skillful |
| Attitudes toward condom use | Parents' permissive attitudes about sex | Skills | Girls and boys expressed that condoms were the responsibility of the other gender |
| Experience with condom use: don't like condoms | Community perceptions of gender inequality in sex | Outcome expectations | Perception of no risk of HIV with only one partner (mistook "serial monogamy" for monogamy) |
| Gender: males do not want to use condoms | Nonopen communication | | |
| Lack of salience—not knowing someone with AIDS | Neighborhood characteristics, such as high unemployment | | |
| Lack of confidence in using condoms | Lack of access to family planning services | | |
| | Lack of parental supervision | | |
| | Parental trust | | |
| | Association with deviant peers | | |
| | Coercive parenting | | |

For this preliminary list, there is no reason for health educators to favor one explanation over another; however, in the subsequent processes, they should take into account two criteria for good answers: (1) an explanation should describe a process (an explanation of causation) and (2) an explanation should be plausible. For example, socioeconomic status on the students' list may be an important contextual factor or root cause of lack of condom use, but it may need to be explored further to describe a process that explains behavior better. A useful aid is to represent the explanation in a logic model schematic that shows causation (Earp & Ennett, 1991). A plausible explanation is one that can survive when it is depicted visually and examined critically, using logic to evaluate the relationships among the various elements in the model.

## Reviewing Findings From Published Research

The next core process is to support or refute provisional answers to the questions that the planning group has asked. We suggest a simple process here, but urge the reader to consult the many expert sources in the burgeoning field of systematic review and evidence-based public health. Basic how-to guidance is available from many sources (Briss, Mullen, & Hopkins, 2005; Cochrane, 2014; Community Preventive Services Task Force, 2015; Cooper, Hedges, & Valentine, 2009; Higgins & Green, 2008, 2011; Peters, 2014). Not every literature review need be a formal systematic study; however, every literature review should be clearly linked to a question, should specify parameters so that the nature of the numerator (what studies are used in the evidence summary) is understood in terms of the denominator (what studies were conducted or reported), and should specify what variation exists in the quality of evidence. The following questions will help guide a basic review:

1. What question(s) do you want to answer?
2. What evidence will address the questions?
3. What are the inclusion and exclusion criteria for the evidence?
4. How will you find the evidence you want? What is the search strategy?
5. Which evidence from the search process meets your criteria?
6. How will you document answers to your question(s)?
7. What metric will you use to judge strength of the evidence?
8. How will you summarize the findings and draw conclusions based on the data and the limitations?

The review in Table 1.1 generated evidence supporting both theory-informed and nontheoretical answers to the question at hand. This may be described as a topical approach to theory. The question that the students asked for their initial literature review was not about theory but was about the topic at hand—adolescent unprotected sex. When the students approached the literature, they found some issues related to unprotected sex that were not explicitly theory-informed such as not perceiving condoms as pregnancy prevention (Bobrova, Sergeev, Grechukhina, & Kapiga, 2005), perceiving condoms as embarrassing (Bell, 2009), not taking personal responsibility for having condoms (Parkes, Henderson, & Wight, 2005), low family connectedness and parents' permissive attitudes about sex (Kao & Manczak, 2013), perceptions of gender inequality in sex (Bauman, Karasz, & Hamilton, 2007), and closed communication (Crosby et al., 2000). The group also found a number of studies that reported the relation of theoretical constructs to unsafe sex, including intention to use condoms and perceived social norms (Bobrova et al., 2005; Villarruel, Jemmott, Jemmott, & Ronis, 2007) and self-efficacy for negotiating and discussing condom use with partners (Bell, 2009; Black, Sun, Rohrbach, & Sussman, 2011).

From the literature review, the group of students also became interested in information on the wider social context of why adolescents might not protect against pregnancy and STIs. They found that researchers had demonstrated that community characteristics—such as proportion of families living below the poverty line, low levels of education, and high unemployment—were highly related to birthrates among young teenagers (Penman-Aguilar, Carter, Snead, & Kourtis, 2013). They also discovered that other neighborhood characteristics, such as neighborhood economic disadvantage, high unemployment (Bauermeister, Zimmerman, & Caldwell, 2011), and access to family planning services had been linked to adolescent contraceptive use (Averett, Rees, & Argys, 2002; Smith, Novello, & Chacko, 2011). This broader search located evidence that parental monitoring, parental trust, and unsupervised time were associated with sexual activity (Borawski, Ievers-Landis, Lovegreen, & Trapl, 2003).

Sometimes evidence in response to a well-defined question may be scarce. For example, another student working group was interested in the question: "What factors predict cervical cancer screening in young women in Ghana?" The students were disappointed that they could find only three references directly related to the specific question in their defined priority population. They broadened their search in two ways: (1) research studies in populations that were arguably similar (sharing demographic and cultural characteristics) to young women in Ghana—young women in other West African countries—and (2) research studies about similar behaviors—other cancer screenings.

## Accessing and Using Theory

When reviewing the literature by topic as described above, planners will encounter theory. In addition, planners can find useful information by specifically searching theories. Table 1.2 presents examples of types of theories that might be applied for the various questions. Notice that these theories do not apply equally to all steps and that adequate use of the core processes enables a planning group to apply multiple theories or models throughout the planning process. In a problem-driven context, all theories, theoretical models, and constructs are potentially useful within the parameters that the theory describes (Buunk & Van Vugt, 2013; Kok, Schaalma, Ruiter, van Empelen, & Brug, 2004). One challenge is to find the best theory or combination of theoretical constructs first to understand, and then to solve, the problem at hand. Limiting the pool of candidate theories too soon may lead to an inadequate solution of a practical problem or, worse, to conclusions that are counterproductive. A theory that is helpful in making one decision might not be very helpful for making another.

Both brainstorming and searching the literature will have turned up theoretical constructs. The next core process task is to continue to refine, add to, and discard provisional answers based on theoretical concepts, and the planning group will need to look specifically for theory-related answers. The student group first searched the literature using the topic approach pertaining to adolescent sexual behavior, condom use, and the

**Table 1.2**   Examples of Theories for Intervention Mapping Steps and Questions

| Intervention Mapping Step | Decision (Sample Question) | Examples of Theories |
|---|---|---|
| Step 1 | Needs assessment (What quality-of-life issues are related to [a specific] health problem?) | Quality-of-life theories |
| Step 2 | Behaviors (What behaviors benefit [a specific] health outcome?) Environmental conditions (What agents control harmful or health promoting environmental conditions?) Personal determinants (What factors influence the risk behavior or the health promoting behavior?) | Self-regulatory theories Power theories Value-expectancy theories |
| Step 3 | Change methods and practical applications (What strategies have been shown to influence [specific] determinants and behavior?) | Persuasive communication theories |
| Step 4 | Messages (What factors have been shown to influence comprehension and retention of messages?) | Theories of Information Processing |
| Step 5 | Implementation (What factors have been shown to influence implementation of similar interventions?) | Diffusion theories Dissemination and implementation models |

prevention of HIV, STIs, and pregnancy. However, even when searching the literature through the health problem or behavioral topic, the group discovered theoretical ideas, as depicted in Table 1.1.

A second approach to accessing theoretical ideas is through concepts that turn up during brainstorming. Even though the ideas from the brainstorming are usually initially stated in lay terms, there may be some advantage to relabeling them with their theoretical labels. The information that can be garnered about a theoretical construct can be somewhat more precise than that related to a simple lay concept. For example, on the students' original list, the idea of lack of confidence appeared. This concept might also be labeled as the theoretical construct of self-efficacy, giving the students the opportunity to find out more about the construct by reading what Bandura has to say about self-efficacy (Bandura, 1986; Mulvihill, 1996). When group members explored the construct of self-efficacy in the literature, they found two kinds of self-efficacy—self-efficacy for negotiating condom use as separate from self-efficacy in applying a condom.

Accessing theory from a construct approach can also lead to considering the parent theory and to a general theories approach to accessing theory. A general theories approach is simply perusing a theory that might offer insight into one's question. The student group might have used the general theories approach to access Social Cognitive Theory (Kelder, Hoelscher, & Perry, 2015). As it turned out, the group approached this theory through the construct of self-efficacy and also followed the construct of intention back to the parent theory, the Theory of Planned Behavior (see Chapter 2; Montaño & Kasprzyk, 2015). As the group members explored these theories, they found that self-efficacy is closely related to skills, perceived norms, and outcome expectations, so they added perceived norms and skills for negotiating condom use and applying a condom to the list (Table 1.1). Further, they encountered methods for influencing self-efficacy and began to think ahead about the intervention. None of this useful information would have been available if the group had not looked beyond the concept of confidence.

## Identifying and Addressing the Need for New Research

The previous core processes are important before the planners jump into research so that they are clear about what questions to ask. With the previous core processes, the planners will have assembled a set of answers from both the theoretical and the empirical literature that fit with, suggest changes to, or add to the provisional explanations. In some cases this information provides insight into the exact processes of the provisional answers. The information may, at the same time, raise questions that the planning team had not thought of before. For example, the planners would want to know whether certain theoretical constructs that look promising were actually explanatory in their population. They would also want to know the particular way an explanation found in published research is operating in their population.

Often, health promotion planners use a combination of qualitative and quantitative techniques to explore the questions of interest in their population (Bryman, 2006; Creswell, 2013; de Vries, Weijts, Dijkstra, & Kok, 1992; Morgan, 2006; Steckler, McLeroy, Goodman, Bird, & McCormick, 1992; see Chapter 4). For example, for a question regarding determinants, planners first search the available theoretical and empirical literature on the cause of the behavior or environmental condition of interest to find theories and data. They might then use a qualitative method to find out the population's ideas about determinants of their behavior and then conduct a quantitative study using a structured questionnaire with questions that are based on the results of the qualitative phase. Some factors cannot be measured just by asking members of the population because perceptions may be different from reality; planners may need information from key observers. In some situations qualitative methods are used later in the research process to better understand the findings from a quantitative approach (Curry et al., 2013; Morgan, 2006, 2007; Östlund, Kidd, Wengström, & Rowa-Dewar, 2011; Steckler et al., 1992).

For example, the student working group needed more information from their priority population about the items on the provisional list to determine whether the proposed factors were valid in their population. The group conducted individual interviews and focus groups with both boys and girls from their local area. They learned a lot about youth experiences with protected and unprotected sex and the reasons for both occurrences. The new data called into question the adolescents' lack of knowledge about HIV or STIs in their population. The adolescents also felt that the argument that condoms don't work is more of an excuse and less of a belief about effectiveness. The adolescents who had tried condoms expressed some embarrassment with the process of using condoms and a need for a greater level of skills and self-efficacy. With this new information the group was able to move on to the next core process.

## Formulating the Working List of Answers

At this point the planning team is ready to summarize and complete its provisional list of answers into a working list for which the evidence is sufficient. The planners will consider the criteria of plausibility and process and also judge their answers for relevance or importance (strength of association) and changeability. Relevance is the strength of the evidence for the causal relationship between the determinant and the behavior (unprotected sex). Changeability is the strength of the evidence that the proposed change can be realized by an intervention. The latter criterion requires health educators to consider that some determinants may be changed by interventions directed at the individual, and other determinants by interventions directed at the environment. For questions regarding determinants, answers that remain on the list will be factors that are both important and changeable. For a solutions or methods question, answers that remain on the list will be methods that have been shown to produce significant change in similar situations. After this process, the planning group will have enough information to finalize a list of important determinants and depict the causal model as a simple logic model (Earp & Ennett, 1991).

## The Role of Culture in Intervention Planning

A theme that appears in each step of Intervention Mapping is the need to create culturally relevant programs for diverse groups (see Chapters 4 and 7). Often health educators work with groups of people who are members of a cultural group different from their own; often these are underserved groups. Program planning must be conducted with an awareness of the roles of cultural and power differences and with what some professional fields now label cultural humility (Tervalon, 2003; Tervalon & Murray-Garcia, 1998). The idea of cultural humility arose in the context of physician training when Tervalon (2003) and Tervalon and Murray-Garcia (1998) asserted that the idea of competency-based education does not map well to culture. *Competency* implies that it is possible to fully know another culture whereas *humility* indicates that it is impossible to do so (Levi, 2009). Because we can never become fully competent in another culture, an appropriate goal may be lifelong self-evaluation and self-critique. Although Tervalon and Murray-Garcia's (1998) approach was originally proposed to redress the power imbalances in patient-physician relationships, it is equally applicable to health promotion (DeLemos et al., 2007; Minkler, 2004; Tervalon, 2003; Tervalon & Murray-Garcia, 1998; Wallerstein & Duran, 2006). The recognition that one is never fully competent in this domain should lead to the firm intention to develop communication skills that demonstrate flexibility, openness, and self-reflection so that cultural learning is possible (Hixon, 2003).

There are several important reasons for planners to be able to develop effective programs across cultures, including the expanding diversity within countries, the reality of globalization and global health promotion practice, and the critical issue of health disparities (Braveman, Egerter, & Williams, 2011; Fiscella, Franks, Gold, & Clancy, 2000; National Center for Health Statistics, 2012; Pamuk, Makuc, Heck, Reuben, & Lochner, 1998; Phelan, Link, & Tehranifar, 2010; Richardson & Norris, 2010; Thomas, Quinn, Butler, Fryer, & Garza, 2011; Work Group for Community Health and Development, University of Kansas, n.d.-a, n.d.-b). The U.S. Healthy People 2010 objectives highlighted the health disparities between racial and ethnic groups, with particular emphasis on eliminating those dispari-ties in infant mortality, cancer screening and management, cardiovascular disease, diabetes, HIV/AIDS, and childhood and adult immunizations (U.S. Department of Health and Human Services, 2001), whereas the 2020 report set even more aggressive objectives for the elimination of disparities (Elliot, 2008; Secretary's Advisory Committee on National Health Promotion and Disease Prevention Objectives for 2020, 2010). The authors of *The Com-munity Tool Box* (Work Group for Community Health and Development, University of Kansas, n.d.-a, n.d.-b) suggested that understanding culture is important for community builders and health promoters because attaining significant change requires people working together to build communi-ties that are powerful enough to attain change; working effectively across cultures allows incorporation of the unique strengths and perspectives of many groups; cultural sensitivity can help overcome racial and ethnic divi-sions, which result in lost opportunities; full involvement of diverse groups in decision making can result in more effective programs; appreciation of cultural diversity goes hand in hand with a just and equitable society; and if we do not learn about the influences of cultural groups, we are missing an accurate view of our society and communities. See the *Com-munity Tool Box* websites regarding cultural adaptation of interventions at http://ctb.ku.edu/en/tablecontents/section_1163.htm (Work Group for Community Health and Development, University of Kansas, n.d.-b) and regarding cultural competence at http://ctb.ku.edu/en/table-of-contents/culture/cultural-competence (Work Group for Community Health and Development, University of Kansas, n.d.-a).

Each planning step requires a specific aspect of a culturally relevant approach conducted by a self-aware planner and planning group. In Step 1, needs assessment (Chapter 4), the planner must be aware of the roles culture can play in both the causation and the outcomes of health prob-lems. In Step 1, planners also conduct community, including cultural, assessments as a part of defining the priority population for the program. In Step 2, program outcomes and objectives (Chapter 5), culture can be an important aspect of defining performance objectives and of understanding their determinants. Without the culturally correct matrix components, program materials are unlikely to be salient to the intended cultural group. In Steps 3 and 4, program components, change methods, and applications (Chapters 6 and 7), planners must maintain the participation of the intended audience in the development of materials and understand their responses to program materials.

## Navigating the Book

The process of Intervention Mapping is essentially unchanged from the third edition text. However, we have rearranged the presentation of some aspects of the process. We also have tried to simplify some explanations and discard terms that have caused confusion.

## Organization of the Book

The book has two sections. The first section, Foundations, contains an introductory chapter and two chapters that are reviews of theories often used in health education and promotion. Chapter 2 provides an overview of behavior-oriented theories, and Chapter 3 provides an overview of environment-oriented theories. The next six chapters explain the Intervention Mapping steps and include a case study example that runs at the end of each chapter. Further case studies can be found at the book's website, www.wiley.com/go/bartholomew4e. The final chapter explains how to use Intervention Mapping to adapt evidence-based interventions for new populations and settings.

## Changes From the Previous Editions

Readers familiar with the previous editions of Intervention Mapping will find several changes that may have an impact on their practice and teaching. We have made two changes that will be of interest to previous users of the book and of the Intervention Mapping process. For the fourth edition of the book, we have increased the focus on logic models in both Steps 1 and 2. The other change parses material between steps differently, with the inclusion of characteristics of the intervention, such as scope and sequence, with the choice of methods and practical applications in Step 3. This reshuffling enables more emphasis in Step 4 on the how-tos of writing and producing communications. These slight changes resulted in revised step names (Figure 1.1).

Chapter 10 offers a simplified process for using Intervention Mapping to adapt evidence-based interventions for new settings and populations.

# Important Repeating Concepts in the Book

Throughout the book, several key concepts are repeated in different contexts. These are planning matrices, iterative planning, logic models, and evaluation.

## Matrices as a Foundation for Intervention Planning

In Intervention Mapping, matrices that combine performance objectives with their determinants are the basis for program development. They are used in both planning a program (Step 2) and planning its implementation (Step 5). If a change method or practical application used in an intervention is not intended to change the objectives in the matrices, then either it does not belong in the program or the matrix is not adequate and should be revisited.

## Planning as an Iterative Process

To describe program development, we have laid out a series of steps. This orderly presentation may suggest to the reader that every step is completed only once and in a rigid order. This is not the case. Each step provides the basis for the next; each step also generates new information that may suggest revision or embellishment of a previous step. With increasing ideas about the program, knowledge about the intended beneficiaries, community participation, and research and theory, a planner often needs to revisit and fine-tune a previous step. In addition to the process of revisiting prior steps, some processes are repeated in many of the steps. For example, using the core processes to access relevant theory and evidence, planning evaluation, involving stakeholders, and thinking about implementation all begin in the needs assessment and continue in each step. Also, each step provides information for generating an evaluation plan.

## Logic Models

We described the use of logic models above in the descriptions of Steps 1 and 2. In the process of Intervention Mapping, the planner will build a logic model of the health problem causation in Step 1 and begin a logic model of change in Step 2. In Step 3, the planner will add change methods to the logic model of change. These are the only logic models that are necessary components of Intervention Mapping. However, in addition to the logic model that is pieced together as intervention development progresses, we present a number of models to help clarify relations among concepts, such as theoretical constructs (Chapters 2 and 3). We also use other graphic devices that do not imply causal relations, such as Figure 1.1, a depiction of the steps involved in Intervention Mapping. When a figure is a logic model, that is, implies causal relations, we clearly label it as such.

## Program Evaluation

Program evaluation begins with a thorough description of the program to be evaluated and its proposed causal pathways for change. This description is accomplished step-by-step in Intervention Mapping. First, in the needs assessment, the planner begins to formulate goals for program outcomes. These become part of the plan for evaluating effects (Chapter 9). In Step 2, the planner specifies desired changes in behavior and environment as well as their determinants, which again become further outcomes for evaluating effects. Steps 3, 4, and 5 guide the specification of program components and implementation plans that link closely to process evaluation. Step 4 also contains discussion of pretesting and pilot testing or formative evaluation of the program.

## Planning With Limited Resources

Finally, we encourage health promotion planners to use Intervention Mapping regardless of the time or resources available. We point this out because we often hear people say that Intervention Mapping is not practical for use in the "real world." We have also seen people belabor the importance of following the Intervention Mapping steps sequentially and to the "letter of the law" at the cost of losing constituent buy-in. To avoid these pitfalls, the planning group's health promotion practitioner often works behind the scenes to draft end products for each IM step, for example, the matrices of change objectives. This can take an afternoon, a weekend, or a month, depending on the time available. Other time- and resource-saving strategies include using a rapid assessment approach to complete the needs assessment in Step 1, or having longer workshop-type meetings so that planning groups do not forget what has been accomplished between meetings. Above all, simply posing the key questions for each Intervention Mapping step, for example, "Why do adolescents have sexual intercourse without using condoms?" will result in a more well-defined program based in theory and evidence, and increase the potential for effective behavioral and environmental change.

## Summary

Intervention Mapping is a series of steps, tasks, and processes to help health promotion and health education planners develop theory- and evidence-based programs. Well-designed and effective interventions should be guided by theory and informed by empirical evidence regarding the targets for change. For example, meta-analyses of cancer-screening interventions have found that larger effect sizes are achieved when interventions are based on theory (Stone et al., 2002; Yabroff & Mandelblatt, 1999; Yabroff, O'Malley, Mangan, & Mandelblatt, 2001). However, no one theoretical model completely predicts or explains health behaviors or environmental changes (Institute of Medicine, Committee on Health Literacy, 2004; Rakowski & Breslau, 2004; Rimer, 2002). Therefore, a system is needed to help intervention developers choose useful theories and integrate relevant constructs from multiple theories to describe health problems and develop health promotion and health education solutions (Kok et al., 2004; van Bokhoven, Kok, & van der Weijden, 2003). Intervention Mapping ensures that theoretical models and empirical evidence guide planners in two areas:

- The identification of determinants of behavioral and environmental causes related to a health problem

- The selection of the most appropriate change methods and applications to address the identified determinants to achieve changes in behavioral and environmental outcomes related to a health problem

Intervention Mapping has been used to develop many programs, and Table 1.3 presents some examples. Intervention Mapping is also being used to further the description of intervention characteristics and to deconstruct why interventions were effective or not (Bluethmann, Bartholomew, Murphy, & Vernon, 2014; Brug et al., 2010). Further, Intervention Mapping is being used to help health promoters find and adapt evidence-based interventions (see Chapter 10; Leerlooijer et al., 2011) and to evaluate the quality of planning that has been used to create interventions (Kok et al., 2015). For example, the Netherlands has a system whereby organizations can ask for accreditation of their programs (Brug et al., 2010), and others have used Intervention Mapping as a checklist to evaluate the quality of program planning of existing programs (Gagnon, Godin, Alary, Levy, & Otis, 2007; Schaafsma, Stoffelen, Kok, & Curfs, 2013).

Even though Intervention Mapping has not been directly compared to other processes for developing interventions, planners of the referenced projects and others considering guidance for intervention development think that the systematic process has been useful and flexible and that continued use will strengthen future program development (Aro & Absetz, 2009; Belansky et al., 2011; Hoelscher, Evans, Parcel, & Kelder, 2002).

**Table 1.3**    Programs Developed Using Intervention Mapping

| Topic | Intervention Title | References |
|---|---|---|
| Acute Stroke Therapy | The T.L.L. Temple Foundation Stroke Project | Morgenstern et al. (2002) <br> Morgenstern et al. (2003) |
| Adolescent Reproductive Health | Project Community-Embedded Reproductive Health Care for Adolescents (CERCA) | Decat et al. (2013) |
| Alcohol Abuse Prevention | Preventing Alcohol Abuse Among Undergraduates | Whittingham, Ruiter, Castermans, Huiberts, & Kok (2008) |
| Asthma Self-Management | Watch, Discover, Think, and Act | Bartholomew et al. (2000b) <br> Bartholomew et al. (2000c) <br> Shegog et al. (2001) |
| Asthma Management in Hispanic Children | Familias | Fernández et al. (2000a) <br> Fernández et al. (2000b) |
| Breast Cancer (going to provider with symptoms) | Promoting Early Presentation of Breast Cancer | Burgess et al. (2008) |
| Breast Cancer Screening | Mammography Barriers for Underserved African American Women | Highfield, Bartholomew, Hartman, Ford, & Balihe (2014) |
| Breast Cancer Screening | Project Healthy Outlook on the Mammography Experience (HOME) | Vernon et al. (2008) |
| Breast and Cervical Cancer Screening | Cultivando La Salud | Fernández, Gonzales, Tortolero-Luna, Partida, & Bartholomew (2005) |
| Breastfeeding | Early Postnatal Breastfeeding Support | Kronborg, Væth, Olsen, Iversen, & Harder (2007) |
| Blood Pressure Dissemination | Improving Blood Pressure Treatment in the Community | Bartholomew et al. (2009) |
| Cancer and Work | Work-Related Guidance Tool for Those Diagnosed With Cancer | Munir, Kalawsky, Wallis, & Donaldson-Feilder (2013) |
| Cervical Cancer Prevention | Cervical Cancer Prevention Among Latina Immigrants | Scarinci, Bandura, Hidalgo, & Cherrington (2012) |
| Cervical Cancer Screening | Love Yourself Before You Take Care of Your Family | Hou, Fernández, Baumler, & Parcel (2002) <br> Hou, Fernández, & Parcel, (2004) |
| Childhood Obesity Prevention | Healthy and Active Parenting Program for Early Years (HAPPY) | Taylor et al. (2013) |
| Childhood Obesity Prevention | Identification and Prevention of Dietary- and Lifestyle-Induced Health Effects in Children and Infants (IDEFICS) | De Henauw et al. (2011) <br> Verbestel et al. (2011) |
| Childhood Obesity Prevention | ToyBox | De Craemer et al. (2014) <br> De Decker et al. (2014) <br> Duvinage et al. (2014) |
| Childhood Overweight Prevention | Training Program for Nurses and Physicians | Dera-de Bie, Gerver, & Jansen (2013) |
| *Chlamydia trachomatis* Testing | SafeFriend | Theunissen et al. (2013) |

**Table 1.3** *(Continued)*

| Topic | Intervention Title | References |
|---|---|---|
| Chronic Disease Management | Chronic Disease Self-Management Program (CDSMP) | Detaille, van der Gulden, Engles, Heerkens, & van Dijk (2010) |
| Colorectal Cancer Screening | Tailored Interactive Intervention to Increase CRC Screening | Vernon et al. (2011) |
| Cyberbullying | Stop Online Bullying | Jacobs, Völlink, Dehue, & Lechner (2014) |
| Cystic Fibrosis | Cystic Fibrosis Family Education Program | Bartholomew, Czyzewski, Swank, McCormick, & Parcel (2000a) Bartholomew et al. (1997) |
| Diabetes Self-Management | Persian Diabetes Self-Management Education Program | Shakibazadeh, Bartholomew, Rashidian, & Larijani (2015) |
| Diet and Physical Activity | Waste the Waist | Gillison et al. (2012) |
| Flu Vaccination | A Program to Increase Influenza Vaccine Uptake Among Workers in Health Care Settings | Looijmans-van den Akker et al. (2011) |
| Flu Vaccination | Deliberately Vaccinated for You | Riphagen-Dalhuisen et al. (2013) |
| Fruit and Vegetable Promotion | The Pro Children Intervention | Pérez-Rodrigo et al. (2005) |
| Forgetfulness | Determining the Psychosocial Determinants of Forgetfulness | Mol, Ruiter, Verhey, Dijkstra, & Jolles (2008) |
| Global Health | School-Based Sexuality and HIV/AIDS Education Program in Tanzania | Mkumbo et al. (2009) |
| Healthy Lifestyle Promotion | Prescribe Vida Saludable | Sanchez et al. (2009) |
| Hepatitis B Screening | HBV Screening Programme Aimed at Turkish Immigrants | Van Der Veen, van Empelen, & Richardus (2012) |
| HIV Management | Intervention to Promote Sexual Health | van Kesteren, Kok, Hospers, Schippers, & de Wildt (2006) |
| HIV Prevention | AIDS Risk Reduction Program for Dutch Drug Users | van Empelen, Kok, Schaalma, & Bartholomew (2003) |
| HIV Prevention | Gay Cruise | Kok, Harterink, Vriens, de Zwart, & Hospers (2006) |
| HIV Prevention | Queermasters: The Online Gay Health Show | Mikolajczak, Kok, & Hospers (2008) |
| HIV Prevention | Project Growing, Reaching, Advocating for Change and Empowerment (GRACE) | Corbie-Smith et al. (2010) |
| HIV Treatment | Self-Management Program to Optimize Long-Term Adherence to Antiretroviral Therapy Among Persons Living With HIV | Côté, Godin, Garcia, Gagnon, & Rouleau (2008) |
| Injection Drug Users | Efficacy of a Computer-Tailored Intervention to Promote Safer Injection Practices Among Drug Users | Gagnon, Godin, Alary, Bruneau, & Otis (2010) |
| Injury Prevention | iPlay | Collard, Chinapaw, van Mechelen, & Verhagen (2009) |

*(continued)*

**Table 1.3**    (*Continued*)

| Topic | Intervention Title | References |
|---|---|---|
| Internet-Delivered Interventions | Understanding and Improving Adolescents' Exposure to Internet-Delivered Interventions | Crutzen et al. (2008) |
| Leg Ulcers | Lively Legs | Heinen, Bartholomew, Wensing, van de Kerkhof, & van Achterberg (2006) |
| Low Back Pain | Enhancing Implementation of Physical Therapy Guidelines for Management of Patients With Low Back Pain | Rutten et al. (2014) |
| Medical Communication Skills | Communication Skills Training Programme for Specialists With Patients With Medically Unexplained Physical Symptoms | Weiland et al. (2013) |
| Medication Adherence | Program to Improve Medication Adherence Among Rheumatoid Arthritis Patients | Zwikker et al. (2012) |
| Medication Guidelines | Strategy to Implement the Insurance Medicine Guidelines for Depression | Zwerver, Schellart, Anema, Rammeloo, & van der Beek (2011) |
| Mental Disorders | Workplace Intervention for Sick-Listed Employees With Common Mental Disorders | van Oostrom et al. (2007) van Oostrom et al. (2008) |
| Mental Health | Program to Increase Effective Behaviors by Patients and Clinicians in Psychiatric Services | Koekkoek, van Meijel, Schene, & Hutschemaekers (2010) |
| Mental Health Service Delivery | Online Mental Health Continuing Education Program for Pharmacy Staff | Wheeler, Fowler, & Hattingh (2013) |
| Nutrition | Conscious Eating, How Do You Do It? | Springvloet, Lechner, & Oenema (2014) |
| Nutrition | Fruit and Vegetable Nutrition Program | Cullen, Bartholomew, & Parcel (1997) Cullen, Bartholomew, Parcel, & Kok (1998) Hoelscher et al. (2002) |
| Nutrition | School-Based Interventions to Increase Fruit and Vegetable Intake | Reinaerts, de Nooijer, & de Vries (2008) |
| Obesity Prevention | GRIPP Program Focused on Weight Maintenance Among Overweight Adults | van Genugten, van Empelen, Flink, & Oenema (2010) |
| Obesity Prevention | Text-Driven and a Video-Driven, Web-Based, Computer-Tailored Intervention to Prevent Obesity | Walthouwer, Oenema, Soetens, Lechner, & de Vries (2013) |
| Overweight Prevention | Balance@Work | Verweij, Proper, Weel, Hulshof, & van Mechelen (2009) |
| Overweight Management | Minimal Intervention Strategy (MIS) to Address Overweight and Obesity | Fransen et al. (2008) |
| Overweight Prevention | Dutch Obesity Intervention in Teenagers | Singh et al. (2006) |
| Overweight Prevention | Netherlands Research Programme Weight Gain Prevention (NHF-NRG) | Kremers et al. (2005) Kwak et al. (2007) |
| Overweight Prevention | FATaintPHAT | Ezendam, Oenema, van de Looij-Jansen, & Brug (2007) |

**Table 1.3**   *(Continued)*

| Topic | Intervention Title | References |
|---|---|---|
| Parent–Child Communication | What Should We Tell the Children About Relationships and Sex? | Newby, Bayley, & Wallace (2011) |
| Physical Activity | Active *plus* | van Stralen et al. (2008) |
| Physical Activity | Healthy Ageing—Physical Activity Program (HA-PAP) | Van Schijndel-Speet, Evenhuis, van Empelen, van Wijck, & Echteld (2013) |
| Physical Activity | I Move | Friederichs et al. (2014) |
| Physical Activity | Stages of Change for Moderate-Intensity Physical Activity in Deprived Neighborhoods | Kloek, van Lenthe, van Nierop, Schrijvers, & Mackenbach (2006) |
| Physical Activity | Worksite Physical Activity Intervention | McEachan, Lawton, Jackson, Conner, & Lunt (2008) |
| Physical Activity | YouRAction | Prins, van Empelen, Beenackers, Brug, & Oenema (2010) |
| Quality Improvement | Designing a Quality Improvement Intervention | van Bokhoven et al. (2003) |
| Relationship and Sex Education | Positive Relationships: Eliminating Coercion and Pressure in Adolescent Relationships (PR:EPARe) | Arnab et al. (2013) |
| Return-to-Work | Participatory Return-to-Work Intervention for Temporary Agency Workers and Unemployed Workers Sick-Listed due to Musculoskeletal Disorders | Vermeulen, Anema, Schellart, van Mechelen, & van der Beek (2009) |
| Return-to-Work | Designing a Return-to-Work Program for Occupational Low Back Pain | Ammendolia et al. (2009) |
| Safety Programs | Randomized, Controlled Intervention of Machine Guarding and Related Safety Programs in Small Metal Fabrication Businesses. | Brosseau, Parker, Samant, & Pan (2007) Parker et al. (2009) |
| School-Based Obesity Prevention | Healthy Lifestyles Programme (HeLP) | Lloyd, Logan, Greaves, & Wyatt (2011) Wyatt et al. (2013) |
| School Health Promotion | SchoolBeat | Leurs, Jansen, Schaalma, Mur-Veeman, & de Vries (2005) |
| Service Utilization | Promoting Access to Health Services (PATHS) | Suzuki et al. (2012) |
| Smoking Cessation | Happy Ending | Brendryen, Kraft, & Schaalma (2010) |
| STI/HIV Prevention | Uma Tori! | Bertens, Eiling, van den Borne, & Schaalma (2009) Bertens, Schaalma, Bartholomew, & van den Borne (2008) |
| STI/HIV Prevention | Programme to Prevent Sexually Transmittable Infections | Wolfers, van den Hoek, Brug, & de Zwart (2007) |
| STI Testing | ROsafe | Wolfers, de Zwart, & Kok (2012) |
| Stroke Prevention | Teaching Others to Live With Stroke (TOOLS) | Schmid, Andersen, Kent, Williams, & Damush (2010) |

*(continued)*

**Table 1.3**    *(Continued)*

| Topic | Intervention Title | References |
|---|---|---|
| Sun Protection | Sun Protection Is Fun! | Tripp, Herrmann, Parcel, Chamberlain, & Gritz (2000) |
| Teen Motherhood | The Teenage Mothers Project | Leerlooijer et al. (2013) |
| Urinary Incontinence | Program to Promote Adherence to Pelvic Floor Muscle Exercise | Alewijnse, Mesters, Metsemakers, & van den Borne (2002) |
| Violence | Padres Trabajando por la Paz | Murray, Kelder, Parcel, & Orpinas (1998) |
| Vitality in Older Adults | Vital@Work | Strijk, Proper, van der Beek, & van Mechelen (2009) |
| Work-Related Health Problems | Be Active and Relax "Vitality in Practice" (VIP) | Coffent et al. (2012) |
| Worksite Health | An Intervention at the Worksite for Older Construction Workers | OudeHengel, Joling, Proper, van der Molen, & Bongers (2011) |
| Worksite Wellness | Working on Wellness (WOW) | Kolbe-Alexander et al. (2012) |

## Discussion Questions and Learning Activities

1.  Why is it important to apply a systematic approach to the development of health promotion programs? What are the risks if a systematic approach is not used for health promotion program development?

2.  Explain what is meant by ecological and systems approaches to intervention development. Give examples of how factors at different ecological levels can have an impact on health.

3.  Discuss why so many health promotion programs focus only on behavior change of individuals at risk for a health problem and do not address environmental influences.

4.  Using tobacco control as an example, describe the types of interventions that have been used at the individual, organizational, community, and societal levels.

5.  When using core processes for Intervention Mapping, the planners first pose a question, then brainstorm answers to the question. They also gather evidence from the literature, theory, or new data. To access theories three approaches can be used: the topic-related approach, the concept-related approach, and the general theories approach. Discuss how a planning group can identify theories to answer planning questions using each of these three approaches.

6.  Access the website for Diffusion of Effective Behavioral Interventions at www.effectiveinterventions.org/ (Centers for Disease Control and Prevention, 2015) or the website for Cancer Control P.L.A.N.E.T. at cancercontrolplanet.cancer.gov/ (National Cancer Institute, Division

of Cancer Control and Population Sciences, n.d.), and select three different health promotion/prevention intervention programs to review. Determine which ecological level the program is addressing for change, and describe how the intervention will make a change to improve health or prevent a health problem.

# References

ActKnowledge & Aspen Institute Roundtable on Community Change. (2003, July). *Making sense: Reviewing program design with theory of change.* Retrieved from http://www.theoryofchange.org/pdf/making_sense.pdf

Alewijnse, D., Mesters, I. E., Metsemakers, J. F., & van den Borne, B. H. (2002). Program development for promoting adherence during and after exercise therapy for urinary incontinence. *Patient Education and Counseling, 48*(2), 147–160.

*American Journal of Community Psychology.* (2007). [Systems thinking issue]. *American Journal of Community Psychology, 39*(3–4).

Ammendolia, C., Cassidy, D., Steensta, I., Soklaridis, S., Boyle, E., Eng, S., . . . Côté, P. (2009). Designing a workplace return-to-work program for occupational low back pain: An intervention mapping approach. *BMC Musculoskeletal Disorders, 10,* 65.

Arnab, S., Brown, K., Clarke, S., Dunwell, I., Lim, T., Suttie, N., . . . de Freitas, S. (2013). The development approach of a pedagogically-driven serious game to support relationship and sex education (RSE) within a classroom setting. *Computers & Education, 69,* 15–30.

Aro, A. R., & Absetz, P. (2009). Guidance for professionals in health promotion: Keeping it simple—but not too simple. *Psychology & Health, 24*(2), 125–129.

Averett, S. L., Rees, D. I., & Argys, L. M. (2002). The impact of government policies and neighborhood characteristics on teenage sexual activity and contraceptive use. *American Journal of Public Health, 92*(11), 1773–1778.

Bandura, A. (1986). *Social foundations of thought and action: A Social Cognitive Theory.* Englewood Cliffs, NJ: Prentice-Hall.

Bartholomew, L. K., Cushman, W. C., Cutler, J. A., Davis, B. R., Dawson, G., Einhorn, P. T., . . . ALLHAT Collaborative Research Group. (2009). Getting clinical trial results into practice: Design, implementation, and process evaluation of the ALLHAT Dissemination Project. *Clinical Trials, 6*(4), 329–343.

Bartholomew, L. K., Czyzewski, D. I., Parcel, G. S., Swank, P. R., Sockrider, M. M., Mariotto, M. J., . . . Seilheimer, D. K. (1997). Self-management of cystic fibrosis: Short-term outcomes of the Cystic Fibrosis Family Education Program. *Health Education & Behavior, 24*(5), 652–666.

Bartholomew, L. K., Czyzewski, D. I., Swank, P. R., McCormick, L., & Parcel, G. S. (2000a). Maximizing the impact of the Cystic Fibrosis Family Education Program: Factors related to program diffusion. *Family & Community Health, 22*(4), 27–47.

Bartholomew, L., Gold, R., Parcel, G., Czyzewski, D., Sockrider, M., Fernández, M., . . . Swank, P. (2000b). Watch, Discover, Think, and Act: Evaluation of computer-assisted instruction to improve asthma self-management in inner-city children. *Patient Education and Counseling, 39*(2), 269–280.

Bartholomew, L. K., & Mullen, P. D. (2011). Five roles for using theory and evidence in the design and testing of behavior change interventions. *Journal of Public Health Dentistry, 71*(S1), S20–S33.

Bartholomew, L., Shegog, R., Parcel, G., Gold, R., Fernández, M., Czyzewski, D., . . . Berlin, N. (2000c). Watch, Discover, Think, and Act: A model for patient education program development. *Patient Education and Counseling, 39*(2), 253–268.

Bauermeister, J. A., Zimmerman, M. A., & Caldwell, C. H. (2011). Neighborhood disadvantage and changes in condom use among African American adolescents. *Journal of Urban Health, 88*(1), 66–83.

Bauman, L. J., Karasz, A., & Hamilton, A. (2007). Understanding failure of condom use intention among adolescents completing an intensive preventive intervention. *Journal of Adolescent Research, 22*(3), 248–274.

Becker, A. B., Israel, B. A., & Allen, A. (2005). Strategies and techniques for effective group process in community-based participatory research partnerships. In B. A. Israel, E. Eng, A. J. Schultz, & E. Parker (Eds.), *Methods in community-based participatory research for health* (pp. 52–72). San Francisco, CA: Jossey-Bass.

Belansky, E. S., Cutforth, N., Chavez, R. A., Waters, E., & Bartlett-Horch, K. (2011). An adapted version of intervention mapping (AIM) is a tool for conducting community-based participatory research. *Health Promotion Practice, 12*(3), 440–455.

Bell, J. (2009). Why embarrassment inhibits the acquisition and use of condoms: A qualitative approach to understanding risky sexual behaviour. *Journal of Adolescence, 32*(2), 379–391.

Berkman, L. F., Kawachi, I., & Glymour, M. M. (Eds.). (2014). *Social epidemiology* (2nd ed.). New York, NY: Oxford University Press.

Bertens, M. G., Eiling, E. M., van den Borne, B., & Schaalma, H. P. (2009). Uma Tori! Evaluation of an STI/HIV-prevention intervention for Afro-Caribbean women in the Netherlands. *Patient Education and Counseling, 75*(1), 77–83.

Bertens, M. G., Schaalma, H. P., Bartholomew, L. K., & van den Borne, B. (2008). Planned development of culturally sensitive health promotion programs: An intervention mapping approach. In P. Swanepoel & H. Hoeken (Eds.), *Adapting health communication to cultural needs: Optimizing documents in South-African health communication on HIV/AIDS prevention* (pp. 11–30). Amsterdam, Netherlands: John Benjamins.

Black, D. S., Sun, P., Rohrbach, L. A., & Sussman, S. (2011). Decision-making style and gender moderation of the self-efficacy–condom use link among adolescents and young adults: Informing targeted STI/HIV prevention programs. *Archives of Pediatrics & Adolescent Medicine, 165*(4), 320–325.

Bluethmann, S., Bartholomew, L. K., Murphy, C. C., & Vernon, S. W. (2014). Analysis of behavior theory use in physical activity intervention development for breast cancer survivors. *Annals of Behavioral Medicine, 47*(S1), S193.

Bobrova, N., Sergeev, O., Grechukhina, T., & Kapiga, S. (2005). Social-cognitive predictors of consistent condom use among young people in Moscow. *Perspectives on Sexual and Reproductive Health, 37*(4), 174–178.

Borawski, E. A., Ievers-Landis, C. E., Lovegreen, L. D., & Trapl, E. S. (2003). Parental monitoring, negotiated unsupervised time, and parental trust: The role of perceived parenting practices in adolescent health risk behaviors. *Journal of Adolescent Health, 33*(2), 60–70.

Braveman, P., Egerter, S., & Williams, D. R. (2011). The social determinants of health: Coming of age. *Annual Review of Public Health, 32*, 381–398.

Brendryen, H., Kraft, P., & Schaalma, H. (2010). Looking inside the black box: Using intervention mapping to describe the development of the automated smoking cessation intervention "Happy Ending." *Journal of Smoking Cessation, 5*(1), 29–56.

Briss, P. A., Mullen, P. D., & Hopkins, D. P. (2005). Methods used for reviewing evidence and linking evidence to recommendations in the community guide. In P. A. Zaza, P. A. Briss, & K. W. Harris (Eds.), *The guide to community preventive services: What works to promote health?* (pp. 431–448). New York, NY: Oxford University Press.

Brosseau, L. M., Parker, D., Samant, Y., & Pan, W. (2007). Mapping safety interventions in metalworking shops. *Journal of Occupational and Environmental Medicine, 49*(3), 338–345.

Brug, J., Oenema, A., & Ferreira, I. (2005). Theory, evidence and Intervention Mapping to improve behavior nutrition and physical activity interventions. *International Journal of Behavioral Nutrition and Physical Activity, 11*, 2.

Brug, J., van Dale, D., Lanting, L., Kremers, S., Veenhof, C., Leurs, M., . . . Kok, G. (2010). Towards evidence-based, quality-controlled health promotion: The Dutch recognition system for health promotion interventions. *Health Education Research, 25*(6), 1100–1106.

Bryman, A. (2006). Integrating quantitative and qualitative research: How is it done? *Qualitative Research, 6*(1), 97–113.

Burgess, C. C., Bish, A. M., Hunter, H. S., Salkovskis, P., Michell, M., Whelehan, P., & Ramirez, A. J. (2008). Promoting early presentation of breast cancer: Development of a psycho-educational intervention. *Chronic Illness, 4*(1), 13–27.

Buunk, A. P., & Van Vugt, M. (2013). *Applying social psychology: From problems to solutions* (2nd ed.). London, United Kingdom: Sage.

Cavanuagh, N., & Cheney, K. S. W. D. (2002). Community collaboration—A weaving. *Journal of Public Health Management & Practice 8*(1), 13–20.

Centers for Disease Control and Prevention. (1999). Framework for program evaluation in public health. *Morbidity and Mortality Weekly Report, 48*, 1–40. Retrieved from http://www.cdc.gov/mmwr/preview/mmwrhtml/rr4811a1.htm

Centers for Disease Control and Prevention. (2011, October). *Introduction to program evaluation for public health programs: A self-study guide.* Retrieved from http://www.cdc.gov/eval/guide/CDCEvalManual.pdf

Centers for Disease Control and Prevention. (2015). *Effective interventions: HIV prevention that works.* Retrieved from https://effectiveinterventions.cdc.gov/

Chen, H. T. (2014). *Practical program evaluation: Theory-driven evaluation and the integrated evaluation perspective* (2nd ed.). Los Angeles, CA: Sage.

Cochrane Collaboration. (2014). *Cochrane Reviews.* Retrieved from http://www.cochrane.org/cochrane-reviews

Coffent, J. K., Hendriksen, I. J. M., Duijts, S. F., Proper, K. I., van Mechelen, W., & Boot, C. R. L. (2012). The development of the Be Active & Relax "Vitality in Practice" (VIP) project and design of an RCT to reduce the need for recovery in office employees. *BMC Public Health, 12,* 592.

Collard, D. C. M., Chinapaw, M. J. M., van Mechelen, W., & Verhagen, E. A. L. M. (2009). Design of the iPlay study: Systematic development of a physical activity injury prevention programme for primary school children. *Sports Medicine, 39*(11), 889–901.

Community Preventive Services Task Force. (2015, July). *The guide to community preventive services.* Retrieved from http://www.thecommunityguide.org/index.html

Connell, J. P., & Kubisch, A. C. (1996). Applying a theories of change approach to the evaluation of comprehensive community initiatives: Progress, prospects, and problems. In K. Fulbright-Anderson, A. C. Kubisch, & J. P. Connell (Eds.), *New approaches to evaluating community initiatives: Vol. 2. Theory, measurement, and analysis* (pp. 15–44). Washington, DC: The Aspen Institute.

Cooper, H., Hedges, L. V., & Valentine, J. C. (2009). *The handbook of research synthesis and meta-analysis* (2nd ed.). New York, NY: Russell Sage Foundation.

Corbie-Smith, G., Akers, A., Blumenthal, C., Council, B., Wynn, M., Muhammad, M., & Stith, D. (2010). Intervention mapping as a participatory approach to developing an HIV prevention intervention in rural African American communities. *AIDS Education & Prevention, 22*(3), 184–202.

Côté, J., Godin, G., Garcia, P. R., Gagnon, M., & Rouleau, G. (2008). Program development for enhancing adherence to antiretroviral therapy among persons living with HIV. *AIDS Patient Care and STDs, 22*(12), 965–975.

Creswell, J. W. (2013). *Research design: Qualitative, quantitative, and mixed methods approaches* (4th ed.). Los Angeles, CA: Sage.

Crosby, R. A., DiClemente, R. J., Wingood, G. M., Sionéan, C., Cobb, B. K., & Harrington, K. (2000). Correlates of unprotected vaginal sex among African American female adolescents: Importance of relationship dynamics. *Archives of Pediatrics & Adolescent Medicine, 154*(9), 893–899.

Crosby, R. A., Salazar, L. F., & DiClemente, R. J. (2011). Ecological approaches in the new public health. In R. J. DiClemente, L. Salazar, & R. A. Crosby (Eds.), *Health behavior theory for public health: Principles, foundations, and applications* (pp. 231–251). Burlington, MA: Jones & Bartlett Learning.

Crutzen, R., de Nooijer, J., Brouwer, W., Oenema, A., Brug, J., & de Vries, N. K. (2008). Internet-delivered interventions aimed at adolescents: A Delphi study on dissemination and exposure. *Health Education Research, 23*(3), 427–439.

Cullen, K. W., Bartholomew, L. K., & Parcel, G. S. (1997). Girl scouting: An effective channel for nutrition education. *Journal of Nutrition Education, 29*, 86–91.

Cullen, K. W., Bartholomew, L. K., Parcel, G. S., & Kok, G. (1998). Intervention mapping; Use of theory and data in the development of a fruit and vegetable nutrition program for Girl Scouts. *Journal of Nutrition Education, 30*, 188–195.

Curry, L. A., Krumholz, H. M., O'Cathain, A., Plano Clark, V. L., Cherlin, E., & Bradley, E. H. (2013). Mixed methods in biomedical and health services research. *Circulation. Cardiovascular Quality and Outcomes, 6*(1), 119–123.

Decat, P., Nelson, E., De Meyer, S., Jaruseviciene, L., Orozco, M., Segura, Z., ... Degomme, O. (2013). Community embedded reproductive health interventions for adolescents in Latin America: Development and evaluation of a complex multi-centre intervention. *BMC Public Health, 13*, 31.

De Craemer, M., De Decker, E., De Bourdeaudhuij, I., Verloigne, M., Duvinage, K., Koletzko, B., ... Cardon, G. (2014). Applying the Intervention Mapping protocol to develop a kindergarten-based, family-involved intervention to increase European preschool children's physical activity levels: The ToyBox-Study. *Obesity Reviews, 15*(S3), S14–S26.

De Decker, E., De Craemer, M., De Bourdeaudhuij, I., Verbestel, V., Duvinage, K., Iotova, V., ... Cardon, G. (2014). Using the Intervention Mapping protocol to reduce European preschoolers' sedentary behavior, an application to the ToyBox-Study. *International Journal of Behavioral Nutrition and Physical Activity, 11*, 19–35.

De Henauw, S., Verbestel, V., Mårild, S., Barba, G., Bammann, K., Eiben, G., ... Pigeot, I. (2011). The IDEFICS community-oriented intervention programme: A new model for childhood obesity prevention in Europe? *International Journal of Obesity, 35*(S1), S16–S23.

DeLemos, J., Rock, T., Brugge, D., Slagowski, N., Manning, T., & Lewis, J. (2007). Lessons from the Navajo: Assistance with environmental data collection ensures cultural humility and data relevance. *Progress in Community Health Partnerships, 1*(4), 321–326.

Dera-de Bie, E., Gerver, W. J., & Jansen, M. (2013). Training program for overweight prevention in the child's first year: Compilation and results. *Nursing & Health Sciences, 15*(3), 387–397.

Detaille, S. I., van der Gulden, J. W. J., Engels, J. A., Heerkens, Y. F., & van Dijk, F. J. H. (2010). Using Intervention Mapping (IM) to develop a self-management programme for employees with a chronic disease in the Netherlands. *BMC Public Health, 10*, 353.

de Vries, H., Weijts, W., Dijkstra, M., & Kok, G. (1992). The utilization of qualitative and quantitative data for health education program planning, implementation, and evaluation: A spiral approach. *Health Education & Behavior, 19*(1), 101–115.

DiClemente, R. J., Salazar, L., & Crosby, R. A. (2011). *Health behavior theory for public health: Principles, foundations, and applications.* Burlington, MA: Jones & Bartlett Learning.

Duvinage, K., Ibrügger, S., Kreichauf, S., Wildgruber, A., De Craemer, M., De Decker, E., . . . Koletzko, B. (2014). Developing the intervention material to increase physical activity levels of European preschool children: The ToyBox-study. *Obesity Reviews, 15*(S3), S27–S39.

Earp, J. A., & Ennett, S. T. (1991). Conceptual models for health education research and practice. *Health Education Research, 6*(2), 163–171.

Economos, C. D., & Irish-Hauser, S. (2007). Community interventions: A brief overview and their application to the obesity epidemic. *The Journal of Law, Medicine & Ethics, 35*(1), 131–137.

Elliot, V. S. (2008, June). Healthy people 2020: National agenda shifts to risks, roots of disease. *American Medical News.* Retrieved from http://www.amednews.com/article/20080602/health/306029976/2/

Ezendam, N. P., Oenema, A., van de Looij-Jansen, P. M., & Brug, J. (2007). Design and evaluation protocol of "FATaintPHAT," a computer-tailored intervention to prevent excessive weight gain in adolescents. *BMC Public Health, 7,* 324.

Faridi, Z., Grunbaum, J. A., Gray, B. S., Franks, A., & Simoes, E. (2007). Community-based participatory research: Necessary next steps. *Preventing Chronic Disease, 4*(3). Retrieved from http://www.cdc.gov/pcd/issues/2007/jul/06_0182.htm

Fernández, M. E., Bartholomew, K., Linares, A., Lopez, A., Sockrider, M., Czyzewski, D., . . . Parcel, G. S. (2000a). *Qualitative research in the planning of a school-based asthma intervention: The FAMILIAS Project.* Paper presented at the Prevention Research Center Conference, Centers for Disease Control and Prevention, Atlanta, GA.

Fernández, M. E., Bartholomew, L. K., Lopez, A., Tyrrell, S., Czyzewski, D., Sockrider, M. M., & Abramson, S. (2000b). *Using Intervention Mapping in the development of a school-based asthma management intervention for Latino children and families: The FAMILIAS Project.* Paper presented at the meeting of the American Public Health Association, Boston, MA.

Fernández, M. E., Gonzales, A., Tortolero-Luna, G., Partida, S., & Bartholomew, L. K. (2005). Using intervention mapping to develop a breast and cervical cancer screening program for Hispanic farmworkers: Cultivando La Salud. *Health Promotion Practice, 6*(4), 394–404.

Fiscella, K., Franks, P., Gold, M. R., & Clancy, C. M. (2000). Inequality in quality: Addressing socioeconomic, racial, and ethnic disparities in health care. *Journal of the American Medical Association, 283*(19), 2579–2584.

Foster-Fishman, P. G., Nowell, B., & Yang, H. (2007). Putting the system back into systems change: A framework for understanding and changing organizational and community systems. *American Journal of Community Psychology, 39*(3–4), 197–215.

Fransen, G. A., Hiddink, G. J., Koelen, M. A., van Dis, S. J., Drenthen, A. J., van Binsbergen, J. J., & van Woerkum, C. M. (2008). The development of a minimal intervention strategy to address overweight and obesity in adult primary care patients in the Netherlands. *Family Practice, 25*(S1), i112–i115.

Frechtling, J. A. (2007). *Logic modeling methods in program evaluation.* San Francisco, CA: Jossey-Bass.

Friederichs, S. A. H., Oenema, A., Bolman, C., Guyaux, J., van Keulen, H. M., & Lechner, L. (2014). I Move: Systematic development of a web-based computer tailored physical activity intervention, based on motivational interviewing and Self-Determination Theory. *BMC Public Health, 14,* 212.

Gagnon, H., Godin, G., Alary, M., Bruneau, J., & Otis, J. (2010). A randomized trial to evaluate the efficacy of a computer-tailored intervention to promote safer injection practices among drug users. *AIDS and Behavior, 14*(3), 538–548.

Gillison, F., Greaves, C., Stathi, A., Ramsay, R., Bennett, P., Taylor, G.,... Chandler, R. (2012). "Waste the waist": The development of an intervention to promote changes in diet and physical activity for people with high cardiovascular risk. *British Journal of Health Psychology, 17*(2), 327–345.

Glanz, K., & Bishop, D. B. (2010). The role of behavioral science theory in development and implementation of public health interventions. *Annual Review of Public Health, 31,* 399–418.

Glanz, K., Rimer, B. K., & Viswanath, K. (Eds.). (2015). *Health behavior: Theory, research, and practice* (5th ed.). San Francisco, CA: Jossey-Bass.

Godin, G., Gagnon, H., Alary, M., Levy, J. J., & Otis, J. (2007). The degree of planning: An indicator of the potential success of health education programs. *Promotion & Education, 14*(3), 138–142.

Grant, A., Treweek, S., Dreischulte, T., Foy, R., & Guthrie, B. (2013). Process evaluations for cluster-randomised trials of complex interventions: A proposed framework for design and reporting. *Trials, 14,* 15.

Green, L. W., & Kreuter, M. W. (1999). *Health promotion planning: An educational and ecological approach* (3rd ed.). Mountain View, CA: Mayfield.

Green, L. W., & Kreuter, M. W. (2005). *Health program planning: An educational and ecological approach* (4th ed.). New York, NY: McGraw-Hill Professional.

Green, L. W., & Mercer, S. L. (2001). Can public health researchers and agencies reconcile the push from funding bodies and the pull from communities? *American Journal of Public Health, 91*(12), 1926–1929.

Hawe, P., Shiell, A., & Riley, T. (2009). Theorising interventions as events in systems. *American Journal of Community Psychology, 43*(3–4), 267–276.

Heinen, M. M., Bartholomew, L. K., Wensing, M., van de Kerkhof, P., & van Achterberg, T. (2006). Supporting adherence and healthy lifestyles in leg ulcer patients: Systematic development of the Lively Legs program for dermatology outpatient clinics. *Patient Education and Counseling, 61*(2), 279–291.

Higgins, J. P. T., & Green, S. (Eds.). (2008). *Cochrane handbook for systematic reviews of interventions.* Chichester, England: Wiley-Blackwell.

Higgins, J. P. T., & Green, S. (Eds.). (2011). *Cochrane handbook for systematic reviews of interventions: Version 5.1.0.* Retrieved from www.cochrane-handbook.org

Highfield, L., Bartholomew, L. K., Hartman, M. A., Ford, M. M., & Balihe, P. (2014). Grounding evidence-based approaches to cancer prevention in the community: A case study of mammography barriers in underserved African American women. *Health Promotion Practice, 15*(6), 904–914.

Hixon, A. L. (2003). Beyond cultural competence. *Academic Medicine, 78*(6), 634.

Hochbaum, G. M., Sorenson, J. R., & Lorig, K. (1992). Theory in health education practice. *Health Education Quarterly, 19*(3), 295–313.

Hoelscher, D. M., Evans, A., Parcel, G. S., & Kelder, S. H. (2002). Designing effective nutrition interventions for adolescents. *Journal of the American Dietetic Association, 102*(S3), S52–S63.

Horn, K., McCracken, L., Dino, G., & Brayboy, M. (2008). Applying community-based participatory research principles to the development of a smoking-cessation program for American Indian teens: "Telling our story." *Health Education & Behavior, 35*(1), 44–69.

Hou, S. I., Fernández, M. E., Baumler, E., & Parcel, G. S. (2002). Effectiveness of an intervention to increase Pap test screening among Chinese women in Taiwan. *Journal of Community Health, 27*(4), 277–290.

Hou, S. I., Fernández, M. E., & Parcel, G. S. (2004). Development of a cervical cancer educational program for Chinese women using Intervention Mapping. *Health Promotion Practice, 5*(1), 80–87.

Institute of Medicine, Committee on Health Literacy. (2004). *Health literacy: A prescription to end confusion.* Washington, DC: National Academies Press.

Israel, B. A., Schulz, A. J., Parker, E. A., & Becker, A. B. (1998). Review of community-based research: Assessing partnership approaches to improve public health. *Annual Review of Public Health, 19*, 173–202.

Israel, B. A., Schultz, A. J., Parker, E. A., Becker, A. B., Allen, A. J., III, & Guzman, J. R. (2008). Critical issues in developing and following community based participatory research principles. In M. Minkler & N. Wallerstein (Eds.), *Community-based participatory research for health: From process to outcomes* (2nd ed., pp. 47–66). San Francisco, CA: Jossey-Bass.

Israel, B. A., Parker, E. A., Rowe, Z., Salvatore, A., Minkler, M., López, J., ... Halstead, S. (2005). Community-based participatory research: Lessons learned from the Centers for Children's Environmental Health and Disease Prevention Research. *Environmental Health Perspectives, 113*(10), 1463–1471.

Jacobs, N. C., Völlink, T., Dehue, F., & Lechner, L. (2014). Online Pestkoppenstoppen: Systematic and theory-based development of a web-based tailored intervention for adolescent cyberbully victims to combat and prevent cyberbullying. *BMC Public Health, 14*, 396.

Jones, S. C., & Donovan, R. J. (2004). Does theory inform practice in health promotion in Australia? *Health Education Research, 19*(1), 1–14.

Kao, T. A., & Manczak, M. (2013). Family influences on adolescents' birth control and condom use, likelihood of sexually transmitted infections. *The Journal of School Nursing, 29*(1), 61–70.

Kass, N. E. (2001). An ethics framework for public health. *American Journal of Public Health, 91*(11), 1776–1782.

Kelder, S., Hoelscher, D., & Perry, C. L. (2015). How individuals, environments, and health behaviour interact: Social Cognitive Theory. In K. Glanz, B. K. Rimer, & K. Viswanath (Eds.), *Health behavior: Theory, research, and practice* (5th ed., pp. 285–325). San Francisco, CA: Jossey-Bass.

Kirby, D. (2004, August). BDI logic models: A useful tool for designing, strengthening and evaluating programs to reduce adolescent sexual risk-taking, pregnancy, HIV and other STDs. Retrieved from http://recapp.etr.org/recapp/documents/BDILOGICMODEL20030924.pdf

Kloek, G. C., van Lenthe, F. J., van Nierop, P. W., Schrijvers, C., & Mackenbach, J. P. (2006). Stages of change for moderate-intensity physical activity in deprived neighborhoods. *Preventive Medicine, 43*(4), 325–331.

Koekkoek, B., van Meijel, B., Schene, A., & Hutschemaekers, G. (2010). Development of an intervention program to increase effective behaviours by patients and clinicians in psychiatric services: Intervention Mapping study. *BMC Health Services Research, 10,* 293.

Kok, G., Gottlieb, N. H., Commers, M., & Smerecnik, C. (2008). The ecological approach in health promotion programs: A decade later. *American Journal of Health Promotion, 22*(6), 437–442.

Kok, G., Gottlieb, N., Peters, G., Mullen, P. D., Parcel, G. S., Ruiter, R. A. C., ... Bartholomew, L. K. (2015). A taxonomy of behavior change methods: An intervention mapping approach. *Health Psychology Review.* Advance online publication. doi: 10.1080/17437199.2015.1077155

Kok, G., Harterink, P., Vriens, P., de Zwart, O., & Hospers, H. J. (2006). The gay cruise: Developing a theory- and evidence-based Internet HIV-prevention intervention. *Sexuality Research and Social Policy, 3*(2), 52–67.

Kok, G., Schaalma, H., Ruiter, R. A. C., van Empelen, P., & Brug, J. (2004). Intervention mapping: Protocol for applying health psychology theory to prevention programmes. *Journal of Health Psychology, 9*(1), 85–98.

Kolbe-Alexander, T., Proper, K. I., Lambert, E. V., van Wier, M. F., Pillay, J. D., Nossel, C., ... Van Mechelen, W. (2012). Working on wellness (WOW): A worksite health promotion intervention programme. *BMC Public Health, 12,* 372.

Kremers, S. P. J., Visscher, T. L. S., Brug, J., Chin, A. P., Schouten, E. G., Schuit, A. J., ... Kromhout, D. (2005). Netherlands research programme weight gain prevention (NHF-NRG): Rationale, objectives and strategies. *European Journal of Clinical Nutrition, 59*(4), 498–507.

Kreuter, M. W., De Rosa, C., Howze, E. H., & Baldwin, G. T. (2004). Understanding wicked problems: A key to advancing environmental health promotion. *Health Education & Behavior, 31*(4), 441–454.

Krieger, J., Allen, C., Cheadle, A., Ciske, S., Schier, J. K., Senturia, K., & Sullivan, M. (2002). Using community-based participatory research to address social determinants of health: Lessons learned from Seattle Partners for Healthy Communities. *Health Education & Behavior, 29*(3), 361–382.

Kronborg, H., Væth, M., Olsen, J., Iversen, L., & Harder, I. (2007). Effect of early postnatal breastfeeding support: A cluster-randomized community based trial. *Acta Paediatrica, 96*(7), 1064–1070.

Kwak, L., Kremers, S. P. J., Werkman, A., Visscher, T. L. S., van Baak, M. A., & Brug, J. (2007). The NHF-NRG In Balance-project: The application of Intervention Mapping in the development, implementation and evaluation of weight gain prevention at the worksite. *Obesity Reviews, 8*(4), 347–361.

Leerlooijer, J. N., Ruiter, R. A. C., Reinders, J., Darwisyah, W., Kok, G., & Bartholomew, L. K. (2011). The World Starts With Me: Using intervention mapping for the systematic adaptation and transfer of school-based sexuality education from Uganda to Indonesia. *Translational Behavioral Medicine, 1*(2), 331–340.

Leerlooijer, J. N., Weyusya, J., Ruiter, R. A. C., Bos, A. E. R., Rijsdijk, L. E., Nshakira, N., . . . Kok, G. (2013). Empowering teenage mothers in Uganda: The development of a community based intervention to improve psychological and social well-being of unmarried teenage mothers. *BMC Public Health, 13*, 816.

Leurs, M. T. W., Jansen, M. W. J., Schaalma, H. P., Mur-Veeman, I. M., & de Vries, N. K. (2005). The tailored schoolBeat-approach: New concepts for health promotion in schools in the Netherlands. In S. Clift & B. B. Jensen (Eds.), *The Health promoting school: International advances in theory, evaluation and practice* (pp. 89–107). Retrieved from http://www.euro.who.int/__data/assets/pdf_file/0012/111117/E90358.pdf?ua=1#page=88

Levi, A. (2009). The ethics of nursing student international clinical experiences. *Journal of Obstetric, Gynecologic, & Neonatal Nursing, 38*(1), 94–99.

Lloyd, J., Logan, S., Greaves, C., & Wyatt, K. (2011). Evidence, theory and context—Using intervention mapping to develop a school-based intervention to prevent obesity in children. *International Journal of Behavioral Nutrition and Physical Activity, 8*, 73–87.

Looijmans-van den Akker, I., Hulscher, M. E., Verheij, T. J. M., Riphagen-Dalhuisen, J., van Delden, J. J. M., & Hak, E. (2011). How to develop a program to increase influenza vaccine uptake among workers in health care settings? *Implementation Science, 6*, 47–55.

Marmot, M. (2000). Social determinants of health: From observation to policy. *The Medical Journal of Australia, 172*(8), 379–382.

McEachan, R. R., Lawton, R. J., Jackson, C., Conner, M., & Lunt, J. (2008). Evidence, theory and context: Using intervention mapping to develop a worksite physical activity intervention. *BMC Public Health, 8*, 326.

McLeroy, K. (2006). Thinking of systems. *American Journal of Public Health, 96*(3), 402.

Mikolajczak, J., Kok, G., & Hospers, H. J. (2008). Queermasters: Developing a theory- and evidence-based Internet HIV-prevention intervention to promote HIV-testing among men who have sex with men (MSM). *Applied Psychology, 57*(4), 681–697.

Minkler, M. (2004). Ethical challenges for the "outside" researcher in community based participatory research. *Health Education & Behavior, 31*(6), 684–697.

Minkler, M. (2005). Community-based research partnerships: Challenges and opportunities. *Journal of Urban Health, 82*(S2), ii3–ii12.

Minkler, M., Thompson, M., Bell, J., Rose, K., & Redman, D. (2002). Using community involvement strategies in the fight against infant mortality: Lessons from a multisite study of the national Healthy Start experience. *Health Promotion Practice, 3*(2), 176–187.

Mkumbo, K., Schaalma, H., Kaaya, S., Leerlooijer, J., Mbwambo, J., & Kilonzo, G. (2009). The application of Intervention Mapping in developing and implementing school-based sexuality and HIV/AIDS education in a developing country context: The case of Tanzania. *Scandinavian Journal of Public Health, 37*(S2), 28–36.

Mol, M. E., Ruiter, R. A. C., Verhey, F. R., Dijkstra, J., & Jolles, J. (2008). A study into the psychosocial determinants of perceived forgetfulness: Implications for future interventions. *Aging and Mental Health, 12*(2), 167–176.

Montaño, D. E., & Kasprzyk, D. (2015). Theory of Reasoned Action, Theory of Planned Behavior, and the Integrated Behavioral Model. In K. Glanz, B. K. Rimer, & K. Viswanath (Eds.), *Health behavior: Theory, research, and practice* (5th ed., pp. 168–222). San Francisco, CA: Jossey-Bass.

Morgan, D. L. (2006). Practical strategies for combining qualitative and quantitative methods: Applications to health research. In C. N. Hesse-Biber & P. Leavy (Eds.), *Emergent methods in social research* (pp. 165–182). Thousand Oaks, CA: Sage.

Morgan, D. L. (2007). Paradigms lost and pragmatism regained: Methodological implications of combining qualitative and quantitative methods. *Journal of Mixed Methods Research, 1*(1), 48–76.

Morgenstern, L. B., Bartholomew, L. K., Grotta, J. C., Staub, L., King, M., & Chan, W. (2003). Sustained benefit of a community and professional intervention to increase acute stroke therapy. *Archives of Internal Medicine, 163*(18), 2198–2202.

Morgenstern, L. B., Staub, L., Chan, W., Wein, T. H., Bartholomew, L. K., King, M., ... Grotta, J. C. (2002). Improving delivery of acute stroke therapy: The TLL Temple Foundation Stroke Project. *Stroke: A Journal of Cerebral Circulation, 33*(1), 160–166.

Mulvihill, C. K. (1996). AIDS education for college students: Review and proposal for a research-based curriculum. *AIDS Education and Prevention, 8*(1), 11–25.

Munir, F., Kalawsky, K., Wallis, D. J., & Donaldson-Feilder, E. (2013). Using intervention mapping to develop a work-related guidance tool for those affected by cancer. *BMC Public Health, 13*, 6.

Murray, N., Kelder, S., Parcel, G., & Orpinas, P. (1998). Development of an intervention map for a parent education intervention to prevent violence among Hispanic middle school students. *Journal of School Health, 68*(2), 46–52.

National Cancer Institute. (2007). *Greater than the sum: Systems thinking in tobacco control* (Publication no. 06-6085, Tobacco Control Monograph No. 18). Bethesda, MD: U.S. Department of Health and Human Services, National Institutes of Health, Author.

National Cancer Institute, Division of Cancer Control and Population Sciences. (n.d.). *Cancer control P.L.A.N.E.T.* Retrieved from http://cancercontrolplanet .cancer.gov/

National Center for Health Statistics. (2012). *Health, United States, 2011: With special feature on socioeconomic status and health.* Hyattsville, MD: U.S. Department of Health and Human Services.

Newby, K., Bayley, J., & Wallace, L. M. (2011). "What should we tell the children about relationships and sex?": Development of a program for parents using intervention mapping. *Health Promotion Practice, 12*(2), 209–228.

Östlund, U., Kidd, L., Wengström, Y., & Rowa-Dewar, N. (2011). Combining qualitative and quantitative research within mixed method research designs: A methodological review. *International Journal of Nursing Studies, 48*(3), 369–383.

Oude Hengel, K. M., Joling, C. I., Proper, K. I., van der Molen, H. F., & Bongers, P. M. (2011). Intervention Mapping as a framework for developing an intervention at the worksite for older construction workers. *American Journal of Health Promotion, 26*(1), e1–e10.

Pamuk, E., Makuc, D., Heck, K., Reuben, C., & Lochner, K. (1998). *Socioeconomic status and health chartbook. Health, United States, 1998.* Hyattsville, MD: National Center for Health Statistics.

Parker, D. L., Brosseau, L. M., Samant, Y., Xi, M., Pan, W., Haugan, D., & Study Advisory Board. (2009). A randomized, controlled intervention of machine guarding and related safety programs in small metal-fabrication businesses. *Public Health Reports, 124*(S1), 90–100.

Parkes, A., Henderson, M., & Wight, D. (2005). Do sexual health services encourage teenagers to use condoms? A longitudinal study. *The Journal of Family Planning and Reproductive Health Care, 31*(4), 271–280.

Patton, M. Q. (2008). *Utilization-focused evaluation* (4th ed.). Los Angeles, CA: Sage.

Patton, M. Q. (2012). *Essentials of utilization-focused evaluation.* Los Angeles, CA: Sage.

Penman-Aguilar, A., Carter, M., Snead, M. C., & Kourtis, A. P. (2013). Socioeconomic disadvantage as a social determinant of teen childbearing in the U.S. *Public Health Reports, 128*(S1), 5–22.

Pérez-Rodrigo, C., Wind, M., Hildonen, C., Bjelland, M., Aranceta, J., Klepp, K., & Brug, J. (2005). The pro children intervention: Applying the intervention mapping protocol to develop a school-based fruit and vegetable promotion programme. *Annals of Nutrition & Metabolism, 49*(4), 267–277.

Peters, G. Y. (2014). A practical guide to effective behavior change: How to identify what to change in the first place. *European Health Psychologist, 16*(5), 142–155.

Phelan, J. C., Link, B. G., & Tehranifar, P. (2010). Social conditions as fundamental causes of health inequalities: Theory, evidence, and policy implications. *Journal of Health and Social Behavior, 51*(S), S28–S40.

Prins, R. G., van Empelen, P., Beenackers, M. A., Brug, J., & Oenema, A. (2010). Systematic development of the YouRActionprogram, a computer-tailored physical activity promotion intervention for Dutch adolescents, targeting personal motivations and environmental opportunities. *BMC Public Health, 10*, 474.

Rakowski, W., & Breslau, E. S. (2004). Perspectives on behavioral and social science research on cancer screening. *Cancer, 101*(S5), S1118–S1130.

Reinaerts, E., de Nooijer, J., & de Vries, N. K. (2008). Using intervention mapping for systematic development of two school-based interventions aimed at increasing children's fruit and vegetable intake. *Health Education, 108*(4), 301–320.

Richard, L., Gauvin, L., & Raine, K. (2011). Ecological models revisited: Their uses and evolution in health promotion over two decades. *Annual Review of Public Health, 32*, 307–326.

Richardson, L. D., & Norris, M. (2010). Access to health and health care: How race and ethnicity matter. *Mount Sinai Journal of Medicine, 77*(2), 166–177.

Rimer, B. K. (2002). Perspectives on intrapersonal theories of health behavior. In K. Glanz, B. K. Rimer, & F. M. Lewis (Eds.), *Health behavior and health education: Theory, research, and practice* (3rd ed., pp. 144–159). San Francisco, CA: Jossey-Bass.

Riphagen-Dalhuisen, J., Frijstein, G., van der Geest-Blankert, M., Danhof-Pont, M., de Jager, H., Bos, N., . . . Hak, E. (2013). Planning and process evaluation of a multi-faceted influenza vaccination implementation strategy for health care workers in acute health care settings. *BMC Infectious Diseases, 13*, 235.

Rossi, P. H., Lipsey, M. W., & Freeman, H. E. (2004). *Evaluation: A systematic approach* (7th ed.). Thousand Oaks, CA: Sage.

Ruiter, R. A. C., Massar, K., van Vugt, M., & Kok, G. (2012). Applying social psychology to understanding social problems. In A. G. de Zavala & A. Cichocka (Eds.), *Social psychology of social problems: The intergroup context* (pp. 337–362). London, United Kingdom: Palgrave Macmillan.

Rutten, G. M., Harting, J., Bartholomew, L. K., Braspenning, J. C., van Dolder, R., Heijmans, M. F., . . . Oostendorp, R. A. (2014). Development of a theory- and evidence-based intervention to enhance implementation of physical therapy guidelines for the management of low back pain. *Archives of Public Health, 72*, 1.

Sanchez, A., Grandes, G., Cortada, J. M., Pombo, H., Balague, L., & Calderon, C. (2009). Modelling innovative interventions for optimising healthy lifestyle promotion in primary health care: "*Prescribe Vida Saludable*" phase I research protocol. *BMC Health Services Research, 9*, 103.

Scarinci, I. C., Bandura, L., Hidalgo, B., & Cherrington, A. (2012). Development of a theory-based (PEN-3 and Health Belief Model), culturally relevant intervention on cervical cancer prevention among Latina immigrants using intervention mapping. *Health Promotion Practice, 13*(1), 29–40.

Schaafsma, D., Stoffelen, J. M. T., Kok, G., & Curfs, L. M. G. (2013). Exploring the development of existing sex education programmes for people with intellectual disabilities: An intervention mapping approach. *Journal of Applied Research in Intellectual Disabilities, 26*(2), 157–166.

Schmid, A. A., Andersen, J., Kent, T., Williams, L. S., & Damush, T. M. (2010). Using intervention mapping to develop and adapt a secondary stroke prevention program in Veterans Health Administration medical centers. *Implementation Science, 5,* 97–107.

Secretary's Advisory Committee on National Health Promotion and Disease Prevention Objectives for 2020. (2010, July). *Healthy People 2020: An opportunity to address social determinants of health.* Retrieved from http://www.healthypeople.gov/sites/default/files/SocietalDeterminantsHealth.pdf

Shakibazadeh, E., Bartholomew, L. K., Rashidian, A., & Larijani, B. (2015). Persian Diabetes Self-Management Education (PDSME) program: Evaluation of effectiveness in Iran. *Health Promotion International.* Advance online publication. doi:10.1093/heapro/dav006

Shegog, R., Bartholomew, L. K., Parcel, G. S., Sockrider, M. M., Mâsse, L., & Abramson, S. L. (2001). Impact of a computer-assisted education program on factors related to asthma self-management behavior. *Journal of the American Medical Informatics Association, 8*(1), 49–61.

Simons-Morton, D. G., Simons-Morton, B. G., Parcel, G. S., & Bunker, J. F. (1988). Influencing personal and environmental conditions for community health: A multilevel intervention model. *Family & Community Health, 11*(2), 25–35.

Singh, A. S., Chin A Paw, M. J. M., Kremers, S. P. J., Visscher, T. L. S., Brug, J., & van Mechelen, W. (2006). Design of the Dutch Obesity Intervention in Teenagers (NRG-DOiT): Systematic development, implementation and evaluation of a school-based intervention aimed at the prevention of excessive weight gain in adolescents. *BMC Public Health, 6,* 304.

Smith, P., Novello, G., & Chacko, M. R. (2011). Does immediate access to birth control help prevent pregnancy? A comparison of onsite provision versus off campus referral for contraception at two school-based clinics. *Journal of Applied Research on Children, 2*(2), 8.

Society for Public Health Education. (n.d.). *Ethics: Code of ethics for the health education profession.* Retrieved from http://www.sophe.org/ethics.cfm

Springvloet, L., Lechner, L., & Oenema, A. (2014). Planned development and evaluation protocol of two versions of a web-based computer-tailored nutrition education intervention aimed at adults, including cognitive and environmental feedback. *BMC Public Health, 14,* 47.

Steckler, A., & Linnan, L. A. (Eds.). (2002). *Process evaluation for public health interventions and research.* San Francisco, CA: Jossey-Bass.

Steckler, A., McLeroy, K. R., Goodman, R. M., Bird, S. T., & McCormick, L. (1992). Toward integrating qualitative and quantitative methods: An introduction. *Health Education Quarterly, 19*(1), 1–8.

Stokols, D. (1996). Translating social ecological theory into guidelines for community health promotion. *American Journal of Health Promotion, 10*(4), 282–298.

Stone, E. G., Morton, S. C., Hulscher, M. E., Maglione, M. A., Roth, E. A., Grimshaw, J. M.,...Shekelle, P. G. (2002). Interventions that increase use of adult immunization and cancer screening services: A meta-analysis. *Annals of Internal Medicine, 136*(9), 641–651.

Strijk, J. E., Proper, K. I., van der Beek, A. J., & van Mechelen, W. (2009). The Vital@Work Study. The systematic development of a lifestyle intervention to improve older workers' vitality and the design of a randomised controlled trial evaluating this intervention. *BMC Public Health, 9,* 408.

Suzuki, R., Peterson, J. J., Weatherby, A. V., Buckley, D. I., Walsh, E. S., Kailes, J. I., & Krahn, G. L. (2012). Using intervention mapping to promote the receipt of clinical preventive services among women with physical disabilities. *Health Promotion Practice, 13*(1), 106–115.

Taylor, N. J., Sahota, P., Sargent, J., Barber, S., Loach, J., Louch, G., & Wright, J. (2013). Using intervention mapping to develop a culturally appropriate intervention to prevent childhood obesity: The HAPPY (Healthy and Active Parenting Programme for Early Years) study. *International Journal of Behavioral Nutrition and Physical Activity, 10,* 142–172.

Tervalon, M. (2003). Components of culture in health for medical students' education. *Academic Medicine, 78*(6), 570–576.

Tervalon, M., & Murray-Garcia, J. (1998). Cultural humility versus cultural competence: A critical distinction in defining physician training outcomes in multicultural education. *Journal of Health Care for the Poor and Underserved, 9*(2), 117–125.

Theunissen, K. A. T. M., Hoebe, C. J. P. A., Crutzen, R., Kara-Zaïtri, C., de Vries, N. K., van Bergen, J. E. A. M., . . . Dukers-Muijrers, H. T. M. (2013). Using intervention mapping for the development of a targeted secure web-based outreach strategy named SafeFriend, for *Chlamydia trachomatis* testing in young people at risk. *BMC Public Health, 13,* 996.

Thomas, J. C., Sage, M., Dillenberg, J., & Guillory, V. J. (2002). A code of ethics for public health. *American Journal of Public Health, 92*(7), 1057–1059.

Thomas, S. B., Quinn, S. C., Butler, J., Fryer, C. S., & Garza, M. A. (2011). Toward a fourth generation of disparities research to achieve health equity. *Annual Review of Public Health, 32,* 399–416.

Tripp, M. K., Herrmann, N. B., Parcel, G. S., Chamberlain, R. M., & Gritz, E. R. (2000). Sun Protection Is Fun! A skin cancer prevention program for preschools. *Journal of School Health, 70*(10), 395–401.

Trochim, W. M., Cabrera, D. A., Milstein, B., Gallagher, R. S., & Leischow, S. J. (2006). Practical challenges of systems thinking and modeling in public health. *American Journal of Public Health, 96*(3), 538–546.

U.S. Department of Health and Human Services. (2001, January). *Healthy People 2010: Understanding and improving health.* Retrieved from http://www.health .gov/healthypeople/Document/html/uih/uih_2.htm#obj

van Bokhoven, M. A., Kok, G., & van der Weijden, T. (2003). Designing a quality improvement intervention: A systematic approach. *Quality & Safety in Health Care, 12*(3), 215–220.

Van Der Veen, Y. J. J., van Empelen, P., & Richardus, J. H. (2012). Development of a culturally tailored internet intervention promoting hepatitis B screening in the Turkish community in the Netherlands. *Health Promotion International, 27*(3), 342–355.

van Empelen, P., Kok, G. Schaalma. H. P., & Bartholomew, L. K. (2003). An AIDS risk reduction program for Dutch drug users: An intervention mapping approach to planning. *Health Promotion Practice, 4*(4), 402–412.

van Genugten, L., van Empelen, P., Flink, I., & Oenema, A. (2010). Systematic development of a self-regulation weight-management intervention for overweight adults. *BMC Public Health, 10,* 649.

van Kesteren, N. M., Kok, G., Hospers, H. J., Schippers, J., & de Wildt, W. (2006). Systematic development of a self-help and motivational enhancement intervention to promote sexual health in HIV-positive men who have sex with men. *AIDS Patient Care & STDs, 20*(12), 858–875.

van Oostrom, S. H., Anema, J. R., Terluin, B., de Vet, H. C. W., Knol, D. L., & van Mechelen, W. (2008). Cost-effectiveness of a workplace intervention for sick-listed employees with common mental disorders: Design of a randomized controlled trial. *BMC Public Health, 8,* 12.

van Oostrom, S. H., Anema, J. R., Terluin, B., Venema, A., de Vet, H. C. W., & van Mechelen, W. (2007). Development of a workplace intervention for sick-listed employees with stress-related mental disorders: Intervention Mapping as a useful tool. *BMC Health Services Research, 7,* 127.

van Schijndel-Speet, M., Evenhuis, H. M., van Empelen, P., van Wijck, R., & Echteld, M. A. (2013). Development and evaluation of a structured programme for promoting physical activity among seniors with intellectual disabilities: A study protocol for a cluster randomized trial. *BMC Public Health, 13,* 746.

van Stralen, M. M., Kok, G., de Vries, H., Mudde, A. N., Bolman, C., & Lechner, L. (2008). The Active *plus* protocol: Systematic development of two theory- and evidence-based tailored physical activity interventions for the over-fifties. *BMC Public Health, 8,* 399.

Verbestel, V., De Henauw, S., Maes, L., Haerens, L., Mårild, S., Eiben, G., ... De Bourdeaudhuij, I. (2011). Using the intervention mapping protocol to develop a community-based intervention for the prevention of childhood obesity in a multi-centre European project: The IDEFICS intervention. *International Journal of Behavioral Nutrition and Physical Activity, 8,* 82–96.

Vermeulen, S. J., Anema, J. R., Schellart, A. J. M., van Mechelen, W., & van der Beek, A. J. (2009). Intervention mapping for development of a participatory return-to-work intervention for temporary agency workers and unemployed workers sick-listed due to musculoskeletal disorders. *BMC Public Health, 9,* 216.

Vernon, S. W., Bartholomew, L. K., McQueen, A., Bettencourt, J. L., Greisinger, A., Coan, S. P., ... & Myers, R. E. (2011). A randomized controlled trial of a tailored interactive computer-delivered intervention to promote colorectal cancer screening: Sometimes more is just the same. *Annals of behavioral medicine, 41*(3), 284–299.

Vernon, S. W., del Junco, D. J., Tiro, J. A., Coan, S. P., Perz, C. A., Bastian, L. A., ... DiClemente, C. (2008). Promoting regular mammography screening II. Results from a randomized controlled trial in US women veterans. *Journal of the National Cancer Institute, 100*(5), 347–358.

Verweij, L. M., Proper, K. I., Weel, A. N. H., Hulshof, C. T. J., & van Mechelen, W. (2009). Design of the Balance@Work project: Systematic development, evaluation and implementation of an occupational health guideline aimed at the prevention of weight gain among employees. *BMC Public Health*, *9*, 461.

Villarruel, A. M., Jemmott, J. B., III, Jemmott, L. S., & Ronis, D. L. (2007). Predicting condom use among sexually experienced Latino adolescents. *Western Journal of Nursing Research*, *29*(6), 724–738.

Wallerstein, N. B., & Duran, B. (2006). Using community-based participatory research to address health disparities. *Health Promotion Practice*, *7*(3), 312–323.

Walthouwer, M. J. L., Oenema, A., Soetens, K., Lechner, L., & de Vries, H. (2013). Systematic development of a text-driven and a video-driven web-based computer-tailored obesity prevention intervention. *BMC Public Health*, *13*, 978.

Weiland, A., Blankenstein, A. H., Willems, M. H. A., Van Saase, J. L. C. M., Van der Molen, H. T., Van Dulmen, A. M., & Arends, L. R. (2013). Post-graduate education for medical specialists focused on patients with medically unexplained physical symptoms; Development of a communication skills training programme. *Patient Education and Counseling*, *92*(3), 355–360.

Weiss, B. D., & Coyne, C. (1997). Communicating with patients who cannot read. *The New England Journal of Medicine*, *337*(4), 272–274.

Wheeler, A., Fowler, J., & Hattingh, L. (2013). Using an intervention mapping framework to develop an online mental health continuing education program for pharmacy staff. *Journal of Continuing Education in the Health Professions*, *33*(4), 258–266.

Whittingham, J. R., Ruiter, R. A. C., Castermans, D., Huiberts, A., & Kok, G. (2008). Designing effective health education materials: Experimental pre-testing of a theory-based brochure to increase knowledge. *Health Education Research*, *23*(3), 414–426.

Windsor, R., Clark, N., Boyd, N. R., & Goodman, R. M. (2003). *Evaluation of health promotion, health education and disease prevention programs* (3rd ed.). New York, NY: McGraw-Hill.

W. K. Kellogg Foundation. (2006, February). *W. K. Kellogg Foundation logic model development guide*. Retrieved from https://www.wkkf.org/resource-directory/resource/2006/02/wk-kellogg-foundation-logic-model-development-guide

W. K. Kellogg Foundation. (2010). *W. K. Kellogg Foundation evaluation handbook*. Retrieved from https://www.wkkf.org/resource-directory/resource/2010/w-k-kellogg-foundation-evaluation-handbook

Wolfers, M. E. G., van den Hoek, C., Brug, J., & de Zwart, O. (2007). Using Intervention Mapping to develop a programme to prevent sexually transmittable infections, including HIV, among heterosexual migrant men. *BMC Public Health*, *7*, 141.

Wolfers, M., de Zwart, O., & Kok, G. (2012). The systematic development of ROsafe: An intervention to promote STI testing among vocational school students. *Health Promotion Practice*, *13*(3), 378–387.

Work Group for Community Health and Development, University of Kansas. (n.d.-a.). *Chapter 27. Cultural competence in a multicultural world.* Retrieved from http://ctb.ku.edu/en/table-of-contents/culture/cultural-competence

Work Group for Community Health and Development, University of Kansas. (n.d.-b.). *Section 4. Adapting community interventions for different cultures and communities.* Retrieved from http://ctb.ku.edu/en/tablecontents/section_1163.htm

World Health Organization. (2011). *Standards and operational guidance for ethics review of health-related research with human participants.* Geneva, Switzerland: Author.

Wyatt, K. M., Lloyd, J. J., Abraham, C., Creanor, S., Dean, S., Densham, E., . . . Logan, S. (2013). The healthy lifestyles programme (HeLP), a novel school-based intervention to prevent obesity in school children: Study protocol for a randomised controlled trial. *Trials, 14,* 95.

Yabroff, K. R., & Mandelblatt, J. S. (1999). Interventions targeted toward patients to increase mammography use. *Cancer Epidemiology, Biomarkers & Prevention, 8*(9), 749–757.

Yabroff, K. R., O'Malley, A., Mangan, P., & Mandelblatt, J. (2001). Inreach and outreach interventions to improve mammography use. *Journal of the American Medical Women's Association (1972), 56*(4), 166–173, 188.

Yoo, S., Weed, N. E., Lempa, M. L., Mbondo, M., Shada, R. E., & Goodman, R. M. (2004). Collaborative community empowerment: An illustration of a six-step process. *Health Promotion Practice, 5*(3), 256–265.

Zwerver, F., Schellart, A. J. M., Anema, J. R., Rammeloo, K. C., & van der Beek, A. J. (2011). Intervention mapping for the development of a strategy to implement the insurance medicine guidelines for depression. *BMC Public Health, 11,* 9.

Zwikker, H., van den Bemt, B., van den Ende, C., van Lankveld, W., den Broeder, A., van den Hoogen, F., . . . van Dulmen, S. (2012). Development and content of a group-based intervention to improve medication adherence in non-adherent patients with rheumatoid arthritis. *Patient Education and Counseling, 89*(1), 143–151.

# BEHAVIOR-ORIENTED THEORIES USED IN HEALTH PROMOTION

## Competency

• Use behavior-oriented theories to understand health problems and to plan interventions.

The purpose of this and the next chapter is to identify theories that are applicable to health education and promotion problems and solutions. The primary focus is health-related behavior, the supporting social and physical environments for this behavior, and the environments related directly to health. We review theories that help explain or change the health-related behavior of the at-risk group or the behavior of individuals who are responsible for health-related aspects of environments.

In Chapter 1 we explained that health promoters start with an assessment of health and quality-of-life problems, describe who has the problem and who is at risk for it, and explore behavioral and environmental conditions that contribute to the problem. Planners then must search for causes of the behaviors or environmental conditions and choose change methods to influence those determinants. In this process the health educator can look to theory for help with the following planning tasks:

• Describing the at-risk and intervention groups

• Understanding the health-promoting behaviors and environmental conditions

• Describing possible determinants of both risk and healthful behavior and environments

## LEARNING OBJECTIVES AND TASKS

• Identify and use behavior-oriented theories and theoretical constructs to explain behavior of at-risk individuals, environmental agents, and program users at each ecological level

• Select behavior-oriented theoretical constructs to inform methods to change determinants of behaviors at each ecological level

• Apply the core processes to make theory-informed decisions

**Table 2.1**    Examples of When to Use Theory in Intervention Planning

| Task | Examples |
| --- | --- |
| Describing the at-risk and intervention groups | Stage theories<br>Diffusion of Innovations Theory<br>Agenda-Building Theory |
| Understanding the health-promoting behaviors | Theories of self-regulation<br>Self-Determination Theory<br>Organizational development theories<br>Diffusion of Innovations Theory |
| Understanding the health-promoting environmental conditions | Social Cognitive Theory<br>Theories of social support<br>Organizational development theories |
| Describing possible determinants of both risk and health behavior and environments | Reasoned Action Approach<br>Social Cognitive Theory<br>Health Belief Model |
| Finding methods to promote change in the determinants, behavior, and environmental conditions | Communication-Persuasion Matrix<br>Organizational development theories<br>Conscientization |
| Identifying relevant program adopters, implementers, and maintainers, describing determinants of program adoption and implementation, and identifying methods for change | Diffusion of Innovations Theory<br>Reasoned Action Approach<br>Interactive Systems Framework<br>Consolidated Framework for Implementation Research |

- Finding methods to promote change in the determinants, behavior, and environmental conditions
- Describing determinants of program adoption and implementation among important stakeholders and identifying methods for change

An understanding of theoretical frameworks and constructs applicable to health promotion can broaden the planner's ability to complete the planning tasks. Table 2.1 presents some uses of theory in health promotion planning and examples of theories for each use.

## Perspectives

In this chapter, we focus on the importance of an ecological understanding of health problems and their solutions. We encourage planners to break away from their habitual approaches that use single theories when developing programs and instead use a variety of theories to enhance their practice. We also encourage planners to consider the cultural sensitivity of theories and the common constructs that many theories share.

## Eclectic Use of Theory

In discussions of theory, several authors have described the limitations of current theories and how they have been used in epidemiological research and intervention design (Head & Noar, 2014; Resnicow & Page, 2008; Resnicow & Vaughan, 2006; Sniehotta, Presseau & Araújo-Soares, 2014). Other authors have responded that increasing the sophistication of our models and measurement procedures will show the usefulness of our current health behavior theories (Baranowski, 2006; Brug, 2006; Kok & Ruiter, 2014). We agree that current health behavior theories, along with environmental change theories, provide a basis for understanding and predicting behavior change and designing interventions. However, we encourage planners to break away from their habitual (theory-driven) approaches that use single theories when developing programs and instead use a variety of theories to enhance their practice. That is, one theory will never explain all aspects of a real-life problem. Using a multitheories approach encourages the planner to consider the complexity of designing behavior change interventions (Schaalma & Kok, 2009). As a consequence, we use various theories when planning behavior change, each of which focuses on one aspect of the behavior or the behavior change. Some theories are especially relevant in terms of identifying the determinants of behavior (e.g., Reasoned Action Approach, Dual Systems Theory); others are more useful with regard to choosing and applying behavior change methods (e.g., Social Cognitive Theory, Precaution-Adoption Process Model). The unique skill of the well-trained behavioral scientist is to link the relevant elements of a given problem to useful theories (Buunk & van Vugt, 2013; Crosby & Noar, 2010; Ruiter, Massar, van Vugt, & Kok, 2012), which emphasizes a benefit of including behavioral scientists and their unique expertise on an intervention planning team (Kok, 2014).

## Ecological Interventions

As mentioned in Chapter 1, Intervention Mapping acknowledges that human behaviors happen in complex ecological systems. Individuals live and work in many different kinds of multilevel environments, including interpersonal, organizational, community, and societal environments (Kok, Gottlieb, Commers, & Smerecnik, 2008). Changing people's health behaviors (e.g., the behavior of a group of employees) therefore also involves changing the relevant environmental conditions (e.g., the workplace). These environments are often not under the control of the individual, but rather under the control of agents or decision makers (e.g., a manager). Thus, changing an environmental condition for health purposes means changing the behavior of the environmental agent. On the one hand, environmental agents are individuals and may be addressed with individual-level behavior change methods; on the other hand, they also function at the environmental level and may be addressed with behavior change methods that are effective at that level, for example, organizational change methods or community development methods (Kok, 2014; Kok, Zijlstra, & Ruiter, 2015). Intervention Mapping is a tool to design behavior change interventions that use change methods to affect theoretical variables from multiple levels within an ecological system. Not only should health educators understand a health problem, including behavioral causes, environmental conditions, and their determinants, but they should also make informed choice of the level(s) of intervention, which can be one or more of the individual, interpersonal, organizational, community, societal, or supranational environment levels (Crosby & Noar, 2010; Kok, Gottlieb, Panne, & Smerecnik, 2012; Richard, Potvin, Kishchuk, Prlic, & Green, 1996). Table 2.2 presents theories by ecological level.

Health promoters need to look at the determinants of the behavior of the at-risk population; of the agents who influence the environmental conditions related to the at-risk individuals' behavior, health, and quality of life; and of those who bring the program to the populations at risk by adopting and using the program. Figure 2.1 depicts the determinants of the at-risk group and environmental agents. Questions regarding what influences the behavior of individuals, decision makers, and program users at different environmental levels will help increase understanding of the determinants of these behaviors and inform future interventions, as illustrated in the following nutrition example.

At the individual level, the planner might ask: What influences the individual to eat more fruits and vegetables? At the higher levels, the planner might ask: What influences the decision-making agent to promote environmental conditions that facilitate the healthful decision? Why, for example, do the decision-making agents buy fruits and vegetables for the home, purchase or modify healthful foods for the school cafeteria, develop feature articles in the newspaper about how families are changing the way they eat for health and well-being, or pass legislation subsidizing healthful school meals for low-income children? As with individual health behavior, personal determinants and environmental conditions influence agent decision making. At the higher-order system levels, however, complexity increases, and different factors come into play. For example, decisions related to environmental changes are often made by individuals within groups, such as school boards or legislatures, who are referred to as environmental agents. Emergent processes unique to each level constrain the behavior of individual agents, and the action by the group changes the environmental condition. Also, individuals at the higher levels act within roles

**Table 2.2**    Theories Arrayed by Level

| Intervention Levels | Theories |
|---|---|
| **Chapter 2** | |
| Individual | Learning theories |
| | Theories of information Processing |
| | Health Belief Model |
| | Protection Motivation Theory and Extended Parallel Process Model |
| | Theory of Reasoned Action, Theory of Planned Behavior, Integrated Behavioral Model, Reasoned Action Approach |
| | Goal-setting theory, Theories of goal-directed behaviors |
| | Theories of automatic behavior and habits |
| | Transtheoretical Model of Behavior Change |
| | Precaution-Adoption Process Model and risk communication |
| | Attribution theory and relapse prevention |
| | Communication-Persuasion Matrix |
| | Elaboration Likelihood Model |
| | Theories of self-regulation |
| | Self-Determination Theory |
| Interpersonal environment | Social Cognitive Theory |
| | Theories of stigma and discrimination |
| | Diffusion of Innovations Theory |
| **Chapter 3** | |
| Multilevel theories | Systems theory |
| | Theories of power |
| | Empowerment theories |
| Interpersonal environment | Social networks and social support theories |
| Organization | Theories of organizational change |
| | Theories of organizational development |
| | Stakeholder theory |
| Community | Coalition theory |
| | Social capital theory |
| | Social norms theories |
| | Conscientization |
| | Community organization theories |
| Society and government | Multiple Streams Theory |
| | Advocacy Coalition Framework |

(e.g., school principal, medical director, and health care provider) with certain expectations and responsibilities. See Chapter 3.

Figure 2.1 presents a logic model for the relationships among theory- and evidence-based change methods, personal determinants, environmental conditions, behaviors, and health. As planners ask the questions pertinent to each step in the logic model, theories will be one

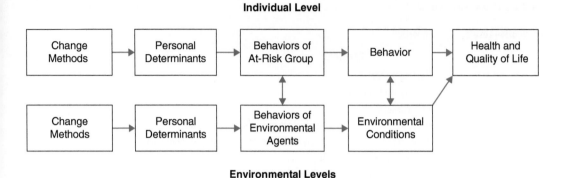

**Figure 2.1**   Logic Model for Methods, Determinants, Behaviors, Environmental Conditions, and Health

source for answers. Among the contributors to health are the behavior of the at-risk group and environmental conditions. Planners search for personal determinants and environmental conditions influencing the at-risk group's behavior. They also identify agents that could act on the environmental condition(s) and identify the personal determinants and environmental conditions that influence the agents' behavior. Finally, they identify change methods and practical applications that may influence these sets of determinants.

## Cultural Sensitivity of Theories

With respect to applying theories across cultures, our position is that theories are descriptions of processes that can be generalized over groups and over cultures. The weight of each different variable in a theory may vary over cultures as it varies over subpopulations. For example, researchers have used the constructs in the Health Belief Model (HBM) to describe health behavior in various cultures, even though the relative importance of the variables may differ from culture to culture (Champion & Skinner, 2008). The specific content of the variables within theories—surface as well as deep structure variables—may be very different. For instance, the meaning of health, environmental factors, lifestyles, determinants of behaviors, media characteristics, or settings may differ across cultural groups. In other words, the construct outcome *beliefs* may influence attitude, which in turn determines the behavioral response, but the content of the belief may vary across cultures. Likewise, self-efficacy expectations may vary across groups for a specific behavior, but they will still predict behavior change. The role models used in interventions will reflect the cultural background of the intended audience, but modeling should be a useful method for change in any culture. Self-management of diseases will take different forms in different cultural settings, but the process of monitoring, evaluating, and moving to action is the same Leerlooijer et al., 2011; Leerlooijer et al., 2014a; Leerlooijer et al., 2014b; Shilubane et al., 2013; Sialubanje, Massar, Hamer, & Ruiter, 2014; Nyembezi et al., 2014). Pasick et al. (2009) argued that our theories are not culture-free; however, finding specific details that are not part of a general theory does not in itself invalidate the usefulness of the theory (see also Fishbein, 2000). Other scholars described the importance of selecting a theory that is specific for the context where it is applied (Head & Noar, 2014). They thus prefer utility of a theory—that is, the degree to which the theory fits the intervention context—over generalizability across different populations, behaviors, and diseases. In our view the challenge of applying theories across cultures is in determining the content and the application of selected theories through systematic qualitative and quantitative research among intervention group members, program users, and experts, not in deciding whether the use of theory in general is advantageous or having specific theories for specific contexts (Kok & Ruiter, 2014).

## Theories and Common Constructs

Because theories are intended to reflect reality, many of the ones we discuss have similar elements but use different names for the constructs. Some agreement is emerging in the health promotion and behavioral health fields regarding important theoretical constructs across theories. For example, in 2001, five major behavioral science theorists (Albert Bandura, Marshall Becker, Martin Fishbein, Frederick Kanter, and Harry Triandis) agreed on a set of eight variables as key determinants of behavior (Committee on Communication for Behavior Change in the 21st Century: Improving the Health of Diverse Populations, 2002; Fishbein et al., 2001; Montaño & Kasprzyk, 2015):

1. The person has formed a strong positive intention (or made a commitment) to perform the behavior.

2. No environmental constraints make it impossible for the behavior to occur (barriers).

3. The person has the skills necessary to perform the behavior.

4. The person believes that the advantages of performing the behavior outweigh the disadvantages (attitude).

5. The person perceives more social (normative) pressure to perform the behavior than not to do so.

6. The person perceives that performing the behavior is more consistent than inconsistent with his or her own self-image (personal norms, personal standards).

7. The person's emotional reaction to performing the behavior is more positive than negative.

8. The person perceives that he or she has the capability to perform the behavior under a number of different circumstances (perceived self-efficacy, perceived behavioral control).

The five theorists saw the first three constructs as necessary and sufficient to determine behavior and the remaining five as influencing the strength and direction of intention. Many of these eight key variables have different names in different theories (see Noar & Zimmerman, 2005). For example, theorists have termed attitudes as outcome expectations and expectancies in Social Cognitive Theory, benefits and barriers in the Health Belief Model, behavioral beliefs and values in the Theory of Planned Behavior, and pros and cons in the Transtheoretical Model. When we discuss a theory, we point out similar or related constructs from other theories.

## BOX 2.1. MAYOR'S PROJECT

The mayor's planning committee finds itself in a predicament. All the group members have their favorite recipes for intervention. The group members have brainstormed some determinants of obesity-related behaviors, diet and exercise, and they used the core processes (Chapter 1) to access theory and evidence; however, the health promoter seems hard-pressed to get the group members to see beyond their own pet theories. What to do? She is determined to help the group construct a useful model of the problem from multiple theoretical perspectives. She wants to help the group develop a hypothetical causal model of the problem and then think about what behaviors and environmental conditions should change, what intervention levels might be appropriate, and which change methods would influence determinants. But how will she get the group to make progress?

The health promoter approaches the group management problem as she would any other planning process question. What are the determinants of the group members' behavior? What is holding them back from really working with theory? She considers that perhaps some group members know only one theory; some want a venue for theory testing; others just want to get the intervention done and aren't sure that theory is helpful at all. Looking at this short list, the health educator decides that if the group members have better knowledge of multiple theories and of ways to apply them to the problem of obesity, they may be more willing to continue with the planning process. She decides to sort all the literature that the group had gathered by the theories used in the research and by whether the articles present causes of obesity or interventions to decrease obesity. To each set of obesity-related articles, the health promoter attaches an article that reviews the relevant theory. She then assigns small groups from the task force to summarize a set of articles and present them to the larger group. The small groups are to answer the following questions: Does the article address causation of the behavior and environmental conditions or solutions? What do these articles say about the determinants of obesity-related behavior? Which of these causes are psychosocial determinants of individual behavior, and which are environmental conditions? If the causes are environmental, does the article contain data or theories that suggest the determinants of the environmental cause? Eager to know, the health educator awaits the results.

## Overview of Theories

This and the next chapter organize theories by ecological levels. This chapter covers major behavior-oriented theories used in health promotion, in which understanding and changing human behavior are the processes of interest. In Chapter 3, the focus is on environment-oriented theories, in which understanding and changing environmental conditions for health are the major processes of interest (see Table 2.2).

The chapters present brief reviews of selected theories to give the reader an overview of the use of theories in understanding and changing behavior at the individual and higher-order ecological levels. More than anything else, both chapters should alert the reader to the need to delve further into theories by consulting the references provided with the descriptions of the theories and searching for applications of the theory using the core processes (see Chapter 1; Buunk & van Vugt, 2013; Kok, Schaalma, de Vries, Parcel, & Paulussen 1996; Ruiter et al., 2012). A description of each theory is followed by a summary of the theory's use in health promotion to indicate the contribution to the following, if applicable:

- Intervention groups: How and why do we differentiate members of a group of program participants into subgroups?

- Behaviors: How can we describe relevant behaviors for intervention?

- Environments: What are relevant environmental conditions for interventions?

- Determinants: What are the personal factors that have been shown to predict or change behavior and environments?

- Change methods: What are appropriate methods to create change in determinants of behavior and environment?

Theories often link different ecological levels. For example, Social Cognitive Theory includes determinants from the social and physical environments, and the Theory of Planned Behavior has as a key predictor of behavior the normative expectations of others (in the environment) as the individual perceives them. In addition, many theories are potentially applicable to all ecological levels. The Theory of Planned Behavior, for example, is often applied to individual health behavior (Godin & Kok, 1996) but can be applied to explain the behavior of environmental agents, such as politicians (Flynn et al., 1998; N. Gottlieb et al., 2003), and program implementers, as well (Paulussen, Kok, Schaalma, & Parcel, 1995). Also, some theories are primarily explanatory (theory of understanding behavior, e.g., Theory of Planned Behavior); some are primarily about methods of change (theory of changing behavior, e.g., goal-setting theory); and others have elements of both types (e.g., Social Cognitive Theory). Explanatory theories suggest what needs to change; theories of change ideally tell how to change it. In practice, the jump from objectives about what to change to methods for creating change may sometimes be difficult. If applicable, we present in the current chapter first the theory's contribution to understanding behavior and then its contribution to change.

## Learning Theories

Learning theory is the foundation of most behavioral science theories. Learning refers to any enduring change in the way an organism responds based on its experience (Kazdin, 2012; Robbins, Schwartz, & Wasserman, 2001). Learning theories assume that experiences shape behavior and that learning is adaptive. Two major learning theory perspectives are classical conditioning and operant conditioning (McSweeney & Murphy, 2014).

### Classical Conditioning

Classical, or Pavlovian, conditioning is the learning of an association between a biologically relevant (appetitive or aversive), unconditioned stimulus (UCS) and a neutral, conditioned stimulus (CS; D. Gottlieb & Begej, 2014). A UCS produces an unconditioned response (UR), which is a response that does not have to be learned (e.g., pleasure as a result of being with friends). A conditioned response (CR) is a learned response that is qualitatively similar to the UR, which people learn as a result of the paired association of a neutral stimulus (called the conditioned stimulus, CS) with the UCS (e.g., pleasure as a result of drinking beer in the company of friends). In general, the association CS–UCS is most effective in producing a CR when the time interval is short, the CS precedes the UCS, and CS and UCS are repeatedly paired. People generalize from one CS to another, in case of similar CSs (e.g., pleasure when drinking alcohol with friends but also when drinking coffee with friends), but they also discriminate between

CSs (e.g., pleasure when drinking beer with your boss but not when drinking coffee with your boss). Discrimination between similar CSs or extinction of the learned association will occur when the stimuli are unpaired, such as when the CS (beer) is repeatedly presented without the UCS (drinking alone), although unlearning the CS–CR relationship is difficult even if the CR is punished (a hangover the day after).

Attitudes toward an appetitive or aversive stimulus (UCS) may become more positive or negative when that stimulus is spatiotemporally paired with a positively or negatively valued other stimulus (CS), which is called evaluative conditioning. This may be due to implicit misattribution in which people experience a positive feeling because of the CS and misattribute that feeling to the UCS (Jones, Fazio, & Olson, 2009). Evaluative conditioning can be effective in practice. For example, women with high body concern completed a conditioning procedure in which pictures of their bodies were selectively linked to positive social feedback: smiling faces (Martijn, Vanderlinden, Roefs, Huijding, & Jansen, 2010). The result was an increase in body satisfaction, compared with a control group without the conditioning. Or in the case of the alcohol drinking example, alcohol addicts in a rehabilitation program who in four sessions of 20 minutes each pushed away (UCS; avoidance behavior) pictures with alcohol contents (CS) and pulled pictures without alcohol toward them reported drinking less alcohol at one-year follow-up, presumably through the learning of a new inhibitory CS–UCS association in which alcohol stimuli are devalued to resolve the emerging response conflict between previous approach behavior and newly learned avoidance behavior (Houben, Havermans, Nederkoorn, & Jansen, 2012; Wiers, Gladwin, Hofmann, Salemink, & Ridderinkhof, 2013).

## Operant Conditioning

Like classical conditioning, operant conditioning is a form of associative learning in which the behavioral act becomes associated with its outcome: reward or punishment resulting in more or less frequent occurrence of the behavior (Murphy & Lupfer, 2014). Whether the behavior increases or decreases in frequency depends on how a person experiences the outcome of the behavior. Presentation of a stimulus that is rewarding (e.g., a valued gift) is positive reinforcement and makes a behavior more likely to occur, whereas the removal of a stimulus that is punishing (e.g., silencing a loud noise) is negative reinforcement but has the same positive effect of making the behavior more likely to occur. Punishment, on the other hand, decreases the probability that a behavior will recur either through the application of an unpleasant stimulus (positive punishment) or the removal of a pleasant stimulus (negative punishment).

There are several important characteristics of reinforcement:

• Reinforcement can be internal to the individual. For example, a person may have positive feelings in response to performing a behavior.

• The more continuous the reinforcement schedule is, the faster the learning. However, the more intermittent the reinforcement schedule is, the stronger the resistance to extinction of the learned behavior.

• The shorter the time interval between the behavior and the reinforcement is, the faster is the learning.

• As judged by the receiver, the value, size, and quality of a reinforcer lead to faster learning.

• The value of stimuli that serve as reinforcers varies among individuals and among cultures, but more-preferred stimuli result in higher rates of responding than less-preferred stimuli.

People learn to discriminate between situations that lead to reinforcement and situations that do not. People also learn to discriminate between behaviors that are reinforced immediately and those for which reinforcement is delayed (Robbins et al., 2001). Most people will prefer a smaller immediate reward (tasty food) over a large delayed reward (good health). Interestingly, when forced to make a choice between an immediate small reward versus a larger delayed reward far in advance of a situation, most people will choose the larger delayed reward. Therefore change methods might include helping people make an early commitment to healthy choices and helping them develop self-control and skills to follow through. This training should preferably start early in development, as correlational findings show that the ability or tendency to delay gratification in early childhood (preschool age) is associated with better life and health outcomes in adolescence and adulthood. For example, a study by Schlam, Wilson, Shoda, Mischel, and Ayduk (2013) found an association between the ability at the age of 4 to forego a smaller immediate reward (e.g., one cookie) in preference for a larger delayed reward (two cookies) and a lower body mass index 30 years later.

The reinforcing effects of positive feelings form the basis for social cognitive theories, such as the Theory of Planned Behavior and Social Cognitive Theory (discussed in more detail later in this chapter). The basic assumption of social cognitive theories is that the perception of the environmental stimulus rather than the stimulus itself is crucial to learning. Perceptions of environmental stimuli include, for instance, negative and positive evaluations of behavioral outcomes (outcome expectations) and the feasibility of behavior in a given context (self-efficacy expectations; Bandura, 1986; Kelder, Hoelscher, & Perry, 2015).

## Mere Exposure

Learning occurs in forms other than responses to reinforcing stimuli. For example, people become more positive about stimuli to which they are repeatedly exposed, even if they are not consciously aware of the process (Zajonc, 1980, 2001). This mere exposure effect is probably limited to stimuli to which a person has a relatively neutral attitude at the start. One method to change people's attitudes in a positive direction would be to expose them repeatedly to the new behavior or object. For instance, educators could show condoms repeatedly in classroom HIV-prevention education; parents and teachers could expose children to new foods. A related form of learning, referred to as social or vicarious learning, comes from observing and imitating others' behavior. Albert Bandura (1965, 1969) demonstrated vicarious learning, which requires the presence of a role model, in the classic Bobo doll experiments. In these studies, preschool children observed an adult model who kicks, hits, and throws things at an inflatable punching doll and then copied the aggressive behavior of the model when left alone with the doll. The effect of vicarious learning may be stronger when the social model is liked and respected and if the model's behavior is positively reinforced (Bandura, 1977).

## Summary: Learning Theories

Groups of people with the same learning history may have different behaviors, environmental conditions, and determinants and may need different methods to change. Learning theory applies to all human behavior. Many stimuli originate in the physical and social environment. Determinants include association of conditioned stimuli with uncondi- tioned stimuli, responses to short-term positive reinforcement, negative reinforcement, punishment, and attitude. Methods derived from learning theories are classical conditioning, feedback and reinforcement, short-term positive reinforcement for healthy behaviors, removal of punishing stim- uli for healthy behaviors, punishment of unhealthy behaviors, contingent rewards, early commitment, deconditioning, direct experience, modeling, and repeated exposure.

Feedback and reinforcement are effective methods to create changes in various determinants and behavior (Bandura, 1986; Kazdin, 2012). Feedback is information given to the learner regarding the extent to which the learner is accomplishing learning or performance (e.g., demonstrating better skills to mobilize social support) or the extent to which change is having an impact (e.g., an increase in physical activity leading to a reduction in blood pressure and weight). Feedback is a method for the learner to become aware of learning and performance, but it can also function to raise the learner's awareness regarding risk. Reinforcement is any component of the intervention that rewards or punishes the learner for the behavior (after the learner has enacted the behavior). Kazdin (2012) suggested that in a behavior modification program, punishment should be avoided because it may result in negative side effects, such as escaping or avoiding the source of the punishment. If punishment is used as a last resort, emphasis should first be placed on positive reinforcement for healthy behavior. Bandura (1986) distinguished among three types of directly applied reinforcement:

- Social reinforcement: praise from other people
- Vicarious reinforcement: observation of reinforcement of another
- Self-reinforcement: giving oneself a reward

Another relevant prediction of learning theory is that people learn behaviors through positive reinforcement, but they very slowly unlearn them through lack of reinforcement (Robbins et al., 2001). Deconditioning, letting people experience a lack of reinforcement or even negative outcomes, will not immediately lead to their unlearning a behavior. People accept, for instance, losing a number of sports games (punishment) if they sometimes win (positive reinforcement). Experiencing that an unhealthy behavior sometimes has negative consequences may not have much influence as long as these behaviors sometimes lead to positive reinforcement. Unlearning a behavior may require a continuous lack of positive reinforcement. In many cases this is practically impossible. For example, smoking will result in relaxation, and unsafe sex will result in immediate pleasure. A more effective approach is to learn new associations between recommended behavior and positive outcomes, for example through evaluative conditioning as illustrated above (Houben et al., 2012) or through direct experience (Maibach & Cotton, 1995). One caution is advisable when using direct experience as a method: Although it may enhance positive outcome expectations, direct experience may also enhance negative outcome expectations in the presence of unpleasant results from the behavior (punishment), such as discomfort during a mammogram or decreased sensation during condom use. Modeling, as a form of indirect experience, is also powerful, especially if it is clear that the model's behavior resulted in a lower risk and positive health or other attributes.

## Theories of Information Processing

Conventional wisdom has long held that giving people information could help them change their behavior and thereby solve health and social problems. However, knowledge does not generally lead directly to behavior change (McGuire, 1985). Furthermore, ensuring that people attain knowledge is not necessarily an easy task. Theories of Information Processing, such as Semantic Network Theory (Kintsch & van Dijk, 1978) and Mental Model Theory (Mayer, 1989), provide several concepts that suggest methods for successfully conveying information. Health promoters can benefit from incorporating evidence-based principles to improve the presentation and coherence of textual material to enhance message comprehension (Kools, Ruiter, van de Wiel, & Kok, 2004).

## Memorizing Through Chunking

Theories of Information Processing are concerned with how information is perceived, stored, and retrieved. Drawing from the Gestalt school of psychology (Koffka, 1935), these theories suggest that the senses perceive information in the context of what people already know. People perceive information actively to make sense of incomplete stimuli. For instance, someone who sees only eyes and a forehead will tend to perceive a face in order to complete the expected pattern. Theorists in perception, learning, and cognition suggest that people use their short-term memory, also called working memory, to complete the pattern. Working memory is a small "space," and its effectiveness can be increased by a method called chunking (Garrison, Anderson, & Archer, 2001; Smith, 2008). A chunk combines smaller pieces of information that have strong associations with one another to create one meaningful unit of information (Gobet et al., 2001). Chunking is typically employed by expert decision makers (as compared with novices). For example, Dutch chess master and psychologist Adriaan de Groot (1946/1978, as cited in Gobet et al., 2001) introduced chunking to explain the enhanced ability of expert chess players (as compared with novice chess players) to recall briefly presented positions from a tournament game. People might use chunking to promote learning by assigning an acronym or a summary slogan to a process so that the entire process can be encoded into memory (Gobet, 2005). For example, children in an asthma self-management program learned a rap song with the words "Watch, discover, think, and act" for the stages of self-management (Bartholomew et al., 2000a; Bartholomew et al., 2000b). Other examples of the use of chunking to enhance learning are "Stop, drop, and roll" for burn prevention; "Slip, slap, and slop" for use of hats and sunscreen; and "Stop, look, and listen" for traffic safety.

## Text Comprehension and Learning

When readers try to comprehend a text, they need to cognitively encode the incoming information by linking concepts from the text to the knowledge they already have. Some cognitive psychologists view knowledge as an associative network stored in long-term memory (Kintsch, 1988). Nodes in this network represent concepts, whereas the connections between the nodes represent the kinds and strengths of associations among concepts. Thus, a person assigns meaning to a concept based on its position in the network and by the strength of its connections to both neighboring and more distant concepts. Learners transfer information from working memory to long-term memory, integrate it into existing knowledge networks, and create nodes or change existing connections among nodes. In short, comprehension takes place.

The encoding (comprehension) of a text can take place on a textbase level (memory) and on a situation model level (learning; Kintsch, 1994; van Dijk & Kintsch, 1983). Textbase comprehension refers to a relatively superficial form of understanding; readers will be able to memorize the text from long-term memory rather literally, without necessarily having a thorough understanding of its content. In contrast, readers who have formed a situation model representation of a text have elaborated on the information by actively integrating it with their prior knowledge. Based on this more extensive representation of the information in the text, learning takes place, and readers will be able to generalize the acquired knowledge to other situations.

The coherence of text, at the macro level and at the micro level, influences comprehension (van Dijk & Kintsch, 1983). Coherence at the macro level means that the sections of the text have a logical order and are clearly related to each other and to the overall topic. Writers establish coherence by using headings that flag content for the reader and by structuring main parts (sections) as distinguished from subparts (paragraphs; Kools, Ruiter, van de Wiel, & Kok, 2007, 2008). They also make sure that first and last sentences in paragraphs explain how the information relates to previous and upcoming information, respectively (Kools, 2012). Coherence at the micro level means that each sentence is explicitly related to the next. The following principles of text development can be helpful: using a linking word from the previous sentence to maintain argument overlap, using demonstrative pronouns (*this, that, these, those*) only when they have only one possible referent, using sentence connectives (*furthermore, however*) to clarify relationships between sentences, maintaining an order of old information before new, and explicitly stating the actor and the action in each sentence (Kools, 2012; J. Williams & Bizup, 2015).

The use of imagery, the encoding of pictures with concepts to be stored in long-term memory, also improves memory and learning (Wright, 2012). Kools, van de Wiel, Ruiter, Crüts, and Kok (2006) show that graphic organizers, a graphic representation that conveys important relations between concepts in the text and thus helps in activating relevant knowledge networks, could improve the learning of health education materials substantially.

## Elaboration

To enhance learning and memory, learners must add to the meaning of the material presented to them—they must elaborate. Learners are particularly likely to elaborate if they have the ability to process information (e.g., sufficient time) and are motivated to do so (e.g., message relevance). Elaboration is effective if it helps tie the information together so that it can be consolidated into more durable and stronger memory representations (Bayliss, Bogdanovs, & Jarrold, 2015). Methods to encourage effective elaboration include group discussion and rehearsal of information. Van Blankenstein, Dolmans, van der Vleuten, and Schmidt (2011) tested the effects on short-term and long-term memory by having subjects either provide explanations or simply listen during small-group discussion. Contributing to the discussion did not increase immediate recall of a text that participants studied following the discussion, but contributing did increase recall 1 month later. Rehearsal of information may help make the information more salient for people (Smith, 2008). Rehearsal is even more effective in promoting remembering when the learner adds something to the information being learned. Hamilton and Ghatala (1994) related rehearsal to the ancient Greek method of *loci*, in which orators mentally attached parts of long speeches to landmarks on well-known travel routes. One might imagine a patient educator helping a learner memorize a long self-care process by attaching the steps in the procedure to landmarks on a familiar daily route. Verbal images or analogies are also helpful for encoding information to long-term memory. If material is too foreign or discrepant, it will not be learned. Therefore, analogies to more common events, concepts, or processes may be a helpful method, especially if learners can be guided to create their own analogies (cf. Foer, 2011). Promoting skills for information processing is a relevant issue in the Elaboration Likelihood Model (ELM; Petty, Barden, & Wheeler, 2009), which provides determinants and change methods for increasing these skills and for increasing motivation to process information more carefully (see Elaboration Likelihood Model section).

## Cues

Getting information into long-term memory is only the first part of learning. Usually, the learner must also get the information back out of long-term memory. People retrieve information from memory more easily when the memory is a strong one, and they make stronger memories when encoding requires effort as described above.

Health promoters can provide cues as a method for helping people retrieve information. For a cue to be effective, it should be present at the time of encoding and at the time of retrieval. For example, for teens who are learning to negotiate condom use, the cues present during learning and practice, such as what the partner says and the situation or setting, should be as similar as possible to what teens will encounter when they try to retrieve and apply the steps of negotiation in the real situation (Evans, Getz, & Raines, 1991; Godden & Baddeley, 1975; Tulving & Thomson, 1973). Cues work best when people systematically select and provide their own cues and in processes that are typically found in individuals with high (as opposed to low) working memory capacity (Unsworth, Brewer, & Spillers, 2013).

## Summary: Theories of Information Processing

Theories of Information Processing are concerned with how information is perceived, stored, and retrieved, making a distinction between long-term and short-term memory. Preexisting knowledge in long-term memory may facilitate information processing in short-term memory, thus enhancing successful encoding and retrieval of information. Methods derived from information processing theories that support encoding and retrieval include chunking, advance organizers, imagery, elaboration, rehearsal, group discussion, and cues.

## Theories of Health Behavior

Historically, a number of theories have focused directly on health and risk-related behavior (Brewer & Rimer, 2015; Conner & Norman, 2005; Glanz & Bishop, 2010). Most of these models are based on psychological expectancy-value models, which hypothesize that human behavior depends mainly on the value individuals place on a particular goal and their estimate of the likelihood that a specific action will achieve that goal. With respect to health, the components are typically the desire to avoid illness or to get well and the belief that a specific behavior will prevent or reduce illness.

### Health Belief Model

The Health Belief Model (HBM) has been used in a wide range of health-related contexts (Abraham & Sheeran, 2005; Skinner, Tiro, & Champion, 2015). The original HBM comprises the following four psychological constructs (Janz & Becker, 1984):

- Perceived susceptibility: a person's perception of the risk of contracting a particular condition or illness

- Perceived severity: a person's evaluation of the seriousness of contracting an illness

- Perceived benefits: a person's beliefs regarding the effectiveness of actions available to reduce the threat of a disease

- Perceived barriers: a person's beliefs regarding the potential negative aspects of a particular health action

Individuals decide to engage in a health action based on their perceptions of personal susceptibility to, and the severity of, a particular condition or illness balanced against benefits and barriers ascribed to taking the health action. According to the HBM, this decision making is triggered by a cue to action, which may be internal (e.g., symptoms of a disease) or external (e.g., a health education message or a friend with the disease). The HBM may be most helpful in understanding relatively simple health behaviors, such as mammography screening or immunization.

Although an impressive body of research findings has linked HBM dimensions to health actions, research has also demonstrated the importance of factors that were not originally examined as a part of the model. For example, people undertake many health-related behaviors for non-health reasons, suggesting that their analysis includes barriers and benefits that are not health related (Ajzen, 1988). Current social psychological models suggest that an individual's behavior, including health-related behavior, is also determined by perceptions of social influences and behavioral control (Fishbein & Ajzen, 2010; Montaño & Kasprzyk, 2015). In later applications of the HBM, researchers incorporated these variables, self-efficacy specifically and the role of social influences more generally (Skinner et al., 2015).

## Protection Motivation Theory and Extended Parallel Process Model

Protection Motivation Theory (PMT) has the same basic ingredients as the HBM (Norman, Boer, & Seydel, 2005; R. Rogers, 1983; Ruiter & Kok, 2012). PMT suggests that threat messages instigate two mediating cognitive processes (threat appraisal and coping appraisal) that, together, promote responses to the threat (referred to as danger control responses) rather than to the evoked fear (referred to as fear control responses). Threat appraisal includes assessments of threat seriousness and personal susceptibility, whereas coping appraisal includes assessments of the effectiveness of potential responses (response efficacy) and one's ability to undertake these successfully (self-efficacy). Together these appraisals generate protection motivation that is measured as an intention to adopt the protective recommendations (R. Rogers, 1983). PMT incorporates two additional constructs: rewards or reinforcement associated with maladaptive responses (e.g., smoking and relaxation) and costs or punishment associated with adaptive responses (e.g., not smoking and gaining weight).

Witte (1992) and Witte, Meyer, and Martell (2001) argued that it is important to understand both fear control and danger control responses. She proposed the Extended Parallel Process Model (EPPM), which suggests that threat perception initially instigates danger control processes (Ruiter & Kok, 2012; Witte, 1992; Witte et al., 2001). As in PMT, EPPM suggests that when people perceive a threat, they evaluate a recommended action based on its effectiveness and feasibility and that their response to the threat depends on the outcome of this coping appraisal. If they think the recommended action is effective and feasible, then they formulate intentions to perform the action. However, if they think the recommended action is ineffective or impossible, then the continuing perception of threat will result in emotional and, in particular, fear arousal. At this point, they may use fear control processes, such as denial and avoidance coping, to reduce unpleasant feelings of fear.

PMT and EPPM have been extensively tested (de Hoog, Stroebe, & de Wit, 2007; Floyd, Prentice-Dunn, & Rogers, 2000; Milne, Orbell, & Sheeran, 2002; Ruiter, Abraham, & Kok, 2001; Witte & Allen, 2000). Although the support for the impact of response efficacy and especially self-efficacy is strong, the support for the impact of susceptibility and severity is weak (Ruiter, Kessels, Peters, & Kok, 2014). PMT and EPPM suggest that threatening health information may be used to raise awareness and increase risk perceptions, but only if coping information can be successfully applied to enhance self-efficacy perceptions to deal with the health threat (Peters, Ruiter, & Kok, 2013).

## Fear

Fear arousal—vividly showing people the negative health consequences of life-endangering behaviors—has been suggested as a method to raise awareness of risk behavior and to change the risk behavior into health-promoting behavior. Using fear may be intuitively appealing to the health educator, and research on fear-arousing communication has a long tradition in social psychology and public health education (Peters, Ruiter, & Kok, 2014; ten Hoor et al., 2012). Most relevant theories and the available empirical data suggest that fear, as a result of subjective appraisals of personal susceptibility and severity, motivates an individual to action; however, the type of action depends on both outcome expectations and self-efficacy expectations (Peters et al., 2013). For instance, smokers may become afraid of cancer when they recognize their own susceptibility to cancer and the severity of the disease. Their fear may motivate them to stop smoking but only when they are convinced that quitting is effective in preventing cancer (response efficacy or outcome expectation) and when they feel confident that they are able to quit (self-efficacy). In this example, low self-efficacy may be the most important barrier to quitting for most smokers. What happens when people are afraid but are not convinced of the effectiveness of the alternative behavior or of their own self-efficacy? Most data suggest that under those conditions, the resulting behavior may be defensive, in essence, oriented toward avoidance of the fear message rather than health-promoting action, especially when the threat is highly personally relevant (Kessels, Ruiter, & Jansma, 2010; Ruiter et al., 2014).

What does this mean for the use of fear-arousing communication as a change method? First, fear is a motivator for behavior change; that is: no fear, no action. Second, fear motivates health-promoting behavior but only if the individual has high outcome and self-efficacy expectations. In cases in which people are not aware of their risk, health promoters may be able to provide confrontation with undeniable negative consequences of the risky behavior; however, to be effective, the messages probably should not be emotionally arousing (de Hoog et al., 2007). In situations in which people are aware of their risk but lack self-efficacy for engaging in a health-promoting alternative behavior, messages should focus on improving self-efficacy (Peters et al., 2013; Ruiter et al., 2014).

Self-Affirmation Theory has been applied to make people less defensive in the face of threatening health messages (Epton, Harris, Kane, van Koningsbruggen, & Sheeran, 2014; Harris, Mayle, Mabbott, & Napper, 2007; Schüz, Schüz, & Eid, 2013; Sherman, Nelson, & Steele, 2000). Self-Affirmation Theory suggests that fear appeals cause defensive reactions because they threaten people's self-image. Therefore, affirming a person's self-image would increase the acceptance of the risk information and motivate engagement with the healthy behavior. Recent empirical evidence extends the effect of self-affirmation and suggests that this technique increases sensitivity to the self-relevance of health information (Griffin & Harris, 2011; Kessels, Harris, Ruiter, & Klein, 2015). Examples of applications for self-affirmation include a writing exercise in which people write about their previously measured highest ranking values or record as many of their desirable characteristics as they can think of. Interestingly, self-affirmation can also be applied in fields other than health, for example as a method for promoting interpersonal relationships and enhancing student performance in threatening classroom settings (Cohen & Sherman, 2014).

## Message Framing

Health messages may be framed in terms of the beneficial consequences of healthy behavior (gain-framed messages) or the detrimental consequences of unhealthy behavior (loss-framed messages). For example, "Missing early detection of cancer by not getting a Pap test every year can cost you your life" (loss frame); "Getting a Pap test every year may enable you to live longer" (gain frame). A loss frame is not the same as a fear-arousing message; loss frames do not automatically lead to an emotional response (de Hoog et al., 2007). A large, and still-growing, body of literature is dedicated to investigating which type of frame is more effective under which circumstances and why. The single most influential explanation of message framing effects has been the notion that the relative effectiveness of gain- versus loss-framed information is dependent on the risk that is associated with the advocated behavior (risk-framing hypothesis). According to the risk-framing hypothesis, gain-framed messages are especially effective in promoting behaviors that prevent disease or promote health, such as exercising and healthy eating, and loss-framed messages are more effective in promoting behaviors that entail the "risk" of detecting a disease, such as undergoing a screening test for cancer (Rothman & Salovey, 1997). However, the evidence for the risk-framing hypothesis is weak and inconsistent (O'Keefe & Jensen, 2006, 2007, 2009; van't Riet et al., 2014). Werrij, Ruiter, van't Riet, and de Vries (2012) summarized the evidence and recommended using a gain frame because these messages are more easily processed and are therefore more readily accepted by the message receiver (see also Brüll, Ruiter, & Jansma, 2015).

## Summary: Theories of Health Behavior

Groups may be identified according to their perceptions of susceptibility and seriousness. Theories of health behavior recognize perceived environmental barriers in relation to perceived benefits. Determinants include perceived susceptibility, perceived severity, perceived benefits, and perceived barriers. Methods from the HBM, PMT, and EPPM are consciousness raising (cues to action), self-affirmation, framing, and methods to increase self-efficacy.

## Theories of Reasoned Action

Once there was a theory, the Theory of Reasoned Action (TRA), the original TRA (Fishbein & Ajzen, 1975). Then, there was an extension of the TRA, the Theory of Planned Behavior (TPB; Ajzen, 1988; Conner & Sparks, 2005). Then there was an extension of the TPB, the Integrated Behavioral Model (IBM; Montaño & Kasprzyk, 2015). And, finally there is the new and revitalized Theory of Reasoned Action, the Reasoned Action Approach (RAA; Fishbein & Ajzen, 2010). RAA is also an extension of the TPB but is more parsimonious than the IBM. All of these theories focus primarily on determinants of behavior and can be seen as expectancy-value theories. Although they do not give specific methods for behavior change, these theories help health promoters understand the specific constructs that need to be changed (Fishbein & Ajzen, 2010; Witte, 1995). Research with these theories has almost solely focused on the TPB.

## Theory of Planned Behavior

The TPB has successfully been applied to understand many types of health and other behaviors, such as blood donation (Bagot, Masser, & White, 2015), helmet use (Brijs et al., 2014), and energy conservation (Abrahamse & Steg, 2011). The TPB postulates that intention, the most important determinant of behavior, is in turn influenced by three constructs: attitude, subjective norms, and perceived behavioral control. Perceived behavioral control is comparable to self-efficacy in Social Cognitive Theory, which is discussed later in the chapter (Bandura, 1986; Fishbein & Ajzen, 2010, p. 160).

Health promoters are concerned mostly about attitude toward a behavior, "the individual's positive or negative evaluation of performing the particular behavior of interest" (Ajzen, 1988, p. 117). To understand attitudes toward a behavior, there must be correspondence, meaning that attitudes may predict behavior when both concepts are assessed at identical levels of action, context, and time. The attitude toward the behavior is determined by salient beliefs about that behavior. Each behavioral belief links the behavior to a certain outcome or to an attribute (e.g., "Going on a low-fat diet reduces my blood pressure"). Beliefs are weighted by the evaluations of those outcomes ("Reducing my blood pressure is very good for me").

Subjective norms (perceived social expectations) are a function of beliefs by people that specific, important individuals or groups (social referents) approve or disapprove of their performing a behavior and how important that opinion is to them. Beliefs about specific social referents, such as "my partner thinks..." or "my mother thinks..." are termed normative beliefs. Relative to normative beliefs, some authors distinguish between social expectations and social pressure, describing the latter as a much stronger influence (de Vries, Backbier, Kok, & Dijkstra, 1995). Not in the TPB, but integrated into the RAA, is the construct of descriptive norms: the behavior of relevant others (see Social Cognitive Theory section).

Perceived behavioral control (Ajzen, 1988), or self-efficacy (Bandura, 1986), refers to the subjective probability that a person is capable of executing a certain course of action (e.g., "For me to go on a low-fat diet would be [easy versus difficult]"). Ajzen (1988) described perceived behavioral control as influencing behavior through intention and as influencing behavior directly.

Although most often applied at the individual level, the TPB can be applied to other ecological levels as well. For example, investigators used the TPB to examine the voting intentions of state legislators in North Carolina, Vermont, and Texas (Flynn et al., 1998; N. Gottlieb et al., 2003). Legislators' general attitudes and norms concerning cigarette tax increases were predictive of their intentions to vote for a cigarette tax. Normative influences were perceived interests of the tobacco industry, constituents, the legislature, and the health sector. Legislators who intended to vote for enforcement of minors' access legislation held strong outcome beliefs and evaluations about the public health impact of the legislation. Furthermore, their intention to vote for the bill was also influenced by their perceived impact of the cigarette tax legislation on retail sales, public health, and loss of political support for the next election and their perceived behavioral control for getting the bill out of committee, voting for it, and passing it. These types of TPB findings can provide guidance to health educators who plan messages for advocacy efforts.

The TPB has also been used to plan the implementation of health education program innovations. For example, differences in beliefs, perceived social expectations, and self-efficacy were associated with teachers' different rates of diffusion, adoption, and implementation of an HIV-prevention program (Paulussen, Kok, & Schaalma, 1994; Paulussen et al., 1995; Schutte et al., 2014). Diffusion was associated with the social influence of colleagues through professional networks; adoption with outcome expectations, such as expected student satisfaction; and implementation with self-efficacy expectations about the proposed teaching strategies and with teachers' moral opinions on sexuality. Surprisingly, knowledge of the effectiveness of the program had no influence on teachers' implementation decisions.

## Anticipated Regret

Some authors have suggested determinants in addition to the three that are currently in the TPB. One suggestion is the addition of personal moral norms: people's judgments as to whether they themselves think they should or should not perform a certain behavior (Godin, Fortin, Michaud, Bradet, & Kok, 1997). Personal moral norms related to condom use are measured, for example, as "I personally think I should always use a condom." Another suggested addition is anticipated regret: having people imagine how they would feel after they behaved in a risky way contrary to their own intentions (Koch, 2014). Anticipated regret would be measured as "How would you feel afterward if you had unprotected sex?" Health promoters can use anticipated regret as a method for attitude change by having people imagine how they would feel after they behaved in a risky way to help them to refrain from that behavior. Anticipated regret and other anticipated feelings and emotions (e.g., shame or positive affect) are different from anticipatory affective feelings, as postulated by the risk-as-feelings hypothesis (Loewenstein, Weber, Hsee, & Welch, 2001). Whereas anticipated affective feelings are part of the expected outcomes of behavior in the future, anticipatory affective feelings, such as worry, fear, dread, or anxiety, result directly from thinking about risks and uncertainties. Following the risk-as-feelings hypothesis, these anticipatory feelings directly influence decision making and behavior. Indeed, studies by Janssen and colleagues suggest that affective risk beliefs (i.e., reported feelings about a risk) are more strongly related to health behavior than cognitive risk beliefs (i.e., reported thoughts about a risk; Janssen, van Osch, de Vries, & Lechner, 2011; Janssen, van Osch, Lechner, Candel, & de Vries, 2012; Janssen, Waters, van Osch, Lechner, & de Vries, 2014).

## Integrated Behavioral Model

The Integrated Behavioral Model (IBM) states that behavior is determined by variables besides intention (e.g., knowledge and skills to perform the behavior) and that intention is determined by attitude, subjective norms, and perceived behavioral control (Montaño & Kasprzyk, 2015). The two-step idea, in which certain variables determine intention and then another set of variables determine behavior, is also reflected in other theories, such as the Information-Motivation-Behavioral Skills model (IMB; Fisher, Fisher, Amico, & Harman, 2006), Social Cognitive Theory (Kelder et al., 2015; see Social Cognitive Theory section), and the Transtheoretical Model (TTM; Brug et al., 2005; see Transtheoretical Model of Behavior Change), as well as in theorizing about the intention-behavior relation (Webb & Sheeran, 2006).

## Reasoned Action Approach

In their book, Fishbein and Ajzen (2010) explained that after their early collaboration on the TRA, both authors independently developed new theoretical ideas and later discovered that those ideas were comparable, resulting in the Reasoned Action Approach (RAA). They selected constructs for the new model very carefully and intended for it to succeed the TPB. In the RAA, behavior is determined by intention, as far as people have actual control over their behavior. Actual control is determined by environmental factors and skills to deal with these factors. Intention is determined by attitude, perceived norm, and perceived behavioral control, which in turn are all determined by salient beliefs (behavioral beliefs, normative beliefs, and control beliefs). Compared with the TPB, the RAA includes the affective part of attitude, descriptive norm along with injunctive norm, self-efficacy along with perceived behavioral control, and environmental constraints.

## Measuring TPB and RAA Determinants

The TPB and RAA give very clear guidelines for measuring the determinants of behavior. The theories suggest starting with qualitative methods, such as interviews and focus groups, to find the salient factors, the prevalence and strength of which are then determined with quantitative methods (de Vries, Weijts, Dijkstra, & Kok, 1992). Based on this elicitation procedure, structured questionnaires are developed to measure the TPB concepts (Ajzen, 2006; Francis et al., 2004). Fishbein and Ajzen (2010) have provided an extensive appendix on measurement of RAA constructs (pp. 449–464).

## Changing Intentions and Behavior

In the RAA there is a distinction between goals (e.g., avoiding HIV infection), behaviors (e.g., condom use), intentions, and beliefs (Fishbein & Ajzen, 2010). Change is seen as a planned process in three phases: eliciting the relevant beliefs, changing intentions by changing salient beliefs, and changing behavior by changing intentions and increasing skills or decreasing environmental constraints. The basic idea behind selecting any potential change method is that the salient beliefs are to be changed, and therefore it is important that the salient beliefs are identified and measured correctly (for a practical guide, see Peters, 2014).

In a project to design an intervention to get people who are about to turn 50 to obtain a colonoscopy, pilot work identified the following four primary beliefs as targets for the intervention (Fishbein & Ajzen, 2010, p. 345):

- My getting a colonoscopy in the next two months would be embarrassing (attitude).
- My getting a colonoscopy in the next two months would be painful (attitude).
- My doctor thinks I should get a colonoscopy in the next two months (perceived norm).
- My health insurance won't cover my getting a colonoscopy in the next two months (perceived control).

Based on these beliefs, Fishbein & Ajzen (2010) suggested that, whatever intervention method one chooses, the essential message should be: "Your getting a colonoscopy in the next two months will be neither embarrassing nor painful; it is recommended by your doctor, and there are ways to have the cost of a colonoscopy paid for even if you don't have health insurance." The message should be formulated at the personal level and should be truthful. Of course this message will need supporting information and strong arguments that are directly tied to the behavior of interest. Fishbein and Ajzen (2010) recognized methods such as persuasive communication, use of arguments, framing, active participation, modeling, and group discussion but indicated that these methods will have an effect only when salient behavioral, normative, or control beliefs are changed (pp. 321–368). Witte (1995) suggested organizing the results of a determinants analysis into a list of relevant categories (e.g., beliefs, social influences, self-efficacy, and values) and then deciding which determinants need to be changed, which need to be reinforced, and which need to be introduced. For example, in a program for HIV prevention in Hispanic men, the men's belief that condoms were unclean needed to be *changed*; the importance of family values needed to be *reinforced*; and the belief that condoms could prevent HIV infection needed to be *introduced*.

## Shifting Perceived Norms

Thinking about how to shift subjective norms requires an understanding of the construct. The perceived norm is a special case of social influence: the impact of others on people's perceptions and behaviors (Forsyth, 2014). The TPB focuses on the perceived expectations of others, whereas Social Cognitive Theory focuses on vicarious learning or modeling, the observation of the behavior of others, and the RAA combines both types of norms.

There are three ways to influence the perceived norms in the TPB and RAA:

1. Influence normative beliefs by making peer expectations or peer behaviors visible (only if those expectations or behaviors are supportive of the health promoting behavior; if not, use injunctive norms; Mollen, Ruiter, & Kok, 2010).

2. Influence motivation to comply by building resistance to social pressure to engage in risk behavior.

3. Finally, if we are unable to shift either the perceived norm or the motivation to comply, we can advise the person to hide the behavior or shift attention from the behavior: shifting focus.

Upward and downward social comparison of patients with other patients has been described in the area of patient education (Suls & Wheeler, 2000). Upward comparison with patients who are perceived to do better than oneself will provide information on how to cope with the disease; downward comparison with patients who do worse will make you feel better about your own situation. Use of a patients' self-help group may serve both purposes in addition to providing social support (see Chapter 3).

Methods for changing social influences and for improving self-efficacy are sometimes the same, relating both to self-efficacy and to skills. Resistance to social pressure, for instance, can be seen as a skill. How can we teach people to resist social pressure? A summary of the literature (McGuire, 1985) suggested five methods: training refusal skills, modeling resistance, committing to earlier intention and behavior, relating intended behavior to values, and executing a psychological inoculation against pressure.

## Summary: Theories of Reasoned Action

Groups can be identified according to their beliefs and intentions. Theories of reasoned action are useful for understanding health risk behaviors when people are aware of the negative outcomes associated with continuing the behavior. The most recent formulation, the RAA, recognizes environmental constraints in relation to perceived behavioral control; all constructs can be used to explain the behavior of agents at every ecological level. Determinants of intention are salient beliefs, instrumental attitudes, experiential attitudes, perceived social expectations, descriptive norms, perceived behavioral control, and self-efficacy. Determinants of behavior are intentions, skills, and environmental constraints. Theories of reasoned action do not directly suggest methods but refer to methods from other theories. Essential is the change in salient beliefs based on belief selection (Fishbein & Ajzen, 2010, pp. 100–103). Other theories suggest anticipated regret, information about others' approval, providing opportunities for social comparison, mobilizing social support, resistance to social pressure, and shifting focus as methods of behavior change.

## Theories of Goal-Directed Behavior

A central tenet of theories of goal-directed behavior is that people hold personal goals, which represent desired states or outcomes to be achieved or avoided (Gollwitzer, 1999). Goals are reference points against which people compare current states or outcomes. Theorists distinguish two aspects of goals, goal content and goal process.

Goal content refers to people having simultaneous goals that can differ in their importance and compatibility. For goals to be useful in acquiring behavioral change, people must ensure that their health goals are salient and must shield them from other potentially conflicting goals. For health promoters to successfully use goal setting as a change method, they must consider possible conflicts (Stroebe, van Koningsbruggen, Papies, & Aarts, 2013). For instance, Stroebe, Mensink, Aarts, Schut, and Kruglanski (2008) described the food intake of dieters as characterized by two conflicting and incompatible goals, eating enjoyment and weight control. Dieters would have to make major efforts to shield their weight control goal against the chronic stimulation of the eating enjoyment goal, and health promoters would need to design programs with this in mind.

Goal processes relate to mental processes and behaviors of goal striving. These goal processes follow a sequence: (1) establishment, (2) planning, (3) striving and monitoring, and (4) attainment, revision, and persistence (Austin & Vancouver, 1996). Gollwitzer (1993) described the sequence as wishing, planning, acting, and evaluating. Theories of goal-directed behavior suggest that successful behavioral changes are the result of these goal-striving processes (not necessarily in a fixed order). In addition to these processes, people have to engage in a series of subgoals in order to attain the overall health goal (see the introduction of performance objectives in Chapter 5).

## Goal-Setting Theory

Goal-setting theory is clearly a theory of change and describes a particular method for behavior change involving an action sequence described above (Austin & Vancouver, 1996; Carver & Scheier, 1998). Goal setting leads to better performance because people with goals exert themselves to a greater extent, persevere in their tasks, concentrate more, and develop strategies for carrying out the behavior (Latham & Locke, 2007; Locke & Latham, 1990; 2002; 2005). Goal-setting theory thus helps close what is referred to as "the intention-behavior gap," which arises because people with positive intentions to act often fail to perform the behavior (Sheeran, 2002). For example, de Bruin and colleagues (2012) studied HIV medication adherence and found that when patients monitored goal progress by keeping track of medication intake, identified discrepancies with their goal, and developed concrete action plans to manage the discrepancies, the intention-behavior relationship was strengthened (de Bruin et al., 2012).

Pyne et al. (2013) used Intervention Mapping to develop an intervention to help patients and their mental health providers improve antipsychotic medication adherence. The patients and providers worked together to bridge the gap in their mutual understanding of the patient's perceived barriers, facilitators, and motivators (BFM) for taking antipsychotic medications. Performance objectives for the mental health providers followed goal-setting theory and included using progress notes of current patient medication adherence, identifying the top three patient BFM, clarifying patient questions, and developing actionable adherence tips to address patient-identified barriers. Based on these objectives, the intervention provided an information feedback system in which BFM data were collected from the patient, summarized, and delivered to the provider using the electronic medical record to enable real-time feedback and facilitate discussion.

## Characteristics of Goals

A goal should be behaviorally specific and measurable or observable. Strecher et al. (1995) advised that goals should therefore be stated in terms of behavior (e.g., exercise behavior and food intake) instead of health outcomes (e.g., weight loss). Setting a challenging goal, a goal that is feasible though somewhat difficult, leads to a better performance than does setting an easy goal or simply urging people to do their best (Locke & Latham, 1990, 2002, 2013). This positive effect of difficult goals occurs only if a person accepts the challenge and has sufficient goal commitment, experience, self-efficacy, and feedback to be able to perform adequately. The rewards for reaching the goal are not only the expected outcomes but also a sense of self-satisfaction. Goal setting probably will not be effective when the task is too complex. In that case, the health promoter can help the client set subgoals and suggest strategies for attainment (e.g., not to quit smoking permanently but first to abstain for one week and then set a new goal (Brown & Latham, 2002). Another method is to focus on the acquisition of knowledge and skills rather than on an increase in effort and performance by setting learning goals—that is, a goal to acquire the requisite skills—as opposed to performance goals (Seijts & Latham, 2005; Seijts, Latham, Tasa, & Latham, 2004).

## Implementation Intentions

Gollwitzer (1999) distinguished between goal intentions and implementation intentions. Goal intentions ("I intend to pursue X," as in the TPB) result in a commitment to realize a wish or desire. Implementation intentions ("I intend to initiate behavior X when conditions Y are met") connect a certain goal-directed behavior with an anticipated situation (Sheeran, Milne, Webb, & Gollwitzer, 2005). The purpose of an implementation intention is to lay down a specific plan to promote the initiation and efficient execution of goal-directed activity. By forming implementation intentions, people pass the control of the behavior over to the environment (Gollwitzer, 1999). Situations and means are turned into cues to action that are hard to forget, ignore, or miss. For example, when the goal is to effectively regulate one's emotions when going for a mammography, an implementation intention may look like: "As soon as I feel concerned about attending my appointment, then I will ignore that feeling and tell myself this is perfectly understandable" (regulate the information value of feelings), or "... then I will talk about it with somebody I can trust" (seek social support), or

"... then I will think about all the good things I stand for" (self-affirmation), or "... then I will look at things from the perspective of a wise friend" (detached perspective). Participants select the response that they think will work best for them (P. Sheeran, 2015, personal communication). It appears that forming an implementation intention is a conscious cognitive act that has automatic consequences.

Several studies have supported the usefulness of implementation intentions for behavior change. Based on a meta-analysis of 94 studies, Gollwitzer and Sheeran (2006) concluded that forming an implementation intention makes an important difference as to whether people achieve their goals. This finding was robust across variations in study design, in outcome measurements, and in the domain of goal attainment. If-then planning facilitated goal striving no matter what self-regulatory problem was at hand. Studies obtained medium to large effects in relation to initiating goal striving, shielding goals from unwanted influences, disengaging from failing goals, and preserving self-regulatory capacity for future goal striving. There was also strong support for the if-then process: People who form implementation intentions are in a good position to recognize and respond to opportunities to act. In a study of the effects of text messages, Prestwich, Perugini, and Hurling (2009) showed that the effect of forming implementation intentions may be enhanced via reminders about the plan.

Forming implementation intentions may also help in goal shielding, in that people can identify cues that may result in relapse and describe adequate responses in advance of exposure (Achtziger, Gollwitzer, & Sheeran, 2008). Whereas earlier implementation intention studies have been directed at specific situations, later studies have examined their effectiveness in relation to motivational cues (such as feeling bored and negative mood) and have shown promising effects on behavioral maintenance, including dietary behaviors (Adriaanse, de Ridder, & de Wit, 2009) and preventing risky decision making (Webb et al., 2012).

In a critical empirical and theoretical review, Sniehotta (2009) argued that implementation intentions are effective only when striving for a behavior in a specific situation. However, changes in health behaviors are often complex, with the desired behavior occurring in all kinds of possible situations. Thus, implementation intentions are most effective in changing behavior if the situational cue is frequent and the behavior appears exclusively in this situation. For many health promotion behaviors, however, the behavior appears in various kinds of situations and not always frequently. Sniehotta (2009) distinguished between action plans that describe when, where, and how to act in line with the goal intention and coping plans that describe how a person will overcome obstacles by anticipating personal risk situations and planning coping responses in detail (Sniehotta, Schwarzer, Scholz, & Schüz, 2005). Sniehotta (2009) also suggested that action planning and coping planning need to go beyond implementation intentions, and interventions that involve both action and coping planning seem to be more efficacious than action plans only (Kwasnicka, Presseau, White, & Sniehotta, 2013). In line with the study by Pyne et al. (2013; above), coping planning seems to be most effective in realizing behavior change if people are supported in the process of forming coping plans (Kwasnicka et al., 2013). A recent overview of the literature on implementation intention and action planning studies suggested that effective behavior change interventions include if-then plans, make sure participants have access to salient and relevant cues, are guided rather than user defined, and include boosters (Hagger & Luszczynska, 2014).

## Unconscious Goal Pursuit

Goals can operate outside of conscious awareness. Cues in the environment may activate goals that are then unconsciously pursued, suggesting that conscious intention is not necessarily the starting point of goal pursuit (Dijksterhuis & Aarts, 2010). For example, participants in one study talked more softly when looking at a picture of a library on the wall (Aarts & Dijksterhuis, 2003). The operation of unconscious goal pursuit may be mediated by positive affect. Cues that are presented in the environment—even at the subconscious level—may activate a behavioral goal, which is then pursued if the person has the necessary actions and resources to attain the goal and the mental representation of this goal is associated with positive affect. This goal-directed behavior may happen fully unconsciously, without the person being aware of it (Custers & Aarts, 2010). Similarly, ongoing, automatic goal-directed behavior may cease if the goal becomes associated with negative affect (Aarts, Custers, & Holland, 2007).

## Summary: Theories of Goal-Directed Behavior

Goal-setting theory suggests a positive linear relationship between goal difficulty and performance. Determinants are goal commitment, self-efficacy, and skills. Goal setting may be applied to all behaviors in which feedback is feasible. Methods include goal setting, selecting a somewhat difficult goal, match of goal complexity and difficulty with skills, and provision of feedback. Goal-directed behavior theories focus on people who are motivated for change but also on habitual behaviors and behavior influenced by environmental stimuli. Determinants for these theories are habits and environmental influences. Methods include implementation intentions, cue altering, mastery experiences, planning coping responses, and feedback.

# Theories of Automatic Behavior, Impulsive Behavior, and Habits

Much of health promotion research and theory is based on the assumption that people are consciously and systematically processing information in order to interpret their world and to plan and engage in courses of action. In contrast, Chartrand and Bargh (1999) argued that most of our moment-to-moment psychological life occurs through nonconscious means (Hassin, Uleman, & Bargh, 2005). They presented evidence that goal-directed behavior may start consciously but may become automatic over time. An example is driving style: During the first lessons, the aspiring driver is fully aware of the actions required to perform the most basic driving activities, for example, starting a car. For the experienced driver, however, driving a car is largely automatic, and drivers are able to do other activities at the same time.

Environmental cues may also guide people's behavior outside their awareness. An example can be found in the effects of priming, in which people are exposed to a stimulus—often subconsciously—and later their actions are congruent with the stimulus. For example, in one series of studies, participants were invited to a behavioral laboratory and seated either in a cubicle that contained a hidden bucket with lukewarm water mixed with citrus-scented all-purpose cleaner or in a cubicle in which no scent was diffused. Participants previously exposed to the cleaning scent showed greater cognitive access to cleaning-related words and activities in experimental tasks than those assigned to the control condition. They also behaved more in line with the concept of cleaning by keeping their table cleaner while eating a round biscuit that usually produces crumbs when one bites into it (Holland, Hendriks, & Aarts, 2005). In social interaction, people tend to change their behavior as a function of other people's behavior. For instance, participants in a study better liked other participants (who were in fact confederates of the experimenter) who deliberately mimicked the participants' mannerisms and body postures. In all these cases, the participants were not aware of these behavioral influences. Automatic behavior, as Chartrand and Bargh (1999) pointed out, is a necessity for living. If all life's simple decisions and actions involved deliberate thought, people would simply not have enough time and resources for the demands of daily life. Because a large part of behavior is conducted on automatic pilot, people are, for instance, able to do two things at the same time.

Attitudes can also be activated automatically, without a person's being aware (Fazio, 2001). In a first demonstration of this phenomenon,

Fazio (1986) found that the mere presentation of an attitude object that possessed a strong evaluative association (e.g., cockroach, baby) facilitated the latency with which subjects could indicate whether a subsequently presented target adjective had a positive or a negative connotation (e.g., dirty, lovely). The implications of these findings is that exposure to an attitude object may evoke a negative or positive automatic evaluative reaction that subsequently influences how a person categorizes objects or people. When a person later encounters members of the category, the related knowledge and attitudes may be activated and influence behavioral responses. This is, for example, the case in stereotyping whereby people assign a person to a group, access knowledge about that group, and then enact prejudice and discrimination toward the person (Devine, 1989). In other words, automatically activated attitudes impose selectivity in the perception of behavioral choices. For example, people who habitually drive to work and who readily access representations of car use in memory will, when asked about a way to travel to a holiday destination, automatically activate a positive car use attitude and may have difficulty even considering alternative ways of transportation (Danner, Aarts, & de Vries, 2008).

## Impulsive Behavior: Dual-Systems Models

Dual-systems models explain social cognitions and behavior as a joint function of two interconnected mental faculties that operate according to different principles. The Reflective-Impulsive Model (RIM) is an example of dual-systems models (Deutsch & Strack, 2006; Strack & Deutsch, 2004). The RIM distinguishes between a reflective system and an impulsive system. The impulsive system directs behavior by linking perceptual stimuli to behavioral schemata based on previously learned associations of pleasure or pain. With the reflective system features, complementary to the impulsive system, people generate judgments, decisions, and intentions. Together, these two systems result in behavior. The impulsive system is always active, while the reflective system acts on intentions. Often, health-promoting behavior entails a conflict between feeling and knowing, between the impulsive system and the reflective system. For example, a person may have an urge to smoke even while having an awareness of the negative consequences of smoking. People with strong preferences for snack foods and low inhibitory capacity are more susceptible to the temptations of palatable foods, eat more, and are more often overweight and obese (Nederkoorn, Houben, Hofmann, Roefs, & Jansen, 2010). In the case of conflicting systems, interventions must help people suppress impulses or seek distractions. The reflective system has less power to suppress the impulsive system when available cognitive resources are reduced under the following circumstances (Hofmann, Friese, & Strack, 2009):

* High cognitive load, ego depletion (see Theories of Self-Regulation section), alcohol consumption, or substance abuse

* A dispositional low capacity for self-control

* Low working memory capacity

* A habitual behavior

* A positive mood

* A focus on affective reactions (e.g., sexual arousal)

The RIM suggests that interventions directed at changing health behaviors should simultaneously attempt to change people's reflective reactions (which health promoters often do) and their impulsive reactions (which is difficult). Interventions should also create situational circumstances and skills that are conducive for effective self-regulation, including improving cues, self-efficacy, coping skills, and control motivation (Hofmann, Friese, & Wiers, 2008; Wiers & Hofmann, 2010). One other method to inhibit impulsive, unhealthy behavior is public commitment in which a person pledges in front of others to perform the healthful behavior (Ajzen, Czasch, & Flood, 2009; Conn, Valentine, & Cooper, 2002).

A dual-systems approach may also explain why adolescents and young adults take more risks than younger or older individuals. Research in developmental neuroscience suggests a temporal gap between puberty, which impels adolescents toward thrill seeking, and the slow maturation of the cognitive control system that regulates these impulses (Crone & Dahl, 2012; Steinberg, 2008). This temporal gap makes adolescence a time of heightened vulnerability for risky behavior. Interventions such as preventing teens from driving in the presence of other teens to reduce crash rates are based on this view (Chein, Albert, O'Brien, Uckert, & Steinberg, 2011; Gardner & Steinberg, 2005; Keating, 2007; Ross et al., 2014).

## Training Executive Function

One behavior change method to help people keep their impulses in check is impulse or inhibitory control. This method can help people control attention, behavior, thoughts, and emotions to override strong internal predispositions or external lures and make it more likely that they can instead do what is appropriate or needed (Diamond, 2013). Inhibitory control, one of the main processes in executive function, is the top-down mental control that people use when going on automatic pilot or relying on instinct or intuition would be ill-advised, insufficient, or impossible (Diamond, 2013, p. 136). Along with inhibitory control, executive functions comprise working memory (working with information no longer perceptually present) and cognitive flexibility (thinking outside the box, taking different perspectives, and quickly and flexibly adapting to changed circumstances). Executive functions predict social, emotional, and physical health. Stress, lack of sleep, and loneliness negatively influence executive function.

Executive functions can be trained and improved with practice. For example, executive function in children has been improved by computerized training, a combination of computerized and interactive games, task-switching computerized training, and Taekwondo traditional martial arts (Diamond & Lee, 2011). The evidence on other approaches, such as aerobics, mindfulness, and yoga, is less strong. Recent reviews of computerized training with adults are cautiously optimistic (Diamond, 2013). For all these approaches, the parameters for effectiveness are that the task has to be challenging and that substantial repetition is required (Jurado & Rosselli, 2007).

## Habits

Habits are a special case of automatic behavior. "Habits are learned sequences of acts that have become automatic responses to specific cues and are functional in obtaining certain goals or end-states" (Verplanken & Aarts, 1999, p. 104). The most prominent characteristics of habits are that they are efficient and occur without much awareness. Habits predict intentions and future behaviors, especially when individuals repeatedly perform the behaviors and when the habit is strong. Intentions predict behavior only if habits are weak, meaning they have a low frequency or the context is unstable. Habits overrule intentions when the representation of the habitual behavior can be easily accessed from memory (Danner et al., 2008). For example, when people have an intention to eat healthy foods but a habit of eating fatty foods, their eating pattern will often be unhealthy.

Habits are difficult to change, and they are not particularly influenced by information for two reasons (Verplanken & Aarts, 1999). First, information influences attitude and intentions, but these do not change behavior when they have to compete with a strong habit. Second, people with strong habits are usually not very interested in new information. Therefore, forming new habits may be the best method to change old habits. Forming implementation intentions (see the earlier discussion of goal-directed behavior) may be a useful start to creating new habits to replace old ones. With enough repetition, people can form new cue-response links, and these new behaviors may turn into new habits. However, the new cue-response links may not be as rewarding as the earlier ones. Thus, applying implementation intentions as a method for changing habits needs to be paralleled by applying other methods, such as relapse prevention (see the discussion of attribution theory and relapse prevention later in this chapter) and ongoing positive reinforcement of new behavior (i.e., reinforcement that surpasses the initial incentives for changing behavior). A recent example of the latter is an unpublished study in the city of Utrecht in the Netherlands in which commuters received a financial incentive to use public transportation to get to work and continued the practice after the initial financial incentive was removed because they perceived the advantages of the new behavior as greater than the advantages of the old habit.

Wood and Neal (2007) listed possible interventions for habit change. First, people can break habits after exposure to relevant contextual cues by actively inhibiting the cued response. Such inhibition appears to be effortful, to draw on limited regulatory resources, and to be unlikely to be sufficient to bring about long-term change in habits. Avoidance may help, as may counterconditioning. Most promising is to combine inhibition with learning and performing a new desired response. Second, people can try to alter or disrupt the exposure to relevant contextual cues. Avoidance is one strategy, cue altering another. An example of cue altering is to use smaller sizes of plates, spoons, and glasses to reduce the amounts of food and drink that people serve and consume (Sobal & Wansink, 2007). However, individuals' efforts to control habit cueing are only as strong as their self-control resources. Wood and Neal (2007) expected the most success when changes in context occurred naturally as a function of life events, such as changing jobs, moving to a new home, or transferring to a new university. If people are best able to act on their intentions when related habits are disrupted, then it is during these times that people's overt reactions are most likely to change through behavior change interventions. Wood and Neal (2007) suggested that interventions to break habits should be directed to people when they are best able to respond, for instance, as new residents in a neighborhood.

## Nudging

A nudge is a simple change in the presentation of alternatives that makes the desired behavior the easy, automatic, or default choice (Thaler & Sunstein, 2008). The nudge approach advocates libertarian paternalism: It respects freedom of choice (libertarian) but suggests sensible choices at the same time (paternalistic). Persuasive communication, based on reasoned action, has limited effect on health behavior. In comparison, nudges are a new idea that fits with the insight that many behaviors are automatic, impulsive, or habitual (de Ridder, 2014). Applying nudges requires that health promoters respect the autonomy of the decision maker by encouraging freedom of choice and a sense of awareness and by making the healthy choice the default choice (easy and attractive). An example of nudging is to increase the distance to unhealthy food in a buffet-style presentation. In a study by Maas, de Ridder, de Vet, and de Wit (2012), increasing the distance as little as 25 cm decreased intake without any aftereffects on craving for food. In another successful intervention to encourage people to use stairs instead of elevators, health promoters placed 12 orange footsteps (cues or prompts) leading to the stairs from both sides of a hallway (van Nieuw-Amerongen, Kremers, de Vries, & Kok, 2009).

In a recent study of nudging, Lehmann, Chapman, Kok, and Ruiter (2015a) sought to increase influenza vaccination uptake among health care workers from a specialist center for patients with chronic organ failure in the Netherlands. Despite World Health Organization and other agency guidelines, the rate of influenza vaccination among health care workers has been low in Europe (Amodio et al., 2014; Lehmann, Ruiter, van Dam, Wicker, & Kok, 2015b; Voirin, Barret, Metzger, & Vanhems, 2009). In the Netherlands and most other countries, influenza vaccination is offered to health care workers through an opt-in strategy. Lehmann and colleagues compared an opt-in strategy against an opt-out strategy to promote influenza vaccination. They delivered e-mails from a pulmonary physician explaining free influenza vaccinations were available. One group was instructed to schedule an appointment if they wanted to get vaccinated while the other group received an appointment and had to opt out by cancelling (i.e., making the vaccination appointment the default option—the option that comes into effect if the decision making does not actively decide against it; Goldstein, Johnson, Herrmann, & Heitmann, 2008; Li & Chapman, 2013). Results indicated an 11.5 percent increase in vaccination rate.

An essential parameter for successful use of nudging is that recipients feel respected in their sense of autonomous decision making (see also Self-Determination Theory later in this chapter). Lehmann and colleagues (2015a) implemented an intervention similar to the one described above in a general hospital setting. However, that intervention failed because representatives of the health care workers successfully objected to the intervention with the board of directors because the change from opting in to opting out was perceived as a violation of the freedom of choice. Indeed, nudging is probably most effective in decision-making situations where the advocated behavior is positively evaluated.

## Summary: Theories of Automatic Behavior and Habits

Behaviors explained by these theories are automatic, unconscious, impulsive behaviors: those behaviors that could become habitual. Automatic behaviors are often guided by external stimuli or context cues with reduced cognitive resources. Determinants are habits, environmental influences, and automatic activation of attitudes. Methods include implementation intentions, cue altering, counterconditioning, stimulus control, public commitment, training executive functions, nudging, and methods for improving self-efficacy and skills.

## Stage Theories

Stage theories suggest that people in different stages need different methods to help them move through the stages and ultimately change (N. D. Weinstein, 1988). People who have decided not to act are a particularly difficult group in which to promote change because they may be well informed but dispute or ignore information that challenges their decision. One relevant factor in deciding not to act may be that people systematically underestimate their own risk (see Unrealistic Optimism section later in this chapter).

## Transtheoretical Model of Behavior Change

The Transtheoretical Model of Behavior Change (TTM) has two major sets of constructs, stages of change and processes of change, and the model has been used by health promoters to tailor change methods to stages (Prochaska, Redding, & Evers, 2015). Researchers have used this model to describe cessation of addictive behaviors and to predict uptake of health-promoting behaviors.

The TTM stages are as follows:

- Precontemplation, in which people have no intention of changing their behavior within the next six months

- Contemplation, in which people are thinking about changing the problem behavior in the next six months

- Preparation, in which people are planning to change this behavior in the short term (one month) and are taking steps to get ready for the change

- Action, in which people have recently (less than six months) changed the behavior

- Maintenance, in which people have performed the new behavior for more than six months

- Termination, in which there is no temptation to relapse and people have 100 percent confidence in maintaining the new behavior

There is ongoing debate among scholars on the validity of the TTM. Brug and colleagues (2005) suggested that distinguishing only between two larger stages of motivation is well supported, in essence, precontemplation, contemplation, and preparation on the one hand and action, maintenance, and termination on the other. Armitage (2009) concluded that critical evaluations of the TTM focus too much on the stages and ignore other aspects of the theory, such as the processes of change. He argued that the processes of change (consciousness raising, dramatic relief, environmental reevaluation, self-reevaluation, self-liberation, helping relationships, counterconditioning, contingency management, and stimulus control) are excellent methods for improving health behavior independent of the stages (Prochaska et al., 2015; see the tables with behavior change methods in Chapter 6). Brug and colleagues (2005) added that longer-term behavioral changes need interventions that go beyond health messages to incorporate methods for changing environmental conditions, such as social liberation, a process of change from the TTM (see Chapter 6). However, these environment-directed change methods have seldom been incorporated in intervention studies based on the TTM.

## Precaution-Adoption Process Model and Risk Communication

Another stage theory, the Precaution-Adoption Process Model (PAPM), pays more attention to the issue of awareness of the risk and to the difficulty of reaching high-resistant groups as compared with the TTM (N. D. Weinstein, 1988; N. D. Weinstein, Sandman, & Blalock, 2008). The PAPM incorporates determinants and methods for change that other health promotion theories, especially Social Cognitive Theory, support (Bandura, 1997). Table 2.3 presents the seven stages and factors or issues that are likely to determine progress through the stages (N. D. Weinstein et al., 2008).

### *Unrealistic Optimism*

People often underestimate their risk, a condition that risk-perception theorists call unrealistic optimism: People think they are less at risk than comparable others (Chapin, 2014; Harris, Griffin, & Murray, 2008; Shepperd, Klein, Waters, & Weinstein, 2013). The main reasons for unrealistic optimism are that people underestimate what techniques others undertake to protect themselves and that they have stereotypes of people who run high risks. To illustrate, adolescents may refrain from condom use because they think that other adolescents have multiple partners whereas they have regular partners, and they think that only adolescents who often change partners are at risk for contracting HIV. Health educators can help make each person's risks clear by making comparisons to an absolute and a normative standard (the risks of others), preferably using undeniable

**Table 2.3**   The Precaution-Adoption Process Model

| Stage Transitions | Factors or Issues |
| --- | --- |
| Stage 1: Unaware of the problem to Stage 2: Aware but not thinking about changing | Media messages about the hazards and precautions |
| Stage 2 to Stage 3: Thinking about changing | Communications from significant others <br> Personal experience with the hazard |
| Stage 3 to Stage 4: Decided not to act or Stage 5: Decided to act | Beliefs about hazard likelihood and severity <br> Beliefs about personal susceptibility <br> Beliefs about precaution effectiveness and difficulty <br> Behaviors and recommendations of others <br> Perceived social norms <br> Fear and worry |
| Stage 5 to Stage 6: Action <br> Stage 7: Maintenance | Time, effort, and resources needed to act <br> Detailed how-to information <br> Reminders and other cues to action <br> Assistance in carrying out action |

feedback. They should also indicate that risk is a matter of risk behavior rather than of the risk groups to which the person belongs. The following methods for changing risk-perception variables are suggested (Skinner et al., 2015):

- Define the risk levels of the population at risk

- Personalize risk based on a person's behavior

- Make perceived susceptibility more consistent with the individual's actual risk

- Specify consequences of the risk

### *Risk Communication*

There are various methods to effectively communicate risks (Holtgrave, Tinsley, & Kay, 1995). Health educators can, for example, compare risks on the same dimensions (dread, control, catastrophic potential, equity, and novelty) or compare risks with similar dimensional profiles. However, sometimes people become angry when a risk over which they have no control, such as air pollution, is compared to a risk over which they do have control, such as smoking (Visschers, Meertens, Passchier, & de Vries, 2007). Visschers, Meertens, Passchier, and de Vries (2009) summarized the empirical evidence on the effects of risk communication, especially probability information. Their recommendations include the following:

1. Use the same denominator in probability information throughout the risk message.

2. Use step-by-step probability descriptions that are easy to understand and are likely to result in adequate risk estimates.

3. Be careful about presenting relative risk reduction, as this may be mistaken for absolute risk reduction.

4. Take the context of the risk communication into account (setting, frame, and severity).

5. Present both numerical and verbal probability information in a risk message.

6. Use graphs to present probability of harm.

When trying to increase perceived susceptibility for sexually transmitted infections (STIs), scenario-based risk information was the most effective method, especially when people generated their own scenarios and when multiple risk scenarios were provided. When people find it very difficult to imagine the risk situation, scenario information is ignored (Mevissen, Meertens, Ruiter, Feenstra, & Schaalma, 2009; Mevissen, Meertens, Ruiter, & Schaalma, 2012). Communicating risk seems to induce defensive reactions. It is therefore advisable to pilot test messages carefully before using them on a large scale. Personalized probability-based risk information is promising, especially in combination with behavioral recommendations and information tailored to motivation and skills.

### *Raising Awareness*

Awareness is often described as the first step in the change process. In the theories of self-regulation and coping, the first step in an intervention is some form of need recognition or problem appraisal. However, these theories do not provide clear methods for stimulating need recognition. Often, self-regulatory and coping theories are applied in situations in which people have a disease, such as asthma, cystic fibrosis, or AIDS, and they already perceive a need (Wenzel, Glanz, & Lerman, 2002). For example, individuals are taught appraisal skills to detect a problem related to disease or self-management and other skills with which to solve the problem (Bartholomew et al., 1993). Without these additional problem-solving skills to raise self-efficacy and outcome expectations, avoidance of thinking about the risk may ensue. For people who are not motivated to perform appraisal, methods for awareness may be applied, such as risk information, confrontation, and fear arousal.

Messages to promote awareness should focus on self-evaluation related to risk and reevaluation of outcome expectations, rather than on action (Maibach & Cotton, 1995). Messages could include personalization by reminding someone of recent episodes of the risk behavior and the potential consequences of the person's risk behavior on significant others. At a higher ecological level, mass media gatekeepers must also become aware of an issue as a necessary condition for featuring health-promoting issues (McGrath, 1995).

## Summary: Stage Theories

Based on the TTM, different groups can be identified: people in precontemplation, contemplation, preparation, action, and maintenance. Behaviors have different determinants for each stage. However, most researchers suggest only two stages: motivation and action. Methods derived from the TTM include tailoring (to stages), individualization, and methods guided by processes of change: consciousness raising, dramatic relief, environmental reevaluation, self-reevaluation, self-liberation, helping relationships, counterconditioning, contingency management, and stimulus control. The PAPM identifies people in different stages of precaution adoption and may be applied to all health behaviors, but especially to risk behaviors of which people are unaware. The PAPM describes lack of environmental resources as barriers for change. Determinants are different in different stages. Methods from the PAPM are tailoring to stages, consciousness raising, personalizing risk, specifying consequences of the risk, comparing risks on the same dimension, using step-by-step probability descriptions, presenting both numerical and verbal probability information, and providing scenario-based risk information.

## Attribution Theory and Relapse Prevention

An important construct in many models that try to explain determinants of behavior is self-efficacy, the self-confidence for performing a particular behavior. But what are the determinants of self-efficacy? Weiner (1986) suggested that self-efficacy, or expectancy of success as he calls it, is determined by the perceived stability of the attributions for success and failure. Attribution theory describes the impact of the way people attribute the outcomes of behavior on their future cognition and behavior across the three dimensions of stability, locus, and controllability (Weiner, 1986).

Stability is the relevant dimension for the understanding of success expectations for health behavior change. A person attributing a failure to a stable cause (e.g., ability) will have a lower expectancy of success for performing the same task again, as compared with somebody who attributes a failure on the same task to an unstable cause (e.g., bad luck). In the case of success, this effect is reversed. If a person succeeds, attributing the success to a stable cause (e.g., talent) will be associated with a higher expectation of success than if the person attributes the success to an unstable cause (e.g., fortunate circumstances). Furthermore, attribution theory suggests that lower success expectancy leads to less adaptive task behavior; people will invest less energy in the task at hand. Hospers, Kok, and Strecher (1990) found that success of participants in a weight reduction program was positively related to the participants' self-efficacy at the start of the program. Self-efficacy was inversely related to stability of attributions for earlier failures, and both relationships were independent of the number of failures.

## Attributional Retraining and Relapse Prevention

One method for changing attributions to improve self-efficacy is called attributional retraining, or reattribution (Kok et al., 1992). The health educator or counselor tries to help people reinterpret previous failures in terms of unstable attributions ("You were in a very difficult situation there") and previous successes in terms of stable attributions ("You are the type of person who has been able to stay off cigarettes during your whole pregnancy").

Attributional retraining is often used in attempts to prevent relapse (Marlatt & Donovan, 2005). Relapses are caused when a person lapses in a high-risk situation due to a lack of coping response. Self-efficacy expectations and perceived skills are relevant not only for new behavior but also for the maintenance of behavior changes. Relapse prevention theory describes the process of lapses, attributions, self-efficacy estimations, coping, craving, emotional states, and successes and failures in maintaining the behavior change. The major distinction between success and failure is the presence or absence of a coping response for high-risk situations (Marlatt & Donovan, 2005). High-risk situations are those situations that invite or pressure people to take up their risk behavior again. For instance, a worker who has quit smoking goes to the coffee shop, where colleagues are smoking. If the worker has an adequate coping response, she will be more likely to maintain her health-promoting behavior and may develop an even higher estimation of self-efficacy. However, if she does not have an adequate coping response to the high-risk situation at the coffee shop, she may lapse into her earlier risk behavior and experience a sense of failure. She may attribute this failure to stable and uncontrollable causes and develop lower self-efficacy and a higher chance of complete relapse as a result. Marlatt and Donovan (2005) stressed that their relapse prevention model is not linear but dynamic. Relapses are a complex phenomenon and seemingly insignificant changes in one risk factor may kindle a downward spiral resulting in a major relapse.

How can health promotion programs help people prevent relapse? The theory suggests a series of primarily face-to-face or group methods that involve helping the person at risk identify high-risk situations, plan coping responses, and practice the responses until they become automatic (Marlatt & Donovan, 2005). It also suggests reattribution training for incidental lapses so that the at-risk person attributes failure to an unstable cause.

## Summary: Attribution Theory and Relapse Prevention

People may be differentiated as those who make stable versus unstable attributions for failure for all behaviors with success or failure characteristics. There may exist real barriers in the environment that may make maintenance of behavior change too difficult even with high self-efficacy. Determinants are stable versus unstable attributions for failure. Methods include reattribution training, relapse prevention, planning coping responses, and methods to train skills and self-efficacy.

# Theories of Persuasive Communication

Theories of persuasive communication are applicable to any behavior that communication can influence. Persuasive communication typically aims to change attitudes by making appeals to logic and reasoning.

## Communication-Persuasion Matrix

One general theory for attitude and behavior change is McGuire's (1985; 2001) Communication-Persuasion Matrix (CPM). Health educators use this model somewhat differently from the way McGuire originally intended by including variables from Social Cognitive Theory (attitude, social influences, and self-efficacy) and stage theories (maintenance; Kok et al., 1996). The model combines seven steps describing the effects of persuasive communication with four communication variables in a matrix. The first steps posit that successful communication should result in the receiver's attention and comprehension. The subsequent steps refer to the receiver's changes in attitudes, social influences, self-efficacy, and behavior; the last step refers to the maintenance of that behavior change. McGuire (1985) argued that educational interventions should match each step. Choices related to the communication variables, message content, program audience, communication channels, and message source depend on the step that is addressed. For instance, certain mass media messages, such as statements by famous sports heroes, may attract a lot of attention but may have negative effects on self-efficacy. An important contribution of the CPM is that every method that uses communication will have to go through the steps for successful communication in order to have any effect at all. Protocols for pretesting of educational materials should apply these steps, and in practice most of them do (U.S. Department of Health and Human Services, Office of Cancer Communications, National Cancer Institute, 2002). Applying the CPM to all program communications is a basic method for change.

The CPM can accommodate a host of social psychological variables that have been found to influence attitude and behavior (McGuire, 1985, 2001). However, for many of these variables, the relationship to attitude and behavior change is ambiguous. McGuire explained this ambiguity by distinguishing differential effects on reception of the message (that is, successful communication) and yielding to the message (that is, attitude and behavior change). For instance, as mentioned before, the use of celebrities in persuasive messages can have a positive effect on reception but may have a negative effect on yielding.

## Cultural Similarity

The CPM may be applied to analyze the role of culture as a factor in enhancing the effects of health communication. Kreuter and McClure (2004) addressed message source, context, and communication channel because these three aspects are modifiable by communication. Cultural similarity between source and receivers leads to greater message recall and favorable attitudes, especially among receivers who identify strongly with their cultural group. With respect to message content, using surface characteristics of the intervention group, such as preferred language, enhances receptivity. Using deep structure, such as social-cultural characteristics, leads to a more positive processing of the message. With respect to message channel, at the most basic level, an intervention must reach the intended group. Different cultural groups use different media, because they have different needs and contexts for sense of community, cohesiveness, and culturally relevant information. Exposure to minority newspapers, for instance, gives people a more culturally relevant agenda (see Advocacy Coalition Framework section in Chapter 3). For example, Larkey, Ogden, Tenorio, and Ewell (2008) gave examples of culturally relevant messages directed at Latinos for cancer prevention and screening trials.

## Elaboration Likelihood Model

The Elaboration Likelihood Model (ELM) is another perspective on persuasion effects (Petty, Barden, & Wheeler, 2002; Petty, Briñol, & Priester, 2009; Petty & Cacioppo, 1986a; 1986b). The basic idea of the ELM is that people differ in the ability and motivation for thoughtful information processing. Petty and Cacioppo (1986a, 1986b) explained two ways of processing information: central and peripheral. Central processing occurs when a person carefully considers a message and compares it against other messages and beliefs. Peripheral processing occurs when a person processes a message without thoughtful consideration or comparison. For example, students learning about self-efficacy for the first time can process the information centrally by comparing their own self-efficacy for performing several different behaviors. They can continue the central processing by searching for situations wherein self-efficacy seems to be important in their decisions to attempt a behavior or to maintain effort.

Pollay et al. (1996) suggested that advertisers use peripheral cues in advertisements for youth because these cues tend to bypass logical analysis. A variable—for instance, the source credibility of a sports hero as a role model—may have a positive effect when receivers process the message through the peripheral route but a negative effect when they follow the central route. In the case of the sports hero, people realize that their behavioral capabilities are different from those of the sports hero. For example, a well-intentioned health promoter might invite a famous cyclist to be in a mass media campaign to promote physical activity among youth. With peripheral processing, overweight, sedentary teens might admire the athlete and react favorably to the ad for a brief time. However, with central processing, the same teens might compare the attributes of the athlete to their own fitness and have lower self-efficacy for physical activity than before the campaign. The same variable, source credibility, may also influence the motivation and ability to think, thus shifting people from the peripheral route to the central route or vice versa (Petty & Wegener, 1998).

Successful communication is a prerequisite for any other change method (McGuire, 1985). A program cannot have any effect if the population is not exposed, does not pay attention to the program, or does not understand the message. Any program that includes methods for changing determinants and behavior should also include methods to achieve successful communication. Research findings suggest that thoughtful information processing relates to stronger persistence of attitude change, resistance to counter persuasion, and consistency between attitude and behavior (Petty & Cacioppo, 1986b). Health educators should thus promote thoughtful information processing as much as possible. The ELM suggests three ways to stimulate motivation to think about a message: Make the message personally relevant, unexpected, and repeated. An illustration is the program Sex, Games, and Videotapes, an HIV-prevention program for homeless, mentally ill men in a New York shelter, which made messages personally relevant, surprising, and repeated by embedding them in activities that were salient pastimes in the shelter, such as playing competitive games, storytelling, and watching videos (Susser, Valencia, & Torres, 1994). Additional methods that improve skills for information processing are media that allow self-pacing, environments without distractions, and the use of language that people easily understand. Anticipation of interaction over the message and direct instructions to process the message carefully can help centralize the processing (Petty & Wegener, 1998). When the intervention group has the time and the behavioral capability, health promoters can use active learning to promote central information processing—making individuals search for answers to questions they pose.

### Persuasive Arguments

One of the most widely used intervention methods for attitude change is the presentation of arguments in a persuasive message. The ELM predicts that high-quality arguments are effective only when the receivers process the message through the central route, not when they use the peripheral route. A higher number of arguments does not ensure quality and, in fact, may negatively affect attitude change (Petty & Wegener, 1998). A greater number of arguments may be convincing for people who process the information through the peripheral route, but they will be less convincing for people who process through the central route. Petty and Wegener (1998) suggested that the following characteristics determine the quality of arguments, that is, their effectiveness after careful processing:

- Expectancy value: People like outcomes that are likely and desirable and avoid outcomes that are unlikely and undesirable.
- Causal explanations: A causal explanation will convince receivers of the likelihood of the outcome.
- Functionality: Arguments that match the way people look at the world are more convincing.
- Importance: The relevance of outcomes determines the argument's effectiveness.
- Novelty: An unfamiliar or unique argument has more impact than does a familiar argument.

Health promoters may use carefully crafted persuasive arguments at the individual level to encourage people to adopt healthful behaviors, and they may use them to influence agents at higher ecological levels. For example, viewing a television broadcast on the health consequences to children from environmental tobacco smoke and the benefits of protecting children from smoke may influence a mother to declare her home smoke free. Seeing other legislators receive media attention for promoting a healthy policy may lead legislators to vote for health legislation. In either of these cases, the receivers must both expect positive health outcomes and value the outcomes for persuasion to be effective. For example, a city council must be persuaded both that fluoridation prevents dental caries and that the prevention of dental caries is something to value because of its effect on children's health. A persuasive argument about the extent of dental disease in children in the community and the outcome to their overall health that uses facts and personalized models might influence the council to accept both beliefs and to change the way it votes.

## Summary: Theories of Persuasive Communication

Communication receivers are at different stages of awareness, attitude change, and behavior change and have different tendencies to process the messages with either high or low elaboration likelihood. Determinants will be different by stage. Information processing may be disturbed by information complexity and external factors. Methods from the CPM include persuasive communication, active processing of information (active learning), tailoring (to stage), arguments, and cultural similarity. Methods derived from the ELM are persuasive communication, elaboration, discussion, active processing of information, tailoring to the individual's stage, and strong arguments.

## Theories of Self-Regulation

Self-regulatory concepts explain how individuals function to self-correct behavior (Baumeister & Vohs, 2004; Boekaerts, Pintrich, & Zeidner, 2000; Mann, de Ridder, & Fujita, 2013). Creer (2000) argued that self-management, the term that has often been used in the health domain, and self-regulation, the term used in psychology (Cleary & Zimmerman, 2004; Zimmerman, 2000) and in education (Schunk & Ertmer, 2000), refer to the same phenomenon. Self-management is an active, iterative process of observing oneself, making judgments based on observation (as opposed to judgments based on habit, fear, or tradition), setting a goal, choosing strategies, reacting appropriately in light of one's goal, and revising one's strategy accordingly (Clark, 2003). The process is iterative, because feedback loops, through which one sees discrepancies between goals and outcomes and feels dissatisfaction, play an essential part in self-regulation (Scheier & Carver, 2003). Various authors' descriptions of self-regulation processes make a distinction between awareness and action. In the awareness phase people monitor themselves and, after an evaluation of the outcomes, decide they want to change. In the action phase people make plans, implement plans, and revise plans if necessary. After implementation people again self-monitor their behavior and decide whether their goals have been reached and, in case they have not, what other plans may be helpful (Mann et al., 2013).

Rothman, Baldwin, and Hertel (2004) have extended the self-management stages to include continuation, maintenance, and habit formation. They also pointed out that the determinants for change and the methods to promote change vary over these stages, comparable to the other stage models that we described earlier. Alberts (2007) explained:

> Rosenbaum (2000) states that peoples' general repertoire of self-regulatory skills is essential for goal accomplishments. He uses the term "learned resourcefulness" to indicate the acquired regulatory skills that help people to control their behavior. By repetition, the employment of self-control strategies may become internalized and automatic, thereby contributing to overall improved self-control abilities. (p. 106)

Muraven and Baumeister (2000) suggested a "strength model" of self-management in which a person's capacity to exert self-control is defined by personal restrictions. The restrictions exist because people have limited resources on which self-control can be drawn in the same way they have limited energy or strength. After an act of self-control, a person's resources decrease, and performance on a subsequent self-control act can be impaired (Alberts, 2007; Schmeichel & Baumeister, 2004). For instance, Muraven, Collins, and Nienhaus (2002) showed that individuals whose self-control was depleted through the prior exertion of self-control consumed more alcohol than individuals whose self-control was not depleted. Self-control becomes tired after use and, like a muscle, needs rest to recover and can become stronger with repeated practice. Strengthening through repeated practice may offer a strategy to counter regulatory failure (Alberts, 2007; Muraven et al., 2002; Oaten & Cheng, 2006). Activation of persistence has been shown to help people overcome the effects of ego depletion and to lead to stable self-control performance (Alberts, Martijn, Greb, Merckelbach, & de Vries, 2007).

## Interventions Based on Self-Regulation

Self-regulatory theory is useful for designating health-promoting behaviors for the self-management of chronic disease. For example, in a family-oriented pediatric asthma self-management program, Bartholomew et al. (2000a) conceptualized both asthma-specific skills (e.g., taking control medications) and self-regulatory skills (e.g., monitoring for symptoms of asthma). Shegog and colleagues (2013) also used self-regulation models (Bandura, 1986; Clark, 2003) among other theories to develop the Management Information Decision-Support Epilepsy Tool (MINDSET), a tablet-based program to provide real-time self-management decision support to patients living with epilepsy and their health care providers (see

Web-based case study at www.wiley.com/go/bartholomew4e). Another excellent example of an intervention based on self-management is a program to promote therapy adherence with HIV-positive patients by de Bruin and colleagues (2010). In a review of 13 successful theory-based interventions for disease management, Clark (2003) noted that eight of the programs used self-regulatory approaches, which encourage the executive cognitive processes of setting goals, observing behavior, and revising goals. Other reviews showed positive effects of self-management on pain reduction (Reid et al., 2008), health of patients with osteoarthritis (Devos-Comby, Cronan, & Roesch, 2006), and diabetes adherence and dietary behavior (Hill-Briggs & Gemmell, 2007). Self-management through the Internet has been shown to improve the health condition of children with a chronic illness (Stinson, Wilson, Gill, Yamada, & Holt, 2009). However, many other reviews and meta-analyses suffer from a lack of clarity about the criteria for including self-management interventions and do not provide clear descriptions of the included interventions in terms of the earlier mentioned self-management steps: monitoring, evaluation, planning, and implementation (see for instance Warsi, Wang, LaValley, Avorn, & Solomon, 2004).

## Self-Determination Theory

Self-Determination Theory (SDT) contributes to understanding of health behavior and in the design of behavior change methods. SDT examines the degree to which an individual's behavior is self-motivated or self-determined. SDT studies individual, social, and cultural factors that affect the impetus to act in a particular way in given situations and how in turn personal well-being is affected (Ryan & Deci, 2000). This theory differentiates motivation between individuals who act from a sense of personal commitment toward certain behaviors and those whose behavior is driven by fear of pressure from external sources. The two types of motivational orientations (autonomous and controlled) lie on a continuum called perceived locus of causality. In intrinsic and autonomous types of motivation, individuals engage in behaviors for interest, enjoyment, and satisfaction or to achieve outcomes that are important to them. In health-related behaviors, individuals with autonomous orientations act with interest in pursuing important life goals for psychological and physical well-being; whereas in extrinsic and controlled motivations, engagement in behavior is based on others' wants and needs, which are placed above the individual's own needs (Ng et al., 2012). Those individuals with higher controlled motivation orientation succumb to social pressure and have increased public self-consciousness and defensive responses. These findings have been demonstrated in explaining adolescent alcohol abuse and risky sexual behavior (Patrick & Williams, 2012; G. Williams, Hedberg, Cox, & Deci, 2000).

SDT posits that the three basic needs at the core of human motivation should be met to facilitate growth and development. These are autonomy (versus control), competence, and relatedness (Deci & Ryan, 2002; Ryan & Deci, 2000). Autonomy requires an environment that enables freedom, agency, initiative, and control over decision making without burden from external pressures (Ryan & Deci, 2006). Autonomy in sexual contexts provides women the opportunity to protect their own health, while oppressive cultural norms diminish that right (Sanders-Phillips, 2002). Autonomy has been shown to be an important predictor of health-promoting behaviors, as it determines whether decisions and beliefs are internalized and therefore will be sustained in the long term (Ng et al., 2012; Ryan & Deci, 2006). Competence forms the foundation for self-esteem and self-confidence and involves feelings of being effective in ongoing interactions with one's external environment. The competence need has been defined as very similar to self-efficacy. However, competence refers to a psychological need being met that has more to do with general feelings about self and working efficiently or having a sense of motivation while self-efficacy is more about the ability to attain a specific goal (Bandura, 1997). Finally, relatedness can be defined as feeling connected to a partner, feeling secure, and having a sense of belonging with others and to the social environment. If the need of relatedness is satisfied, a person will have a sense of control in interpersonal spaces, including sexual relationships. When these three needs are met, they yield increased motivation, well-being, and mental health, and thus people may feel more efficacious to protect their physical health (Milyavskaya & Koestner, 2011; Patrick, Knee, Canevello, & Lonsbary, 2007; N. Weinstein & Ryan, 2011). The resulting behavior can be said to be self-determined and is more likely to be continued. SDT has successfully been applied to predict performance and motivation not only at the individual level but also at the organizational level (Gagné, 2014).

## Motivational Interviewing

Motivational Interviewing (MI) is a counseling approach that originated in clinical psychology but has been proved effective also in motivating behavior change in the context of public health (Miller & Rollnick, 1991, 2002, Op de Coul, Spijker, van Aar, van Weert, & de Bruin, 2013; van Eijk-Hustings, Daemen, Schaper, & Vrijhoef, 2011). MI recognizes that people have different levels of readiness to change and often have ambivalent feelings and emotions about potential change-related decisions. MI works together with clients by helping them develop intrinsic motivation, think about how change may happen, deal with difficulties along the way, and align specific behavior change with personal values. MI originated in in clinical practice without guidance from an underlying theoretical framework (Miller & Rose, 2009). Because of the conceptual overlap in regard to processes of internalization and needs satisfaction, SDT and MI have been linked. An integration of the two frameworks may provide theorists and practitioners with a good, practical theory for both understanding and changing health behavior (Patrick & Williams, 2012; Rutten et al., 2014; Vansteenkiste & Sheldon, 2006).

## Summary: Theories of Self-Regulation

Theories of self-regulation may be used with people who are trying to incorporate complex behaviors into their lifestyles. These theories identify performance objectives for self-regulatory behaviors, that is, planning, monitoring, evaluation, and action. The learner is helped to explicitly consider the role of the environment in the performance of certain behaviors, for example, to appraise the environment in the monitoring phase. Self-regulation can be seen as a determinant of behavioral capability. For human behavior to be intrinsically motivated and thus continued, SDT puts emphasis on needs satisfaction. Methods from theories of self-regulation and self-determination include goal setting, self-monitoring, feedback, Motivational Interviewing, and methods to change self-efficacy and skills.

## Social Cognitive Theory

Bandura's Social Cognitive Theory (SCT; 1986) is an interpersonal theory that covers both determinants of behavior and methods for behavior change (Bandura, 1997; Kelder et al., 2015; Luszczynska & Schwarzer, 2005). SCT explains human behavior as a model of reciprocal determinism in which behavior, cognitive, and other personal factors and environmental events interact (Bandura, 1986). Major determinants of behavior SCT describes are outcome expectations, outcome expectancies, self-efficacy, behavioral capability, perceived behavior of others, and environment.

### Outcome Expectations, Self-Efficacy, and Behavioral Capability

An outcome expectation is a person's judgment of the likely consequence of a behavior ("When I use a condom consistently, I will prevent sexually transmitted infections"). Outcome expectancies, on the other hand, are the values that individuals place on a certain outcome ("Preventing sexually transmitted infections is something I value"; Kelder et al., 2015). Outcome expectations are comparable to behavioral beliefs in the TPB, and outcome expectancies are comparable to evaluations.

Self-efficacy is an individual's judgment of his or her capability to accomplish a certain level of performance ("I am confident that I can use a condom consistently"). Bandura (1986) was explicit about the interrelation between outcome expectations and self-efficacy: Judgments of ability to perform a behavior greatly influence expected outcomes. For example, when people are not confident that they can use a condom consistently, they may also not expect to prevent STIs. Some studies have found an interaction effect between self-efficacy and outcome expectations. When a person is in a situation in which outcome expectations are positive and strong but self-efficacy for that behavior is low, a situation of avoidance or denial may occur; and the person is unlikely to attempt the behavior (Bandura, 1986). In addition to personal self-efficacy, Bandura (1997) described perceived collective efficacy, belief in the performance capability of a social system as a whole (see also Chapter 3).

The concept of behavioral capability is that if people are to perform a particular type of behavior, they must know what the behavior is (knowledge of the behavior) and how to perform the behavior (skills for the behavior). Self-efficacy is a person's perception; capability is the real thing. Health promotion programs should go beyond providing knowledge to providing behavioral capability, which is closer to actual performance. The development of behavioral capability is the result of the individual's training, intellectual capacity, and learning style. Enactive mastery experiences provide procedural knowledge of the activities to perform, practice in performing those activities, and feedback about successful performance.

## Observational Learning and Environment

Most human behavior is learned through observation of models (vicarious learning). By observing others, a person can form rules for behavior; and on future occasions this coded information can serve as a guide for action. Four constituent processes govern modeling:

- Attention to and perception of the relevant aspects of modeled activities (including characteristics of the observer and the model)

- Retention and representation of learned knowledge and remembering

- Production of appropriate action

- Motivation as a result of observed positive incentives and reinforcement

When providing models to encourage the learning of certain behaviors, the health educator should find a role model from the community or at-risk group that will encourage identification among the intervention group. The model should present a coping model (e.g., "I tried to quit smoking several times and was not successful. Then I tried again... Now I have been off cigarettes for...") rather than a mastery model (e.g., "I just threw my pack away, and that was it"). Learners should be able to observe models being reinforced for their behavior (e.g., being congratulated by friends for staying off cigarettes or having a partner say how fresh the ex-smoker smells). Perceived behavior of others is distinguishable from perceived social expectations: Smoking parents (behavior of the parents) may be contributing to their child's taking up smoking while they expect their child not to smoke (perceived social expectation).

In addition to focusing on individuals, planners should focus on creating environments that facilitate health-promoting change. The term *environment* refers to an objective notion of all the factors that can affect a person's behavior but that are physically external to that person. The social environment includes family members, peers, and neighbors. The physical environment includes availability of certain foods, indoor and outdoor air quality, restrictions for smoking, and so on. All learning has to be complemented by facilitation, the provision of means for the learner to take action or means to reduce barriers to action (Bandura, 1986; Mullen & DiClemente, 1992; Mullen, Green, & Persinger, 1985). Facilitation often means creating a change in the environment (Golden & Earp, 2012). For instance, a program that targets improvement in drug users' self-efficacy for using clean needles must also facilitate clean needles being easily accessible. People with higher self-efficacy will exert more effort, although actual barriers ultimately mediate what the effect will be. Individuals may or may not be aware of the strong influence that the environment has on their behavior. Likewise, health promoters may underuse the role of environment in their program planning. Keeping the concept of reciprocal determinism in mind will help planners avoid this pitfall.

## SCT and Behavior Change

SCT integrates determinants of behavior with methods for behavior change (Clark & Zimmerman, 2014; Stacey, James, Chapman, Courneya, & Lubans, 2014; Young, Plotnikoff, Colling, Callister, & Morgan, 2015). All SCT interventions are based on active learning that promotes performance during the learning process. Perceived behavior of others is not only a determinant of behavior but also a very effective method for behavior change through modeling. Reinforcement is a general method of SCT. Modeling, in which a person experiences vicarious reinforcement, is a special case of reinforcement. A person may experience vicarious reinforcement by observing a model receiving reinforcement. Reinforcements may be external (such as receiving money) or internal (such as doing something that one perceives as right). Self-efficacy and behavioral capability may be improved through the following (Bandura, 1997):

- Enactive mastery experiences: enabling the person to succeed in attainable but increasingly challenging performances of desired behaviors

- Vicarious experiences (modeling): showing the person that others like that person can do it, including detailed demonstrations of the small steps taken in the attainment of a complex objective

- Verbal persuasion: telling the person that he or she can do it; strong encouragement can boost confidence enough to induce the first efforts toward behavior change

- Improving physical and emotional states: making sure people are well rested and relaxed before attempting a new behavior; including efforts to reduce stress and depression while building positive emotions, such as when fear is relabeled as excitement

### *Tailoring, Relevance, and Individualization*

Relevance, tailoring, and individualization have all been shown to be effective basic methods in health education interventions, and they can be traced to a number of theories, especially Social Cognitive Theory. Adapting the program to the knowledge, beliefs, circumstances, and prior experience of the learner, as assessed by pretesting or other means, can create relevance. Computer programs enable one to tailor interventions to measured characteristics of the individual, such as beliefs, attitude, and self-efficacy (Lustria, Cortese, Noar, & Glueckauf, 2009; Peels et al., 2013; Portnoy, Scott-Sheldon, Johnson, & Carey, 2008). Tailoring will be effective only when there is a clear link between characteristics of the person and the messages that are supposed to address those characteristics. Tailoring the message to salient beliefs of the intervention group increases people's motivation and ability to process the message carefully, thereby increasing the chance of persistent changes in attitudes and behavior (Witte, 1995).

Individualization is the provision of opportunities for learners to have personal questions answered or instructions paced according to their individual progress. It may also include the ability to offer instruction that is geared to specific needs and disease characteristics. The Watch, Discover, Think, and Act asthma computer application individualizes instruction to each child's asthma triggers and symptoms based on information the child types in (Bartholomew et al., 2000a; Bartholomew et al., 2000b).

## Summary: Social Cognitive Theory

SCT may be applied to any behavior, but is usually applied to behaviors that are complex and require considerable behavioral capability. Actual barriers are recognized as difficult even with high self-efficacy, and there is a strong impact of the social and the physical environment. Determinants include outcome expectations, self-efficacy expectations, behavioral capability, perceived behavior of others, and social and physical environment. Methods derived from SCT are active learning, reinforcement, graded tasks, enactive mastery experiences, modeling, guided practice, verbal persuasion, improving physical and emotional states, and facilitation.

# Theories of Stigma and Discrimination

A stigma is defined as an "attribute that is deeply discrediting" and that reduces the bearer "from a whole and usual person to a tainted, discounted one" (Goffman, 1963, p. 3). The immediate reaction to a stigma seems to be avoidance as if physical contact or even proximity to the stigmatized person can result in some form of contamination (Pryor, Reeder, Yeadon, & Hesson-McInnis, 2004). The origin of stigmatization lies in the perception and cognitive representation of people with a deviant condition. These conditions may subsequently trigger perceivers' emotional and behavioral reactions (Dijker & Koomen, 2003, 2007). Deviant conditions may relate to many circumstances, such as ethnicity and sexual preference, but also to illness, including AIDS, mental illness, and physical conditions or handicaps.

## Social-Psychological and Sociological Views on Stigma

Dijker and Koomen (2003, 2007) extended attribution theory's explanation of people's tendency to stigmatize persons with illnesses or handicaps. They distinguished four determinants of stigmatization and three resulting emotional reactions to stigmatization. Bos, Schaalma, and Pryor (2008) applied these to AIDS-related stigma. The four determinants are the perception of contagiousness of the disease, seriousness of the disease, personal responsibility of the patient, and norm-violating behavior of the patient in terms of having the disease. The three emotional reactions are fear, leading to more stigmatization and avoidance; pity, leading to less stigmatization and avoidance; and anger, leading to more stigmatization and avoidance. Perceived contagiousness leads to fear and to avoidance behavior. Perceived seriousness leads to fear but also to pity, which in turn leads to less avoidance. High perceived responsibility leads to anger, but low perceived responsibility to pity. If the disease is associated with perceived norm-violating behavior (e.g., drug use, homosexuality), anger increases; if it is not, pity increases. Most reactions to AIDS patients are negative, but some determinants lead to increased pity, resulting in less stigmatization.

Reactions to the stigmatized are not always negative, as Pryor et al. (2004) explained by applying a dual-systems approach (see previous discussion of dual-systems models). A stigma may evoke reflexive and reflective reactions. Reflexive reactions are immediate, emotional, and negative; reflective reactions are rule-based, thoughtful, and often more positive. Pryor and colleagues (2004) showed that initial reactions to stigma are governed by the reflexive system, whereas subsequent reactions are governed by the reflective system. People show more positive reactions, for instance, to a person with an uncontrollable stigma (low responsibility) when they are given time to consider their responses than when they are asked for an immediate response. An emotion such as pity may be derived from a reflective process and may be slower to emerge than an emotion such as fear or anger (Frijda, 2007).

Bos, Pryor, Reeder, and Stutterheim (2013) distinguished four types of stigma: public stigma, self-stigma, stigma by association, and structural stigma. Being stigmatized has a detrimental impact on self-esteem because of stress and loss of social support. Persons with a concealable stigma, such as mental illness, sexual diversity, or HIV, encounter the dilemma of disclosure (Bos, Kanner, Muris, Janssen, & Mayer, 2009; Meyer, 2003; Stutterheim et al., 2009). Sociologists point to stereotypes that label human differences with undesirable characteristics that separate "us" from "them" (Link & Phelan, 2001). These labels and stereotypes create status hierarchies and inequalities based on power. Often these inequalities result from institutional discrimination, accumulated institutional practices that work to the disadvantage of stigmatized groups even in the absence of individual discrimination. Stereotypes, status hierarchies, and inequalities reduce a person's life chances. Thus, members of a potentially stigmatized group may engage in "label avoidance" so that they are not identified with the group and thus escape the negative effects of public stigma (Corrigan & Wassel, 2008).

## How to Reduce Stigmatization

There are a number of possible methods for stigma reduction (Bos et al., 2008). Interpersonal contact with members of a stigmatized group may change stereotypes when the contact is sustained and personal between members of equal status who share important goals and is supported by the institution within which it occurs (Paluck & Green, 2009; see Pettigrew & Tropp, 2006). For instance, HIV-positive speakers in AIDS education may decrease fear and stigmatization among the audience (Markham et al., 2000;

Paxton, 2002). Instructions to be empathic and shifting perspective by imagining oneself in the situation of the stigmatized person have been shown to be effective in reducing stigmatizing reactions (Batson et al., 1997a; Batson et al., 1997b; Batson, Chang, Orr, & Rowland, 2002; Paluck & Green, 2009). In classroom settings, cooperative learning lessons can be engineered so that students must learn from one another to reduce stigmatization (Paluck & Green, 2009). Teachers in the Jigsaw classroom, a cooperative learning technique that reduces racial conflict among schoolchildren, give each student one piece of the lesson plan so that good comprehension requires students to collaborate (Aronson, 2008, 2015).

Conscious repression of stereotypes may be effective in changing stereotypes when people are highly motivated and when they have some experience with suppressing stereotypic thoughts (Monteith, Ashburn-Nardo, Voils, & Czopp, 2002). Otherwise, attempts at conscious repression may lead to rebound effects (Macrae, Bodenhausen, Milne, & Jetten, 1994; Paluck & Green, 2009). Presenting stereotype-inconsistent information may also be ineffective because people may see the stereotype-inconsistent individuals as exceptions that confirm the rule. Presenting stereotype-inconsistent information may have positive effects when stereotype-disconfirming attributes are present among a large number of group members and when these attributes do not differ too extremely from people's preexisting stereotypes (Kunda & Oleson, 1995, 1997).

AIDS-related stigma has many causes and outcomes and thus has to be tackled at different levels: social, political, and economic (Bos et al., 2008; Parker & Aggleton, 2003). Unfortunately, stigma intervention developers often have limited possibilities to establish macrosocial changes. Link and Phelan (2001) recognized that stigmatized groups actively use available resources to resist the stigmatizing tendencies. However, if one mechanism is changed, it will be easily replaced by another. An approach to change must, in their view, address the fundamental cause of stigma. Either it must change the deeply held attitudes and beliefs of powerful groups that have led to labeling, stereotyping, setting apart, devaluing, and discriminating, or it must change circumstances as to limit the power of such groups to make their cognitions the dominant ones (see Mahajan et al., 2008). Corrigan and Kosyluk (2013) reviewed three processes for erasing public stigma under the title "Where Science Meets Advocacy," focusing on the stigma of mental illness. Protest strategies highlight the injustice of stigma, but may have little or negative impact on public attitudes. Educational approaches challenge inaccurate stereotypes and replace these with facts, but their effect is short-lived. Interpersonal contact, mentioned earlier, has shown to be promising, but subtyping (seeing the contact as an exception) may diminish contact effects. Nevertheless, Corrigan and Kosyluk (2013) saw interpersonal contact as the most effective strategy and provided five conditions for use:

- The contact must be in vivo
- The contact needs to be addressing key groups, usually people in power
- Local contact programs are more effective
- Contacts must be credible, in essence, similar in roles
- Contacts must be continuous

## Summary: Theories of Stigma and Discrimination

These theories focus on stigmatized groups and people who stigmatize. People who are stigmatized may learn to cope with stigma or resist stigma. People who stigmatize may learn to reduce stigmatizing. Relevant elements in the environment are power differences and institutionalized stigma. Determinants of stigma include perceived contagiousness, severity, responsibility, norm violation, reflexive and reflective reactions, and power. The main determinant of coping with stigma is self-efficacy. These theories suggest methods for stigma reduction: stereotype-inconsistent information with stereotype-disconfirming attributes present, interpersonal contact, empathy training, shifting perspective, cooperative learning, conscious regulation of impulsive stereotyping and prejudice, and at the societal level, methods for reducing power differences.

## Diffusion of Innovations Theory

An innovation is an idea, practice, or product that is new to the adopter, which may be an individual or an organization (Brownson, Glanz, Tabak, & Stamatakis, 2015). Healthy behavior, for example, physical activity, cessation of smoking, and use of contraceptives, may be innovations for individuals. Health promotion programs to encourage these behaviors may be innovations in an organization and for the implementers. For example, patient self-management programs may be an innovation in an organization because they change the power relationship between patients and providers.

For many years E. Rogers (2003) studied the process of diffusion, beginning with a focus on individual adopters of new technology. Rogers's individual model is useful for health promotion because it describes decision making not only of individuals but also of change agents and program implementers. The Diffusion of Innovations Theory (DIT) can be applied to any new behavior, but in the context of Intervention Mapping, the main focus is on diffusion of a (new) health promotion program; see Chapter 8. Implementers may be compared to agents in the environment, and the Intervention Mapping steps guide planners to develop a separate intervention for implementation (see Schutte et al., 2014).

Diffusion is seen as happening in phases. The most often used distinction in health promotion is between dissemination, adoption, implementation, and maintenance (Wiecha et al., 2004):

- Dissemination: the planned systematic efforts designed to make a program or innovation more widely available, with diffusion as the result

- Adoption: uptake and commitment to initiate the program or innovation

- Implementation: the active planned efforts to implement an innovation within a defined setting

- Maintenance, sustainability, and institutionalization: the ongoing use of an intervention after initial resources are expended; incorporation of the program into the routines of an organization

## Characteristics of Adopters and Innovations

Of course, potential adopters can decide not to adopt an innovation. This decision can be either an active process or simply a passive failure to become familiar with the innovation and to decide. Classic diffusion theory has dealt with characteristics of both adopters and innovations. Adopters adopt at different times following the introduction of the innovation into their social system; and the population can be segmented into innovators, early adopters, early majority, late majority, and laggards, based on the point in time at which they adopt the innovation. E. Rogers (2003) described the process of adoption as a normal, bell-shaped distribution that places majority adopters within one standard deviation on either side of the mean of the curve, early adopters and laggards two standard deviations away, and innovators three standard deviations away. These categories of adopters have different characteristics: Innovators are venturesome; early adopters are opinion leaders; early majority are deliberators; late majority are skeptical; and the laggards are traditional.

Innovations are often communicated through two different channels: media and interpersonal communication. Initially, media increase awareness of the innovation. As people hear about the innovation and begin to adopt it, they talk with others about their interest and experience. The interpersonal channel thus becomes more important as more members of the population adopt the innovation. More potent outreach and incentives are needed for late adopters and laggards, who have not adopted even though the innovation has been communicated through the media and the majority of members of the population have adopted the innovation. Thus, for intervention planning, it is important to know the adopter category (Green, Gottlieb, & Parcel, 1991; E. Rogers, 2003).

SCT provides explanations of the psychological mechanisms by which diffusion occurs (Bandura, 1997). For implementers to adopt, implement, and maintain a new program, they must be aware of the program, hold positive outcome expectations and expectancies for it, and have sufficient self-efficacy and behavioral capability for both adoption and implementation. Teachers adopting a new sex education program, for example, must know the program is available, see benefits of the program for themselves, find the program practical and easy to use, and believe that others appreciate and support their use of the program (Schutte et al., 2014). In Chapter 3 we discuss adoption, implementation, and sustainability at the organizational and community levels, and in Chapter 8 we focus on diffusion of health promotion programs.

Also important in the consideration of interventions to promote diffusion of behavior change is the characteristics of innovations (Brownson et al., 2015; E. Rogers, 2003). These characteristics are the potential adopters' perceptions of what the innovation is like. They include the following:

- Relative advantage of the innovation compared with what is being used
- Compatibility with the intended users' current behavior
- Complexity
- Observability of the results
- Impact on social relations
- Reversibility in case of discontinuation
- Communicability
- Required time
- Risk and uncertainty
- Required commitment
- Ability to be modified

Each of these characteristics of an innovation must be considered as either a predictor of or a barrier to adoption and implementation, both in innovation design and in the creation of an intervention to aid diffusion.

DIT suggests methods and applications to influence the determinants and accomplish the performance objectives for adoption, implementation, and sustainability of new behavior (E. Rogers, 2003). Communication within the community about the innovation is essential for the diffusion process; the health promoter will want to stimulate communication and mobilize social support for the innovation. One effective method is to speed this process by using the mass media to communicate the stories of people who have been successful in adopting the new behavior. These early adopters then serve as role models for the early majority in the intervention community, and the early majority serve as models for the late majority. One way to do this is through behavioral journalism (McAlister et al., 1995; van Empelen et al., 2003). Combining DIT with SCT, behavioral journalism includes the use of appropriate role-model stories (e.g., those of early adopters) based on authentic interviews with members of the at-risk group and the use of mass media and networks within the community to distribute those role-model stories to the larger population (e.g., the early majority).

## Implementation Frameworks

The Diffusion of Innovations Theory is often applied in Step 5 of Intervention Mapping when planning for dissemination, adoption, implementation, and maintenance of the program. Dissemination and implementation frameworks can help inform Step 5 by helping the planner think carefully about implementation outcomes, consider who the adopters and implementers may be, what may influence their actions (personal and contextual factors), and what types of capacity building may be required. In Chapter 8 we present three examples of frameworks of influences on and outcomes of dissemination and implementation. The RE-AIM framework (Gaglio, Shoup, & Glasgow, 2013; Glasgow, Vogt, & Boles, 1999) can be used to help the planner identify implementation targets for developed programs and for thinking through the potential impact of programs during development. The Interactive Systems Framework (ISF; Fernández et al., 2014; Wandersman et al., 2008) helps researchers and practitioners to better understand the process of implementation and the varying levels and actors involved. The Consolidated Framework for Implementation Research (Damschroder et al. 2009; Zulman et al., 2013) describes constructs in the following five domains: intervention characteristics (e.g., cost, complexity), outer setting (e.g., external policy and incentives, patient needs and resources), inner setting (e.g., implementation climate, available resources), characteristics of individuals (e.g., self-efficacy, knowledge and beliefs about the intervention), and implementation process (e.g., planning, reflecting, and evaluating). However, none of these frameworks provides guidance for how to design interventions that specifically address the factors included in the models. There are only a few examples in the literature of the systematic planning of dissemination interventions (see Chapter 8).

## Summary: Diffusion of Innovations Theory

Intervention groups can be distinguished by adopter category: innovators, early adopters, early majority, late majority, and laggards. Relevant performance objectives are adoption, implementation, and sustainability. DIT may be applied to any behavior that is new to the person: at-risk individuals, environmental agents, or program users. Determinants include the characteristics of adopters, such as being venturesome individuals, opinion leaders, deliberators, skeptical, or traditional, and the characteristics of the innovation, such as relative advantage, compatibility, complexity, observability, impact on social relations, reversibility, communicability, time, risk and uncertainty, commitment, and ability to be modified. Methods are increasing the rate of diffusion by linkage (participation), persuasive communication about the innovation, mobilizing social support, and modeling.

## Summary

The purpose of this chapter is to identify individual-oriented theories and models that are useful for planning health promotion interventions, including three theories at the interpersonal level. We first present learning theories, then theories of information processing; theories of health behavior; theories of reasoned action; goal-setting theory; theories of automatic, impulsive, and habitual behavior; stage theories; attribution theory and relapse prevention; theories of persuasive communication; and theories of self-regulation. Finally, we present Social Cognitive Theory, theories of stigma and discrimination, and Diffusion of Innovations Theory. Each theory is summarized in terms of its contribution to problem analysis and intervention development.

## Discussion Questions and Learning Activities

1. Give examples for all six Intervention Mapping tasks of how to use theory for program planning.

2. Describe what is meant by an eclectic, or problem-focused, approach to theory, and explain why this approach is useful in planning health promotion programs.

3. Select a theory that explains behavior at the individual level, and describe how the theory could be used to understand or predict behavior at the organizational, community, or societal levels.

4. Describe eight variables that are considered important determinants of behavior across five different theories. Which variables are considered necessary and sufficient to explain behavior?

5. Describe a method from Social Cognitive Theory that can be used to improve self-efficacy for changing a behavior.

6. Sometimes health promotion campaigns use sports heroes as role models to influence people to practice a health behavior (such as eating fruits and vegetables) or not to do a health risk behavior (such as not using drugs). Use Social Cognitive Theory to explain why sports heroes may not be the best role models to influence a change in health-related behavior for most community members.

7. When considering the Elaboration Likelihood Model, give examples of what that theory says about effective ways to stimulate central processing of information.

8. List ways to reduce stigma. How much evidence is there for each of these methods?

## References

Aarts, H., Custers, R., & Holland, R. W. (2007). The nonconscious cessation of goal pursuit: When goals and negative affect are coactivated. *Journal of Personality and Social Psychology, 92*(2), 165–178.

Aarts, H., & Dijksterhuis, A. (2003). The silence of the library: Environment, situational norm, and social behavior. *Journal of Personality and Social Psychology, 84*(1), 18–28.

Abraham, C., & Sheeran, P. (2005). The Health Belief Model. In M. Conner & P. Norman (Eds.), *Predicting health behaviour: Research and practice with social cognition models* (2nd ed., pp. 28–80). Maidenhead, Berkshire, United Kingdom: Open University Press, McGraw-Hill Education.

Abrahamse, W., & Steg, L. (2011). Factors related to household energy use and intention to reduce it: The role of psychological and socio-demographic variables. *Human Ecology Review, 18*(1), 30–40.

Achtziger, A., Gollwitzer, P. M., & Sheeran, P. (2008). Implementation intentions and shielding goal striving from unwanted thoughts and feelings. *Personality and Social Psychology Bulletin, 34*(3), 381–393.

Adriaanse, M. A., de Ridder, D. T., & de Wit, J. B. F. (2009). Finding the critical cue: Implementation intentions to change one's diet work best when tailored to personally relevant reasons for unhealthy eating. *Personality and Social Psychology Bulletin, 35*(1), 60–71.

Ajzen, I. (1988). *Attitudes, personality and behavior*. Chicago, IL: Dorsey Press.

Ajzen, I. (2006). *Constructing a TPB questionnaire: Conceptual and methodological considerations*. Unpublished manuscript.

Ajzen, I., Czasch, C., & Flood, M. G. (2009). From intentions to behavior: Implementation intention, commitment, and conscientiousness. *Journal of Applied Social Psychology, 39*(6), 1356–1372.

Alberts, H. J. E. M. (2007). *Carrying on or giving in: Processes of self-control and ego-depletion.* Retrieved from dissertaties.ub.unimaas.nl

Alberts, H. J. E. M, Martijn, C., Greb, J., Merckelbach, H., & de Vries, N. K. (2007). Carrying on or giving in: The role of automatic processes in overcoming ego depletion. *British Journal of Social Psychology, 46*(Pt 2), 383–399.

Amodio, E., Restivo, V., Firenze, A., Mammina, C., Tramuto, F., & Vitale, F. (2014). Can influenza vaccination coverage among healthcare workers influence the risk of nosocomial influenza-like illness in hospitalized patients? *Journal of Hospital Infection, 86*(3), 182–187.

Armitage, C. J. (2009). Is there utility in the transtheoretical model? *British Journal of Health Psychology, 14*(Pt 2), 195–210.

Aronson, E. (2008). *The social animal* (10th ed.). New York, NY: Worth/Freeman.

Aronson, E. (2015). *Jigsaw classroom.* Retrieved from http://www.jigsaw.org/

Austin, J. T., & Vancouver, J. B. (1996). Goal constructs in psychology: Structure, process, and content. *Psychological Bulletin, 120*(3), 338–375.

Bagot, K. L., Masser, B. M., & White, K. M. (2015). Using an extended Theory of Planned Behavior to predict a change in the type of blood product donated. *Annals of Behavioral Medicine, 49*(4), 510–521.

Bandura, A. (1965). Influence of models' reinforcement contingencies on the acquisition of imitative responses. *Journal of Personality and Social Psychology, 1*(6), 589.

Bandura, A. (1969). Social-learning theory of identificatory processes. In D. A. Goslin (Ed.), *Handbook of socialization theory and research* (pp. 213–262). Chicago, IL: Rand McNally.

Bandura, A. (1977). *Social learning theory.* Englewood Cliffs, NJ: Prentice Hall.

Bandura, A. (1986). *Social foundations of thought and action: A Social Cognitive Theory.* Englewood Cliffs, NJ: Prentice Hall.

Bandura, A. (1997). *Self-efficacy: The exercise of control.* New York, NY: W.H. Freeman.

Baranowski, T. (2006). Crisis and chaos in behavioral nutrition and physical activity. *International Journal of Behavioral Nutrition and Physical Activity, 3*, 27.

Bartholomew, L., Gold, R., Parcel, G., Czyzewski, D., Sockrider, M., Fernández, M., ... Swank, P. (2000a). Watch, Discover, Think, and Act: Evaluation of computer-assisted instruction to improve asthma self-management in inner-city children. *Patient Education and Counseling, 39*(2), 269–280.

Bartholomew, L., Shegog, R., Parcel, G., Gold, R., Fernández, M., Czyzewski, D., ... Berlin, N. (2000b). Watch, Discover, Think, and Act: A model for patient education program development. *Patient Education and Counseling, 39*(2), 253–268.

Bartholomew, L. K., Sockrider, M. M., Seilheimer, D. K., Czyzewski, D. I., Parcel, G. S., & Spinelli, S. H. (1993). Performance objectives for the self-management of cystic fibrosis. *Patient Education and Counseling, 22*(1), 15–25.

Batson, C. D., Chang, J., Orr, R., & Rowland, J. (2002). Empathy, attitudes, and action: Can feeling for a member of a stigmatized group motivate one to help the group? *Personality and Social Psychology Bulletin, 28*(12), 1656–1666.

Batson, C. D., Early, S., & Salvarani, G. (1997a). Perspective taking: Imagining how another feels versus imaging how you would feel. *Personality and Social Psychology Bulletin, 23*(7), 751–758.

Batson, C. D., Polycarpou, M. P., Harmon-Jones, E., Imhoff, H. J., Mitchener, E. C., Bednar, L. L., . . . Highberger, L. (1997b). Empathy and attitudes: Can feeling for a member of a stigmatized group improve feelings toward the group? *Journal of Personality and Social Psychology, 72*, 105–118.

Baumeister, R. F., & Vohs, K. D. (Eds.). (2004). *Handbook of self-regulation: Research, theory, and applications.* New York, NY: Guilford Press.

Bayliss, D. M., Bogdanovs, J., & Jarrold, C. (2015). Consolidating working memory: Distinguishing the effects of consolidation, rehearsal and attentional refreshing in a working memory span task. *Journal of Memory and Language, 81*, 34–50.

Boekaerts, M., Pintrich, P. R., & Zeidner, M. (Eds.). (2000). *Handbook of self-regulation.* San Diego, CA: Academic Press.

Bos, A. E. R., Kanner, D., Muris, P., Janssen, B., & Mayer, B. (2009). Mental illness stigma and disclosure: Consequences of coming out of the closet. *Issues in Mental Health Nursing, 30*(8), 509–513.

Bos, A. E. R., Pryor, J. B., Reeder, G. D., & Stutterheim, S. E. (2013). Stigma: Advances in theory and research. *Basic and Applied Social Psychology, 35*, 1–9.

Bos, A. E. R., Schaalma, H. P., & Pryor, J. B. (2008). Reducing AIDS-related stigma in developing countries: The importance of theory- and evidence-based interventions. *Psychology, Health & Medicine, 13*(4), 450–460.

Brewer, N. T., & Rimer, B. K. (2015). Introduction to health behavior theories that focus on individuals. In K. Glanz, B. K. Rimer, & K. Viswanath (Eds.), *Health behavior: Theory, research, and practice* (5th ed., pp. 115–130). San Francisco, CA: Jossey-Bass.

Brijs, K., Brijs, T., Sann, S., Trinh, T. A., Wets, G., & Ruiter, R. A. C. (2014). Psychological determinants of motorcycle helmet use among young adults in Cambodia. *Transportation Research Part F: Traffic Psychology and Behaviour, 26*(Pt A), 273–290.

Brown, T. C., & Latham, G. P. (2002). The effects of behavioural outcome goals, learning goals, and urging people to "do their best" on an individual's teamwork behaviour in a group problem-solving task. *Canadian Journal of Behavioural Science, 34*(4), 276–285.

Brownson, R., Glanz, K., Tabak, R., & Stamatakis, K. (2015). Implementation, dissemination, and diffusion of public health interventions. In K. Glanz, B. K. Rimer, & K. Viswanath (Eds.), *Health behavior: Theory, research, and practice* (5th ed., pp. 544–592). San Francisco, CA: Jossey-Bass.

Brug, J. (2006). Order is needed to promote linear or quantum changes in nutrition and physical activity behaviors: A reaction to "A chaotic view of behavior change" by Resnicow and Vaughan. *The International Journal of Behavioral Nutrition and Physical Activity, 3*, 29.

Brug, J., Conner, M., Harré, N., Kremers, S., McKellar, S., & Whitelaw, S. (2005). The transtheoretical model and stages of change: A critique: Observations by five commentators on the paper by Adams, J. and White, M. (2004) Why don't stage-based activity promotion interventions work? *Health Education Research, 20*(2), 244–258.

Brüll, P., Ruiter, R. A. C., & Jansma, B. M. (2015). *Frame it right—Straightforward affirmative message framing predicts recognition memory performance.* Manuscript in preparation.

Buunk, A. P., & van Vugt, M. (2013). *Applying social psychology: From problems to solutions* (2nd ed.). London, United Kingdom: Sage.

Carver, C. S., & Scheier, M. F. (1998). *On the self-regulation of behavior.* New York, NY: Cambridge University Press.

Champion, V. L., & Skinner, C. S. (2008). The Health Belief Model. In K. Glanz, B. K. Rimer, & K. Viswanath (Eds.), *Health behavior and health education: Theory, research, and practice* (4th ed., 45–65). San Francisco, CA: Jossey-Bass.

Chapin, J. (2014). Adolescents and cyber bullying: The precaution adoption process model. *Education and Information Technologies, 19.*

Chartrand, T. L., & Bargh, J. A. (1999). The chameleon effect: The perception–behavior link and social interaction. *Journal of Personality and Social Psychology, 76*(6), 893–910.

Chein, J., Albert, D., O'Brien, L., Uckert, K., & Steinberg, L. (2011). Peers increase adolescent risk taking by enhancing activity in the brain's reward circuitry. *Developmental Science, 14*(2), F1–F10.

Clark, N. M. (2003). Management of chronic disease by patients. *Annual Review of Public Health, 24*(1), 289–313.

Clark, N. M., & Zimmerman, B. J. (2014). A social cognitive view of self-regulated learning about health. *Health Education & Behavior, 41*(5), 485–491.

Cleary, T. J., & Zimmerman, B. J. (2004). Self-regulation empowerment program: A school-based program to enhance self-regulated and self-motivated cycles of student learning. *Psychology in the Schools, 41*(5), 537–550.

Cohen, G. L., & Sherman, D. K. (2014). The psychology of change: Self-affirmation and social psychological intervention. *Annual Review of Psychology, 65*, 333–371.

Committee on Communication for Behavior Change in the 21st Century: Improving the Health of Diverse Populations. (2002). *Speaking of health: Assessing health communication strategies for diverse populations.* Washington, DC: National Academies Press.

Conn, V. S., Valentine, J. C., & Cooper, H. M. (2002). Interventions to increase physical activity among aging adults: A meta-analysis. *Annals of Behavioral Medicine, 24*(3), 190–200.

Conner, M., & Norman, P. (2005). *Predicting health behaviour: Research and practice with social cognition models* (2nd ed.). Maidenhead, Berkshire, United Kingdom: Open University Press, McGraw-Hill Education.

Conner, M., & Sparks, P. (2005). Theory of Planned Behavior and health behavior. In M. Conner & P. Norman (Eds.), *Predicting health behavior* (2nd ed., pp. 170–222). London, UK: Open University Press.

Corrigan, P. W., & Kosyluk, K. A. (2013). Erasing the stigma: Where science meets advocacy. *Basic and Applied Social Psychology, 35*, 131–140.

Corrigan, P. W., & Wassel, A. (2008). Understanding and influencing the stigma of mental illness. *Journal of Psychosocial Nursing and Mental Health Services, 46*(1), 42–48.

Creer, T. L. (2000). Self-management of chronic illness. In M. Boekaerts, P. R. Pintrich, & M. Zeidner (Eds.), *Handbook of self-regulation* (pp. 601–629). San Diego, CA: Academic Press.

Crone, E. A., & Dahl, R. E. (2012). Understanding adolescence as a period of social–affective engagement and goal flexibility. *Nature Reviews Neuroscience, 13*(9), 636–650.

Crosby, R., & Noar, S. M. (2010). Theory development in health promotion: Are we there yet? *Journal of Behavioral Medicine, 33*(4), 259–263.

Custers, R., & Aarts, H. (2010). The unconscious will: How the pursuit of goals operates outside of conscious awareness. *Science, 329*(5987), 47–50.

Damschroder, L. J., Aron, D. C., Keith, R. E., Kirsh, S. R., Alexander, J. A., & Lowery, J. C. (2009). Fostering implementation of health services research findings into practice: A consolidated framework for advancing implementation science. *Implementation Science, 4*, 50.

Danner, U. N., Aarts, H., & de Vries, N. K. (2008). Habit vs. intention in the prediction of future behaviour: The role of frequency, context stability and mental accessibility of past behaviour. *British Journal of Social Psychology, 47*(Pt 2), 245–265.

de Bruin, M., Hospers, H. J., van Breukelen, G. J., Kok, G., Koevoets, W. M., & Prins, J. M. (2010). Electronic monitoring-based counseling to enhance adherence among HIV-infected patients: A randomized controlled trial. *Health Psychology, 29*(4), 421.

de Bruin, M., Sheeran, P., Kok, G., Hiemstra, A., Prins, J. M., Hospers, H. J., & van Breukelen, G. J. (2012). Self-regulatory processes mediate the intention-behavior relation for adherence and exercise behaviors. *Health Psychology, 31*(6), 695–703.

Deci, E. L., & Ryan, R. M. (Eds.). (2002). *Handbook of self-determination research.* Rochester, NY: University of Rochester Press.

de Hoog, N., Stroebe, W., & de Wit, J. B. (2007). The impact of vulnerability to and severity of a health risk on processing and acceptance of fear-arousing communications: A meta-analysis. *Review of General Psychology, 11*(3), 258–285.

de Ridder, D. (2014). Nudging for beginners: A shortlist of issues in urgent needs research. *The European Health Psychologist, 16*(1), 1–6.

Deutsch, R., & Strack, F. (2006). Duality models in social psychology: From dual processes to interacting systems. *Psychological Inquiry, 17*(3), 166–172.

Devine, P. G. (1989). Stereotypes and prejudice: Their automatic and controlled components. *Journal of Personality and Social Psychology, 56*, 5–18.

Devos-Comby, L., Cronan, T., & Roesch, S. C. (2006). Do exercise and self-management interventions benefit patients with osteoarthritis of the knee? A metaanalytic review. *The Journal of Rheumatology, 33*(4), 744–756.

de Vries, H., Backbier, E., Kok, G., & Djikstra, M. (1995). The impact of social influences in the context of attitude, self-efficacy, intention, and previous behavior as predictors of smoking onset. *Journal of Applied Social Psychology, 25*(3), 237–257.

de Vries, H., Weijts, W., Dijkstra, M., & Kok, G. (1992). The utilization of qualitative and quantitative data for health education program planning, implementation, and evaluation: A spiral approach. *Health Education & Behavior, 19*(1), 101–115.

Diamond, A. (2013). Executive functions. *Annual Review of Psychology, 64*, 135–168.

Diamond, A., & Lee, K. (2011). Interventions shown to aid executive function development in children 4 to 12 years old. *Science, 333*(6045), 959–964.

Dijker, A. J., & Koomen, W. (2003). Extending Weiner's attribution-emotion model of stigmatization of ill persons. *Basic and Applied Social Psychology, 25*, 51–68.

Dijker, A. J. M., & Koomen, W. (2007). *Stigmatization, tolerance and repair: An integrative psychological analysis of responses to deviance.* In K. Oatley & A. Manstead (Series Eds.), Studies in Emotion and Social Interaction. Cambridge, United Kingdom: Cambridge University Press.

Dijksterhuis, A., & Aarts, H. (2010). Goals, attention, and (un)consciousness. *Annual Review of Psychology, 61*, 467–490.

Epton, T., Harris, P. R., Kane, R., van Koningsbruggen, G. M., & Sheeran, P. (2014). The impact of self-affirmation on health-behavior change: A meta-analysis. *Health Psychology, 34*(3), 187–196.

Evans, R., Getz, J., & Raines, B. (1991). *Theory-guided models on prevention of AIDS in adolescents.* Paper presented at the Science Weekend of the American Psychological Association, San Francisco, CA.

Fazio, R. H. (1986). How do attitudes guide behavior? In R. M. Sorrentino & E. T. Higgins (Eds.), *Handbook of motivation and cognition: Volume 1: Foundations of social behavior* (pp. 204–243). New York, NY: Guilford Press.

Fazio, R. H. (2001). On the automatic activation of associated evaluations: An overview. *Cognition & Emotion, 15*(2), 115–141.

Fernández, M. E., Melvin, C. L., Leeman, J., Ribisl, K. M., Allen, J. D., Kegler, M. C., . . . Hebert, J. R. (2014). The cancer prevention and control research network: An interactive systems approach to advancing cancer control implementation research and practice. *Cancer Epidemiology, Biomarkers & Prevention, 23*(11), 2512–2521.

Fishbein, M. (2000). The role of theory in HIV prevention. *AIDS Care, 12*(3), 273–278.

Fishbein, M., & Ajzen, I. (1975). *Belief, attitude, intention and behavior: An introduction to theory and research.* Reading, MA: Addison Wesley.

Fishbein, M., & Ajzen, I. (2010). *Predicting and changing behaviour: The Reasoned Action Approach*. New York, NY: Psychology Press.

Fishbein, M., Triandis, H. C., Kanfer, F. H., Becker, M., Middlestadt, S. E., & Eichler, A. (2001). Factors influencing behavior and behavior change. In A. S. Baum, T. A. Revenson, & J. E. Singer (Eds.), *Handbook of health psychology* (pp. 1–17). Mahwah, NJ: Lawrence Erlbaum.

Fisher, J. D., Fisher, W. A., Amico, K. R., & Harman, J. J. (2006). An information-motivation-behavioral skills model of adherence to antiretroviral therapy. *Health Psychology, 25*(4), 462–473.

Floyd, D. L., Prentice-Dunn, S., & Rogers, R. W. (2000). A meta-analysis of research on Protection Motivation Theory. *Journal of Applied Social Psychology, 30*(2), 407–429.

Flynn, B. S., Goldstein, A. O., Solomon, L. J., Bauman, K. E., Gottlieb, N. H., Cohen, J. E., . . . Dana, G. S. (1998). Predictors of state legislators' intentions to vote for cigarette tax increases. *Preventive Medicine, 27*(2), 157–165.

Foer, J. (2011). *Moonwalking with Einstein: The art and science of remembering everything*. New York, NY: Penguin.

Forsyth, D. R. (2014). *Group dynamics* (6th ed.). Belmont, CA: Wadsworth Cengage Learning.

Francis, J. J., Eccles, M. P., Johnston, M., Walker, A., Grimshaw, J., Foy, R., . . . Bonetti, D. (2004). *Constructing questionnaires based on the Theory of Planned Behavior: A manual for health services researchers*. Newcastle upon Tyne, United Kingdom: Centre for Health Services Research, University of Newcastle.

Frijda, N. H. (2007). *The laws of emotion*. New York, NY: Psychology Press.

Gaglio, B., Shoup, J. A., & Glasgow, R. E. (2013). The RE-AIM framework: A systematic review of use over time. *American Journal of Public Health, 103*(6), e38–e46.

Gagné, M. (2014). *The Oxford handbook of work engagement, motivation, and Self-Determination Theory*. In P. E. Nathan (Series Ed.), Oxford Library of Psychology. Oxford, United Kingdom: Oxford University Press.

Gardner, M., & Steinberg, L. (2005). Peer influence on risk taking, risk preference, and risky decision making in adolescence and adulthood: An experimental study. *Developmental Psychology, 41*(4), 625.

Garrison, D. R., Anderson, T., & Archer, W. (2001). Critical thinking, cognitive presence, and computer conferencing in distance education. *American Journal of Distance Education, 15*, 7–23.

Glanz, K., & Bishop, D. B. (2010). The role of behavioral science theory in development and implementation of public health interventions. *Annual Review of Public Health, 31*, 399–418.

Glasgow, R. E., Vogt, T. M., & Boles, S. M. (1999). Evaluating the public health impact of health promotion interventions: The RE-AIM framework. *American Journal of Public Health, 89*(9), 1322–1327.

Gobet, F. (2005). Chunking models of expertise: Implications for education. *Applied Cognitive Psychology, 19*(2), 183–204.

Gobet, F., Lane, P. C., Croker, S., Cheng, P. C., Jones, G., Oliver, I., & Pine, J. M. (2001). Chunking mechanisms in human learning. *Trends in Cognitive Sciences, 5*(6), 236–243.

Godden, D. R., & Baddeley, A. D. (1975). Context-dependent memory in two natural environments: On land and underwater. *British Journal of Psychology, 66*(3), 325–331.

Godin, G., Fortin, C., Michaud, F., Bradet, R., & Kok, G. (1997). Use of condoms: Intention and behaviour of adolescents living in juvenile rehabilitation centres. *Health Education Research, 12*(3), 289–300.

Godin, G., & Kok, G. (1996). The Theory of Planned Behavior: A review of its applications to health-related behaviors. *American Journal of Health Promotion, 11*(2), 87–98.

Goffman, E. (1963). *Stigma: Notes on the management of spoiled identity.* Englewood Cliffs, NJ: Prentice Hall.

Golden, S. D., & Earp, J. A. (2012). Social ecological approaches to individuals and their contexts: Twenty years of health education & behavior health promotion interventions. *Health Education & Behavior, 39*(3), 364–372.

Goldstein, D. G., Johnson, E. J., Herrmann, A., & Heitmann, M. (2008). Nudge your customers toward better choices. *Harvard Business Review, 86*(12), 99–105.

Gollwitzer, P. M. (1993). Goal achievement: The role of intentions. *European Review of Social Psychology, 4,* 141–185.

Gollwitzer, P. M. (1999). Implementation intentions: Strong effects of simple plans. *American Psychologist, 54*(7), 493–503.

Gollwitzer, P. M., & Sheeran, P. (2006). Implementation intentions and goal achievement: A meta-analysis of effects and processes. *Advances in Experimental Social Psychology, 38,* 69–119.

Gottlieb, D. A., & Begej, E. L. (2014). Principles of Pavlovian conditioning: Description, content, function. In F. K. McSweeney & E. S. Murphy (Eds.), *The Wiley Blackwell handbook of operant and classical conditioning* (pp. 3–26). Chichester, United Kingdom: John Wiley & Sons.

Gottlieb, N. H., Goldstein, A. O., Flynn, B. S., Cohen, E. J., Bauman, K. E., Solomon, L. J., . . . McMorris, L. E. (2003). State legislators' beliefs about legislation that restricts youth access to tobacco products. *Health Education & Behavior, 30*(2), 209–224.

Green, L. W., Gottlieb, N., & Parcel, G. (1991). Diffusion theory extended and applied. In W. B. Ward & F. M. Lewis (Eds.), *Advances in health education and promotion* (Vol. 3, pp. 91–117). Philadelphia, PA: Jessica Kingsley.

Griffin, D. W., & Harris, P. R. (2011). Calibrating the response to health warnings: Limiting both overreaction and underreaction with self-affirmation. *Psychological Science, 22*(5), 572–578.

Hagger, M. S., & Luszczynska, A. (2014). Implementation intention and action planning interventions in health contexts: State of the research and proposals for the way forward. *Applied Psychology: Health and Well-Being, 6*(1), 1–47.

Hamilton, R. J., & Ghatala, E. (1994). *Learning and instruction.* New York, NY: McGraw-Hill.

Harris, P. R., Griffin, D. W., & Murray, S. (2008). Testing the limits of optimistic bias: Event and person moderators in a multilevel framework. *Journal of Personality and Social Psychology, 95*(5), 1225–1237.

Harris, P. R., Mayle, K., Mabbott, L., & Napper, L. (2007). Self-affirmation reduces smokers' defensiveness to graphic on-pack cigarette warning labels. *Health Psychology, 26*(4), 437.

Hassin, R. R., Uleman, J. S., & Bargh, J. A. (Eds.). (2005). *The new unconscious.* In R. R. Hassin (Series Ed.), Oxford series in social cognition and social neuroscience. New York, NY: Oxford University Press.

Head, K. J., & Noar, S. M. (2014). Facilitating progress in health behaviour theory development and modification: The Reasoned Action Approach as a case study. *Health Psychology Review, 8*(1), 34–52.

Hill-Briggs, F., & Gemmell, L. (2007). Problem solving in diabetes self-management and control: A systematic review of the literature. *The Diabetes Educator, 33*(6), 1032–1050.

Hofmann, W., Friese, M., & Strack, F. (2009). Impulse and self-control from a dual-systems perspective. *Perspectives on Psychological Science, 4*(2), 162–176.

Hofmann, W., Friese, M., & Wiers, R. W. (2008). Impulsive versus reflective influences on health behavior: A theoretical framework and empirical review. *Health Psychology Review, 2,* 111–137.

Holland, R. W., Hendriks, M., & Aarts, H. (2005). Smells like clean spirit. Nonconscious effects of scent on cognition and behavior. *Psychological Science, 16*(9), 689–693.

Holtgrave, D. R., Tinsley, B. J., & Kay, L. S. (1995). Encouraging risk reduction: A decision-making approach to message design. In E. Maibach & R. L. Parrott (Eds.), *Designing health messages: Approaches from communication theory and public health practice* (pp. 24–40). Thousand Oaks, CA: Sage.

Hospers, H. J., Kok, G., & Strecher, V. J. (1990). Attributions for previous failures and subsequent outcomes in a weight reduction program. *Health Education Quarterly, 17*(4), 409–415.

Houben, K., Havermans, R. C., Nederkoorn, C., & Jansen, A. (2012). Beer à no-go: Learning to stop responding to alcohol cues reduces alcohol intake via reduced affective associations rather than increased response inhibition. *Addiction, 107*(7), 1280–1287.

Janssen, E., van Osch, L., de Vries, H., & Lechner, L. (2011). Measuring risk perceptions of skin cancer: Reliability and validity of different operationalizations. *British Journal of Health Psychology, 16*(Pt 1), 92–112.

Janssen, E., van Osch, L., Lechner, L., Candel, M., & de Vries, H. (2012). Thinking versus feeling: Differentiating between cognitive and affective components of perceived cancer risk. *Psychology & Health, 27*(7), 767–783.

Janssen, E., Waters, E. A., van Osch, L., Lechner, L., & de Vries, H. (2014). The importance of affectively-laden beliefs about health risks: The case of tobacco use and sun protection. *Journal of Behavioral Medicine, 37*(1), 11–21.

Janz, N. K., & Becker, M. H. (1984). The Health Belief Model: A decade later. *Health Education Quarterly, 11*(1), 1–47.

Jones, C. R., Fazio, R. H., & Olson, M. A. (2009). Implicit misattribution as a mechanism underlying evaluative conditioning. *Journal of Personality and Social Psychology, 96*(5), 933–948.

Jurado, M. B., & Rosselli, M. (2007). The elusive nature of executive functions: A review of our current understanding. *Neuropsychology Review, 17*(3), 213–233.

Kazdin, A. E. (2012). *Behavior modification in applied settings* (7th ed.). Long Grove, IL: Waveland Press.

Keating, D. P. (2007). Understanding adolescent development: Implications for driving safety. *Journal of Safety Research, 38*(2), 147–157.

Kelder, S., Hoelscher, D., & Perry, C. L. (2015). How individuals, environments, and health behaviour interact: Social Cognitive Theory. In K. Glanz, B. K. Rimer, & K. Viswanath (Eds.), *Health behavior: Theory, research, and practice* (5th ed., pp. 285–325). San Francisco, CA: Jossey-Bass.

Kessels, L. T. E., Harris, P. R., Ruiter, R. A. C., & Klein, W. M. P. (2015). *Early implicit effects of self-affirmation in attending to graphic anti-smoking images.* Unpublished manuscript.

Kessels, L.T.E., Ruiter, R.A.C., & Jansma, B. M. (2010). Increased attention but more efficient disengagement: Neuroscientific evidence for defensive processing of threatening health information. *Health Psychology, 29*, 346–354.

Kintsch, W. (1988). The role of knowledge in discourse comprehension: A construction-integration model. *Psychological Review, 95*(2), 163–182.

Kintsch, W. (1994). Text comprehension, memory, and learning. *American Psychologist, 49*(4), 294–303.

Kintsch, W., & van Dijk, T. A. (1978). Toward a model of text comprehension and production. *Psychological Review, 85*(5), 363–394.

Koch, E. J. (2014). How does anticipated regret influence health and safety decisions? A literature review. *Basic and Applied Social Psychology, 36*(5), 397–412.

Koffka, K. (1935). *Principles of Gestalt psychology.* New York, NY: Harcourt Brace.

Kok, G. (2014). A practical guide to effective behavior change: How to apply theory- and evidence-based behavior change methods in an intervention. *European Health Psychologist, 16*(5), 156–170.

Kok, G., den Boer, D. J., de Vries, H., Gerards, F., Hospers, H. J., & Mudde, A. N. (1992). Self-efficacy and attribution theory in health education. In R. Schwarzer (Ed.), *Self-efficacy: Thought control of action* (pp. 245–262). New York, NY: Taylor & Francis.

Kok, G., Gottlieb, N. H., Commers, M., & Smerecnik, C. (2008). The ecological approach in health promotion programs: A decade later. *American Journal of Health Promotion, 22*(6), 437–442.

Kok, G., Gottlieb, N. H., Panne, R., & Smerecnik, C. (2012). Methods for environmental change; An exploratory study. *BMC Public Health, 12*, 1037.

Kok, G., & Ruiter, R. A. C. (2014). Who has the authority to change a theory? Everyone! A commentary on Head and Noar. *Health Psychology Review, 8*(1), 61–64.

Kok, G., Schaalma, H., de Vries, H., Parcel, G., & Paulussen, T. (1996). Social psychology and health education. *European Review of Social Psychology, 7*(1), 241–282.

Kok, G., Zijlstra, F. R. H., & Ruiter, R. A. C. (2015). Changing environmental conditions impacting health: A focus on organizations. In R. J. Burke & A. M. Richardsen (Eds.), *Corporate wellness programs: Linking employee and organizational health* (pp. 28–58). Cheltenham, United Kingdom: Edward Elgar.

Kools, M. (2012). Making written materials easy to use. In C. Abraham & M. Kools (Eds.), *Writing health communication: An evidence-based guide* (pp. 43–62). London, United Kingdom: Sage.

Kools, M., Ruiter, R. A. C., van de Wiel, M. W., & Kok, G. (2004). Increasing readers' comprehension of health education brochures: A qualitative study into how professional writers make texts coherent. *Health Education & Behavior, 31*(6), 720–740.

Kools, M., Ruiter, R. A. C., van de Wiel, M. W., & Kok, G. (2007). Testing the usability of access structures in a health education brochure. *British Journal of Health Psychology, 12*(Pt 4), 525–541.

Kools, M., Ruiter, R. A. C., van de Wiel, M. W. J., & Kok, G. (2008). The effects of headings in information mapping on search speed and evaluation of a brief health education text. *Journal of Information Science, 34*, 833–844.

Kools, M., van de Wiel, M. W., Ruiter, R. A. C., Crüts, A., & Kok, G. (2006). The effect of graphic organizers on subjective and objective comprehension of a health education text. *Health Education & Behavior, 33*(6), 760–772.

Kreuter, M. W., & McClure, S. M. (2004). The role of culture in health communication. *Annual Review of Public Health, 25*, 439–455.

Kunda, Z., & Oleson, K. C. (1995). Maintaining stereotypes in the face of disconfirmation: Constructing grounds for subtyping deviants. *Journal of Personality and Social Psychology, 68*(4), 565–579.

Kunda, Z., & Oleson, K. C. (1997). When exceptions prove the rule: How extremity of deviance determines the impact of deviant examples on stereotypes. *Journal of Personality and Social Psychology, 72*(5), 965–979.

Kwasnicka, D., Presseau, J., White, M., & Sniehotta, F. F. (2013). Does planning how to cope with anticipated barriers facilitate health-related behaviour change? A systematic review. *Health Psychology Review, 7*(2), 129–145.

Larkey, L. K., Ogden, S. L., Tenorio, S., & Ewell, T. (2008). Latino recruitment to cancer prevention/screening trials in the Southwest: Setting a research agenda. *Applied Nursing Research, 21*(1), 30–39.

Latham, G. P., & Locke, E. A. (2007). New developments in and directions for goal-setting research. *European Psychologist, 12*(4), 290–300.

Leerlooijer, J. N., Kok, G., Weyusya, J., Bos, A. E. R., Ruiter, R. A. C., Rijsdijk, L. E.,...Bartholomew, L. K. (2014a). Applying Intervention Mapping to develop a community-based intervention aimed at improved psychological and social well-being of unmarried teenage mothers in Uganda. *Health Education Research, 29*(4), 598–610.

Leerlooijer, J. N., Ruiter, R. A. C., Damayanti, R., Rijsdijk, L. E., Eiling, E., Bos, A. E. R., & Kok, G. (2014b). Psychosocial correlates of the motivation to abstain from sexual intercourse among Indonesian adolescents. *Tropical Medicine & International Health, 19*(1), 74–82.

Leerlooijer, J. N., Ruiter, R. A. C., Reinders, J., Darwisyah, W., Kok, G., & Bartholomew, L. K. (2011). The World Starts With Me: Using intervention mapping for the systematic adaptation and transfer of school-based sexuality education from Uganda to Indonesia. *Translational Behavioral Medicine, 1*(2), 331–340.

Lehmann, B. A., Chapman, G., Kok, G., & Ruiter, R. A. C. (2015a). *Changing the default to promote influenza vaccination in health care workers*. Unpublished manuscript.

Lehmann, B. A., Ruiter, R. A. C., van Dam, D., Wicker, S., & Kok, G. (2015b). Sociocognitive predictors of the intention of healthcare workers to receive the influenza vaccine in Belgian, Dutch and German hospital settings. *Journal of Hospital Infection, 89*(3), 202–209.

Li, M., & Chapman, G. B. (2013). Nudge to health: Harnessing decision research to promote health behavior. *Social and Personality Psychology Compass, 7*(3), 187–198.

Link, B. G., & Phelan, J. C. (2001). Conceptualizing stigma. *Annual Review of Sociology, 27*, 363–385.

Locke, E. A., & Latham, G. P. (1990). *A theory of goal setting & task performance*. Englewood Cliffs, NJ: Prentice Hall.

Locke, E. A., & Latham, G. P. (2002). Building a practically useful theory of goal setting and task motivation: A 35-year odyssey. *American Psychologist, 57*(9), 705–717.

Locke, E. A., & Latham, G. P. (2005). Goal setting theory: Theory building by induction. In K. G. Smith & M. A. Hitt (Eds.), *Great minds in management: The process of theory development* (pp. 128–150). Oxford, United Kingdom: Oxford University Press.

Locke, E. A., & Latham, G. P. (Eds.). (2013). *New developments in goal setting and task performance*. New York, NY: Routledge.

Loewenstein, G. F., Weber, E. U., Hsee, C. K., & Welch, N. (2001). Risk as feelings. *Psychological Bulletin, 127*(2), 267–286.

Lustria, M. L. A., Cortese, J., Noar, S. M., & Glueckauf, R. L. (2009). Computer-tailored health interventions delivered over the Web: Review and analysis of key components. *Patient Education and Counseling, 74*(2), 156–173.

Luszczynska, A., & Schwarzer, R. (2005). Social Cognitive Theory. In M. Conner & P. Norman (Eds.), *Predicting health behaviour* (2nd ed., pp. 127–169). London, United Kingdom: Open University Press.

Maas, J., de Ridder, D. T., de Vet, E., & de Wit, J. B. (2012). Do distant foods decrease intake? The effect of food accessibility on consumption. *Psychology & Health, 27*(S2), 59–73.

Macrae, C. N., Bodenhausen, G. V., Milne, A. B., & Jetten, J. (1994). Out of mind but back in sight: Stereotypes on the rebound. *Journal of Personality and Social Psychology, 67*(5), 808–817.

Mahajan, A. P., Sayles, J. N., Patel, V. A., Remien, R. H., Sawires, S. R., Ortiz, D. J.,...Coates, T. J. (2008). Stigma in the HIV/AIDS epidemic: A review of the literature and recommendations for the way forward. *AIDS, 22*(S2), S67–S79.

Maibach, E. W., & Cotton, D. (1995). Moving people to behavior change: A staged social cognitive approach to message design. In E. W. Maibach & R. L. Parrott (Eds.), *Designing health messages: Approaches from communication theory and public health practice* (pp. 41–64). Thousand Oaks, CA: Sage.

Mann, T., de Ridder, D., & Fujita, K. (2013). Self-regulation of health behavior: Social psychological approaches to goal setting and goal striving. *Health Psychology, 32*(5), 487–498.

Markham, C., Baumler, E., Richesson, R., Parcel, G., Basen-Engquist, K., Kok, G., & Wilkerson, D. (2000). Impact of HIV-positive speakers in a multicomponent, school-based HIV/STD prevention program for inner-city adolescents. *AIDS Education and Prevention, 12*(5), 442–454.

Marlatt, G. A., & Donovan, D. M. (Eds.). (2005). *Relapse prevention: Maintenance strategies in the treatment of addictive behaviors* (2nd ed.). New York, NY: Guilford Press.

Martijn, C., Vanderlinden, M., Roefs, A., Huijding, J., & Jansen, A. (2010). Increasing body satisfaction of body concerned women through evaluative conditioning using social stimuli. *Health Psychology, 29*(5), 514–520.

Mayer, R. E. (1989). Models for understanding. *Review of Educational Research, 59*, 43–64.

McAlister, A. L., Fernandez-Esquer, M. E., Ramirez, A. G., Trevino, F., Gallion, K. J., Villarreal, R.,...Zhang, Q. (1995). Community level cancer control in a Texas barrio: Part II—Base-line and preliminary outcome findings. *Journal of the National Cancer Institute. Monographs, 18*, 123–126.

McGrath, J. (1995). The gatekeeping process: The right combinations to unlock the gates. In E. W. Maibach & R. L. Parrott (Eds.), *Designing health messages: Approaches from communication theory and public health practice* (pp. 199–216). Thousand Oaks, CA: Sage.

McGuire, W. J. (1985). Attitudes and attitude change. In G. Lindzey & E. Aronson (Eds.), *Handbook of social psychology: Vol. 2. Special fields and applications* (3rd ed., pp. 233–346). New York, NY: Random House.

McGuire, W. J. (2001). Input and output variables currently promising for constructing persuasive communications. In R. E. Rice & C. K. Atkin (Eds.), *Public communication campaigns* (3rd ed., pp. 22–48). Thousand Oaks, CA: Sage.

McSweeney, F. K., & Murphy, E. S. (Eds.) (2014). *The Wiley Blackwell handbook of operant and classical conditioning*. Chichester, United Kingdom: John Wiley & Sons.

Mevissen, F. E., Meertens, R. M., Ruiter, R. A. C., Feenstra, H., & Schaalma, H. P. (2009). HIV/STI risk communication: The effects of scenario-based risk information and frequency-based risk information on perceived susceptibility to chlamydia and HIV. *Journal of Health Psychology, 14*(1), 78–87.

Mevissen, F. E., Meertens, R. M., Ruiter, R. A. C., & Schaalma, H. P. (2012). Bedtime stories: The effects of self-constructed risk scenarios on imaginability and perceived susceptibility to sexually transmitted infections. *Psychology & Health, 27*(9), 1036–1047.

Meyer, I. H. (2003). Prejudice, social stress, and mental health in lesbian, gay, and bisexual populations: Conceptual issues and research evidence. *Psychological Bulletin, 129*(5), 674–697.

Miller, W. R., & Rollnick, S. (1991). *Motivational interviewing: Preparing people to change addictive behavior*. New York, NY: Guilford Press.

Miller, W. R., & Rollnick, S. (2002). *Motivational interviewing: Preparing people for change* (2nd ed.). New York, NY: Guilford Press.

Miller, W. R., & Rose, G. S. (2009). Toward a theory of motivational interviewing. *American Psychologist, 64*(6), 527–537.

Milne, S., Orbell, S., & Sheeran, P. (2002). Combining motivational and volitional interventions to promote exercise participation: Protection Motivation Theory and implementation intentions. *British Journal of Health Psychology, 7*(Pt 2), 163–184.

Milyavskaya, M., & Koestner, R. (2011). Psychological needs, motivation, and well-being: A test of Self-Determination Theory across multiple domains. *Personality and Individual Differences, 50*(3), 387–391.

Mollen, S., Ruiter, R. A. C., & Kok, G. (2010). Current issues and new directions in *Psychology and Health*: What are the oughts? The adverse effects of using social norms in health communication. *Psychology & Health, 25*(3), 265–270.

Montaño, D. E., & Kasprzyk, D. (2015). Theory of Reasoned Action, Theory of Planned Behavior, and the Integrated Behavioral Model. In K. Glanz, B. K. Rimer, & K. Viswanath (Eds.), *Health behavior: Theory, research, and practice* (5th ed., pp. 168–222). San Francisco, CA: Jossey-Bass.

Monteith, M. J., Ashburn-Nardo, L., Voils, C. I., & Czopp, A. M. (2002). Putting the brakes on prejudice: On the development and operation of cues for control. *Journal of Personality and Social Psychology, 83*(5), 1029–1050.

Mullen, P. D., & DiClemente, C. C. (1992). *Sustaining women's smoking cessation postpartum*. Paper presented at the 8th World Conference on Tobacco or Health, Buenos Aires, Argentina.

Mullen, P. D., Green, L. W., & Persinger, G. S. (1985). Clinical trials of patient education for chronic conditions: A comparative meta-analysis of intervention types. *Preventive Medicine, 14*(6), 753–781.

Muraven, M., & Baumeister, R. F. (2000). Self-regulation and depletion of limited resources: Does self-control resemble a muscle? *Psychological Bulletin, 126*(2), 247–259.

Muraven, M., Collins, R. L., & Neinhaus, K. (2002). Self-control and alcohol restraint: An initial application of the self-control strength model. *Psychology of Addictive Behaviors, 16*(2), 113–120.

Murphy, E. S., & Lupfer, G. J. (2014). Basic principles of operant conditioning. In F. K. McSweeney & E. S. Murphy (Eds.), *The Wiley Blackwell handbook of operant and classical conditioning* (pp. 167–194). Chichester, United Kingdom: John Wiley & Sons.

Nederkoorn, C., Houben, K., Hofmann, W., Roefs, A., & Jansen, A. (2010). Control yourself or just eat what you like? Weight gain over a year is predicted by an interactive effect of response inhibition and implicit preference for snack foods. *Health Psychology, 29*(4), 389–393.

Ng, J. Y. Y., Ntoumanis, N., Thøgersen-Ntoumani, C., Deci, E. L., Ryan, R. M., Duda, J. L., & Williams, G. C. (2012). Self-Determination Theory applied to health contexts a meta-analysis. *Perspectives on Psychological Science, 7*(4), 325–340.

Noar, S. M., & Zimmerman, R. S. (2005). Health Behavior Theory and cumulative knowledge regarding health behaviors: Are we moving in the right direction? *Health Education Research, 20*(3), 275–290.

Norman, P., Boer, H., & Seydel, E. R. (2005). Protection Motivation Theory. In M. Conner & P. Norman (Eds.), *Predicting health behaviour: Research and practice with social cognition models* (pp. 170–222). Maidenhead, Berkshire, United Kingdom: Open University Press, McGraw-Hill Education.

Nyembezi, A., Resnicow, K., Ruiter, R. A. C., van den Borne, B., Sifunda, S., Funani, I., & Reddy, P. (2014). The association between ethnic identity and condom use among young men in the Eastern Cape Province, South Africa. *Archives of Sexual Behavior, 43*(6), 1097–1103.

Oaten, M., & Cheng, K. (2006). Improved self-control: The benefits of a regular program of academic study. *Basic and Applied Social Psychology, 28*, 1–16.

O'Keefe, D. J., & Jensen, J. D. (2006). The advantages of compliance or the disadvantages of noncompliance? A meta-analytic review of the relative persuasive effectiveness of gain-framed and loss-framed messages. *Communication Yearbook, 30*, 1–43.

O'Keefe, D. J., & Jensen, J. D. (2007). The relative persuasiveness of gain-framed loss-framed messages for encouraging disease prevention behaviors: A meta-analytic review. *Journal of Health Communication, 12*(7), 623–644.

O'Keefe, D. J., & Jensen, J. D. (2009). The relative persuasiveness of gain-framed and loss-framed messages for encouraging disease detection behaviors: A meta-analytic review. *Journal of Communication, 59*(2), 296–316.

Op de Coul, E. L. M., Spijker, R., van Aar, F., van Weert, Y., & de Bruin, M. (2013). With whom did you have sex? Evaluation of a partner notification training for STI professionals using motivational interviewing. *Patient Education and Counseling, 93*(3), 596–603.

Paluck, E. L., & Green, D. P. (2009). Prejudice reduction: What works? A review and assessment of research and practice. *Annual Review of Psychology, 60*, 339–367.

Parker, R., & Aggleton, P. (2003). HIV and AIDS-related stigma and discrimination: A conceptual framework and implications for action. *Social Science & Medicine, 57*(1), 13–24.

Pasick, R. J., Burke, N. J., Barker, J. C., Joseph, G., Bird, J. A., Otero-Sabogal, R., . . . Guerra, C. (2009). Behavioral theory in a diverse society: Like a compass on Mars. *Health Education & Behavior, 36*(S5), 11S–35S.

Patrick, H., Knee, C. R., Canevello, A., & Lonsbary, C. (2007). The role of need fulfillment in relationship functioning and well-being: A Self-Determination Theory perspective. *Journal of Personality and Social Psychology, 92*(3), 434–457.

Patrick, H., & Williams, G. C. (2012). Self-Determination Theory: Its application to health behavior and complementarity with motivational interviewing. *International Journal of Behavioral Nutrition and Physical Activity, 9*, 18.

Paulussen, T., Kok, G., & Schaalma, H. (1994). Antecedents to adoption of classroom-based AIDS education in secondary schools. *Health Education Research, 9*(4), 485–496.

Paulussen, T., Kok, G., Schaalma, H., & Parcel, G. S. (1995). Diffusion of AIDS curricula among Dutch secondary school teachers. *Health Education Quarterly, 22*(2), 227–243.

Paxton, S. (2002). The impact of utilizing HIV-positive speakers in AIDS education. *AIDS Education and Prevention, 14*(4), 282–294.

Peels, D. A., de Vries, H., Bolman, C., Golsteijn, R. H., van Stralen, M. M., Mudde, A. N., & Lechner, L. (2013). Differences in the use and appreciation of a web-based or printed computer-tailored physical activity intervention for people aged over 50 years. *Health Education Research, 28*(4), 715–731.

Peters, G.-J. Y. (2014). A practical guide to effective behavior change: How to identify what to change in the first place. *European Health Psychologist, 16*(5), 142–155.

Peters, G.-J. Y., Ruiter, R. A. C., & Kok, G. (2013). Threatening communication: A critical re-analysis and a revised meta-analytic test of fear appeal theory. *Health Psychology Review, 7*(S1), S8–S31.

Peters, G.-J. Y., Ruiter, R. A. C., & Kok, G. (2014). Threatening communication: A qualitative study of fear appeal effectiveness beliefs among intervention developers, policymakers, politicians, scientists, and advertising professionals. *International Journal of Psychology, 49*(2), 71–79.

Pettigrew, T. F., & Tropp, L. R. (2006). A meta-analytic test of intergroup contact theory. *Journal of Personality and Social Psychology, 90*(5), 751–783.

Petty, R. E., Barden, J., & Wheeler, S. C. (2002). The Elaboration Likelihood Model of persuasion: Health promotions that yield sustained behavioral change. In R. J. DiClemente, R. A. Crosby, & M. C. Kegler (Eds.), *Emerging theories in health promotion practice and research: Strategies for improving public health* (pp. 71–99). San Francisco, CA: Jossey-Bass.

Petty, R. E., Barden, J., & Wheeler, S. C. (2009). The Elaboration Likelihood Model of persuasion: Developing health promotions for sustained behavioral change.

In R. J. DiClemente, R. A. Crosby, & M. Kegler (Eds.), *Emerging theories in health promotion practice and research* (2nd ed., pp. 185–214). San Francisco, CA: Jossey-Bass.

Petty, R. E., Briñol, P., & Priester, J. R. (2009). Mass media attitude change: Implications of the Elaboration Likelihood Model of persuasion. In J. Bryant & M. B. Oliver (Eds.), *Media effects: Advances in theory and research* (3rd ed., pp. 125–164). In J. Bryant & D. Zillmann (Series Eds.), Communication. New York, NY: Routledge.

Petty, R. E., & Cacioppo, J. T. (1986a). *Communication and persuasion: Central and peripheral routes to attitude change.* New York, NY: Springer.

Petty, R. E., & Cacioppo, J. T. (1986b). The Elaboration Likelihood Model of persuasion. In L. Berkowitz (Ed.), *Advances in experimental social psychology* (Vol. 19, pp. 123–205). San Diego, CA: Academic Press.

Petty, R. E., & Wegener, D. T. (1998). Attitude change: Multiple roles for persuasive variables. In D. T. Gilbert, S. T. Fiske, & G. Lindzey (Eds.), *The handbook of social psychology* (4th ed., pp. 323–390). Boston, MA: McGraw-Hill.

Pollay, R. W., Siddarth, S., Siegel, M., Haddix, A., Merritt, R. K., Giovino, G. A., & Eriksen, M. P. (1996). The last straw? Cigarette advertising and realized market shares among youths and adults, 1979–1993. *Journal of Marketing, 60*(2), 1–16.

Portnoy, D. B., Scott-Sheldon, L. A. J., Johnson, B. T., & Carey, M. P. (2008). Computer-delivered interventions for health promotion and behavioral risk reduction: A meta-analysis of 75 randomized controlled trials, 1988–2007. *Preventive Medicine, 47*(1), 3–16.

Prestwich, A., Perugini, M., & Hurling, R. (2009). Can the effects of implementation intentions on exercise be enhanced using text messages? *Psychology and Health, 24*(6), 677–687.

Prochaska, J. O., Redding, C. A., & Evers, K. E. (2015). The Transtheoretical Model of stages of change. In K. Glanz, B. K. Rimer, & K. Viswanath (Eds.), *Health behavior: Theory, research, and practice* (5th ed., pp. 168–222). San Francisco, CA: Jossey-Bass.

Pryor, J. B., Reeder, G. D., Yeadon, C., & Hesson-McInnis, M. (2004). A dual-process model of reactions to perceived stigma. *Journal of Personality and Social Psychology, 87*(4), 436–452.

Pyne, J. M., Fischer, E. P., Gilmore, L., McSweeney, J. C., Stewart, K. E., Mittal, D., . . . Valenstein, M. (2013). Development of a patient-centered antipsychotic medication adherence intervention. *Health Education & Behavior, 41*(3), 315–324.

Reid, M. C., Papaleontiou, M., Ong, A., Breckman, R., Wethington, E., & Pillemer, K. (2008). Self-management strategies to reduce pain and improve function among older adults in community settings: A review of the evidence. *Pain Medicine, 9*(4), 409–424.

Resnicow, K., & Page, S. E. (2008). Embracing chaos and complexity: A quantum change for public health. *American Journal of Public Health, 98*(8), 1382–1389.

Resnicow, K., & Vaughan, R. (2006). A chaotic view of behavior change: A quantum leap for health promotion. *International Journal of Behavioral Nutrition and Physical Activity, 3*(1), 25.

Richard, L., Potvin, L., Kishchuk, N., Prlic, H., & Green, L. W. (1996). Assessment of the integration of the ecological approach in health promotion programs. *American Journal of Health Promotion, 10*(4), 318–328.

Robbins, S. J., Schwartz, B., & Wasserman, E. A. (2001). *Psychology of learning and behavior* (5th ed.). New York, NY: W. W. Norton.

Rogers, E. M. (2003). *Diffusion of innovations* (5th ed.). New York, NY: Free Press.

Rogers, R. (1983). Cognitive and physiological processes in fear-based attitude change: A revised theory of protection motivation. In J. T. Cacioppa & R. E. Petty (Eds.), *Social psychophysiology: A sourcebook* (pp. 153–176). New York, NY: Guilford Press.

Rosenbaum, M. (2000). The self-regulation of experience: Openness and construction. In P. Dewe, M. Leiter, & T. Cox (Eds.), *Coping, health and organizations* (pp. 51–67). In T. Cox & A. Griffiths (Series Eds.), Issues in Occupational Health. London, United Kingdom: Taylor and Francis.

Ross, V., Jongen, E. M. M., Wang, W., Brijs, T., Brijs, K., Ruiter, R. A. C., & Wets, G. (2014). Investigating the influence of working memory capacity when driving behavior is combined with cognitive load: An LCT study of young novice drivers. *Accident; Analysis and Prevention, 62*, 377–387.

Rothman, A. J., Baldwin, A. S., & Hertel, A. W. (2004). Self-regulation and behavior change. In R. F. Baumeister & K. D. Vohs (Eds.), *Handbook of self-regulation: Research, theory, and applications* (pp. 130–148). New York, NY: Guilford Press.

Rothman, A. J., & Salovey, P. (1997). Shaping perceptions to motivate healthy behavior: The role of message framing. *Psychological Bulletin, 121*(1), 3.

Ruiter, R. A. C., Abraham, C., & Kok, G. (2001). Scary warnings and rational precautions: A review of the psychology of fear appeals. *Psychology and Health, 16*(6), 613–630.

Ruiter, R. A. C., Kessels, L. T. E., Peters, G.-J. Y., & Kok, G. (2014). Sixty years of fear appeal research: Current state of the evidence. *International Journal of Psychology, 49*(2), 63–70.

Ruiter, R. A. C., & Kok, G. (2012). Planning to frighten people? Think again! In C. Abraham & M. Kools (Eds.), *Writing health communication: An evidence-based guide* (pp. 117-133). London, United Kindgom: Sage.

Ruiter, R. A. C., Massar, K., van Vugt, M., & Kok, G. (2012). Applying social psychology to understanding social problems. In A. Golec de Zavala & A. Cichocka (Eds.), *Social psychology of social problems: The intergroup context* (pp. 337–362). London, United Kingdom: Palgrave Macmillan.

Rutten, G. M., Meis, J. J. M., Hendriks, M. R. C., Hamers, F. J. M., Veenhof, C., & Kremers, S. P. J. (2014). The contribution of lifestyle coaching of overweight patients in primary care to more autonomous motivation for physical activity and healthy dietary behaviour: Results of a longitudinal study. *International Journal of Behavioral Nutrition and Physical Activity, 11*, 86.

Ryan, R. M., & Deci, E. L. (2000). Self-Determination Theory and the facilitation of intrinsic motivation, social development, and well-being. *American Psychologist, 55,* 68–78.

Ryan, R. M., & Deci, E. L. (2006). Self-regulation and the problem of human autonomy: Does psychology need choice, self-determination, and will? *Journal of Personality, 74*(6), 1557–1586.

Sanders-Phillips, K. (2002). Factors influencing HIV/AIDS in women of color. *Public Health Reports, 117*(S1), S151–S156.

Schaalma, H., & Kok, G. (2009). Decoding health education interventions: The times are a-changin'. *Psychology and Health, 24*(1), 5–9.

Scheier, M. F., & Carver, C. S. (2003). Goals and confidence as self-regulatory elements underlying health and illness behavior. In L. D. Cameron & H. Leventhal (Eds.), *The self-regulation of health and illness behavior* (pp. 17–41). New York, NY: Routledge.

Schlam, T. R., Wilson, N. L., Shoda, Y., Mischel, W., & Ayduk, O. (2013). Preschoolers' delay of gratification predicts their body mass 30 years later. *The Journal of Pediatrics, 162*(1), 90–93.

Schmeichel, B. J., & Baumeister, R. F. (2004). Self-regulatory strength. In R. F. Baumeister & K. D. Vohs (Eds.), *Handbook of self-regulation: Research, theory, and applications* (pp. 84–98). New York, NY: Guilford Press.

Schunk, D. H., & Ertmer, P. A. (2000). Self-regulation and academic learning: Self-efficacy enhancing interventions. In M. Boekaerts, P. R. Pintrich, & M. Zeidner (Eds.), *Handbook of self-regulation* (pp. 631–650). San Diego, CA: Academic Press.

Schutte, L., Meertens, R. M., Mevissen, F. E., Schaalma, H., Meijer, S., & Kok, G. (2014). Long Live Love. The implementation of a school-based sex-education program in the Netherlands. *Health Education Research, 29*(4), 583–597.

Schüz, N., Schüz, B., & Eid, M. (2013). When risk communication backfires: Randomized controlled trial on self-affirmation and reactance to personalized risk feedback in high-risk individuals. *Health Psychology, 32*(5), 561–570.

Seijts, G. H., & Latham, G. P. (2005). Learning versus performance goals: When should each be used? *Academy of Management Executive, 19*(1), 124–131.

Seijts, G. H., Latham, G. P., Tasa, K., & Latham, B. W. (2004). Goal setting and goal orientation: An integration of two different yet related literatures. *Academy of Management Journal, 47*(2), 227–239.

Sheeran, P. (2002). Intention–behavior relations: A conceptual and empirical review. In W. Stroebe & M. Hewstone (Eds.), *European review of social psychology* (Vol. 12, pp. 1–36). Chichester, United Kingdom: John Wiley & Sons.

Sheeran, P., Milne, S., Webb, T. L., & Gollwitzer, P. M. (2005). Implementation intentions and health behaviour. In M. Conner & P. Norman (Eds.), *Predicting health behaviour* (2nd ed., pp. 276–323). London, United Kingdom: Open University Press.

Shegog, R., Begley, C. E., Harding, A., Dubinsky, S., Goldsmith, C., Hope, O., Newmark, M. (2013). Description and feasibility of MINDSET: A clinic decision aid for epilepsy self-management. *Epilepsy & Behavior, 29*(3), 527–536.

Shepperd, J. A., Klein, W. M., Waters, E. A., & Weinstein, N. D. (2013). Taking stock of unrealistic optimism. *Perspectives on Psychological Science, 8*(4), 395–411.

Sherman, D. A., Nelson, L. D., & Steele, C. M. (2000). Do messages about health risks threaten the self? increasing the acceptance of threatening health messages via self-affirmation. *Personality and Social Psychology Bulletin, 26*(9), 1046–1058.

Shilubane, H. N., Ruiter, R. A. C., van den Borne, B., Sewpaul, R., James, S., & Reddy, P. S. (2013). Suicide and related health risk behaviours among school learners in South Africa: Results from the 2002 and 2008 national Youth Risk Behaviour Surveys. *BMC Public Health, 13,* 926.

Sialubanje, C., Massar, K., Hamer, D. H., & Ruiter, R. A. C. (2014). Understanding the psychosocial and environmental factors and barriers affecting utilization of maternal healthcare services in Kalomo, Zambia: A qualitative study. *Health Education Research, 29*(3), 521–532.

Skinner, C. S., Tiro, J., & Champion, V. L. (2015). The Health Belief Model. In K. Glanz, B. K. Rimer, & K. Viswanath (Eds.), *Health behavior and health education: Theory, research, and practice* (5th ed., pp. 131–167). San Francisco, CA: Jossey-Bass.

Smith, R. M. (2008). *Conquering the content: A step-by-step guide to online course design.* San Francisco, CA: Jossey-Bass.

Sniehotta, F. F. (2009). Towards a theory of intentional behaviour change: Plans, planning, and self-regulation. *British Journal of Health Psychology, 14*(Pt 2), 261–273.

Sniehotta, F. F., Presseau, J., & Araújo-Soares, V. (2014). Time to retire the theory of planned behaviour. *Health Psychology Review, 8*(1), 1–7.

Sniehotta, F. F., Schwarzer, R., Scholz, U., & Schüz, B. (2005). Action planning and coping planning for long-term lifestyle change: Theory and assessment. *European Journal of Social Psychology, 35*(4), 565–576.

Sobal, J., & Wansink, B. (2007). Kitchenscapes, tablescapes, platescapes, and foodscapes: Influences of microscale built environments on food intake. *Environment and Behavior, 39*(1), 124–142.

Stacey, F. G., James, E. L., Chapman, K., Courneya, K. S., & Lubans, D. R. (2014). A systematic review and meta-analysis of Social Cognitive Theory-based physical activity and/or nutrition behavior change interventions for cancer survivors. *Journal of Cancer Survivorship, 9*(2), 305–338.

Steinberg, L. (2008). A social neuroscience perspective on adolescent risk-taking. *Developmental Review, 28*(1), 78–106.

Stinson, J., Wilson, R., Gill, N., Yamada, J., & Holt, J. (2009). A systematic review of internet-based self-management interventions for youth with health conditions. *Journal of Pediatric Psychology, 34*(5), 495–510.

Strack, F., & Deutsch, R. (2004). Reflective and impulsive determinants of social behavior. *Personality and Social Psychology Review, 8*(3), 220–247.

Strecher, V. J., Seijts, G. H., Kok, G. J., Latham, G. P., Glasgow, R., DeVellis, B., ... Bulger, D. W. (1995). Goal setting as a strategy for health behavior change. *Health Education Quarterly, 22*(2), 190–200.

Stroebe, W., Mensink, W., Aarts, H., Schut, H., & Kruglanski, A. W. (2008). Why dieters fail: Testing the goal conflict model of eating. *Journal of Experimental Social Psychology, 44*, 26–36.

Stroebe, W., Van Koningsbruggen, G. M., Papies, E. K., & Aarts, H. (2013). Why most dieters fail but some succeed: A goal conflict model of eating behavior. *Psychological Review, 120*(1), 110–118.

Stutterheim, S. E., Pryor, J. B., Bos, A. E. R., Hoogendijk, R., Muris, P., & Schaalma, H. P. (2009). HIV-related stigma and psychological distress: The harmful effects of specific stigma manifestations in various social settings. *AIDS, 23*(17), 2353–2357.

Suls, J., & Wheeler, L. (Eds.). (2000). *Handbook of social comparison: Theory and research*. In C. R. Snyder (Series Ed.), Series in Social-Clinical Psychology. New York, NY: Kluwer Academic/Plenum.

Susser, E., Valencia, E., & Torres, J. (1994). Sex, Games, and Videotapes: An HIV-prevention intervention for men who are homeless and mentally ill. *Psychosocial Rehabilitation Journal, 17*(4), 31–40.

ten Hoor, G. A., Peters, G. J., Kalagi, J., de Groot, L., Grootjans, K., Huschens, A., . . . Kok, G. (2012). Reactions to threatening health messages. *BMC Public Health, 12*, 1011.

Thaler, R. H., & Sunstein, C. R. (2008). *Nudge: Improving decisions about health, wealth, and happiness*. New Haven, CT: Yale University Press.

Tulving, E., & Thomson, D. M. (1973). Encoding specificity and retrieval processes in episodic memory. *Psychological Review, 80*(5), 352–373.

U.S. Department of Health and Human Services, Office of Cancer Communications, National Cancer Institute. (2002). *Making health communication programs work: A planner's guide*. Bethesda, MD: U.S. Department of Health and Human Services.

Unsworth, N., Brewer, G. A., & Spillers, G. J. (2013). Working memory capacity and retrieval from long-term memory: The role of controlled search. *Memory & Cognition, 41*(2), 242–254.

van Blankenstein, F. M., Dolmans, D. H. J. M., van der Vleuten, C. P. M., & Schmidt, H. G. (2011). Which cognitive processes support learning during small-group discussion? The role of providing explanations and listening to others. *Instructional Science, 39*, 189–204.

van Dijk, T. A., & Kintsch, W. (1983). *Strategies of discourse comprehension*. San Diego, CA: Academic Press.

van Eijk-Hustings, Y. J., Daemen, L., Schaper, N. C., & Vrijhoef, H. J. (2011). Implementation of motivational interviewing in a diabetes care management initiative in the Netherlands. *Patient Education and Counseling, 84*(1), 10–15.

van Empelen, P., Kok, G., van Kesteren, N. M. C., van den Borne, B., Bos, A. E. R., & Schaalma, H. P. (2003). Effective methods to change sex-risk among drug users: A review of psychosocial interventions. *Social Science & Medicine, 57*(9), 1593–1608.

van Nieuw-Amerongen, M., Kremers, S. P. J., de Vries, N. M., & Kok, G. (2009). The use of prompts, increased accessibility, visibility, and aesthetics of the stairwell to promote stair use in a university building. *Environment and Behavior, 43*(1), 131–139.

Vansteenkiste, M., & Sheldon, K. M. (2006). There's nothing more practical than a good theory: Integrating motivational interviewing and self-determination theory. *British Journal of Clinical Psychology, 45*(Pt 1), 63–82.

Van't Riet, J., Cox, A. D., Cox, D., Zimet, G. D., De Bruijn, G., Van den Putte, B., . . . Ruiter, R. A. C. (2014). Does perceived risk influence the effects of message framing? A new investigation of a widely held notion. *Psychology & Health, 29*(8), 933–949.

Verplanken, B., & Aarts, H. (1999). Habit, attitude, and planned behaviour: Is habit an empty construct or an interesting case of goal-directed automaticity? *European Review of Social Psychology, 10*, 101–134.

Visschers, V. H. M., Meertens, R. M., Passchier, W. F., & de Vries, N. K. (2007). How does the general public evaluate risk information? The impact of associations with other risks. *Risk Analysis, 27*(3), 715–727.

Visschers, V. H. M., Meertens, R. M., Passchier, W. W. F., & de Vries, N. N. K. (2009). Probability information in risk communication: A review of the research literature. *Risk Analysis, 29*(2), 267–287.

Voirin, N., Barret, B., Metzger, M. H., & Vanhems, P. (2009). Hospital-acquired influenza: A synthesis using the Outbreak Reports and Intervention Studies of Nosocomial Infection (ORION) statement. *Journal of Hospital Infection, 71*(1), 1–14.

Wandersman, A., Duffy, J., Flaspohler, P., Noonan, R., Lubell, K., Stillman, L., . . . Saul, J. (2008). Bridging the gap between prevention research and practice: The interactive systems framework for dissemination and implementation. *American Journal of Community Psychology, 41*(3–4), 171–181.

Warsi, A., Wang, P. S., LaValley, M. P., Avorn, J., & Solomon, D. H. (2004). Self-management education programs in chronic disease: A systematic review and methodological critique of the literature. *Archives of Internal Medicine, 164*(15), 1641–1649.

Webb, T. L., & Sheeran, P. (2006). Does changing behavioral intentions engender behavior change? A meta-analysis of the experimental evidence. *Psychological Bulletin, 132*(2), 249–268.

Webb, T. L., Sheeran, P., Totterdell, P., Miles, E., Mansell, W., & Baker, S. (2012). Using implementation intentions to overcome the effect of mood on risky behaviour. *British Journal of Social Psychology, 51*(2), 330–345.

Weiner, B. (1986). *An attributional theory of motivation and emotion.* New York, NY: Springer-Verlag.

Weinstein, N., & Ryan, R. M. (2011). A self-determination theory approach to understanding stress incursion and responses. *Stress & Health, 27*(1), 4–17.

Weinstein, N. D. (1988). The precaution adoption process. *Health Psychology, 7*(4), 355–386.

Weinstein, N. D., Sandman, P. M., & Blalock, S. J. (2008). The Precaution Adoption Process Model. In K. Glanz, B. K. Rimer, & K. Viswanath (Eds.), *Health behavior and health education: Theory, research, and practice* (4th ed., pp. 123–165). San Francisco, CA: Jossey-Bass.

Wenzel, L., Glanz, K., & Lerman, C. (2002). Stress, coping and health behavior. In K. Glanz, B. K. Rimer, & F. M. Lewis (Eds.), *Health behavior and health education: Theory, research and practice* (3rd ed., pp. 121–143). San Francisco, CA: Jossey-Bass.

Werrij, M. Q., Ruiter, R. A. C., Riet, J. V. T., & de Vries, H. (2012). Message framing. In C. Abraham, & M. Kools (Eds.), *Writing health communication: An evidence-based guide* (pp. 134–143). London, United Kingdom: Sage.

Wiecha, J. L., El Ayadi, A. M., Fuemmeler, B. F., Carter, J. E., Handler, S., Johnson, S., . . . Gortmaker, S. L. (2004). Diffusion of an integrated health education program in an urban school system: Planet health. *Journal of Pediatric Psychology, 29*(6), 467–474.

Wiers, R. W., Gladwin, T. E., Hofmann, W., Salemink, E., & Ridderinkhof, K. R. (2013). Cognitive bias modification and cognitive control training in addiction and related psychopathology: Mechanisms, clinical perspectives, and ways forward. *Clinical Psychological Science, 1*, 192–212.

Wiers, R. W., & Hofmann, W. (2010). Implicit cognition and health psychology: Changing perspectives and new interventions. *European Health Psychologist, 12*, 4–6.

Williams, G. C., Hedberg, V. A., Cox, E. M., & Deci, E. L. (2000). Extrinsic life goals and health-risk behaviors in adolescents. *Journal of Applied Social Psychology, 30*(8), 1756–1771.

Williams, J. M., & Bizup, J. (2015). *Style: The basics of clarity and grace* (5th ed.). Boston, MA: Pearson Longman.

Witte, K. (1992). Putting the fear back into fear appeals: The Extended Parallel Process Model. *Communications Monographs, 59*(4), 329–349.

Witte, K. (1995). Fishing for success: Using the persuasive health message framework to generate effective campaign messages. In E. Maibach & R. L. Parrott (Eds.), *Designing health messages: Approaches from communication theory and public health practice* (pp. 145–166). Thousand Oaks, CA: Sage.

Witte, K., & Allen, M. (2000). A meta-analysis of fear appeals: Implications for effective public health campaigns. *Health Education & Behavior, 27*(5), 591–615.

Witte, K., Meyer, G., & Martell, D. (2001). *Effective health risk messages: A step-by-step guide*. Thousand Oaks, CA: Sage.

Wood, W., & Neal, D. T. (2007). A new look at habits and the habit-goal interface. *Psychological Review, 114*(4), 843–863.

Wright, P. (2012). Using graphics effectively in text. In C. Abraham & M. Kools (Eds.), *Writing health communication: An evidence-based guide* (pp. 62–82). London, United Kingdom: Sage.

Young, M. D., Plotnikoff, R. C., Collins, C. E., Callister, R., & Morgan, P. J. (2015). Impact of a male-only weight loss maintenance programme on social–cognitive determinants of physical activity and healthy eating: A randomized controlled trial. *British Journal of Health Psychology*. Advance online publication. doi:10.1111.bjhp. 12137

Zajonc, R. B. (1980). Feeling and thinking: Preferences need no inferences. *American Psychologist, 35*(2), 151.

Zajonc, R. B. (2001). Mere exposure: A gateway to the subliminal. *Current Directions in Psychological Science, 10*(6), 224–228.

Zimmerman, B. J. (2000). Attaining self-regulation: A social cognitive perspective. In K. W. Harris, P. R. Printich, & M. Zeidner (Eds.), *Handbook of self-regulation* (pp. 13–39). San Diego, CA: Academic Press.

Zulman, D. M., Damschroder, L. J., Smith, R. G., Resnick, P. J., Sen, A., Krupka, E. L., & Richardson, C. R. (2013). Implementation and evaluation of an incentivized internet-mediated walking program for obese adults. *Translational Behavioral Medicine, 3*(4), 357–369.

# ENVIRONMENT-ORIENTED THEORIES

## Competency

♦ Use environment-oriented theories to understand health problems and to plan interventions.

The purpose of this chapter is to identify environment-oriented theories and models that are useful for planning health promotion interventions. We first discuss how to describe and select environmental conditions to be changed, and then we suggest how to change these conditions. The theories and models are organized by environmental level: interpersonal, organizational, community, and societal (see Glanz, Rimer, & Viswanath, 2015; Simons-Morton, McLeroy, & Wendel, 2011).

As we discussed in the previous chapters, the individual is embedded within social networks, organizations, community, and society; and each lower level is embedded within higher levels. A facilitating environment that makes the health-promoting behavior the easiest behavior to perform (Milio, 1981) is critical for changing the behavior of the at-risk population, as well as for changing environmental conditions. Examples of environmental conditions include social influences (such as norms, social support, and reinforcement) and structural influences (such as access to resources, organizational climate, and policies). Barriers to performing a health behavior are often structural, such as lack of health insurance, inconvenient clinic hours, lack of transportation, high-fat cafeteria foods, high cost of healthy foods, intense advertising of cigarettes and alcohol, and unsafe neighborhoods for jogging or walking.

## LEARNING OBJECTIVES AND TASKS

- Identify theories to describe environmental conditions that influence behavior and health

- Identify potential environmental agents whose role behavior influences the environmental conditions

- Describe determinants of the behavior of the environmental agents and theoretical methods to change these behaviors

- Explain the differences in intervention methods due to role and power at higher ecological levels of the environment

## Perspectives

In this chapter, we discuss our logic model for the relations among theoretical methods, determinants, agents, environmental conditions, and health as they relate to environmental change and the role of power in influencing environmental change.

## Model for Change of Environmental Conditions

Working to influence change at multiple ecological levels can create synergy between levels to produce and sustain changes in environmental conditions. Figure 2.1, the logic model for the relationships among change methods, determinants, behaviors, environmental conditions, and health that we introduced in Chapter 2, shows the environmental path to change through the environmental agent. The environmental condition is a state of a given environment that influences health either directly or indirectly through behavior. The accessibility of hiking and bicycling trails, for example, is an environmental condition that may facilitate physical activity. The presence of toxic agents in the air acts directly on health. Human agents behave in ways that influence the existence or intensity of each environmental condition. For example, a city council allocates money to build hiking and bicycling trails, and a higher governmental authority may authorize money for use by cities to build such trails. Members of city councils and legislators are environmental agents in this case, and their respective behaviors are proposing and voting to allocate funds. Note that agents and actions at different levels are directed at the same environmental condition in this example. Theories from both Chapters 2 and 3 are needed as the health promoter plans for change in environmental conditions. Once the agents and their behaviors have been identified, the planner can select determinants and methods to change them. In Chapter 2, we presented theoretical constructs that described determinants for behavior and theoretical methods to change specific determinants. These constructs and methods apply to behavior of both the at-risk population and the environmental agent. For example, positive outcome expectations may influence a legislator to vote to allocate funds ("If I vote to allocate funds for trails, people in my district will have more opportunities to exercise"), as well as to influence the at-risk population to jog ("If I jog, I will reduce my level of stress"). Similarly, persuasive communication is a method to influence the outcome expectations of both the population at risk and the environmental agents, the joggers and the legislators.

However, we realize that the perspective of working through environmental agents does not fully capture the process of collective action—how behaviors occur as part of a collective (such as a legislative body, workplace, or social network) or how these collectives are systems in their own right with their own regulatory processes. In a collective, the whole is greater than the sum of its parts. Clearly, a single legislator's vote does not lead to passage of a law. Lawmaking is a complex process, and much goes on behind the scenes in a legislative collective. For example, in the United States, a powerful speaker of the house sometimes assigns the bills to committees in which they will die; key committee chairs schedule hostile hearings; senators make compromise deals in the construction of bills; opposition party members add fatal amendments; and political party leaders bring their legislators' votes in line.

Multilevel interventions that target environmental conditions are still rare; most interventions focus on the individual level plus one environmental level (Golden & Earp, 2012). Better training involving multilevel intervention planning is important (Richard, Gauvin, & Raine, 2011). In this chapter we describe organizational, community, and social change methods that rely on the power and authority vested in organizations, associations of citizens, and government. We examine the change methods and practical applications to address collective action at these higher ecological levels. For example, a health promotion intervention might influence the behavior of the at-risk population directly or indirectly. A legislature may pass a law limiting minors' access to cigarettes or influence a company to go tobacco free; or a social network may support a first-time mother in quitting cigarettes (Kok, Gottlieb, Commers, & Smerecnik, 2008; Randolph, Whitaker, & Arellano, 2012). Alternatively, a legislature might pass a law that companies must reduce emissions of pollutants, which, in turn, influences the environment of the at-risk population (Golden & Earp, 2012). When health educators seek to address these upper ecological levels, they often find general methods for community organization and organizational development, but they may find little guidance on ways to engage in the process. Through an analysis of interviews with health promotion researchers and professionals in the United States and the Netherlands, we discovered that these higher-level methods are frequently bundles of lower-level methods (Kok, Gottlieb, Panne, & Smerecnik, 2012). For example, advocacy includes the methods of persuasion, raising awareness, informing, social comparison, networking, participation, and media exposure. In this chapter, we undertake a careful review of change methods and practical applications that builds on our earlier discussion of the use of individual-level determinants applied to persons in specific roles within social systems, for example, a legislator, school principal, or union official.

## Looking at Healthy Environments as Outcomes

Intervention Mapping considers environmental conditions as they relate to health outcomes directly or through the path of behavior of the at-risk group. Others have looked at creating potentially healthier environments as a desired outcome, irrespective of individual health outcomes. Since the 1986 Ottawa Charter, the World Health Organization has focused on healthy settings where people "learn, work, play and love" (World Health Organization, 1986, p. 4). Healthy settings include nations, cities, communities, workplaces, hospitals, prisons, schools, and universities (Whitelaw et al., 2001). The settings approach is rooted in social ecology and systems thinking (Dooris, 2009, 2013; Green, Poland, & Rootman, 2000; Nutbeam, 1998; Paton, Sengupta, & Hassan, 2005). For example, a healthy city could be characterized as one that has health-promoting policy and characteristics across all sectors (such as a large greenbelt, low population density, recreation facilities, and low unemployment). In addition, a healthy city has explicit political commitment at the highest levels to promote health and investment in formal and informal networking and cooperation to enhance equity and build individual and social competence to deal with issues of importance to the community (Awofeso, 2003; de Leeuw, Tsouros, Dyakova, & Green, 2014; Duhl, 2004).

A healthy worksite would have healthy policies, a health-promoting culture, commitments to self-knowledge and development, respect for individual differences, jobs that foster responsibility and autonomy, safe and healthy working environments, and equitable salaries and promotion opportunities. Health-promoting workplaces balance a focus on customer expectations and organizational targets with a focus on employees' skills and health. This focus extends beyond wellness programs to include broader organizational and environmental issues (Aldana et al., 2012; Chu et al., 2000; Kahn-Marshall & Gallant, 2012; Kok, Zijlstra, & Ruiter, 2015b; O'Donnel, 2014; Paton et al., 2005).

A healthy school would have a coherent, sequential health and physical education curriculum, teacher training, and an ethos that supports student and staff well-being. It would also have health-promoting policies and practices, including those of nutrition and food services, comprehensive health services, counseling, social services, and school–community partnerships, all established with the principles of democracy and equity (Beam, Ehrlich, Black, Block, & Leviton, 2012a, 2012b; Mŭkoma & Flisher, 2004).

# General Environmental-Oriented Theories

This first section provides an overview of general environmental-oriented theories. The following sections provide overviews of theories that pertain to specific levels of the environment—interpersonal, community, societal, and governmental theories.

## Systems Theory

We begin our discussion of environment-oriented theories with a description of systems theory. There are many branches of systems theory, including general systems theory, complexity science, nonlinear dynamics, cybernetics, computational simulation, game theory, and ecology. All share the systems thinking focus on understanding how things work, "a worldview that balances part and whole and focuses on complex interrelationships and patterns from multiple perspectives" (National Cancer Institute, 2007, p. 41). Systems thinking bridges theory and practice and provides an analytic strategy both to address understanding complex systems and to intervene on them. In this regard it is both a theory of the problem and a theory of change.

### *Complex Adaptive Systems*

Through the lens of systems theory, humans are complex adaptive systems made up of other complex adaptive systems (such as organs, cells, and so on) and embedded within other complex adaptive systems (such as dyads, groups, organizations, communities, and societies). Complex adaptive systems (CASs) demonstrate a number of key characteristics listed below (R. Anderson et al., 2013; Goodson, 2009; McDaniel, Jordan, & Fleeman, 2003; Shigayeva & Coker, 2014; Van Beurden, Kia, Zask, Dietrich, & Rose, 2013; B. Zimmerman, Lindberg, & Plsek, 1998):

- Agents, including people and human processes, have the capacity to exchange information with their environment and adjust their behavior accordingly. Diversity of agents increases the likelihood of novel behavior and is necessary for the sustainability of CASs.

- Agents interact and exchange information, creating connections among all agents in the system. Although agents interact locally and no single agent knows the pattern as a whole, global patterns and complexity result as information is spread through the system.

- Interactions are nonlinear; small "causes" can have large effects, and vice versa, large "causes" can have small effects.

- Because of sensitivity to initial conditions, small differences in initial conditions can lead to exponential differences in future conditions.

- CASs are self-organizing as people mutually adjust their behaviors to meet changing internal and external environmental demands. They adapt and evolve over time as spontaneous patterns emerge at the macro level from collective interactions of independent agents at the micro level.

- CASs are open systems, and agents interact with the environment beyond the system's boundaries so that the CAS and systems around it or in which it is embedded coevolve.

Structure, meaning, resources, and power relations have been described as key to understanding social systems, be they groups, organizations, communities, or societies (Naaldenberg et al., 2009). Structure includes agents, their activities, and their relationships. People act on the basis of the meanings that actions or issues have for them and create meaning through interactions with others via an interpretive process that is highly dependent on context. Agents bring resources to the system, and whether they possess or need resources influences power relationships within the system. In the next section we will discuss power as an emergent quality of human interactions.

As we will see throughout this chapter, the health promoter addresses structure, meaning, resources, and power in designing system change efforts. Foster-Fishman, Nowell, and Yang (2007) distinguished deep and apparent, that is, visible, elements of a system. Norms, including attitudes, values, and beliefs, are deep elements of a system and are often found to be root causes of system problems. Regulatory processes—such as policies and procedures; available resources; and dominant operations, especially power and decision-making processes and structures—are apparent elements and are key to change. These elements are interdependent, emerging from interaction and meaning making among system members.

### *Processes for Changing Systems*

The systems change process has been described using the following principles: (1) planning a collective vision, (2) purposeful organizing and participatory self-organizing, (3) facilitating mission leadership, and (4) evaluating and systems learning (National Cancer Institute, 2007). Some techniques, for example, brainstorming, nominal group technique, focus groups, concept mapping, structured conceptualization, and future-search conferences, can be useful for all principles. Others, such as community-based participatory research, participatory action research, empowerment evaluation, appreciative inquiry, total quality management, and the Centers for Disease Control and Prevention evaluation framework, are appropriate primarily for evaluating and systems learning (National Cancer Institute, 2007).

As noted above, successful changes in systems influence multiple elements and relationships within a system, often at multiple levels (Best, 2011). For example, programs to influence healthier diets for children in school focus on the beliefs and behaviors of children and their parents; the purchase of healthful food by the school food service; the cafeteria workers' food preparation methods; and district, city, and perhaps other jurisdictional policy regarding school lunch and vending machines at school. Most antibullying programs also use system approaches (Juvonen & Graham, 2014).

Systems thinking is useful for the dissemination of health promotion programs in addition to their development. The efficacy testing of health promotion is done in highly controlled environments. When these evidence-based programs are disseminated to community settings with a unique context, that is, placed into a complex adaptive system, it is unlikely that implementation will look the same as it did in the original trial or that the same results will be obtained. Systems thinking offers a framework to understand the complex context of dissemination. It provides a model to change the system as needed to ensure program adoption and implementation while maintaining core elements and program sustainability (Green & Glasgow, 2006; Luke & Stamatakis, 2012; Mabry, Milstein, Abraido-Lanza, Livingood, & Allegrante, 2013).

## Summary: Systems Theory

Systems theory is used to define and address all levels of the environment as interrelated social systems. Environmental agents at each level can engage in activities to change the system to facilitate health. The environmental influences of these agents' behavior can include norms, regulatory processes, and resources, whereas methods address social change broadly and include dialogue, planning, organizing, evaluation, and feedback.

## Theories of Power

Power has been defined as the probability that an individual or group will determine what another individual or group will do even if it is contrary to the latter's interests (Orum, 1988). Sociologist Max Weber (1947) defined three sources of power: authority, charisma, and legitimacy. Social psychologists have studied power as an emergent property of relationships.

Each of the ecological levels has different power structures and methods for the change of social influence. In small groups, social influence occurs through interaction and through leadership. The leadership might be shared by members of the group, given over voluntarily to an individual leader by the group, or vested in an individual from a higher authority. At the organizational level, the power of authority comes through the organizational hierarchical structure, that is, who is above whom in the organizational chart. Informal power arises from an individual's charisma, from others' satisfaction with a person's previous leadership activities, or from legitimacy, such as being elected as a chairperson or born into a family business. At the community and societal levels, power is "the social capacity to make binding decisions that have major consequences over the directions in which a society moves" (Orum, 1988, p. 402).

Turner (2005) has developed the three-process theory of power that views power as an emergent quality of human social relationships. In this theory, power is the capacity to exert one's will through other people—that is, using either persuasion or control to get people to do something they are not interested in doing. Control in turn is subdivided into authority, in which group norms have given someone the right to control, or coercion, the attempt to control others against their will.

Group identity can unify people so that they gain the power of collective action to act as a coordinated body. Social change occurs when a subordinate group develops a distinct identity and its own goals and beliefs and can challenge the power of the dominant group. Persuasion, social influence, and coercion, three methods discussed in Chapter 2, are the chief mechanisms for obtaining power, both individually and as a group.

The role of power differs in the three types of social change defined by Rothman (2008) and is discussed in the section on community. In locality development the democratic town hall process distributes power equally; in social planning the power rests with experts; and in social action, disenfranchised people wrest power from the official power structure.

Wallerstein, Minkler, Carter-Edwards, Avila, and Sánchez (2015) have distinguished between the concepts of *power with* and *power over*, using a feminist perspective that views power as a limitless resource. They suggested that community building and capacity building are models of *power with*, whereas empowerment-oriented social action is a model of challenging *power over*. These two types of community organization were argued to lead to community competence, leadership development, and critical awareness.

McCullum, Pelletier, Barr, Wilkins, and Habicht (2004) used a three-dimensional framework of power that is built on core sociological perspectives. The first dimension, participation in decision making, is at first glance simply a determination of whether community members are at the table. In the second dimension, agenda setting, the choice of what issues and decisions are considered, has a bias such that values and beliefs of vested interests determine what is discussed. The third dimension, the shaping of perceived needs, is more insidious. Dominant groups in society frame issues by defining the causes of and solutions for identified problems. Powerless groups have been socialized to accept the frames of reference of the dominant groups and institutions, and they may lack awareness of how their ways of looking at the world have been conditioned. Thus, they may adopt values and interests that are not their own but rather those of the dominant group.

### Using Power to Create Change at Higher Environmental Levels

Power is the key to creating change at the higher environmental levels. Health educators can bring power to play in several ways: They can identify the agent who has the power to carry out the desired change, choose the change method that is most effective given the position and form of power the agent holds and the form of power the person holds. In addition, health promoters must be conscious of the unintended negative effects of power in their work with communities, which can reinforce the status quo and lead to oppression of some groups by others (Hawe & Shiell, 2000; Lehmann & Gilson, 2013; Mendes, Plaza, & Wallerstein, 2014).

## Summary: Power Theories

Power theories are applicable to all environmental levels, and agents at each level with power are able to exert their influence to make environmental changes. The determinants of an agent's power include authority, charisma, legitimacy, group norms, and group identity. Methods for changing the behavior of others and the environmental conditions include persuasion, social influence, coercion, community organizing, and agenda setting.

## Empowerment Theories

Within public health, empowerment has been defined as a "social action process for people to gain mastery over their lives and the lives of their communities" (Wallerstein et al., 2015, p. 284). Empowerment is a multilevel process, focusing on the individual, organizational, and community levels. Empowerment can be viewed as an outcome as well as a process. Empowerment as a process describes how to enable people to take power;

empowerment as an outcome refers to the consequences of this process. An empowering process may result in empowerment as an outcome, but may also result in other desired outcomes, such as improvement of health, relocation of resources, or policy change. M. Zimmerman (2000) and Aiyer, Zimmerman, Morrel-Samuels, and Reischl (2014) have compared empowering processes and empowered outcomes at the individual, organizational, and community levels (Table 3.1). Each level influences and is influenced by empowerment at the other levels.

At the individual level, the results of empowerment are psychological, including increased perception of control over one's destiny, a sense of political efficacy, and motivation to act. This type of empowerment occurs when people take action to understand their environment critically and to gain power and control through organizational and community involvement (see this chapter's discussion of conscientization and social movements). At the organizational and community levels, empowerment involves collective problem solving; shared leadership and decision making; and accessible government, media, and resources (M. Zimmerman, 2000; M. Zimmerman, Stewart, Morrel-Samuels, Franzen, & Reischl, 2011).

Empowerment at the higher ecological levels is a similar concept to collective efficacy, which Bandura (1997) defined as "a group's shared belief in its conjoint capabilities to organize and execute the courses of action required to produce given levels of attainments" (p. 477). Collective efficacy may be applied to the levels of family, organization, community, and nation. For example, perceived organizational efficacy could be employees' beliefs that their organization can accomplish its goals. Although related to personal self-efficacy, it is an emergent group-level attribute that is more

**Table 3.1**    A Comparison of Empowering Processes and Empowered Outcomes Across Levels of Analysis

| Level of Analysis | Process (Empowering) | Outcome (Empowered) |
|---|---|---|
| Individual | Learning decision-making skills | Sense of control |
| | Managing resources | Critical awareness |
| | Working with others | Participatory behavior |
| Organizational | Opportunities to participate in decision making | Effective competition for resources |
| | Shared responsibilities | Networking with other organizations |
| | Shared leadership | Policy influence |
| Community | Access to resources | Coalitions of organizations |
| | Open government structure | Pluralistic leadership |
| | Tolerance for diversity | Social capital |

*Source:* Adapted from "Empowerment Theory: Psychological, Organizational, and Community Levels of Analysis" by Zimmerman, M. A. (2000) in *Handbook of Community Psychology* edited by J. Rappaport & E. Seidman (pp. 43–64). New York, NY: Kluwer Academic/Plenum, p. 47.

than the sum of members' perceived personal efficacies (Woodall, Warwick-Booth, & Cross, 2012). Change in collective efficacy comes through the same mechanisms as change in personal efficacy. The most effective way to enhance a community's collective efficacy is through success at accomplishing a particular goal. A community could experience enhanced efficacy by mounting a successful campaign of lobbying the city council to pass a clean indoor air act. Models of how other communities accomplished similar goals could also enhance efficacy, as might community leaders persuading the community members to take action (Commers, Gottlieb, & Kok, 2005).

## Summary: Empowerment Theories

Empowerment theories address the process by which community members become involved in their communities and take action to gain power and control. Environmental conditions that enable and demonstrate empowerment include collective problem solving, shared leadership and decision making, accessible government, media and resources, and collective efficacy. Methods by which community members become empowered include participation in decision making, enactive mastery experiences and feedback, and modeling.

## Interpersonal-Level Theories

Social relationships are the foundation for human existence, and interpersonal-level theories are key to understanding and intervening on relationships. Relationships at the interpersonal level typically include family members, friends, peers, neighbors, associates, and service providers.

## Social Network Theory

A social network is an analytic framework for understanding relationships among members of social systems. Networks are classified as personal, based on the ties an individual has with other persons, or whole, based on the relationships among a defined group of people. Personal networks are particularly useful for the study of social support. The whole-network approach shows the network in which the personal network is embedded as a larger system, with a view of cliques of individuals and those persons who span the boundaries across networks. Networks can be horizontal (peers) or vertical (hierarchical) and can provide a way to understand types of social capital and power relationships in organizations (McLeroy, Gottlieb, & Heaney, 2001; Valente, 2015).

Social networks consist of nodes (individuals, groups, or organizations) that are joined by ties (the relationships among nodes). Community can be understood as networks of networks in which the nodes of the larger network comprise smaller-scale networks. Networks can be defined by their content—whether they are primarily friendship, kinship, sexual, communication, or task oriented. The network also has a structure, including the number of members, the degree of members' similarity to each other, the way they are connected, and their links to other networks (Valente, 2015). An individual can play several roles in a network: a group member, a linking agent, or an isolate with few ties to other network members. Linking agents are especially important because, as members of multiple networks, they bring information across network boundaries.

## Social Support Theory

The personal social network provides the structure for a variety of social functions, including social influence, control, undermining, comparison, companionship, and support (Simons-Morton et al., 2011; see Chapter 6). We focus here on social support—the help provided through social relationships and interactions (Holt-Lunstad & Uchino, 2015). The four main types of social support are emotional (provision of empathy, love, trust, and caring), instrumental (provision of tangible aid and services), informational (provision of advice, suggestions, and information), and appraisal (provision of feedback useful for self-reevaluation and affirmation). Social support is a positive social interaction. Beets, Cardinal, and Alderman (2010) reviewed parental support for physical activity in youth and reported positive effects. However, negative interactions and modeling for unhealthy or deviant behaviors also occur in relationships. Health educators will need a comprehensive view of relevant social networks, including both support and undermining, with regard to the development of interventions and design of health outcomes studies (Holt-Lunstad & Uchino, 2015).

The extent and nature of social relationships has been linked to health status in a number of studies and physiological processes related to disease outcomes. We refer the reader to comprehensive reviews on social support and health (Berkman & Glass, 2000; Hogan, Linden, & Najarian, 2002; Holt-Lunstad & Uchino, 2015; Smith & Christakis, 2008; Valente, 2015; Wethington & Pillemer, 2014). The mechanisms underlying this epidemiological finding have been hypothesized to include modeling and reinforcement of positive health-related behaviors, buffering of the effects of stress on health, and providing access to resources to cope with stress. Social-structural conditions such as culture, socioeconomic factors, politics, and social change shape social networks. Social networks in turn provide opportunities for social support, norms and social control, social involvement, person-to-person contagion, and access to resources and material goods. For example, distributions of obesity, smoking, eating, exercise, sexually transmitted disease, tuberculosis, suicide, and health care seeking have been shown to vary by networks. Health care interventions, such as treatment of a depressed mother, can also influence others in the treated patient's network; in this case, the child (Berkman & Glass, 2000; Smith & Christakis, 2008).

## Social Support Interventions

Interventions can be directed toward different types of social networks and the specific types of social support they provide. Small, dense, geographically close, intense networks provide emotional and appraisal support. These networks typically do not have access to the larger society or to information outside the network's domain. On the other hand, large, diffuse, and less intense networks provide more informational support and social outreach (McLeroy et al., 2001). Different types of social support are important at different times in the experience of stressors. For example, with the loss of a job, emotional support that the individual is still loved and his or her self is intact is most important at first. Later, the individual needs informational support regarding other job opportunities or possible career changes. Tangible support, such as loans, transportation, or child care, may also help people when he or she is job hunting.

Valente (2012) described four types of social network interventions. The first type uses network data to identify individuals that can act as champions for change. The second type uses segmentation to identify groups of people to change at the same time. The third type uses peer-to-peer interaction to create message diffusion (going viral, snowball effects). The fourth type of intervention tries to alter the network itself by adding or deleting nodes, adding or deleting links, or rewiring existing links.

Holt-Lunstad and Uchino (2015) identified four types of interventions to increase social support: enhancing existing social network linkages, developing new social network linkages, enhancing networks through indigenous natural helpers and community health workers, and enhancing networks at the community level through participatory problem solving. Interventions may also combine these types of interventions.

The enhancement of existing network linkages can be accomplished by training network members in skills for providing support and by training members of the target group to mobilize and maintain their networks.

For example, family members or significant others may be trained to provide support to individuals who are in programs to stop smoking (Palmer, Baucom, & McBride, 2000). At the government and society level, legislation can be enacted to support social networks. Examples of such legislation are family leave acts, policies to promote volunteerism, and funding for child and elder care programs (McLeroy et al., 2001). We describe methods for policy change later in this chapter.

The second type of intervention develops new social network linkages through mentor programs, buddy systems, and self-help groups. For example, youth mentoring programs in which at-risk youth are matched with nonfamilial adults have been found to be effective, although the benefits are modest and results mixed (DuBois, Holloway, Valentine, & Cooper, 2002). Buddies have been used in diverse settings, for example, in smoking cessation programs (Park, Tudiver, Schultz, & Campbell, 2004), for mothers of very preterm infants (Preyde & Ardal, 2003), and in worksite programs (Tessaro et al., 2000). Groups such as Alcoholics Anonymous provide access to new social networks designed to provide cognitive, instrumental, and emotional support for behavioral and life change. Interventions can encourage such networks to reach out to incorporate new members and new information from persons who hold membership in other networks.

Third, indigenous or natural helpers have been employed to enhance networks, particularly around health issues (Mayfield-Johnson, Rachal, & Butler, 2014). Natural helpers are community members to whom other persons turn for advice, emotional support, and tangible aid. Often they agree to become a link between the community and the formal service-delivery system. They may include persons who come into contact with many people in their role, such as hairstylists, shopkeepers, and clergy. They may also be community volunteers and people with similar problems (Eng, Rhodes, & Parker, 2009). Recent comprehensive reviews of lay or community health worker interventions have been conducted by the Cochrane Collaboration (S. Lewin et al., 2005) and the Agency for Healthcare Research and Quality (Viswanathan et al., 2009). Evidence for the effectiveness of these interventions was found for immunizations, appropriate health care utilization, asthma management, cervical cancer screening, mammography, and improving outcomes for acute respiratory infections and malaria.

In addition, Rhodes, Foley, Zometa, and Bloom (2007) did a qualitative systematic review of lay health advisor interventions focused on the Hispanic population that included smoking cessation, cardiovascular health behaviors, condom use, and use of protective eyewear among farmworkers. They concluded that the lay health advisor approach is effective with this population. Rhodes and colleagues (2007) found six roles in their review of lay health advisor interventions in Hispanic communities. The advisors supported participant recruitment and data collection, served as health advisors and referral sources, distributed materials, served as role models, advocated on behalf of community members, and served as coresearchers in participatory research models. Lay health advisors work at the individual, organizational, and community levels to facilitate improved health practices, improved coordination of agency services, and improved community competence (Arvey & Fernández, 2012; Eng et al., 2009; Fernández et al., 2009; Moore, Peele, Simán, & Earp, 2012; Tolli, 2012).

Finally, networks can be enhanced at the community level through participatory problem-solving processes (Martinson & Su, 2012). In the Health, Opportunities, Problem-Solving, and Empowerment (HOPE) Project, young Cambodian girls and women living in Long Beach, California, participated in training sessions, team building, and dialogue (Cheatham-Rojas & Shen, 2008) based on the work of Paulo Freire (1973a, 1973b). Cheatham-Rojas and Shen (2008) developed a program called Community Forum on School Safety that led to the establishment of a community advisory board to work on issues of sexual harassment in the Long Beach schools. Another example is the Healthy Native Communities Fellowship, a technologically innovative and culturally grounded health promotion project that brings together community teams to build an "intentional family" and facilitate change at both the individual and the community levels (Kenneth Jones et al., 2008).

## Summary: Social Network and Social Support Theories

Social network and social support theories address the environmental condition of social networks that provide emotional, instrumental, informational, and appraisal support as appropriate for the context. Environmental agents (including lay health advisors) who are providing this support or who are mobilizing support for individuals from their own networks are the network members. Determinants of the agents' support and mobilization behaviors include knowledge, beliefs and attitudes, self-efficacy and skills, facilitation of policies and culture, availability of self-help groups, and network characteristics of reciprocity, intensity, complexity, density, and homogeneity. Methods for change of these behaviors include enhancement of existing networks by skills training for providing and mobilizing support, use of lay health workers, teaching of participatory problem solving (see methods for community organization later in this chapter), and linking of members to new networks (e.g., mentor programs, buddy systems, and self-help groups).

## Organizational-Level Theories

Health promotion practitioners sometimes work in organizations with the opportunity to serve as internal change agents. They also work as external change agents with community groups seeking to make changes in organizations. In this section we introduce several theories explaining organizational change and present methods to stimulate changes in policy, culture, and other environmental conditions at the organizational level. These theories can also be used to enable the adoption, implementation, and sustaining of health promotion interventions in organizations. Understanding key aspects of organizations and of organizational change is critical to the health promoter's ability to influence change at the organizational level.

## Organizational Change Theories

An organization is a tool people use to coordinate their actions to accomplish an overriding goal. Organizations take inputs from the environment, such as human effort, raw materials, information, and financial and social capital, and transform them to produce goods, services, and value for customers, shareholders, and other stakeholders in the environment. They can be for-profit or not-for-profit, governmental or nongovernmental, and publicly held or privately held. All organizations, however, attempt to manage their complex environments to obtain needed resources and to release valued outputs into the environment. The environment, which includes economic, competitive, technological, political, physical, demographic, cultural, and social forces, is constantly changing, and organizations must change in response to maintain their effectiveness and to survive. Managers design a structure and culture to match the environment, choose technology to convert inputs to outputs, and develop strategies to guide the organization to create value. This planned organizational change can be incremental, using methods such as quality improvement and flexible workgroups, or revolutionary, involving methods such as restructuring, reengineering, and innovation (Boonstra, 2004; Kathryn Jones, Baggott, & Allsop, 2004).

Planned change efforts build on Kurt Lewin's (1947) work on force field analysis. He proposed that organizations exist in a state of quasistationary equilibrium in which two sets of forces—those driving for change and those striving for the status quo—are approximately equal. For change to occur, the forces driving for change could increase, or the forces maintaining the status quo could decrease, or both could occur. Lewin advised that decreasing the status quo forces was less disruptive and more effective than was increasing forces for change. He described the change process as having three phases: unfreezing, moving, and refreezing. Unfreezing reduces the forces that maintain the organization's current behavior, often by showing that the behaviors or conditions that organizational members desire are different from those they currently exhibit. During the moving phase, changes in organizational structures and processes lead to new behaviors, values, and attitudes. In refreezing, the organization puts in place norms, policies, and structures that support the new state of equilibrium (Cummings & Worley, 2014). As a caveat, it should be noted that although planned change is described as a rationally controlled and orderly process, in practice it can be messy and unpredictable!

From an intervention standpoint, the change sequence in a continuous change organization is freezing, rebalancing, and unfreezing. Freezing is making the processes within the organization visible and describing the patterns. Rebalancing involves the reinterpretation, relabeling, and resequencing of patterns so that there are fewer blockages and barriers to them. Leaders do this by modeling the change and inspiring others with their ideas. The last step in the cycle is unfreezing, the resumption of improvisation and learning as the organization continues to meet daily contingencies. The change agent in continuous change is a sense maker who redirects change as opposed to the episodic model's prime mover who creates change (A. Brown, Colville, & Pye, 2014; Weick & Quinn, 1999). Learning replaces control in this model. This view is consonant with a view of the organization as a complex adaptive system that is self-organizing and in a mutual adjustment process with its environment (Cummings & Worley, 2014). Effective managers deal with this unexpectedness by observing, learning in the moment, creating meaning through dialogue, reflecting on experiences, and constructing explanations (McDaniel, 1997). Planned change is more effective in stable than unstable environments.

### Changing Organizational Culture

Changing organizational culture is an example of the continuous change model. Schein (2004, 2010) defined culture as a pattern of basic assumptions invented, discovered, or developed by a given group as it learns to cope with its problems of external adaptation and internal integration. For the pattern to be culture, it must have worked well enough to be considered valid and therefore taught to new members as the way to perceive, think, and feel. Organizational interventions are most effective when they are compatible with the culture, so it is important to understand the culture of the organization in which a health promotion program is being developed and implemented.

It is possible to facilitate changes in organizational culture, although this process is slow and evolutionary. Culture changes with the group's learning and experience over time, as organizational members react to environmental shifts and crises within the organization. Schein (2004) described the importance of leaders' behavior in shaping organizational culture: what leaders pay attention to, how they react to critical incidents, how they model for and coach others, and what criteria they set for allocating rewards and recruiting and promoting personnel. Schein referred to leader behaviors as primary culture-embedding mechanisms. Organizational design, structure, and formal statements reinforce the culture. In a young organization, leaders create the culture, and the organizational systems reinforce it. In mature organizations, the organizational systems become primary and constrain future leaders' behavior.

## Summary: Organizational Change Theory

Health promoters often try to change organizations. Organizational change theories describe the process of change as unfreezing, moving, and refreezing, leading to a new equilibrium. The health promoter as change agent stimulates a process of learning, or sense making, instead of control. Changes are preferably compatible with the organizational culture; changing culture is also possible but difficult.

## Organizational Development Theories

Organizational development, an important method of organizational change, has been defined as "a system-wide application and transfer of behavioral science knowledge to the planned development, improvement and reinforcement of the strategies, structures, and processes that lead to organizational effectiveness" (Cummings & Worley, 2014, pp. 1–2). Growing out of human relations research, it supports the values of human potential, participation, and development.

### *Planned Change Framework*

Steps from contemporary organizational development models can be placed within the planned change framework (Butterfoss, Kegler, & Francisco, 2008; Schein, 2004, 2010). Diagnosis, often conducted using surveys, is equated with K. Lewin's unfreezing (1947). It includes evaluation of an organization's mission, goals, policies, procedures, structures, technologies, and physical setting; social and psychological factors; desired outcomes; and readiness to take action. Action planning is the selection of change strategies. Criteria for selection include the organization's readiness to adopt a particular strategy, the availability of leverage points on which to intervene, and the organizational development consultant's skill in conducting the intervention. Similar to the process that Lewin (1947) called moving, intervention includes the facilitation of problem identification and solving with members of the organization. Group development activities, management building, and structural redesign are among the other intervention elements that can be carried out. Evaluation assesses the planned change effort and the determination of whether additional efforts are needed. Institutionalization, the final step, refreezes the supports for the changes through written plans, goals, job descriptions, and budgets.

Methods used in organizational development to deal with resistance to change include communication, participation and empowerment, facilitation, and bargaining and negotiation. In cases where these methods have not worked, organizations may resort to manipulation and coercion. Organizational development methods to promote change have included counseling, sensitivity training, and process consultation at the individual level; team building and intergroup training at the group level; and organizational confrontation meetings at the level of the whole organization (Kathryn Jones et al., 2004).

## Stage Theory of Organizational Change/Diffusion of Innovation

Stage theory refers to the idea that organizations move through a series of stages as they change and that strategies to promote change must be matched to the stage. K. Lewin's model provided the foundation for this theory, and later theorists, such as Everett Rogers (see Diffusion of Innovations Theory section in Chapter 2) and others, have worked in this tradition (Rogers, 2003). In their work on the establishment of alcohol policy and programs in U.S. government agencies, Beyer and Trice (1978) developed a stage theory of organization change that has been used in health education practice, particularly in the adoption of organizational innovations, such as health promotion interventions (Butterfoss et al., 2008; Hearld & Alexander, 2014). The process of adoption of innovations at the organizational level is more complex than the process at the individual level. Organizational-level factors, such as goals, authority structure, roles, rules and regulations, and informal norms and relationships, must be taken into account (Bonham, Sommerfield, Willging, & Aarons, 2014; Damschroder et al., 2009; Greenhalgh, Robert, Macfarlane, Bate, & Kyriakidou, 2004; Rogers, 1983). However, there are similarities to the Diffusion of Innovations Theory applied to individuals (discussed in Chapter 2). For example, both media and interpersonal channels may need to be used for communicating the innovation to organizational members; organizations can be categorized according to their readiness to adopt; and characteristics of the innovation, such as relative advantage, are important.

In stage theory, an organization is theorized to move sequentially and linearly through seven stages as it adopts and institutionalizes a health promotion innovation. Outside consultants may provide technical assistance to this process. These stages, which are listed below, are similar to those Rogers (1983) described: agenda setting, matching, redefining and restructuring, and clarifying and routinizing.

1. Sensing unsatisfied demands on the system, noting a problem, and bringing it to the surface

2. Searching for possible responses, seeking solutions to the problem

3. Evaluating alternatives, judging potential solutions

4. Deciding to adopt a course of action, selecting one of a number of alternative responses

5. Initiating action within the system, which requires policy changes and resources necessary for implementation

6. Implementing the change, which includes putting the innovation into practice and usually requires some organization members to change their work behaviors and relationships

7. Institutionalizing the change by including the change in strategic plans, job descriptions, and budgets so that it is a routine part of organizational operations (Butterfoss et al., 2008)

The key agents involved in change have been found to differ from stage to stage (Butterfoss et al., 2008; Huberman & Miles, 1984). Senior-level administrators with political skills are important in the early stages, when a problem is recognized and made public, alternative solutions are discussed, and a choice is made and initiated within the organization. These administrators are also important at the institutionalization stage because they have the power to incorporate the changes into organizational structure and routines. Midlevel administrators are active during the adoption and early implementation stages, when administrative skills are critical in order to introduce procedures and provide training on the innovation. The people who need to make changes in their day-to-day practices are the focus of the implementation process. Examples are teachers involved in curriculum innovation or food service workers involved in an innovation in preparing cafeteria food. The focus here is on people's professional and technical skills. Of course, because the agents and behaviors are different at different stages, the determinants change as well. For example, at the decision stage, organizational leaders might be persuaded by their perceptions of an intervention's characteristics, whereas implementation might be determined to a great extent by the implementer's skills and the feedback and reinforcement he or she receives.

Institutionalization focuses on the integration of the innovation into organization functions and routines so that it survives beyond the presence of the original program funding, adopters, or program champions

(Manning et al., 2014; Pluye, Potvin, Denis, & Pelletier, 2004). Institutionalization of an intervention requires mechanisms for becoming embedded in the organization's routines, for example, in the continuing allocation of resources (funding, personnel, materials, facilities, and time), and in the development of objectives, job descriptions, plans, and budgets. In other cases, interventions may be institutionalized outside an organization's boundaries, or the goals of the intervention may be subsumed in other programs. For example, program components may be taken over by community organizations, once the demonstration program is over, as in the historic cases of the Stanford Heart Disease Prevention Program (Jackson et al., 1994) and the Minnesota Heart Health Program (Bracht et al., 1994). Finally, the program continuation goal may be sustainability—to continue the program's effects whether or not the program itself continues intact (Shigayeva & Coker, 2014). For example, in the World Health Organization's historic efforts to eradicate smallpox, the initial program of mass vaccination was followed by surveillance and aggressive follow-up of suspected cases (Fenner, Henderson, Arita, Ježek, & Ladnyi, 1988).

Flaspohler, Duffy, Wandersman, Stillman, and Maras (2008) examined the capacity staff and organizations needed to adopt and implement prevention programs. These elements are also important to consider in general organizational consultation and technical assistance. The Interactive Systems Framework describes support and delivery systems that are needed to increase general and innovation-specific capacity to carry out prevention efforts (Leeman et al., 2014; Wandersman, Chien, & Katz, 2012; Wandersman et al., 2008). Wandersman and colleagues (2012) also proposed an evidence-based system for innovation support (EBSIS) to increase the effectiveness and efficiency of support activities within an organization that is intended to build capacity for implementation (Kreuter, Casey, & Bernhardt, 2012). EBSIS includes four components for innovation-specific and general capacity building: tools, training, technical assistance, and quality assurance/quality improvement (Ray, Wilson, Wandersman, Meyers, & Katz, 2012; Wandersman et al., 2012).

General staff capacity includes intellectual ability, motivation, and tolerance for ambiguity. Innovation-specific capacities include understanding of the innovation, perceived capacity to implement the intervention, and attitude or buy-in toward the innovation. At the organization level, general capacity relates to effectiveness of leadership and management style, organizational structure and climate, availability of resources, and community linkages and support. Innovation-specific capacities include ability to select and adapt innovations to suit the organization's needs; organizational support, resources, and buy-in; technical assistance and training;

and evaluation systems and skills to evaluate innovation implementation and use.

## Summary: Organizational Development and Diffusion Theories

In health promotion, organizational theories focus on the development of health-promoting organizational structures and culture. The environmental agents include upper and middle management, internal change consultants, and other organizational members. Their behaviors are adoption, implementation, and institutionalization of new policies, practices, structures, cultural beliefs, and norms. The determinants of agent behaviors include outcome expectations, attitudes and beliefs, skills, and resources. Methods are at the organizational level, such as sense making, participatory problem solving through organizational diagnosis and feedback, modeling, team building or human relations training, technical assistance, and structural redesign.

## Stakeholder Theory

We include stakeholder theory with organizational theory; however, stakeholders are key agents at the community and societal levels as well. (See also Chapter 4.) Environmental change processes at all levels bring together stakeholders who may differ from each other in their social, political, and ethical paradigms; engagement goals and interests; and types and amounts of power (L. Brown, Bammer, Batliwala, & Kunreuther, 2003). Such diversity is critical to the understanding of an issue from multiple perspectives and to the creation of new meanings and intervention opportunities (McDaniel, 1997). The relationships among stakeholders who cross levels and networks can be particularly important change agents, as they have the potential to produce change in multiple system sectors (Foster-Fishman et al., 2007).

Health promoters, their organizations, and the communities with which they work are frequently external stakeholders of organizations, that is, they exist outside a focal organization but have a direct interest in what the organization does. Stakeholder theory (see Freeman, 1984) has examined how managers can strategically approach relationships with multiple external stakeholders, but more recently theoretical work has focused on strategies of stakeholder influence on organizations, also in the area of health promotion (Kok, Gurabardhi, Gottlieb, & Zijlstra, 2015a).

Stakeholder analysis identifies stakeholders and their interests and prioritizes them based on their characteristics and location in social networks outside the organization (Kok et al., 2015a). The salience of stakeholder participation depends on three attributes: their power (ability to impose their will), legitimacy (perception that their actions are appropriate), and urgency (requirement of immediate attention). Change-focused stakeholder groups, such as community groups seeking to change organizational policies related to environmental conditions, seek to maximize their power, legitimacy, and urgency. They may forge alliances with other stakeholders, and they may use either community development or social action, a more radical approach to change (see Community-Level Theories section). Community development efforts use persuasion, constructive dialogue, and cooperation. In social action, when mass participation is possible, tactics include boycotts, buycotts (buying from preferred companies), letters or e-mails, petitions, marches, and rallies. When there is less dependence on participatory action, blocking of gates, sabotage, Internet activism, lawsuits, shareholder activism, and negative publicity may be useful tactics (Kok et al., 2015a). Social movement theory (discussed later in this chapter) provides insight into legitimacy, framing, and other aspects of stakeholder activism. Berry (2003) provided a case study of an activist community derailing the plans of a multinational chemical company, within the context of stakeholder theory, environmental justice, and community activism.

## Summary: Stakeholder Theory

Stakeholder theory provides guidance to health promoters working through their own organizations or through the community to change an organization's policies and practices. The determinants of agent behaviors, that is, those of the focal organization's decision makers, include outcome expectations, attitudes, and beliefs. Methods include social influence, alliances, community development, and social action.

## Community-Level Theories

Communities may be based on geography; on gender, ethnic, or cultural identity; or on an issue, such as the environment, animal rights, or public health. (See Chapter 4.) A shared reality or identity is key to the construct (Labonte, 2004). We first review community coalition theory, which could also be considered an interorganization network theory. Then we discuss theories of social capital and community capacity. Although social capital can be considered an emergent propriety of social networks, we have included it as a community-level construct because it is so closely intertwined with development of community capacity, which should be a goal of every community change effort. The remainder of this section focuses on social norms, conscientization, and community organization.

## Coalition Theory

Organizations form partnerships to manage their environments. These interactions may be informal and transient or highly structured with shared decision making and leadership. Coalitions have been defined as "an organization of individuals representing diverse organizations, factions or constituencies who agree to work together in order to achieve common goals" (Feighery & Rogers, 1990, p. 1). Community coalitions include a structured arrangement for organizations to work together to achieve a common goal, usually preventing or ameliorating a community problem (Butterfoss & Kegler, 2009, 2012). Thus, coalitions are an important method for facilitating community empowerment, particularly through four processes: enhancing experience and competence, improving group structure and capacity, removing social and environmental barriers, and increasing environmental support and resources (Fawcett et al., 1995).

Over the past two decades, community coalitions, funded by governments and foundations, have become a key approach to community problem solving. This has led to some concern that community coalitions have been coopted by human service organizations and funders, to the detriment of disenfranchised communities (Chavis, 2001). Butterfoss and Kegler (2009) have proposed a theory of action for community coalitions that draws on a large body of empirical research: the Community Coalition Action Theory (Kegler & Swan, 2011). Coalitions develop through three specific stages: formation, maintenance, and institutionalization. Coalitions recycle through these stages with the recruitment of members, renewal of plans, and addition of new issues. Each stage requires a different set of skills and resources and thus different strategies for training and technical assistance by staff and consultants (see Butterfoss & Kegler, 2012, p. 315).

The formation stage is most successful when a convener or lead agency with linkages to the community provides technical assistance, material support, credibility, and valuable contacts. The coalition must also include a deeply committed core group that expands to include community gatekeepers and a broad constituency of participants. The coalition should identify strong staff and member leaders who then develop structures, such as formalized rules, roles, and procedures. During this stage, open and frequent communication, shared and formalized decision-making processes, conflict management, benefits of participation that outweigh the costs, and positive relationships among members will provide a high level of member engagement, pooling of resources, and effective assessment and planning (see Butterfoss & Kegler, 2012, pp. 320–322).

The key tasks of the maintenance stage are sustaining member involvement; pooling member and external resources; and engaging in assessment, planning, and action to achieve coalition goals. There is a synergy in these tasks to promote successful implementation of strategies and community change outcomes. Coalitions are more likely to create community change when they direct interventions at multiple levels. At the institutionalization stage, successful coalitions show an impact on health and social outcomes, as well as increases in capacity that they can apply to other issues (see Butterfoss & Kegler, 2012, pp. 322–325).

Foster-Fishman, Berkowitz, Lounsbury, Jacobson, and Allen (2001) have developed a framework of core competencies and processes needed within coalitions for members, relationships, organizational structures, and the programs they sponsor. Member capacity includes core skills and knowledge about working collaboratively, building effective programs, and developing coalition infrastructure; positive attitudes about collaboration, target issues, other stakeholders, and self as a legitimate member; and access to capacity building and coalition support for member involvement. Relational capacity includes developing a positive working climate, creating a shared vision, promoting power sharing, valuing diversity, and developing positive external relationships with community stakeholders, other communities, and coalitions targeting similar problems. Organizational capacity includes effective leadership, a task-oriented work environment, formalized procedures, effective communication, sufficient resources, and an orientation to continuous improvement. Programmatic capacity includes clear, focused program objectives and realistic goals that are unique, innovative, and ecologically valid.

## Summary: Coalition Theory

A coalition is a method for influencing community and policy environmental conditions. Coalition leaders seek to establish and maintain high-functioning health promotion coalitions. Determinants of these coalition leaders' behaviors include motivation to collaborate, organizational capacity, barriers to collaboration, community capacity, and community resources. Methods to change these determinants include participatory problem solving, technical assistance, skills training for leadership and conflict management, and interlinking organizations and networks.

## Social Capital and Community Capacity

Social capital has been defined variously, for example, as "the ability of actors to secure benefits by virtue of membership in social networks or other social structures" (Portes, 1998, p. 6), as "the processes and conditions among people and organizations that lead to accomplishing a goal of mutual social benefit" (Green & Kreuter, 2005, p. 52), and as "features of social organization such as networks, norms, and social trust that facilitate coordination and cooperation for mutual benefit" (Putnam, 1995, pp. 35–36). The first definition is from the individual perspective and is similar to social support. The latter definitions are from the perspective of the whole network—the collective. High social capital is manifested in high levels of four interrelated constructs: trust, cooperation, civic engagement, and reciprocity (Jin & Lee, 2013).

Three types of social capital have been described: bonding, bridging, and linking. Bonding social capital refers to trust and cooperation between network members with a shared social identity (Szreter & Woolcock, 2004). Bridging social capital occurs between people who are not alike in a sociodemographic or social identity sense and yet have relations of respect and mutuality (Szreter & Woolcock, 2004). Linking social capital, a subset of bridging social capital, comprises norms of respect and trusting relationships between people who are interacting across explicit differences in power (Szreter & Woolcock, 2004).

Kawachi and Berkman (2000) found that social capital, operationalized as interpersonal trust, norms of reciprocity, and per capita membership in voluntary associations aggregated to the state level is directly associated with age-adjusted mortality. Also, when adjusted for individual-level characteristics, social capital is associated with the likelihood of an individual's reporting fair and poor health (Kawachi & Berkman, 2000; Murayama, Fujiwara, & Kawachi, 2012). Although some evidence calls into question the role of social capital in the promotion of health in a cross-national examination (Kennelly, O'Shea, & Garvey, 2003), many researchers agree that it has some role, with the relationship being stronger for countries with high social inequality (Islam, Merlo, Kawachi, Lindström, & Gerdtham, 2006; Kawachi, 2006; Uphoff, Picket, Cabieses, Small, & Wright, 2013). Social capital has also been linked to homicide rates (Lochner, Kawachi, Brennan, & Buka, 2003) and binge drinking (Weitzman & Kawachi, 2000). Stronger bonding ties within deprived communities have been found to be associated with poorer health of residents, as there may be higher expectations to help neighbors, which increases financial and mental strain (Caughy, O'Campo, & Muntaner, 2003; Mitchell & LaGory, 2002). Usher's (2006) explanation, from work in the rural south, is that social capital may be more important as a community than an individual resource and that bridging social ties within poor minority communities is key to breaking the social and economic isolation resulting from segregation.

Community capacity is closely related to and inclusive of social capital. It has been defined as "a set of dynamic community traits, resources, and associational patterns that can be brought to bear for community building and community health improvement" (Wendel et al., 2009, p. 285).

Dimensions of community capacity include skills and resources, the nature of social relations, structures and mechanisms for community dialogue, leadership, civic participation, the value system, and learning culture (Wendel et al., 2009). Central to community capacity are the community's ability to engender leadership and participation, analyze its own thinking processes and change efforts, mobilize resources, experience a sense of connection among people, participate in meaningful rituals, maintain an awareness of previous change efforts and current conditions, and employ power to create change (Flaspohler et al., 2008; Simons-Morton et al., 2011; see Chapter 12).

Community capacity, including social capital, is both a means to achieve community health goals and an end in itself (Wendel et al., 2009). Interventions to increase community capacity include community development and participatory problem solving, which we discuss in the following section (Farquhar, Michael, & Wiggins, 2005; Pronyk et al., 2008). Methods include participatory action research, organizational learning, dynamic systems analysis, consensus building through dialogue, stakeholder consultation and deliberation, and interpersonal and group process. Personal values of the health promoter, such as openness, authenticity, comfort with process and uncertainty, and caring attitudes, are important (Wilson, 1997).

From the perspective of social networks, we emphasize the importance of linking persons to community organizations, such as churches, social clubs, schools, political groups, and work settings, in which individuals can voluntarily associate with others to address issues of community concern. It is also important for residents to have loose ties outside their primary networks to bring in new information and resources, and interorganizational meetings and coalitions can foster such ties (Steckler, Goodman, & Kegler, 2002). For example, statewide meetings of church associations, nonprofit health agency volunteers, political conventions, and joint neighborhood association meetings allow the opportunity for residents to connect with others with similar concerns and interests, to learn about their activities, and to team up to work together.

Democratic management, in which "members share information and power, utilize cooperative decision-making processes, and are involved in the design, implementation, and control of efforts toward mutually defined goals" (Israel, Checkoway, Schulz, & Zimmerman, 1994, p. 152), is essential to the development of community capacity. Deep democracy with roots in action learning, community participation, whole systems theory, social capital, appreciative inquiry, and communitarian thought has been the focus of community interventions in both the United States and the developing world (Wilson & Lowery, 2003).

## Summary: Social Capital Theory

Members and leaders of social and community networks participate in civic affairs, resulting in increased social capital and community competence. The determinants of participation include knowledge, beliefs, attitudes, self-efficacy, and skills; availability of structures and mechanisms for community dialogue; and supportive culture. Methods directed to these determinants include community development and participatory problem solving; linking members to community organizations, interorganizational meetings, and coalitions; skills training for community participation; and technical assistance.

## Social Norms Theories

Social norms, expectations of behavior by members of a social group, are a property of a community. They are the social rules that specify what is appropriate or inappropriate in a particular situation. Norms are the environmental condition that is the basis for perceived social influence, the individual-level variable we discussed earlier. Norms are transmitted to individuals through the process of socialization that occurs primarily in childhood through the family and then continues through institutions, such as churches, voluntary associations, and schools (Smelser, 1998).

Mass media portrayals of role models and reinforcement have been used to shift social norms. A combination of education and entertainment has been used to transmit social norms and culture, using narrative storylines and characters (Hernandez & Organista, 2013; Moyer-Gusé, 2008; Petraglia, 2007; Shen & Han, 2014; Wilkin et al., 2007). In various formats, including soap operas, popular music, films, and comic books, popular characters have modeled norms about health behaviors. Entertainment-education (E-E) programs have been used extensively internationally where nonprofit and governmental agencies can produce and air programs, as well as in the U.S. for-profit television system, where the focus has been on including accurate health information in popular television shows (Wilkin et al., 2007). For example, a fast-paced prime-time crime drama *Jasoos (Detective) Vijay*, produced by the BBC World Service Trust in India, targeted prevention of HIV/AIDS among sexually active men aged 18–34. Those who watched the program had higher awareness and knowledge of HIV/AIDS-related issues; were more likely to discuss condoms, sexually transmitted infections, and AIDS with others; and were more likely to use condoms with sex workers (Chatterjee, Bhanot, Frank, Murphy, & Power, 2009). In the United States, addition of a breast cancer storyline in a Spanish-language telenovela resulted in more calls to a cancer information number, increased knowledge about cancer treatment, and, among men, increased intention to encourage women to have mammograms (Wilkin et al., 2007). Digital games and decision aids are newer modalities using entertainment education (Jibaja-Weiss & Volk, 2007; H. Wang & Singhal, 2009).

Behavioral journalism uses mass media role-model stories of community members and advice from experts to change norms and increase adoption of behaviors (McAlister et al., 2000; Reininger et al., 2010; van Empelen, Kok, Schaalma, & Bartholomew, 2003a; van Empelen et al., 2003b). In behavioral journalism, the health educator interviews potential models for descriptions of reasons for their behavior change, skills used, and ways in which the change has been reinforced. The media materials then use models who are perceived as attractive and similar to members of the at-risk population and model the right kinds of behaviors. Behavioral journalism has also been combined with use of a community network of volunteers who cue people to watch the television documentary stories. Community volunteers, who in some cases are lay health workers, also model behaviors for their contacts and reinforce stated intentions and behaviors. These methods increase the visibility of behaviors of opinion leaders and early adopters, increasing the speed of adoption of the behaviors within the population (McAlister et al., 2000; Ramirez et al., 1999; Reininger et al., 2010).

Mobilizing social networks is another method used to influence social norms. For example, in a natural-helper model intervention Kelly (2004) and Kenneth Jones and colleagues (2008) trained respected and popular patrons of gay bars to adopt protective sexual practices and persuade acquaintances to follow their examples. The researchers considered training 15 percent of the priority population as opinion leaders to be a critical mass to establish new norms among the bar patrons (Kelly, 2004). This intervention led not only to a change in individual behavior but also to increased norms supportive of protective behavior.

## Summary: Social Norm Theories

Community members and opinion leaders at various levels demonstrate and support the health-promoting behavior, resulting in health-promoting social norms. Determinants of their behavior include all the determinants at the individual level and the availability of models and of appropriate social norms. Methods include mass media role modeling, entertainment-education, behavioral journalism, and mobilization of social networks.

## Conscientization

Paulo Freire's work (1973a, 1973b) in liberation education has formed the basis for empowerment models (Wallerstein, Sanchez, & Valarde, 2004;

Wallerstein et al., 2015). In conscientization, facilitators lead individuals in small groups to consider their own realities and constraints. The process moves group members to an understanding of the social forces underlying a problem and an understanding of their responsibility to act.

Critical consciousness, or conscientization, links individual-level and community-level empowerment and is a key method for strengths-based community organization. Using the context of developing literacy in his country, Freire described the method by which critical consciousness emerges. Educators began the process by being with the people in a local community, discovering the words and phrases they used to describe daily life, and observing the way they lived. Educators then selected generative words and integrated them to form codes that represented the life of the people. Program participants discussed these codes, which might be pictures, songs, or words, in cultural circles or in learning groups. They framed the discussion in terms of the participants' lives and the root causes of the conditions of their lives. This reflection on root causes gave rise to a political and social understanding that was accompanied by action to transform this reality. The final step of conscientization was the understanding that oppressive reality is a process that can be overcome. This understanding results in praxis, the unity between a person's understanding and actions (Freire, 1973b; Gadotti, 1994).

The Freirian method has been applied in health education to such areas as women's health; smoking, drug, and alcohol prevention; sexuality and sexual harassment; homelessness; environmental health; youth empowerment; occupational health; and health of the elderly (Cheatham & Shen, 2003; McDonald, Sarche, & Wang, 2004; Roter, Rudd, Keogh, & Robinson, 2006; Wallerstein et al., 2004; Wiggins, 2012). These projects all rely on participatory analysis using critical reflection and dialogue. Questions to encourage a critical stance include the following: "What do you see here? What's really happening here? How does this relate to our lives? Why does this problem, concern or strength exist? What can we do about it?" (C. Wang, 2003, p. 196). Issues, themes, and theories emerge that inform action.

The cycle of reflection-action-reflection continues into the policy realm. For example, the rural Chinese women with whom C. Wang, Yi, Tao, and Carovano (1998) worked presented their concerns to provincial policy makers; adolescents have been involved in peer education, participating in a statewide youth leadership group for policy development and carrying out service projects (Wallerstein et al., 2004); and low-income elderly residents of hotels have formed building tenants' associations, achieved better living conditions, and received compensation for lack of services (Minkler, 2004).

Wallerstein and colleagues (2015) identified three stages through which an individual passes from apathy to a social responsibility to act. The first stage involves individuals beginning to care about the problem, each other, and their ability to act in the world. This stage is accomplished through dialogue and self-disclosure in small groups and through questioning. At the next stage, individual responsibility to act, as well as individuals' self-efficacy to talk and help others, increases as a result of engaging in participatory and caring dialogue with community members who have experienced problems with alcohol or drugs. The final stage, social responsibility to act, involves critical thinking about the social forces that underlie the problem and a commitment to change both self and community. This three-stage transformation results in individual and community empowerment.

## Summary: Conscientization

Community members in groups, especially marginalized populations, become politically and socially active, resulting in the environmental condition of a community empowered to confront larger social and political environments. Determinants of their behavior include understanding of the root causes of social problems and collective self-efficacy. The method of problem-posing education includes reflection-action-reflection, nonjudgmental small-group discussion of learning materials, question posing, and self-disclosure.

## Community Organization

Rothman (2008) developed three models of community organization: locality development, social planning, and social action. Locality development raises consciousness about the underlying causes of problems and identifies strategies for action. It is heavily process oriented, with an emphasis on consensus, cooperation, and development of a sense of community. This model is most akin to the community development tradition in health education. Social planning uses information derived from empirical research. It is heavily task oriented, with an emphasis on expert assistance as a means to solve problems. Social action is based on coercive change and seeks to redress imbalances of power. It relies on conflict methods of change, such as demonstrations and boycotts, and the change agent is both an activist and a partisan. The skillful organizer assesses the context of the community and of the problem at hand and mixes and matches the change models (Longest, 2006).

Wallerstein et al. (2015) extended Rothman's work (2008), presenting a typology of community organization based on change method (consensus versus conflict) and view of the community (needs based versus strengths based; see Minkler & Wallerstein, 2012, p. 43). In their typology, earlier models of community organization—both community development and social action—are viewed as needs based, centering on the organizer's helping the community. Current community organization practice is seen as centered on the community, building on community strengths and assets. The form of practice differs depending on whether consensus or conflict is the change strategy. Community-building approaches use consensus and inclusiveness, a concept of power as *power with*, whereas empowerment-oriented social action uses conflict and challenges *power over*. Both types of community change are directed toward increased community competence, leadership development, and critical awareness within the community. Methods and strategies in their typology include participatory problem solving, grassroots organizing, professionally driven organizing, coalitions, lay health workers, critical awareness and reflection, development of community identity, leadership development, political and legislative actions, and culturally relevant practice (see also Cacari-Stone, Wallerstein, Garcia, & Minkler, 2014).

### *Community Participation*

Community participation is a core method of community work and is one of the bases of the Healthy Cities movement (Bezold & Hancock, 2014; World Health Organization Regional Office for Europe, 2002). The World Health Organization Regional Office for Europe (2002) defined it as:

> a process by which people are enabled to become actively and genuinely involved in defining the issues of concern to them, in making decisions about factors that affect their lives, in formulating and implementing policies, in planning, developing and delivering services and in taking action to achieve change. (p. 10)

Community participation achieves a number of objectives, including increasing democracy, combating exclusion of marginalized and disadvantaged populations, empowering people, mobilizing resources and energy, developing holistic and integrated approaches to problems, achieving better decisions and more effective services, and ensuring the ownership and sustainability of programs. Theorists see community participation as falling along a continuum from no community control to high community control (Minkler, Pies, & Hyde, 2012). Health promoters using community organization methods must decide whether the issue and context make aiming for the highest levels of community participation appropriate. Community organizers may have a greater challenge in aiming for more engagement, but they should not settle for a lower participation level simply because using the more passive processes of providing information and consultation is easier.

Yoo, Butler, Elias, and Goodman (2009), working primarily within a locality development framework, incorporated a social ecological framework in a stepwise process of community empowerment. The facilitation process, which could also be defined as participatory problem solving, involved six steps: entrée into the community, issue identification, prioritization of issues, strategy development, implementation with action plans and feedback, and transition. In the last step responsibility was transferred from the facilitators to community leaders, and an iterative process of action planning using the model continued. This process was first used in African American communities within New Orleans, Louisiana, in 2001 and then was carried out from 2004 to 2006 with primarily Caucasian residents of 12 high-rise buildings for senior citizens in Allegheny County, Pennsylvania. Factors related to success of these projects were a clearly understood and applied sound conceptual framework, consistently well-attended community meetings, available community organization support staff, open communication, focused community leaders, a community network, and regular debriefing among facilitators. Challenges included limited space, time, money, and data; slow process on action steps; difficulty attracting community participation; lack of promotion of the project in the community; and unexpected situations that required responses.

In another example, the Contra Costa County Health Services Department in California, through its Healthy Neighborhoods Project, worked with the El Pueblo neighborhood, a public housing development, to identify and train neighborhood health advocates in health, tobacco use prevention, and nutrition using Freirian popular education methods. The advocates were also trained in aspects of community organization, including door-to-door interviewing, community asset mapping, cross-cultural communication, and media and policy advocacy. The health department coordinator served as a facilitator and broker for resources. The neighborhood health advocates assessed the capacities of residents and residents' perceptions of their community and organized a community-mapping day. Trained adult and youth volunteers mapped the neighborhood's positive and negative physical and institutional features. The group presented its findings at a community forum, and residents who attended developed an action plan and organized the painting of a mural by local children to show the residents' vision for the community (El-Askari & Walton, 2008). To achieve the top priority of installation of speed bumps to slow traffic and reduce drug dealing, an El Pueblo residential council talked with the police chief, lobbied the city council, spoke at public meetings, organized demonstrations, and involved the media. These actions resulted in a consensus decision by the Housing Advisory commissioners to approve the speed bumps. Better street lighting and increased police patrol, two other priorities, were also accomplished. Residents also organized to remove a billboard that advertised cigarettes from the neighborhood and to form a community-based organization offer healthy cooking classes.

Following its initial successes, the El Pueblo residents' council became larger, better organized, and more representative of the residents. Members began to visit other San Francisco Bay Area public housing residents' councils to share their experiences. The council then wrote and received funding for three grants: a tenant opportunities grant to establish computer classes, job training classes, and job search workshops; a drug elimination effort; and a youth sports grant. Over the course of the project, success motivated residents to take leadership roles in addressing other issues, resulting in a strong sense of control. Residents reported increased energy and life satisfaction, and strong social ties developed. Residents also began involvement in broader policy-making initiatives, such as the county's Public and Environmental Health Advisory Board. Since that time, the model has been replicated in the South and West Berkeley communities with a focus on the reduction of health disparities (El-Askari & Walton, 2008).

These two examples clearly show both the health promoter's methods in working to facilitate empowerment in the communities and the communities' methods to achieve the environmental conditions they wanted. As residents achieve success, they increase their collective self-efficacy and empowerment. The latter, however, is contingent on reflection of the action taken and awareness that the action is legitimate and that one's social identity is active and powerful (Drury & Reicher, 2005).

### *Social Action*

Social action organizing, according to Rothman (2008), has as its goal the shifting of power relationships and resources from the haves to the have-nots. Social action as a method achieves change by crystallizing issues and organizing people to take action. Historical examples of this type of community organization practice have included method organizing; the civil rights movement; the United Farm Workers movement; community action programs; and the work of the Students for a Democratic Society (SDS), the Student Nonviolent Coordinating Committee (SNCC), the Black Panthers, the Brown Berets, La Raza Unida (Alinsky, 1972; Fisher, 2008), and Greenpeace actions against genetically engineered ingredients (Frooman & Murrell, 2005). Methods include boycotts, demonstrations, and strikes (see Kok et al., 2015a).

## Social Movements

The study of social movements overlaps considerably with community organization and advocacy that challenges *power over*. It offers insights for understanding the processes of change at the community level. Social movements have been defined as:

> collectivities acting with some degree of organization and continuity outside of institutional or organizational channels for the purpose of challenging or defending extant authority, whether it is institutionally or culturally based, in the group, organization, society, culture or world order of which they are a part. (Snow, Soule, & Kriesi, 2004, p. 11)

Framing is the process of assigning meaning and interpretation to relevant events and conditions in order to mobilize potential constituents, gain bystander support, and demobilize antagonists. Frames focus attention on what is relevant in a situation, create a set of meanings or narratives as to what is going on there, and serve a transformative function for both individuals and groups. Transformation can include altering the meaning of objects and one's relationship to them, including reconfiguring one's biography, and transforming routine grievances into injustices in the context of collective action. This construction of meaning can be viewed as a "politics of signification" (Snow et al., 2004, p. 384), in which social movements, governments at all levels, other authority structures, the media, and interested stakeholder groups seek to establish, among contested frames, the dominant meaning ascribed to persons, experiences, objects, and events. The mass media arena is especially important, as it serves as a public forum, is assumed by all players to have persuasive influence, and signals and diffuses changes in cultural codes, such as language used for framing an issue (Gamson, 2004).

These collective (as opposed to individual) frames are formed within a cultural context, using deeply held cultural values, such as justice, self-reliance, and rights. The culture shapes the framing process; the framing process in turn can shift culture. Movements focused on moderate change act on commonly shared meanings with the available culture, whereas attempts at radical social change require a critique of the current cultural understandings. Thus, the appeals must be different and, for radical change, go beyond cognitive persuasion to embodiment and action. For example, during the civil rights movement, African Americans took action to use facilities that had been designated for "whites only" (R. Williams, 1970; W. Williams, 2004). Social movements use tactics such as persuasion, facilitation, bargaining, and coercion. These have been characterized as either nonconfrontational or insider tactics (such as leafleting, letter-writing campaigns, lobbying, boycotts, lawsuits, and press conferences), and confrontational or outsider tactics (such as sit-ins, demonstrations, vigils, marches, and blockades). Protest tactics may be characterized as conventional (such as lobbying), disruptive (such as boycotts or demonstrations), or violent (such as bombings; Taylor & Van Dyke, 2004).

## *Advocacy*

Advocacy is a primary method used in community organizing and for change at environmental levels, whether sharing *power with* or challenging *power over*. This method addresses many of the processes that social movement theorists have discussed.

Health advocacy has been defined as "the processes by which the actions of individuals or groups attempt to bring about social and/or organizational change on behalf of a particular health goal, program, interest or population" (Galer-Unti, Tappe, & Lachenmayr, 2004). Another definition focuses on using a set of skills to shift public opinion and garner resources to support an issue (Wallack, Dorfman, Jernigan, & Themba, 1993). Some view advocacy as directed primarily to legislative policy, using the strategies of voting, electioneering, direct lobbying, and grassroots lobbying (Christoffel, 2000; Galer-Unti et al., 2004). Others, however, view advocacy as a key component of community organization, with goals other than legislation. An example is forcing New York City to include lead treatment services and its school system to address the hazards of peeling paint in kindergarten classrooms (Klitzman, Kass, & Freudenberg, 2008).

Advocacy seeks to ensure that the rights of disenfranchised individuals are protected, that institutions work the way they should, and that legislation and policy reflect the interests of the people (J. Anderson, Miller, & McGuire, 2012; Blackwell et al., 2012; Dorfman & Gonzalez, 2012). It addresses attitudes and policies at all levels from organizational, through community and state, to the national arena (Webster, Dunford, Kennington, Neal, & Chapman, 2014). In public health advocacy, efforts are made to change community conditions, often pitting consumers against large industry and pitting citizens against city hall. Community activism is rooted in democratic principles and practices, and though often viewed as synonymous with social action, it includes cooperation as well as confrontation. Examples of advocacy groups include local and national groups participating in social movements—such as those for the environment, environmental justice, and tobacco control—and citizen groups that have come together to support issues of importance in their communities. Advocacy groups have different tactics. For example, some are confrontational, such as AIDS Coalition to Unleash Power (ACT UP; an AIDS awareness activist group); others are research based, such as the League of Women Voters (Altman, Balcazar, Fawcett, Seekins, & Young, 1994; Wallack et al., 1993).

It is important that health promoters choose tactics and activities that fit the type of community organizing they are using, the issue, and the community. Groups must decide the ways in which they intend to accomplish goals, and those activities will likely change over time in response to reactions to actions taken and to shifting external forces. Altman and colleagues (1994) listed the following approaches to advocacy: coalition building, community development, coordination, education, networking, public awareness, and policy or legislative change. They suggested the principles of presence (reminding), generosity (praising), shaping (rewarding), escalation (intensifying), accuracy (maintaining credibility), and consistency (being fair) to enhance tactical efforts (Table 3.2). These principles should underlie action, regardless of whether the action flows from a social action, community development, or social planning perspective. Romero, Kwan, and Chavkin (2013) noticed the tension between advocacy and scientific research. They suggested three factors relevant for action-related research: methodological rigor, resources for postresearch evaluation, and acceptance of the combined role of advocate and researcher by the scientific community.

The advocacy process and products have been divided into three stages: research and investigation; strategy, including stakeholder education and mobilization; and direct action (Altman et al., 1994; Christoffel, 2000). In research and investigation, the advocacy group conducts studies of the issue in order to understand it as fully as possible by gathering data on public opinion, obtaining information about the opposition and its strategies and tactics, and acting as a watchdog of target organizations. The advocacy group can also request accountability by formally asking responsible parties for the reasons behind a decision of concern to them, by documenting complaints with evidence, by organizing consumer

**Table 3.2**  Principles Underlying Effective Tactics

| Principle | What to Do |
|---|---|
| Presence | Remind people of the issue by doing something about it frequently |
| Generosity | Praise others for their strengths and actions to gain goodwill and to reinforce their actions |
| Shaping | Reward small steps of those who change toward your goals |
| Escalation | Continue to mobilize more people and increase the intensity of the tactics if the first efforts are unsuccessful |
| Accuracy and honesty | Be scrupulously accurate to maintain credibility and to keep opponents from successfully arguing against the issues raised |
| Consistency | Distribute praise and criticism fairly—if one group is criticized for its position, other groups should be treated the same way |

service audits, and by demonstrating the financial benefits of acting on their issue.

Strategies for encouragement and education include giving personal compliments and public support to reinforce other people's actions, arranging celebrations and publicizing them, developing a detailed proposal for addressing the problem being focused on, and establishing contact with the opposition organization, even to the extent of influencing its decision-making processes. The advocacy group can also prepare fact sheets on the issue (and on the group) to maintain consistency and continuity in public relations, offer public education through mass media and presentations to community groups, and counterattack by explaining the group's point of view.

Interventionists can use direct action strategies to make the group's presence felt, mobilize public support, and use the system (Altman et al., 1994; Blackwell et al., 2012; Dorfman & Gonzalez, 2012). Strategies to make the group's presence felt include postponing action until the issue has matured; establishing alternative programs or finding another source to provide the service; establishing lines of communication with the opponent's traditional allies; criticizing unfavorable actions (first privately and then publicly if there are no results); expressing opposition publicly; reminding those responsible; making complaints (first informally, then formally); and lobbying decision makers. Ways to mobilize public support include sponsoring a conference or public hearing; conducting a letter-writing campaign, a petition drive, or a ballot drive; registering voters; and organizing public demonstrations. For using the system, the advocacy group might file a formal complaint; seek enforcement of existing laws and policies; lobby for new laws, policies, or regulations; use other resources, such as a negotiator, mediator, or fact finder to work with opponents; and initiate legal action if that proves to be the only way to address the issue. Altman and colleagues (1994) also described strategies to use if efforts to work within the system fail. These include arranging a media exposé, overwhelming an unworkable system (e.g., by arranging unmanageable requests for service), organizing a boycott, and using passive resistance. Kok et al. (2015a) described how the use of stakeholders may help health promoters make changes at the organizational and policy level to promote health.

## Media Advocacy

Wallack and his colleagues (2008, 1993) have developed the approach of media advocacy, a set of tactics for community groups to promote social change by using the media. They recognized that the mass media, particularly television, provide a forum for surfacing and discussing issues and setting the agenda for policy makers and the public. Media advocacy seeks to influence the selection and presentation of topics by the media in order to set and achieve a public health agenda (Dorfman & Krasnow, 2014).

Media advocacy is based on three steps: setting the agenda (framing for access), shaping the debate (framing for content), and advancing the policy. In framing for access, the goal is to get the media to select the story. Framing for content involves shifting the view of health from the individual to the social level and dealing with the complexity of health and social problems so that a public health perspective defines the debate. Advancing the policy is a way of framing the content so that it reaches the key decision makers whom the advocacy group is trying to influence.

To gain access, the health promoter needs to understand the various access points of each of the major media outlets. For television these points are news, public affairs, entertainment, editorials, paid advertising, and public service advertising. For newspapers they are the front page; the sports, lifestyle, arts, comics, business, and editorial sections; letters to the editor; and paid advertising. The media advocate needs skills in determining where and how to place the particular issue within the media. Media advocacy strategies focus on earned media (that is, not paid, such as news and talk shows) and on paid placements rather than on public service announcements, in which control over the placement and framing of the story is lost. One can achieve news coverage by targeting journalists who are interested in health issues and providing them accurate information and story ideas. Creating news and piggybacking onto breaking news are also strategies. Elements of newsworthiness include linking the story to the anniversary of an event, a breakthrough, a celebrity, a controversy, injustice, irony, a local point of view, a milestone, a personal angle, and a seasonal theme (Wallack et al., 1993). By monitoring the media, a health promoter can understand which reporters are covering which topics and what the current community concerns are.

To give the public health perspective, the health promoter can frame an individual problem as a social issue, shifting the primary responsibility away from blaming the individual. For example, the advocate can shift the subject from teen drinking to the promotion of alcohol and include a solution with an approach to policy. Story elements to be developed include compelling images, powerful symbols, and social math to show the extent of the problem (e.g., in a year "enough alcohol was consumed by college students to fill 3,500 Olympic-size swimming pools, about 1 on every campus in the United States"; Wallack et al., 1993, p. 108). It is important to use voices of people who are credible because of their experiences but who are also deeply involved in the policy aspects of the issue. For example, a college president who has worked with the college board of trustees to change rules about student alcohol at a campus where a death has occurred due to binge drinking may be a good source for a campaign about student alcohol use. Using sound bites of fewer than 10 seconds to summarize the issue is a valuable skill for the health promoter to learn.

Wallack and colleagues (2008, 1993) also provided practical advice for developing media goals and objectives, pitching the story to journalists, developing media kits, and giving interviews. Their summary rules for working with reporters are to be honest, help the press better understand the issues, comment only on issues that you know about, and remember that everything you say is on the record.

## Summary: Community Organization Theories

All community organization theories are directed to two environmental conditions: a health-promoting environment and community capacity. The agents are community leaders and members who are taking action to change community conditions related to health. The determinants of this behavior include motivation to act, collective efficacy, political efficacy, and community structures that facilitate community action. Methods to influence these determinants include participation and participatory problem solving, organizing (grassroots organizing and professionally driven organizing), forming coalitions, using lay health workers, framing to shift perspectives, media advocacy to build community identity, and culturally relevant practice. The community, in turn, uses the following methods to create a health-promoting environment: participatory problem solving, forming coalitions, advocacy, media advocacy, and framing to shift perspectives.

## Societal and Governmental Theories

For the societal level, we examine theories that relate to public policy and its development. Because public policy is usually set by governments, change in policies will often focus on influencing government action at the local, state, or national levels.

### Theories of Public Policy

Public policy is "a guide to action to change what would otherwise occur, a decision about amounts and allocations of resources, made at any level of government" (Milio, 2001, p. 622). Health policy is directly related to public health and health services. Other public policies directed to issues such as economics, housing, or public safety also have much potential to influence health. Milio (1981) viewed economic policy as acting directly on people's biophysical and socioeconomic environments and indirectly through various areas for public policy, such as environmental safety, energy, income maintenance, and health and human services delivery. This framework shows policy as an environmental determinant of health behavior and of health. *Health in All Policies* is a strategy of the European Union that reflects this close linkage of policy to health (Kickbusch, 2009).

Public policy sets options for organizations and for individuals, both directly and indirectly through organizations. According to Milio (1981, p. 83), policy components should make "the creation and maintenance of healthful environments and personal habits the easiest—the 'cheapest' and most numerous—choices for selections by governmental units and corporations, producers and consumers, among all the options available to them." Policy instruments include direct spending, such as grants and contracts; the production of goods and services; regulation and monitoring; and fiscal incentives, such as subsidies, taxation, and tax deductions.

Policy formation is a cyclical process occurring within a system open to the environment (Freudenberg & Tsui, 2014; Longest, 2006; Themba-Nixon, Minkler, & Freudenberg, 2008). In a rational or economic decision-making model, a policy maker would select the most efficient alternative to maximize the most valuable output. However, policy formation is much more complex than that, with many stakeholders and interest groups with varying power and diverse ideologies, insufficient information about policy problems and solutions, and unique contexts for specific issues. Theorists have endeavored to isolate key constructs and their relationships in this process to create hypotheses that can be tested (B. Jones, 2003). We will discuss several of these theories in the context of a model developed by Longest (2006, p. 108).

Longest (2006) has identified three intertwined phases of the policy process: policy formulation, policy implementation, and policy modification. Policy formulation includes setting the policy agenda and the development of legislation. Policy implementation includes activities associated with rule making that guide operationalization and implementation of a policy. Policy modification is feedback from individuals, organizations, and interest groups on policy formulation and policy implementation. Health advocates and activated communities have opportunities to influence the policy process at each phase.

In a survey of national health consumer groups in the United Kingdom, 82 percent indicated that influencing policy at the national level was "important" or "very important." Three-quarters of the groups had contacted the central government on policy issues within the past three years; almost half had at least quarterly contacts with the Department of Health (DOH) ministers and civil servants and members of parliament.

Sources of strength in the policy process identified were the groups' ability to bring the experience of patients, their relatives, and their caregivers to the table; participation in alliances with other groups with similar concerns; and close relationships with civil servants and ministers. Almost 90% of the groups participated in formal alliances of health consumer groups or linked with other stakeholders, such as other health professionals, in the policy process. Close working relationships with government officials charged with policy implementation and policy making were seen as critical to providing feedback on policy implementation and getting their issues on the policy agenda. Barriers reported were inaccurate coverage in the media, poor communication and feedback on policy developments from the DOH, lack of funding for lobbying activity, and lack of power of consumer groups relative to other policy stakeholders, such as health professionals, commercial interests, and research charities (Kathryn Jones et al., 2004).

The policy process involves the movement from "policy primeval soup" (Kingdon, 2003, p. 116) to the development of legislation. Cobb and Elder (1983) represented the traditional perspective of the policy process in the so-called Agenda-Building Theory. They suggested that the policy process follows clearly distinguishable steps from problem definition, through alternative specification, to resource allocation and implementation. However, Breton and de Leeuw (2011) concluded in their review:

> Although this conceptual framework seems to have served a purpose, it has since become the subject of devastating criticism, predominantly focusing on the fact that the stages heuristic fails to address the dynamics of multiple, interacting, iterative and incremental cycles of action at many different levels of mutual and reciprocal action at the same time. (p. 83)

Breton and de Leeuw cited Sabatier (2007), who defined four parameters to assess appropriate theoretical frameworks of the policy process:

1. Each must do a reasonably good job of meeting the criteria of a scientific theory; that is, its concepts and propositions must be relatively clear and internally consistent, it must identify clear causal drivers, it must give rise to falsifiable hypotheses, and it must be fairly broad in scope (i.e., apply to most of the policy process in a variety of political systems).

2. Each must be the subject of a fair amount of recent conceptual development or empirical testing. A number of currently active policy scholars must view it as a viable way of understanding the policy process.

3. Each must be a positive theory seeking to explain much of the policy process. The theoretical framework may also contain some explicitly normative elements, but these are not required.

4. Each must address the broad sets of factors that political scientists looking at different aspects of public policy making have traditionally deemed important: conflicting values and interests, information flows, institutional arrangements, and variation in the socioeconomic environment (p. 8).

Two theories—the Multiple Streams Theory, and the Advocacy Coalition Framework—are especially useful in understanding how this process occurs (Breton & de Leeuw, 2011; Clavier & de Leeuw, 2013).

## *Multiple Streams Theory*

Kingdon (2003) has also investigated how issues reach systemic or governmental agenda status, inserting an element of chance that explains the fluidity and rapid change of the policy-making process. He views this process in terms of three streams: politics, problems, and policies (Kingdon, 2003; Zahariadis, 2007). The political stream includes changes in administration, party platforms, elections, and national mood regarding government. The problem stream includes issues within the various policy sectors, such as global warming, the national debt, health care costs, teenage pregnancy, specific diseases, and poor housing infrastructure. Science-based information is used to indicate the seriousness and causes of a problem and to provide evaluative information regarding current policies and programs. Policy solutions, such as pollution controls, universal health insurance, school-based clinics, or cooperative housing, "float around in or near government, searching for problems to which to become attached or political events that increase their likelihood of adoption" (Kingdon, 2003, p. 112). In the policy stream, science offers ideas for solutions, legitimates them, and provides information about technical feasibility. Events and ideas in these streams move along independently until there is a change in one stream, such as a change in government, emergence of a large problem, or advocacy of new policies. At this point a window between the streams opens up so that a problem may enter the political stream or a policy may become linked to a problem. The role of the policy advocate is to create, monitor, and capitalize on these opportunities (de Leeuw, Keizer, & Hoeijmakers, 2013).

Policy advocates or entrepreneurs promote their proposals and the associated problems and facilitate coupling between the streams, linking problems, policies, and political opportunities together when the windows are open. Characteristics of effective policy advocates are recognized authority; visibility; strong political, communication, and negotiation skills; ability to engage in strategic planning; creativity; relative independence in resources and structure; and persistence (Kingdon, 2003).

In policy advocacy, as in many other arenas, timing is everything; and opportunity knocks for those advocates who are prepared. Much of the success in placing issues on the systemic and institutional agendas and in achieving policy enactment comes from an understanding of when to act and how to frame the issue. Kingdon's notion of policy windows (2003) provides a framework for timing. Kingdon said that policy is placed on the agenda when the windows between the three streams—politics (including elections, party platforms, and national mood regarding government), problems (all the issues within different policy sectors, including health, housing, and economic sectors), and policy solutions (such as school-based clinics and universal health insurance)—are open so that the policy can be put forward. For example, newly elected officials may focus on certain problems, for which prepared advocates who have networked with the right gatekeepers can present their solutions. Community advocacy groups can work with each of the streams. For instance, they can support candidates for elected office or influence party platforms, build community demand to address particular problems, and develop and promote well-researched and persuasive policy proposals.

Laumann and Knoke (1987) pointed to the importance of organizations in the policy development process. They argued that influential organizations that have specific national policy interests and fluid resources and that are embedded within communication and resource-exchange networks are the main agents in the national policy process. These organizations are typically corporate entities, such as trade associations, professional societies, labor unions, corporations, public interest groups, government bureaus, and congressional committees. The policy process begins when one or more of these organizations recognizes a condition as a problem or an issue and alerts other organizations to it. The interested organizations then generate options, often as solutions in search of issues. The alternative options are then narrowed to get the policy option onto the governmental agenda for consideration. Each step is a product of negotiation and advocacy.

Powerful corporate entities representing industries such as health insurance, pharmaceuticals, processed foods, and tobacco take positions opposed or aligned with those of health promoters. Developing and maintaining strong entities on behalf of public health—such as public health professional associations, associations representing public health officials, and citizens' groups—and carefully creating alliances where appropriate with corporate groups are strategies necessary to represent health promotion in the policy development process.

After policy is enacted into law, it must be operationalized; and advocates, especially strong interest groups, seek to influence this process through lobbying and other forms of influence. Especially important are long-standing working relationships between those implementing policy and the leaders of affected organizations and interest groups. These relationships are marked by the exchange of information and expertise. For complex policies that may affect a number of interest groups, advisory committees and task forces may be set up to help develop the proposed rules. Gaining a seat on these bodies allows for direct input to the process (Kingdon, 2003; Longest, 2006). According to Longest (2006), the success of the operational implementation of the policy rests on the fit between the implementing organizations and policy objectives and on the amount of resources (e.g., authority, fiscal, personnel, information and expertise, and technology) that the organization has. A key consideration is the competence of agency managers related to strategy, leadership, collaboration, and conceptual and technical knowledge and skills. Implementation problems are certain to arise, and management must be able to address these challenges.

The policy-making process is cyclical, and most health policies are the result of modifying previous policies. Policy modification occurs when stakeholders incorporate feedback from policy implementation and consequences into the policy formulation and policy implementation phases. Rules and practices may be changed or the law may be amended, typically in an incremental fashion. Feedback comes from the groups affected by the policies, especially key interest groups, and from those who formulate and take charge of implementation. Pressure to change can be external, from individuals, organizations, and interest groups, and internal, through oversight by the legislative, executive, and judicial branches. Evaluations of policy implementation and outcomes of policy are often crucial to decisions regarding modification.

### Advocacy Coalition Framework

The Advocacy Coalition Framework (Breton, Richard, Gagnon, Jacques, & Bergeron, 2013; Weible, Sabatier, & McQueen, 2009) focuses on the system of policy making. The primary focus is the policy subsystem, the set of agents who follow and seek to influence public policy in a given area across a time frame of a decade or more. Agents can be elected and appointed agency officials at all levels of government, interest group leaders, researchers, and important journalists who cover the issue. The agents engage in coordinated activity through advocacy coalitions. Advocacy coalitions are based on deep and unchangeable shared basic values, causal assumptions, and problem perspectives in the particular policy arena, along with more changeable secondary beliefs about how to implement the policy core. A small number of coalitions within a particular policy subsystem compete, promoting conflicting strategies, and policy brokers within the subsystem attempt to find a reasonable compromise to reduce this conflict so that policy can be enacted.

Stable factors, such as a society's perception of the issue area, distribution of natural resources, cultural values, social structure, and basic legal structure, constrain the options available to the agents. For example, the U.S. cultural values of individualism and capitalism limit the policy options that can be advocated. Dynamic events, such as socioeconomic conditions and technology, large changes in governing coalitions, and decisions and impacts from other subsystems, alter the constraints and opportunities of the subsystem agents. The AIDS epidemic can be viewed as an outside event that enabled the harm reduction coalition to overthrow the well-established abstinence coalition in the drug policy subsystem in Western Europe (Kübler, 2001). Bleach kits and needle exchange programs became policy options.

The Advocacy Coalition Framework provides guidance for carrying out policy advocacy. The framework rejects the notion that there are coalitions of convenience formed by agents motivated by short-term self-interest. Instead, core beliefs or ideologies create a stable lineup of allies and opponents. Advocacy coalitions will negotiate on the secondary beliefs, including decisions on administrative rules, budgets, interpretation of statutes, and information about the problem, before shifting on the fundamental policy core. Because of this, the core attributes of a governmental program are unlikely to change as long as the coalition that instituted that program remains in power. Policy can change through a perturbation from outside the policy subsystem, policy-oriented learning, internal subsystem events that highlight failures in the current subsystem practices, and negotiated agreements between coalitions (Weible et al., 2009). In comparison to Kingdon's Multiple Streams Theory (2003), the Advocacy Coalition Framework sees the policy solution stream as much more integrated with the political stream because of the foundation of core normative and policy beliefs.

The importance of political ideology in public health has been increasingly recognized (Breton, Richard, & Gagnon, 2007; Breton, Richard, Gagnon, Jacques, & Bergeron, 2008; Cohen et al., 2000). Particularly important has been the tension between the views that government has the duty to protect its citizens' health and that individuals have the right to make their own choices. Ideological arguments on both sides have been made regarding pasteurization of milk, fluoridation of public water supplies, use of motorcycle helmets, and tobacco control. Review of newspaper coverage of tobacco issues in the United States from 1985 to 1996 showed that the tobacco industry framed the issue around the core values of freedom, fairness, free enterprise, and autonomy. Tobacco control advocates, on the other hand, framed the issue around the value of health (Menashe & Siegel, 1998).

Joanna E. Cohen and colleagues (2000) have suggested that ideological arguments be used to benefit tobacco control. They and others suggested that advocates use the perspective of the New Right, including its laissez-faire approach, its retreat from state intervention in economic and social affairs, and its belief in market forces; advocates should also use the values of freedom, fairness, and free enterprise to frame the argument for tobacco control (Cohen et al., 2000; McKinlay & Marceau, 2000). This would avoid challenging normative core beliefs so that the focus can be on changing tobacco policy. With regard to framing the issue, freedom could include freedom from the influence of the tobacco industry and from the addiction of tobacco; fairness, treating bar and restaurant workers the same as workers who have protection from secondhand smoke; and free enterprise, that the tobacco industry seeks government tax breaks, trade advantages, and protection of its proprietary information.

Breton and colleagues (2008) analyzed the factors over a 12-year period leading to Quebec's 1998 Tobacco Act, using the Advocacy Coalition Framework and a theory positing coalitions as temporary strategic alliances. Some elements of discourse were relatively stable, such as the lethality of smoking, the difficulty of quitting, the right to a smoke-free environment, and that government intervention in tobacco control is legitimate but must not impede provincial economy. Influential external events included the cigarette contraband crisis, a new minister of health who supported tobacco control, the Supreme Court of Canada's decision overturning federal restrictions on tobacco advertising, the Clinton administration's proposed measures to address youth smoking, and the lawsuits brought by states in the United States against tobacco companies and demanding the release of tobacco industry documents. Their findings were consistent with a broad advocacy coalition from which a strategic alliance of agents emerged. Their work in tobacco control more generally also pointed out that health education played an important advocacy role in sensitizing the public (Breton et al., 2007). They noted the importance of making arguments that take into account the fundamental values in the discourse of policy makers and the public, in addition to the dissemination of scientific arguments.

## Summary: Societal and Governmental Theories

Policy makers are the agents for the environmental condition of health-promoting public policy. They enact health-promoting legislation, regulation, and policy. Determinants of this behavior include motivation and behavioral capability and barriers. Methods include policy advocacy (information, persuasion, and negotiation), agenda setting, and timing for policy windows.

## Summary

The purpose of this chapter is to identify environment-oriented theories and models that are useful for planning health promotion interventions. We discuss how to describe and select environmental conditions to be changed, and then we suggest how to change these conditions. The theories and models are organized by environmental level: interpersonal, organizational, community, and societal level. We first present general environmental-oriented theories: systems theory, theories of power, and empowerment theories; then interpersonal-level theories: social network and social support theories; next organizational-level theories: organizational change theories, organizational development theories, and stakeholder theory; then community-level theories: coalition theory, social capital and community capacity theories, social norms theories, conscientization theory, and community organization theories; finally, societal- and governmental-level theories: public policy theories. Each theory is summarized in terms of its contribution to problem analysis and intervention development.

## Discussion Questions and Learning Activities

1. Discuss why environmental conditions are considered important influences to promote health behavior.

2. Describe three examples of environmental conditions that may influence health outcomes through individual behavior.

3. Explain why agents in the environment are considered an important focus for health promotion programs. Give examples of agents for different types of environmental conditions.

4. Discuss how systems theory can be helpful for health promotion planners to consider for placing a planned intervention in the context of broader social systems.

5. Explain why the role of power in society is an important consideration in planning health promotion programs.

6. Describe how organizational theories could be used to change environmental conditions to promote health behavior and improve health outcomes.

7. How would a community organizer using Freire's conscientization techniques approach the task of organizing a community that was experiencing high incidence rates of HIV?

8. Use one of the policy theories to analyze a health issue of current interest, for example health care reform, HIV prevention, or sexuality education.

## References

Aiyer, S. M., Zimmerman, M. A., Morrel-Samuels, S., & Reischl, T. M. (2014). From broken windows to busy streets: A community empowerment perspective. *Health Education & Behavior, 42*(2), 137–147.

Aldana, S. G., Anderson, D. R., Adams, T. B., Whitmer, R. W., Merrill, R. M., George, V., & Noyce, J. (2012). A review of the knowledge base on healthy worksite culture. *Journal of Occupational and Environmental Medicine, 54*(4), 414–419.

Alinsky, S. D. (1972). *Rules for radicals: A practical primer for realistic radicals.* New York, NY: Random House.

Altman, D. G., Balcazar, F. E., Fawcett, S. B., Seekins, T. M., & Young, J. Q. (1994). *Public health advocacy: Creating community change to improve health.* Palo Alto, CA: Stanford Center for Research in Disease Prevention.

Anderson, J., Miller, M., & McGuire, A. (2012). Organizing for health care reform: National and state-level efforts and perspectives. In M. Minkler (Ed.), *Community organizing and community building for health and welfare* (3rd ed., pp. 386–406). New Brunswick, NJ: Rutgers University Press.

Anderson, R. A., Plowman, D., Corazzini, K., Hsieh, P.-C., Su, H. F., Landerman, L. R., & McDaniel, R. R. (2013). Participation in decision making as a property of complex adaptive systems: Developing and testing a measure. *Nursing Research and Practice, 2013,* 1–16.

Arvey, S. R., & Fernández, M. E. (2012). Identifying the core elements of effective community health worker programs: A research agenda. *American Journal of Public Health, 102*(9), 1633–1637.

Awofeso, N. (2003). The Healthy Cities approach—Reflections on a framework for improving global health. *Bulletin of the World Health Organization, 81*(3), 222–223.

Bandura, A. (1997). *Self-efficacy: The exercise of control.* New York, NY: W.H. Freeman.

Beam, M., Ehrlich, G., Black, J. D., Block, A., & Leviton, L. C. (2012a). Evaluation of the Healthy Schools Program: Part I. *Interim progress. Preventing Chronic Disease, 9.* doi:10.5888/pcd9.110106

Beam, M., Ehrlich, G., Black, J. D., Block, A., & Leviton, L. C. (2012b). Evaluation of the Healthy Schools Program: Part II. *The role of technical assistance. Preventing Chronic Disease, 9.* doi:10.5888/pcd9.110105

Beets, M. W., Cardinal, B. J., & Alderman, B. L. (2010). Parental social support and the physical activity-related behaviors of youth: A review. *Health Education & Behavior, 37*(5), 621–644.

Berkman, L. F., & Glass, T. (2000). Social integration, social networks, social support, and health. In L. F. Berkman & I. Kawachi (Eds.), *Social epidemiology* (pp. 137–173). New York, NY: Oxford University Press.

Berry, G. R. (2003). Organizing against multinational corporate power in cancer alley. The activist community as primary stakeholder. *Organization & Environment, 16*(1), 3–33.

Best, A. (2011). Systems thinking and health promotion. *American Journal of Health Promotion, 25*(4), eix–ex.

Beyer, J. M., & Trice, H. M. (1978). *Implementing change: Alcoholism policies in work organizations.* New York, NY: Free Press.

Bezold, C., & Hancock, T. (2014). The futures of the healthy cities and communities movement. *National Civic Review, 103*(1), 66–70.

Blackwell, A. G., Thompson, M., Freudenberg, N., Ayers, J., Schrantz, D., & Minkler, M. (2012). Using community organizing and community building to influence public policy. In M. Minkler (Ed.), *Community organizing and community building for health and welfare* (3rd ed., pp. 371–385). New Brunswick, NJ: Rutgers University Press.

Bonham, C. A., Sommerfeld, D., Willging, C., & Aarons, G. A. (2014). Organizational factors influencing implementation of evidence-based practices for integrated treatment in behavioral health agencies. *Psychiatry Journal, 2014*(4). doi:10.1155/2014/802983

Boonstra, J. J. (Ed.). (2004). *Dynamics of organizational change and learning.* In P. Herriot (Series Ed.), Handbooks in the Psychology of Management in Organizations. Hoboken, NJ: John Wiley & Sons.

Bracht, N., Finnegan, J. R., Jr., Rissel, C., Weisbrod, R., Gleason, J., Corbett, J., & Veblen-Mortenson, S. (1994). Community ownership and program continuation following a health demonstration project. *Health Education Research, 9*(2), 243–255.

Breton, E., & de Leeuw, E. (2011). Theories of the policy process in health promotion research: A review. *Health Promotion International, 26*(1), 82–90.

Breton, E., Richard, L., & Gagnon, F. (2007). The role of health education in the policy change process: Lessons from tobacco control. *Critical Public Health, 17*(4), 351–364.

Breton, E., Richard, L., Gagnon, F., Jacques, M., & Bergeron, P. (2008). Health promotion research and practice require sound policy analysis models: The case of Quebec's Tobacco Act. *Social Science & Medicine, 67*(11), 1679–1689.

Breton, É., Richard, L., Gagnon, F., Jacques, M., & Bergeron, P. (2013). Coalition advocacy action and research for policy development. In C. Clavier & E. de Leeuw (Eds.), *Health promotion and the policy process* (pp. 43–62). Oxford, United Kingdom: Oxford University Press.

Brown, A. D., Colville, I., & Pye, A. (2014). Making sense of sensemaking in organization studies. *Organization Studies, 36*(2), 265–277.

Brown, L. D., Bammer, G., Batliwala, S., & Kunreuther, F. (2003). Framing practice-research engagement for democratizing knowledge. *Action Research, 1*(1), 81–102.

Butterfoss, F. D., & Kegler, M. C. (2009). The community coalition action theory. In R. J. DiClemente, R. A. Crosby, & M. C. Kegler (Eds.), *Emerging theories in health promotion practice and research* (2nd ed., pp. 237–276). San Francisco, CA: Jossey-Bass.

Butterfoss, F., & Kegler, M. (2012). A coalition model for community action. In M. Minkler (Ed.), *Community organizing and community building for health and welfare* (3rd ed., pp. 309–328). New Brunswick, NJ: Rutgers University Press.

Butterfoss, F. D., Kegler, M. C., & Francisco, V. T. (2008). Mobilizing organizations for health promotion: Theories of organizational change. In K. Glanz, B. K. Rimer, & K. Viswanath (Eds.), *Health behavior and health education: Theory, research, and practice* (4th ed., pp. 335–362). San Francisco, CA: Jossey-Bass.

Cacari-Stone, L., Wallerstein, N., Garcia, A. P., & Minkler, M. (2014). The promise of community-based participatory research for health equity: A conceptual model for bridging evidence with policy. *American Journal of Public Health, 104*(9), 1615–1623.

Caughy, M. O., O'Campo, P. J., & Muntaner, C. (2003). When being alone might be better: Neighborhood poverty, social capital, and child mental health. *Social Science & Medicine, 57*(2), 227–237.

Chatterjee, J. S., Bhanot, A., Frank, L. B., Murphy, S. T., & Power, G. (2009). The importance of interpersonal discussion and self-efficacy in knowledge, attitude, and practice models. *International Journal of Communication, 3*, 28.

Chavis, D. M. (2001). The paradoxes and promise of community coalitions. *American Journal of Community Psychology, 29*(2), 309–320.

Cheatham, A., & Shen, E. (2003). Community based participatory research with Cambodian girls in Long Beach, California. In M. Minkler & N. Wallerstein (Eds.), *Community-based participatory research for health* (pp. 316–331). San Francisco, CA: Jossey-Bass.

Cheatham-Rojas, A., & Shen, E. (2008). CBPR with Cambodian girls in Long Beach, California: A case study. In M. Minkler & N. Wallerstein (Eds.), *Community-based participatory research for health: From process to outcomes* (2nd ed., pp. 121–136). San Francisco, CA: Jossey-Bass.

Christoffel, K. K. (2000). Public health advocacy: Process and product. *American Journal of Public Health, 90*(5), 722–726.

Chu, C., Breucker, G., Harris, N., Stitzel, A., Gan, X., Gu, X., & Dwyer, S. (2000). Health-promoting workplaces—International settings development. *Health Promotion International, 15*(2), 155–167.

Clavier, C., & de Leeuw, E. (Eds.). (2013). *Health promotion and the policy process.* Oxford, United Kingdom: Oxford University Press.

Cobb, R. W., & Elder, C. D. (1983). *Participation in American politics: The dynamics of agenda-building* (2nd ed.). Baltimore, MD: John Hopkins University Press.

Cohen, J. E., Milio, N., Rozier, R. G., Ferrence, R., Ashley, M. J., & Goldstein, A. O. (2000). Political ideology and tobacco control. *Tobacco Control, 9*(3), 263–267.

Commers, M., Gottlieb, N. H., & Kok, G. (2005). *How to change environments for health.* Unpublished manuscript.

Cummings, T. G., & Worley, C. G. (2014). *Organization development and change* (10th ed.). Mason, OH: South-Western Cengage Learning.

Damschroder, L. J., Aron, D. C., Keith, R. E., Kirsh, S. R., Alexander, J. A., & Lowery, J. C. (2009). Fostering implementation of health services research findings into practice: A consolidated framework for advancing implementation science. *Implementation Science, 4,* 50.

de Leeuw, E., Keizer, M., & Hoeijmakers, M. (2013). Health policy networks: Connecting the disconnected. In C. Clavier & E. de Leeuw (Eds.), *Health promotion and the policy process* (pp. 154–173). Oxford, United Kingdom: Oxford University Press.

de Leeuw, E., Tsouros, A. D., Dyakova, M., & Green, G. (Eds.). (2014). *Healthy cities: Promoting health and equity—Evidence for local policy and practice.* Copenhagen, Denmark: World Health Organization Regional Office for Europe.

Dooris, M. (2009). Holistic and sustainable health improvement: The contribution of the settings-based approach to health promotion. *Perspectives in Public Health, 129*(1), 29–36.

Dooris, M. (2013). Expert voices for change: Bridging the silos—Towards healthy and sustainable settings for the 21st century. *Health & Place, 20,* 39–50.

Dorfman, L., & Gonzalez, P. (2012). Media advocacy: A strategy for helping communities change policy. In M. Minkler (Ed.), *Community organizing and community building for health and welfare* (3rd ed., pp. 407–422). New Brunswick, NJ: Rutgers University Press.

Dorfman, L., & Krasnow, I. D. (2014). Public health and media advocacy. *Annual Review of Public Health, 35,* 293–306.

Drury, J., & Reicher, S. (2005). Explaining enduring empowerment: A comparative study of collective action and psychological outcomes. *European Journal of Social Psychology, 35*(1), 35–58.

DuBois, D. L., Holloway, B. E., Valentine, J. C., & Cooper, H. (2002). Effectiveness of mentoring programs for youth: A meta-analytic review. *American Journal of Community Psychology, 30*(2), 157–197.

Duhl, L. (2004). Transitions and paradigms. *Journal of Epidemiology and Community Health, 58*(10), 806–807.

El-Askari, G., & Walton, S. (2008). Local government and resident collaboration to improve health: A case study in capacity building and cultural humility. In M. Minkler (Ed.), *Community organizing and community building for health* (2nd ed., pp. 254–271). New Brunswick, NJ: Rutgers University Press.

Eng, E., Rhodes, S. D., & Parker, E. (2009). Natural helper models to enhance a community's health and competence. In R. J. DiClemente, R. A. Crosby, & M. C. Kegler (Eds.), *Emerging theories in health promotion practice and research* (2nd ed., pp. 303–330). San Francisco, CA: Jossey-Bass.

Farquhar, S. A., Michael, Y. L., & Wiggins, N. (2005). Building on leadership and social capital to create change in 2 urban communities. *American Journal of Public Health, 95*(4), 596–601.

Fawcett, S. B., Paine-Andrews, A., Francisco, V. T., Schultz, J. A., Richter, K. P., Lewis, R. K., . . . Lopez, C. M. (1995). Using empowerment theory in collaborative partnerships for community health and development. *American Journal of Community Psychology, 23*(5), 677–697.

Feighery, E., & Rogers, T. (1990). *How-to guides on community health promotion. Guide 12: Building and maintaining effective coalitions.* Palo Alto, CA: Stanford Health Promotion Resource Center.

Fenner, F., Henderson, D. A., Arita, I., Ježek, Z., & Ladnyi, I. D. (1988). Lessons and benefits. In *History of international public health, Volume 6: Smallpox and its eradication* (pp. 1345–1370). Geneva, Switzerland: World Health Organization.

Fernández, M. E., Gonzales, A., Tortolero-Luna, G., Williams, J., Saavedra-Embesi, M., Chan, W., & Vernon, S. W. (2009). Effectiveness of Cultivando La Salud: A breast and cervical cancer screening education program for low income Hispanic women living in farmworker communities. *Cancer Causes & Control, 99*(5), 936–943.

Fisher, R. (2008). Social action community organizing: Proliferation, persistence, roots and prospects. In M. Minkler (Ed.), *Community organizing and community building for health* (2nd ed., pp. 51–65). New Brunswick, NJ: Rutgers University Press.

Flaspohler, P., Duffy, J., Wandersman, A., Stillman, L., & Maras, M. A. (2008). Unpacking prevention capacity: An intersection of research-to-practice models and community-centered models. *American Journal of Community Psychology, 41*(3–4), 182–196.

Foster-Fishman, P. G., Berkowitz, S. L., Lounsbury, D. W., Jacobson, S., & Allen, N. A. (2001). Building collaborative capacity in community coalitions: A review and integrative framework. *American Journal of Community Psychology, 29*(2), 241–261.

Foster-Fishman, P. G., Nowell, B., & Yang, H. (2007). Putting the system back into systems change: A framework for understanding and changing organizational and community systems. *American Journal of Community Psychology, 39*(3–4), 197–215.

Freeman, R. E. (1984). *Strategic management: A stakeholder approach.* Boston, MA: Pitman.

Freire, P. (1973a). *Education for critical consciousness.* New York, NY: Continuum International.

Freire, P. (1973b). *Pedagogy of the oppressed.* New York, NY: Continuum International.

Freudenberg, N., & Tsui, E. (2014). Evidence, power, and policy change in community-based participatory research. *American Journal of Public Health, 104*(1), 11–14.

Frooman, J., & Murrell, A. J. (2005). Stakeholder influence strategies: The roles of structural and demographic determinants. *Business & Society, 44*(1), 3–31.

Gadotti, M. (1994). Reading Paulo Freire: His life and work. (J. Milton, Trans.). In H. A. Giroux & P. L. McLaren (Series Eds.), *Teacher empowerment and school reform*. New York: State University of New York Press.

Galer-Unti, R. A., Tappe, M. K., & Lachenmayr, S. (2004). Advocacy 101: Getting started in health education advocacy. *Health Promotion Practice, 5*(3), 280–288.

Gamson, W. A. (2004). Bystanders, public opinion, and the media. In D. A. Snow, S. A. Soule, & H. Kriesi (Eds.), *The Blackwell companion to social movements* (pp. 242–261). Oxford, United Kingdom: Blackwell.

Glanz, K., Rimer, B. K., & Viswanath, K. (Eds.). (2015). *Health behavior and health education: Theory, research, and practice* (5th ed.). San Francisco, CA: Jossey-Bass.

Golden, S. D., & Earp, J. A. L. (2012). Social ecological approaches to individuals and their contexts: Twenty years of Health Education & Behavior health promotion interventions. *Health Education & Behavior, 39*(3), 364–372.

Goodson, P. (2009). *Theory in health promotion research and practice: Thinking outside the box*. London, United Kingdom: Jones & Bartlett.

Green, L. W., & Glasgow, R. E. (2006). Evaluating the relevance, generalization, and applicability of research: Issues in external validation and translation methodology. *Evaluation & the Health Professions, 29*(1), 126–153.

Green, L. W., & Kreuter, M. W. (2005). *Health program planning: An educational and ecological approach* (4th ed.). New York, NY: McGraw-Hill Professional.

Green, L. W., Poland, B. D., & Rootman, I. (2000). The settings approach to health promotion. In B. D. Poland, L. W. Green, & I. Rootman (Eds.), *Settings for health promotion: Linking theory and practice* (pp. 1–43). Thousand Oaks, CA: Sage.

Greenhalgh, T., Robert, G., Macfarlane, F., Bate, P., & Kyriakidou, O. (2004). Diffusion of innovations in service organizations: Systematic review and recommendations. *Milbank Quarterly, 82*(4), 581–629.

Hawe, P., & Shiell, A. (2000). Social capital and health promotion: A review. *Social Science & Medicine, 51*(6), 871–885.

Hearld, L. R., & Alexander, J. A. (2014). Governance processes and change within organizational participants of multi-sectoral community health care alliances: The mediating role of vision, mission, strategy agreement and perceived alliance value. *American Journal of Community Psychology, 53*(1–2), 185–197.

Hernandez, M. Y., & Organista, K. C. (2013). Entertainment–education? A fotonovela? A new strategy to improve depression literacy and help-seeking behaviors in at-risk immigrant Latinas. *American Journal of Community Psychology, 52*(3–4), 224–235.

Hogan, B. E., Linden, W., & Najarian, B. (2002). Social support interventions: Do they work? *Clinical Psychology Review, 22*(3), 381–440.

Holt-Lunstad, J., & Uchino, B. N. (2015). Social support and health behavior. In K. Glanz, B. K. Rimer, & K. Viswanath (Eds.), *Health behavior: Theory, research, and practice* (5th ed., pp. 183–204). San Francisco, CA: Jossey-Bass.

Huberman, A. M., & Miles, M. B. (1984). *Innovation up close: How school improvement works.* In L. Susskind (Series Ed.), Environment, Development, and Public Policy. New York, NY: Plenum Press.

Islam, M. K., Merlo, J., Kawachi, I., Lindström, M., & Gerdtham, U. G. (2006). Social capital and health: Does egalitarianism matter? A literature review. *International Journal for Equity in Health, 5,* 3.

Israel, B. A., Checkoway, B., Schulz, A., & Zimmerman, M. (1994). Health education and community empowerment: Conceptualizing and measuring perceptions of individual, organizational, and community control. *Health Education & Behavior, 21*(2), 149–170.

Jackson, C., Fortmann, S. P., Flora, J. A., Melton, R. J., Snider, J. P., & Littlefield, D. (1994). The capacity-building approach to intervention maintenance implemented by the Stanford Five-City Project. *Health Education Research, 9*(3), 385–396.

Jibaja-Weiss, M. L., & Volk, R. J. (2007). Utilizing computerized entertainment education in the development of decision aids for lower literate and naive computer users. *Journal of Health Communication, 12*(7), 681–697.

Jin, B., & Lee, S. (2013). Enhancing community capacity: Roles of perceived bonding and bridging social capital and public relations in community building. *Public Relations Review, 39*(4), 290–292.

Jones, B. D. (2003). Bounded rationality and political science: Lessons from public administration and public policy. *Journal of Public Administration Research and Theory, 13*(4), 395–412.

Jones, K. [Kathryn], Baggott, R., & Allsop, J. (2004). Influencing the national policy process: The role of health consumer groups. *Health Expectations, 7*(1), 18–28.

Jones, K. [Kenneth] T., Gray, P., Whiteside, Y. O., Wang, T., Bost, D., Dunbar, E., ...Johnson, W. D. (2008). Evaluation of an HIV prevention intervention adapted for black men who have sex with men. *American Journal of Public Health, 98*(6), 1043–1050.

Juvonen, J., & Graham, S. (2014). Bullying in schools: The power of bullies and the plight of victims. *Annual Review of Psychology, 65,* 159–185.

Kahn-Marshall, J. L., & Gallant, M. P. (2012). Making healthy behaviors the easy choice for employees: A review of the literature on environmental and policy changes in worksite health promotion. *Health Education & Behavior, 39*(6), 752–776.

Kawachi, I. (2006). Commentary: Social capital and health: Making the connections one step at a time. *International Journal of Epidemiology, 35*(4), 989–993.

Kawachi, I., & Berkman, L. (2000). Social cohesion, social capital, and health. In L. F. Berkman & I. Kawachi (Eds.), *Social epidemiology* (pp. 174–190). New York, NY: Oxford University Press.

Kegler, M. C., & Swan, D. W. (2011). An initial attempt at operationalizing and testing the Community Coalition Action Theory. *Health Education & Behavior, 38*(3), 261–270.

Kelly, J. A. (2004). Popular opinion leaders and HIV prevention peer education: Resolving discrepant findings, and implications for the development of effective community programmes. *AIDS Care, 16*(2), 139–150.

Kennelly, B., O'Shea, E., & Garvey, E. (2003). Social capital, life expectancy and mortality: A cross-national examination. *Social Science & Medicine, 56*(12), 2367–2377.

Kickbusch, I. (2009). Policy innovations for health. In I. Kickbusch (Ed.), *Policy innovations for health* (pp. 1–22). New York, NY: Springer.

Kingdon, J. W. (2003). *Agenda, alternatives, and public policies* (2nd ed.). New York, NY: Longman.

Klitzman, S., Kass, D., & Freudenberg, N. (2008). Coalition building to prevent childhood lead poisoning: A case study from New York City. In M. Minkler (Ed.), *Community organizing and community building for health* (2nd ed., pp. 314–328). New Brunswick, NJ: Rutgers University Press.

Kok, G., Gottlieb, N. H., Commers, M., & Smerecnik, C. (2008). The ecological approach in health promotion programs: A decade later. *American Journal of Health Promotion, 22*(6), 437–442.

Kok, G., Gottlieb, N. H., Panne, R., & Smerecnik, C. (2012). Methods for environmental change; An exploratory study. *BMC Public Health, 12*, 1037.

Kok, G., Gurabardhi, Z., Gottlieb, N. H., & Zijlstra, F. R. H. (2015a). Influencing organizations to promote health: Applying stakeholder theory. *Health Education & Behavior, 42*(1S) 123S–132S.

Kok, G., Zijlstra, F. R. H., & Ruiter, R. A. C. (2015b). Changing environmental conditions impacting health—A focus on organizations. In R. J. Burke & A. M. Richardsen (Eds.), *Corporate wellness programs: Linking employee and organizational health* (pp. 28–58). Cheltenham, United Kingdom: Edward Elgar.

Kreuter, M. E., Casey, C. M., & Bernhardt, J. M. (2012). Enhancing dissemination through marketing and distribution systems: A vision for public health. In R. C. Brownson, G. A. Colditz, & E. K. Proctor (Eds.), *Dissemination and implementation research in health: Translating science to practice* (pp. 213–224). New York, NY: Oxford University Press.

Kübler, D. (2001). Understanding policy change with the Advocacy Coalition Framework: An application to Swiss drug policy. *Journal of European Public Policy, 8*(4), 623–641.

Labonte, R. (2004). Community, community development, and the forming of authentic partnerships: Some critical reflections. In M. Minkler (Ed.), *Community organizing and community building for health* (2nd ed., pp. 82–96). New Brunswick, NJ: Rutgers University Press.

Laumann, E. O., & Knoke, D. (1987). *The organizational state: Social choice in national policy domains.* Madison: University of Wisconsin Press.

Leeman, J., Teal, R., Jernigan, J., Reed, J. H., Farris, R., & Ammerman, A. (2014). What evidence and support do state-level public health practitioners need to address obesity prevention. *American Journal of Health Promotion, 28*(3), 189–196.

Lehmann, U., & Gilson, L. (2013). Actor interfaces and practices of power in a community health worker programme: A South African study of unintended policy outcomes. *Health Policy and Planning*, *28*(4), 358–366.

Lewin, K. (1947). Quasi-stationary social equilibria and the problem of social change. In T. M. Newcomb, & E. L. Hartley (Eds.), *Readings on social psychology* (pp. 73–117). New York, NY: Holt, Rinehart & Winston.

Lewin, S. A., Dick, J., Pond, P., Zwarenstein, M., Aja, G., van Wyk, B., . . . Patrick, M. (2005). Lay health workers in primary and community health care. *Cochrane Database of Systematic Reviews*, *1*, CD004015.

Lochner, K. A., Kawachi, I., Brennan, R. T., & Buka, S. L. (2003). Social capital and neighborhood mortality rates in Chicago. *Social Science & Medicine*, *56*(8), 1797–1805.

Longest, B. B., Jr. (2006). *Health policymaking in the United States* (4th ed.). Chicago, IL: Health Administration Press.

Luke, D. A., & Stamatakis, K. A. (2012). Systems science methods in public health: Dynamics, networks, and agents. *Annual Review of Public Health*, *33*, 357–376.

Mabry, P. L., Milstein, B., Abraido-Lanza, A. F., Livingood, W. C., & Allegrante, J. P. (2013). Opening a window on systems science research in health promotion and public health. *Health Education & Behavior*, *40*(1S), 5S–8S.

Manning, M. A., Bollig-Fischer, A., Bobovski, L. B., Lichtenberg, P., Chapman, R., & Albrecht, T. L. (2014). Modeling the sustainability of community health networks: Novel approaches for analyzing collaborative organization partnerships across time. *Translational Behavioral Medicine*, *4*(1), 46–59.

Martinson, M., & Su, C. (2012). Contrasting organizing approaches: The "Alinksy tradition" and Freirian organizing approaches. In M. Minkler (Ed.), *Community organizing and community building for health and welfare* (3rd ed., pp. 59–77). New Brunswick, NJ: Rutgers University Press.

Mayfield-Johnson, S., Rachal, J. R., & Butler, J., III. (2014). "When we learn better, we do better": Describing changes in empowerment through photovoice among community health advisors in a breast and cervical cancer health promotion program in Mississippi and Alabama. *Adult Education Quarterly*, *64*(2), 91–109.

McAlister, A., Johnson, W., Guenther-Grey, C., Fishbein, M., Higgins, D., & O'Reilly, K. (2000). Behavioral journalism for HIV prevention: Community newsletters influence risk-related attitudes and behavior. *Journalism & Mass Communication Quarterly*, *77*(1), 143–159.

McCullum, C., Pelletier, D., Barr, D., Wilkins, J., & Habicht, J. P. (2004). Mechanisms of power within a community-based food security planning process. *Health Education & Behavior*, *31*(2), 206–222.

McDaniel, R. R., Jr. (1997). Strategic leadership: A view from quantum and chaos theories. *Health Care Management Review*, *22*(1), 21–37.

McDaniel, R. R., Jr., Jordan, M. E., & Fleeman, B. F. (2003). Surprise, surprise, surprise! A complexity science view of the unexpected. *Health Care Management Review*, *28*(3), 266–278.

McDonald, M., Sarche, J., & Wang, C. C. (2004). Using the arts in community organizing and community building. In M. Minkler (Ed.), *Community organizing and community building for health* (2nd ed., pp. 346–364). New Brunswick, NJ: Rutgers University Press.

McKinlay, J. B., & Marceau, L. D. (2000). To boldly go… *American Journal of Public Health, 90*(1), 25–33.

McLeroy, K. R., Gottlieb, N. H., & Heaney, C. A. (2001). Social health in the workplace. In M. P. O'Donnell (Ed.), *Health promotion in the workplace* (3rd ed., pp. 459–486). Albany, NY: Delmar.

Menashe, C. L. & Siegel, M. (1998). The power of a frame: An analysis of newspaper coverage of tobacco issues—United States, 1985–1996. *Journal of Health Communication, 3*(4), 307–325.

Mendes, R., Plaza, V., & Wallerstein, N. (2014). Sustainability and power in health promotion: Community-based participatory research in a reproductive health policy case study in New Mexico. *Global Health Promotion.* Advance online publication. doi:1757975914550255

Milio, N. (1981). *Promoting health through public policy.* Philadelphia, PA: F. A. Davis Company.

Milio, N. (2001). Glossary: Healthy public policy. *Journal of Epidemiology and Community Health, 55,* 622–623.

Minkler, M. (2004). Community organizing with the elderly poor in San Francisco's Tenderloin district. In M. Minkler (Ed.), *Community organizing and community building for health* (2nd ed., pp. 272–288). Piscataway, NJ: Rutgers University Press.

Minkler, M., Pies, C., & Hyde, C. (2012). Ethical issues in community organizing and capacity building. In M. Minkler (Ed.), *Community organizing and community building for health and welfare* (3rd ed., pp. 110–129). New Brunswick, NJ: Rutgers University Press.

Minkler, M., & Wallerstein, N. (2012). Improving health through community organization and community building: Perspectives from health education and social work. In M. Minkler (Ed.), *Community organizing and community building for health and welfare* (3rd ed., pp. 37–58). New Brunswick, NJ: Rutgers University Press.

Mitchell, C. U., & LaGory, M. (2002). Social capital and mental distress in an impoverished community. *City & Community, 1*(2), 199–222.

Moore, A., Peele, P. J., Simán, F. M., & Earp, J. A. (2012). Lay health advisors make connections for better health. *North Carolina Medical Journal, 73*(5), 392–393.

Moyer-Gusé, E. (2008). Toward a theory of entertainment persuasion: Explaining the persuasive effects of entertainment-education messages. *Communication Theory, 18*(3), 407–425.

Mŭkoma, W., & Flisher, A. J. (2004). Evaluations of health promoting schools: A review of nine studies. *Health Promotion International, 19*(3), 357–368.

Murayama, H., Fujiwara, Y., & Kawachi, I. (2012). Social capital and health: A review of prospective multilevel studies. *Journal of Epidemiology, 22*(3), 179–187.

Naaldenberg, J., Vaandrager, L., Koelen, M., Wagemakers, A.-M., Saan, H., & de Hoog, K. (2009). Elaborating on systems thinking in health promotion practice. *Global Health Promotion, 16*(1), 39–47.

National Cancer Institute. (2007). *Greater than the sum: Systems thinking in tobacco control (Publication No.* 06-6085, Tobacco Control Monograph No. 18). Bethesda, MD: U.S. Department of Health and Human Services, National Institutes of Health, National Cancer Institute.

Nutbeam, D. (1998). Health promotion glossary. *Health Promotion International, 13*(4), 349–364.

O'Donnel, M. P. (2014). *Health promotion in the workplace* (4th ed.). North Charleston, SC: CreateSpace Independent Publishing Platform.

Orum, A. M. (1988). Political sociology. In N. J. Smelser (Ed.), *Handbook of sociology* (pp. 393–423). Newbury Park, CA: Sage.

Palmer, C. A., Baucom, D. H., & McBride, C. M. (2000). Couple approaches to smoking cessation. In K. B. Schmaling & T. G. Sher (Eds.), *The psychology of couples and illness: Theory, research, & practice* (pp. 311–336). Washington, DC: American Psychological Association.

Park, E. W., Tudiver, F., Schultz, J. K., & Campbell, T. (2004). Does enhancing partner support and interaction improve smoking cessation? A meta-analysis. *Annals of Family Medicine, 2*(2), 170–174.

Paton, K., Sengupta, S., & Hassan, L. (2005). Settings, systems and organization development: The Healthy Living and Working Model. *Health Promotion International, 20*(1), 81–89.

Petraglia, J. (2007). Narrative intervention in behavior and public health. *Journal of Health Communication, 12*(5), 493–505.

Pluye, P., Potvin, L., Denis, J. L., & Pelletier, J. (2004). Program sustainability: Focus on organizational routines. *Health Promotion International, 19*(4), 489–500.

Portes, A. (1998). Social capital: Its origins and applications in modern sociology. *Annual Review of Sociology, 24,* 1–24.

Preyde, M., & Ardal, F. (2003). Effectiveness of a parent "buddy" program for mothers of very preterm infants in a neonatal intensive care unit. *Canadian Medical Association Journal, 168*(8), 969–973.

Pronyk, P. M., Harpham, T., Busza, J., Phetla, G., Morison, L. A., Hargreaves, J. R., . . . Porter, J. D. (2008). Can social capital be intentionally generated? A randomized trial from rural South Africa. *Social Science & Medicine, 67*(10), 1559–1570.

Putnam, R. D. (1995). Bowling alone: America's declining social capital. *Journal of Democracy, 6*(1), 65–78.

Ramirez, A. G., Villarreal, R., McAlister, A., Gallion, K. J., Suarez, L., & Gomez, P. (1999). Advancing the role of participatory communication in the diffusion of cancer screening among Hispanics. *Journal of Health Communication, 4*(1), 31–36.

Randolph, K. A., Whitaker, P., & Arellano, A. (2012). The unique effects of environmental strategies in health promotion campaigns: A review. *Evaluation and Program Planning*, 35(3), 344–353.

Ray, M. L., Wilson, M. M., Wandersman, A., Meyers, D. C., & Katz, J. (2012). Using a training-of-trainers approach and proactive technical assistance to bring evidence based programs to scale: An operationalization of the interactive systems framework's support system. *American Journal of Community Psychology*, 50(3–4), 415–427.

Reininger, B. M., Barroso, C. S., Mitchell-Bennett, L., Cantu, E., Fernandez, M. E., Gonzalez, D. A.,...McAlister, A. (2010). Process evaluation and participatory methods in an obesity-prevention media campaign for Mexican Americans. *Health Promotion Practice*, 11(3), 347–357.

Rhodes, S. D., Foley, K. L., Zometa, C. S., & Bloom, F. R. (2007). Lay health advisor interventions among Hispanics/Latinos: A qualitative systematic review. *American Journal of Preventive Medicine*, 33(5), 418–427.

Richard, L., Gauvin, L., & Raine, K. (2011). Ecological models revisited: Their uses and evolution in health promotion over two decades. *Annual Review of Public Health*, 32, 307–326.

Rogers, E. M. (1983). *Diffusion of innovations* (3rd ed.). New York, NY: Free Press.

Rogers, E. M. (2003). *Diffusion of innovations* (5th ed.). New York, NY: Free Press.

Romero, D., Kwan, A., & Chavkin, W. (2013). Application of empirical research findings in public health advocacy: Focus on maternal, child, and reproductive health. *Journal of Social Issues*, 69(4), 633–644.

Roter, D. L., Rudd, R. E., Keogh, J., & Robinson, B. (2006). Worker produced health education material for the construction trades. *International Quarterly of Community Health Education*, 27(3), 231–243.

Rothman, J. (2008). Multi modes of community intervention. In: J. Rothman, J. L. Ehrlich, & J. E. Tropman (Eds.), *Strategies of community intervention* (7th ed., pp. 141–170). Peosta, Iowa: Eddie Bowers.

Sabatier, P. A. (2007). The need for better theories. In P. A. Sabatier (Ed.), *Theories of the policy process* (2nd ed., pp. 3–17). Boulder, CO: Westview Press.

Schein, E. H. (2004). *Organizational culture and leadership* (3rd ed.). San Francisco, CA: Jossey-Bass.

Schein, E. H. (2010). *Organizational culture and leadership* (4th ed.). San Francisco, CA: Jossey-Bass.

Shen, F., & Han, J. (2014). Effectiveness of entertainment education in communicating health information: A systematic review. *Asian Journal of Communication*, 24(6), 605–616.

Shigayeva, A., & Coker, R. J. (2014). Communicable disease control programmes and health systems: An analytical approach to sustainability. *Health Policy and Planning*, 30(3), 368–385.

Simons-Morton, B., McLeroy, K. R., & Wendel, M. L. (2011). *Behavior theory in health promotion practice and research*. Burlington, MA: Jones & Bartlett Learning.

Smelser, N. J. (1998). Social structure. In N. J. Smelser (Ed.), *Handbook of sociology* (pp. 103–130). Newbury Park, CA: Sage.

Smith, K. P., & Christakis, N. A. (2008). Social networks and health. *Annual Review of Sociology, 34,* 405–429.

Snow, D. A., Soule, S. A., & Kriesi, H. (2004). Mapping the terrain. In D. A. Snow, S. A. Soule, & H. Kriesi (Eds.), *Blackwell companion to social movements* (pp. 3–16). Oxford, United Kingdom: Blackwell.

Steckler, A., Goodman, R. M., & Kegler, M. (2002). Mobilizing organizations for health enhancement: Theories of organizational change. In K. Glanz, B. K. Rimer, & F. M. Lewis (Eds.), *Health behavior and health education: Theory, research, and practice* (3rd ed., pp. 335–360). San Francisco, CA: Jossey-Bass.

Szreter, S., & Woolcock, M. (2004). Health by association? Social capital, social theory, and the political economy of public health. *International Journal of Epidemiology, 33*(4), 650–667.

Taylor, V., & Van Dyke, N. (2004). "Get up, stand up": Tactical repertoires of social movements. In D. A. Snow, S. A. Soule, & H. Kriesi (Eds.), *Blackwell companion to social movements* (pp. 262–293). Oxford, United Kingdom: Blackwell.

Tessaro, I. A., Taylor, S., Belton, L., Campbell, M. K., Benedict, S., Kelsey, K., & DeVellis, B. (2000). Adapting a natural (lay) helpers model of change for worksite health promotion for women. *Health Education Research, 15*(5), 603–614.

Themba-Nixon, M., Minkler, M., & Freudenberg, N. (2008). The role of CBPR in policy advocacy. In M. Minkler & N. Wallerstein (Eds.), *Community-based participatory research for health: From process to outcomes* (2nd ed., pp. 307–322). San Francisco, CA: Jossey-Bass.

Tolli, M. V. (2012). Effectiveness of peer education interventions for HIV prevention, adolescent pregnancy prevention and sexual health promotion for young people: A systematic review of European studies. *Health Education Research, 27*(5), 904–913.

Turner, J. C. (2005). Explaining the nature of power: A three-process theory. *European Journal of Social Psychology, 35*(1), 1–22.

Uphoff, E. P., Pickett, K. E., Cabieses, B., Small, N., & Wright, J. (2013). A systematic review of the relationships between social capital and socioeconomic inequalities in health: A contribution to understanding the psychosocial pathway of health inequalities. *International Journal for Equity in Health, 12,* 54.

Usher, C. (2006). Social capital and mental health in the urban south, USA: A qualitative study. In K. McKenzie & T. Harpham (Eds.), *Social capital and mental health* (pp. 109–123). Philadelphia, PA: Jessica Kingsley.

Valente, T. W. (2012). Network interventions. *Science, 337*(6090), 49–53.

Valente, T. W. (2015). Social networks and health behavior. In K. Glanz., B. K. Rimer, & K. Viswanath (Eds.), *Health behavior: Theory, research, and practice* (5th ed., pp. 205–222). San Francisco, CA: Jossey-Bass.

Van Beurden, E. K., Kia, A. M., Zask, A., Dietrich, U., & Rose, L. (2013). Making sense in a complex landscape: How the Cynefin Framework from Complex Adaptive Systems Theory can inform health promotion practice. *Health Promotion International, 28*(1), 73–83.

van Empelen, P., Kok, G., Schaalma, H. P., & Bartholomew, L. K. (2003a). An AIDS risk reduction program for Dutch drug users: An intervention mapping approach to planning. *Health Promotion Practice, 4*(4), 402–412.

van Empelen, P., Kok, G., van Kesteren, N. M. C., van den Borne, B., Bos, A. E. R., & Schaalma, H. P. (2003b). Effective methods to change sex-risk among drug users: A review of psychosocial interventions. *Social Science & Medicine, 57*(9), 1593–1608.

Viswanathan, M., Kraschnewski, J., Nishikawa, B., Morgan, L. C., Thieda, P., Honeycutt, A., ... Jonas, D. (2009). *Outcomes of community health worker interventions* (Rep. No. 181). Rockville, MD: Agency for Healthcare Research and Quality (AHRQ).

Wallack, L. (2008). Media advocacy: A strategy for empowering people and communities. In M. Minkler (Ed.), *Community organizing and community building for health* (2nd ed., pp. 419–432). New Brunswick, NJ: Rutgers University Press.

Wallack, L., Dorfman, L., Jernigan, D., & Themba, M. (1993). *Media advocacy and public health: Power for prevention*. Newbury Park, CA: Sage.

Wallerstein, N., Minkler, M., Carter-Edwards, L., Avila, M., & Sánchez, V. (2015). Improving health through community engagement, community organization, and community building. In K. Glanz, B. K. Rimer, & K. Viswanath (Eds.), *Health behavior: Theory, research, and practice* (5th ed., pp. 277–300). San Francisco, CA: Jossey-Bass.

Wallerstein, N., Sanchez, V., & Velarde, L. (2004). Freirian praxis in health education and community organizing: A case study of an adolescent prevention program. In M. Minkler (Ed.), *Community organizing and community building for health* (2nd ed., pp. 218–236). New Brunswick, NJ: Rutgers University Press.

Wandersman, A., Chien, V. H., & Katz, J. (2012). Toward an evidence-based system for innovation support for implementing innovations with quality: Tools, training, technical assistance, and quality assurance/quality improvement. *American Journal of Community Psychology, 50*(3–4), 445–459.

Wandersman, A., Duffy, J., Flaspohler, P., Noonan, R., Lubell, K., Stillman, L., ... Saul, J. (2008). Bridging the gap between prevention research and practice: The interactive systems framework for dissemination and implementation. *American Journal of Community Psychology, 41*(3–4), 171–181.

Wang, C. C. (2003). Using photovoice as a participatory assessment and issue select tool: A case study with the homeless in Ann Arbor. In M. Minkler & N. Wallerstein (Eds.), *Community-based participatory research for health* (pp. 179–196). San Francisco, CA: Jossey-Bass.

Wang, C. C., Yi, W. K., Tao, Z. W., & Carovano, K. (1998). Photovoice as a participatory health promotion strategy. *Health Promotion International, 13*(1), 75–86.

Wang, H., & Singhal, A. (2009). Entertainment-education through digital games. In U. Ritterfield, M. Cody, & P. Vorderer (Eds.), *Serious games: Mechanisms and efforts* (pp. 271–292). New York, NY: Routledge.

Weber, M. (1947). *The theory of social and economic organization* (Vol. 1). New York, NY: Oxford University Press.

Webster, J., Dunford, E., Kennington, S., Neal, B., & Chapman, S. (2014). Drop the salt! Assessing the impact of a public health advocacy strategy on Australian government policy on salt. *Public Health Nutrition, 17*(1), 212–218.

Weible, C. M., Sabatier, P. A., & McQueen, K. (2009). Themes and variations: Taking stock of the Advocacy Coalition Framework. *Policy Studies Journal, 37*(1), 121–140.

Weick, K. E., & Quinn, R. E. (1999). Organizational change and development. *Annual Review of Psychology, 50*, 361–386.

Weitzman, E. R., & Kawachi, I. (2000). Giving means receiving: The protective effect of social capital on binge drinking on college campuses. *American Journal of Public Health, 90*(12), 1936–1939.

Wendel, M. L., Burdine, J. N., McLeroy, K. R., Alaniz, A., Norton, B., & Felix, M. R. J. (2009). Community capacity: Theory and application. In R. J. DiClemente, R. A. Crosby, & M. C. Kegler (Eds.), *Emerging theories in health promotion practice and research* (2nd ed., pp. 277–302). San Francisco, CA: Jossey-Bass.

Wethington, E., & Pillemer, K. (2014). Social isolation among older people. In R. C. Coplan & J. C. Bowker (Eds.), *The handbook of solitude: Psychological perspectives on social isolation, social withdrawal, and being alone* (pp. 242–259). Chichester, United Kingdom: Wiley Blackwell.

Whitelaw, S., Baxendale, A., Bryce, C., MacHardy, L., Young, I., & Witney, E. (2001). "Settings" based health promotion: A review. *Health Promotion International, 16*(4), 339–353.

Wiggins, N. (2012). Popular education for health promotion and community empowerment: A review of the literature. *Health Promotion International, 27*(3), 356–371.

Wilkin, H. A., Valente, T. W., Murphy, S., Cody, M. J., Huang, G., & Beck, V. (2007). Does entertainment-education work with Latinos in the United States? Identification and the effects of a telenovela breast cancer storyline. *Journal of Health Communication, 12*(5), 455–469.

Williams, R. M., Jr. (1970). *American society: A sociological interpretation* (3rd ed.). New York, NY: Alfred A. Knopf.

Williams, W. (2004). The cultural contexts of collective action: Constraints, opportunities and the symbolic life of social movements. In D. A. Snow, S. A. Soule, & H. Kriesi (Eds.), *The Blackwell companion to social movements* (pp. 91–115). Oxford, United Kingdom: Blackwell.

Wilson, P. A. (1997). Building social capital: A learning agenda for the twenty-first century. *Urban Studies, 34*(4–5), 745–760.

Wilson, P. A., & Lowery, C. (2003). Building deep democracy: The story of a grassroots learning organization in South Africa. *Planning Forum, 9*, 47–64.

Woodall, J. R., Warwick-Booth, L., & Cross, R. (2012). Has empowerment lost its power? *Health Education Research, 27*(4), 742–745.

World Health Organization. (1986). Ottawa charter for health promotion. Presented at the International Conference on Health Promotion, Ottawa, Canada. Retrieved from http://www.euro.who.int/__data/assets/pdf_file/0004/129532/Ottawa_Charter.pdf?ua=1

World Health Organization Regional Office for Europe. (2002). Community partici-
pation in local health and sustainable development: Approaches and techniques.
Retrieved from http://www.euro.who.int/__data/assets/pdf_file/0013/101065/
E78652.pdf

Yoo, S., Butler, J., Elias, T. I., & Goodman, R. M. (2009). The 6-step model
for community empowerment: Revisited in public housing communities for
low-income senior citizens. *Health Promotion Practice, 10*(2), 262–275.

Zahariadis, N. (2007). The multiple streams framework: Structure, limitations,
prospects. In P. A. Sabatier (Ed.), *Theories of the policy process* (2nd ed.,
pp. 65–92). Boulder, CO: Westview Press.

Zimmerman, B. J., Lindberg, C., & Plsek, P. E. (1998). *Edgeware: Insights from
complexity science for health care leaders*. Irving, TX: VHA Publishing.

Zimmerman, M. A. (2000). Empowerment theory: Psychological, organizational,
and community levels of analysis. In J. Rappaport & E. Seidman (Eds.),
*Handbook of community psychology* (pp. 43–64). New York, NY: Kluwer
Academic/Plenum.

Zimmerman, M. A., Stewart, S. E., Morrel-Samuels, S., Franzen, S., & Reischl, T. M.
(2011). Youth Empowerment Solutions for Peaceful Communities: Combining
theory and practice in a community-level violence prevention curriculum.
*Health Promotion Practice, 12*(3), 425–439.

PART TWO

# INTERVENTION MAPPING STEPS

# INTERVENTION MAPPING STEP 1

*Logic Model of the Problem*

## Competency

* Develop a logic model of the factors that cause or influence the health problem that will be the focus of the intervention.

The purpose of this chapter is to enable the reader to conduct a needs assessment to create a logic model of the problem and to facilitate participation by those who will be affected by the resulting program. Intervention Mapping or any other health education program planning effort must be based on a thorough assessment of community capacity and needs. This assessment encompasses two components:

1. an epidemiologic, behavioral, and social perspective of a community or population at risk for health-related problems, and

2. an effort to understand the intervention target population, the program setting, and the character of the community, its members, and its strengths.

In the first part of the chapter, we discuss preassessment planning, which includes putting together a work group for intervention development. We touch on essential elements of encouraging participation, work-group management, and culturally sensitive practice.

The needs assessment includes creating a logic model of the problem from data about the health problem, its impact on quality of life, and its behavioral and environmental causes. For this purpose, we present the PRECEDE part of the PRECEDE-PROCEED model (Green & Kreuter, 2005). We also describe how to define the population,

### LEARNING OBJECTIVES AND TASKS

* Establish and work with a planning group

* Conduct a needs assessment to create a logic model of the problem

* Describe the context for the intervention, including the population, setting, and community

* State program goals

potential setting and context for the intervention, and context for the assessment, as well as how to ask questions and choose data sources for each part of the logic model of the problem. Following a focus on the needs or problems, we discuss ways to assess characteristics of the target population and community strengths. Finally, we discuss the postassessment needs, including setting priorities and setting program goals for health and related outcomes.

## Perspectives

Our perspectives in this chapter highlight the importance of needs assessment and a consideration of community strengths as a part of intervention planning.

### Needs Assessment as Part of Intervention Planning

A needs assessment, the first part of intervention planning, is a systematic study of the discrepancy between what is and what should be in a group and situation of interest (Gilmore & Campbell, 2005). A statement of need is a statement of a problem—it does not, either purposefully or inadvertently, suggest a solution (Altschuld & Kumar, 2010). For example, suggesting that a community needs a new gymnasium to facilitate increased physical activity conflates needs and solutions. Gilmore and Campbell (2005) suggest that planners, in addition to focusing on needs rather than solutions, should not worry too much about the difference between "real" need and perceived need because needs are always changing in character and quantity, and because reports and assessments of needs are always interpreted by someone (Gilmore & Campbell, 2005).

Sometimes the term *formative research* is used in literature to describe a needs assessment conducted for the purpose of contributing to the development of a program (Bellows, Anderson, Gould, & Auld, 2008; Vu, Murrie, Gonzalez, & Jobe, 2006; Young et al., 2006; Zapka, Lemon, Estabrook, & Jolicoeur, 2007). Gittelsohn et al. (2006) argue that formative work is important for understanding determinants of health behavior. Formative evaluation can refer specifically to pretesting, or testing the appropriateness of a program or the program materials (see Chapter 7).

A needs assessment helps planners understand "what is" and compare the current status to one that is more desirable in terms of quality of life, health, behavior, and environment. Needs assessments of health problems include an analysis of the physiological risk factors and behavioral and environmental risks to health, even when the actual health problems constitute a possible future event. For example, cardiovascular disease is a health problem with contributing risks of current high-serum cholesterol levels—a physiological risk factor; intake of high-fat foods—a behavioral risk factor; and poor access to healthful foods—an environmental risk factor.

A health-related needs assessment includes the assessment of the determinants of behavior and environmental contributors to health problems or health risks. Determinants are those biological, psychological, and social factors found to be associated with the behavior or environmental condition that has caused or influenced the health problem (Green & Kreuter, 2005). The implication for intervention is that determinants are causally related to the behavior and environmental conditions. However, even though the logic is causal, the empirical evidence may not be, because some studies on determinants are correlational and cross-sectional in nature. Furthermore, determinants should be modifiable. Psychological factors such as thoughts (beliefs) and feelings toward a targeted behavior are typically amenable to change, as they originate from personal experiences and information resources such as formal education, mass media, the Internet, and social interactions with family, friends, and peers. Personality characteristics and biological and social factors (e.g., genetics or demographic characteristics) are generally not changeable or are difficult to change, but they may influence the experiences people have and how they interpret or recall this information. Thus, they are important in the process of selecting and segmenting a target group selection (see Chapter 5; Fishbein & Ajzen, 2010; Green & Kreuter, 2005).

In summary, a needs assessment should present a full description of a problem in as much detail and complexity as can be ascertained within the boundaries of the project. Even though planners may need to narrow their focus at various times during intervention planning, planners should begin by fully analyzing the problem and its multiple causes.

## Partnering With the Community

Studying the strengths of a community can help the health educator keep in mind a community's unique character and its ability to plan its own interventions. An attitude of partnership between health professionals and community members can help prevent a top-down or outsider planning approach (Minkler, 1997, 2012; Minkler, Wallerstein, & Wilson 2008). Furthermore, a focus on community competencies and resources from the outset of program planning, along with the participation of community members, directs attention to the need for enhancing community capacity in program development, implementation, and maintenance (Cargo & Mercer, 2008; Israel et al., 2003; Teufel-Shone, Siyuja, Watahomigie, & Irwin, 2006). All too often, health education and other social programs, especially research and demonstration efforts, have entered communities only to leave them with limited impact on community health status (Goodman & Steckler, 1989; Merzel & D'Afflitti, 2003). Programs that aim to enhance capacity from the start of planning can make this scenario less likely to develop (Hawe, King, Noort, Gifford, & Lloyd, 1998).

## Tasks for Step 1

## Establishing and Working With a Planning Group

### *Ensuring Participation in Program Planning*

The first task in Step 1 is to establish and work with a planning group that includes program stakeholders.

Intervention Mapping draws on many principles already set forth very well by others regarding participation in intervention planning (Belansky, Cutforth, Chavez, Waters, & Bartlett-Horch, 2011; Horn, McCracken, Dino, & Brayboy, 2008; Israel et al., 2003). Participation by community members, potential program implementers, and program beneficiaries helps ensure that a project addresses issues important to the community and the potential program participants, that project outcomes and evaluation findings are locally relevant, and that participating stakeholders develop the capacity for intervention development and evaluation research (Teufel-Shone et al., 2006). All health promotion program development and evaluation should be based on the meaningful participation of stakeholders (Bryant, Altpeter, & Whitelaw, 2006; Centers for Disease and Control and Prevention Program Performance and Evaluation Office, 2012; Israel et al., 2003; Yoo, Butler, Elias, & Goodman, 2009). Meaningful participation can be encouraged in a variety of different planning contexts, which might be described on a continuum where at one end the health educator and planning group work *with* the community and implementers to understand the health problem and its solution, and at the other end the community members *are* the planners and the planning becomes a part of the intervention, as in a community-empowerment model (Blair & Minkler, 2009; Fisher et al., 1994; Hugentobler, Israel, & Schurman, 1992).

Planning should always be earnestly collaborative. Principles of collaboration include the following project characteristics, as described by multiple authors (Cargo & Mercer, 2008; Christopher, Watts, McCormick, & Young, 2008; Green & Kreuter, 2005; Israel et al., 2003; Krieger et al., 2002; Minkler, 2005; Wallerstein & Duran, 2006):

- Acknowledge personal and institutional histories
- Recognize the community as a unit of identity and promote community involvement from the beginning of the project
- Achieve a balance between knowledge generation and intervention in locally important public health problems for mutual benefit of all partners

- Plan from an ecological perspective that recognizes and attends to the multiple determinants of health

- Involve systems development using a cyclical and iterative process

- Disseminate results to all partners and involve them in the dissemination process

- Facilitate collaborative, equitable influence on the direction and activities of the project through all or most phases

- Make sure that the project results in learning, capacity building, and sustainability

- Show respect for the expertise, values, perspectives, contributions, and confidentiality of everyone in the community

- Allot time and resources to group function

- Compensate community participants

Members of the group with the health risk or problem—the priority or at-risk population—are important stakeholders to be included in the planning group. The philosophy of health education is built on the principle of self-determination, an individual's governance of his or her own behavior (Allegrante & Sleet, 2004). Many examples exist of community members participating in all aspects of planning, from documenting needs (Teufel-Shone et al., 2006) to developing program materials (Edgren et al., 2005; Kannan et al., 2008) and implementing programs (Fernández, Gonzales, Tortolero-Luna, Partida, & Bartholomew, 2005a; Lewin et al, 2010).

**Composing and Maintaining Project Work Groups**    At least one well-functioning work group will be necessary to plan and complete a needs assessment, and then to develop, implement, and evaluate a program. Good work-group management is a foundational approach to true participation in program planning. The initiator of such a group may be a community organization, university research team, government agency, or other entity. Most often, the work group comprises stakeholders who have an interest in the health problem, program development, and the expected outcomes of the program. Community stakeholders might be residents, leaders from organizations and government, and service providers (Krieger et al., 2002). Other stakeholders may include professional organizations, third-party payers, media, voluntary health agencies, and academic institutions (Fawcett et al., 2000).

In a guide to engaging stakeholders in program evaluations, Preskill and Jones (2009) present many helpful suggestions for identifying and working with stakeholders, which can apply throughout the life of a project. Table 4.1 presents questions to guide the identification of stakeholders

**Table 4.1**    Questions to Guide Recruitment of Stakeholders

| Planning Group Need | Questions to Consider |
| --- | --- |
| Expertise in the health problem or its causes | Who has content knowledge relative to the health problem or its causes? |
| | What disciplines can be most helpful in describing problems from an ecological perspective? |
| | Who knows about similar problems? |
| | Who is well respected for knowledge of this health problem or ones like it? |
| | Who has worked on a similar needs assessment or program? |
| Diverse perspectives and community participation | Who has needs and perspectives related to the problem? |
| | When programs are developed related to needs and problems, who are the potential clients, participants, or beneficiaries? |
| | Who already works with potential beneficiaries? |
| | Who can help the planning group clarify values related to the needs assessment and intervention development? |
| | Who can help the planning group balance science, social relevance, and cultural relevance? |
| | Who are the potential critics of the program or initiative? |
| Responsibility and authority | Who will manage the needs assessment and program development? |
| | Who is the funder? |
| | Who can become a partner in the assessment and program development? |
| | Who can bring resources to the endeavor? |
| Influence | Who has served as a resource to community members for this problem or related ones? |
| | What policy makers have worked on this type of problem? |
| | Who are opinion leaders who might have an interest in this type of problem? |
| | Who can help the planning team access expertise and other resources of the community? |
| | Who can garner support and buy-in to the project? |
| Commitment to the issue | Who will want to help the needs assessment team develop and disseminate its conclusions? |
| | Who might advocate for the assessment and intervention development? |
| | Who has been working on the problem from a practice perspective? |
| | Who has been working on the problem form a research perspective? |
| | Who could bring creative energy to the project? |

for a needs assessment (Cargo & Mercer, 2008; Preskill & Jones, 2009). Having stakeholders work together can bring a variety of perspectives and knowledge, nurture feelings of project ownership, and contribute to cultural sensitivity. The intended recipients and implementers of a program are best able to interpret the needs and perspectives of the cultural groups to which they belong.

Project leaders may need to reassess and enhance work group membership at various times in the program development process. In beginning each new step of Intervention Mapping, the planning group provides a good opportunity for a quick assessment of whether all the needed stakeholders are "at the table." Planners must keep asking how well they know and are communicating with those whom the intervention is meant to affect, and they must continue to build relationships based on listening and sharing in order to move to ever-higher levels of understanding. Orlandi and colleagues have described a work group as a linkage system between a resource system (program developers), an intermediate-user system (implementers), and an end-user system (participants) (Orlandi, 1986, 1987; Orlandi, Landers, Weston, & Haley, 1990). Especially, as the planning group begins to think about how a program might be delivered, it needs to assess whether all the elements of a linkage system are present in the work group to assure that, once a program is developed, it can be adopted, fully implemented, and maintained.

Many interventions are developed and evaluated with the possibility of wider dissemination once a program is shown to be effective. One aspect of developing programs with an eye to future dissemination is including potential dissemination partners as a part of the initial work group (Glasgow, Marcus, Bull, & Wilson, 2004). For example, in the school-based It's Your Game . . . Keep It Real project, described at the end of this chapter (It's Your Game Box 4.2), and in Chapters 5, 6, 7, 8, and 9, representatives from the local school district administration were included on the initial work group with a view to future dissemination. Once the intervention was proven effective, representatives from additional school districts were invited to join the work group to further scale up implementation.

In addition to at-risk population partnerships, health educators must build linkages with potential program implementers (Bonham, Sommerfild, Willging, & Aarons, 2014; Damschroder, Aron, Keith, Kirsh, Alexander, & Lowery, 2009; Rubenstein & Pugh, 2006). Even though the implementers are not usually the focus of the needs assessment, when the logic model of the problem is being created, they may be an important source of information about both the problem and the community. The person who works with a health problem, rather than the individuals who have the health problem, may be the first contact for the health educator—the physician or nurse for a chronic disease, the emergency medical service for injuries, the HIV counselor for AIDS. These key informants may have very different perspectives on a problem than those of the potential program recipients. For example, in planning health services for the homeless, physicians, workers at homeless shelters, and members of the city council may all be important key informants. These stakeholders are likely to have different viewpoints from each other and from the homeless themselves. We discuss the concept of implementers in more detail in Chapter 8, which covers program adoption and implementation.

## Using Group Management Processes for Productive Groups

Once a work group is put together, it must be managed over time to facilitate successful completion of each step in the Intervention Mapping process. Health promoters will need certain skills, including those used in interpersonal communication and group facilitation. Group process skills are briefly covered here, but the successful health promotion professional will need to pursue further training to learn and practice group skills. To get started, a group will define members' responsibilities, choose a basic structure, decide how to make decisions, agree to tasks, and propose a time line (Centers for Disease Control and Prevention & Oak Ridge Institute for Science and Education, 2003). For some work, groups will function as a whole; for other tasks, members may break into a variety of smaller working and advisory groups.

Effective groups distribute active, two-way communication among group members, rather than strictly to and from group members and the leader (See Table 4.2; Johnson & Johnson, 2012). Leadership and responsibility for group function is also distributed, including group generation of goals and agendas. Furthermore, goals should be fluid and reflect both individual and group needs. Group cohesion is advanced through high levels of problem-solving competence, inclusion, affection, acceptance, support, and trust.

**Facilitation**    Every task group has two necessary types of activities: those related to the work at hand and those related to group process (Bradford, 1976). Project tasks are whatever must be accomplished to do the group's work. However, unless the relationships among group members, feelings of inclusivity, group norms, predictability of procedures, and issues of participation and trust are addressed through group maintenance and team building, the group's work will suffer. The application of good task-management skills can also facilitate group team building and maintenance, which often happen simultaneously with tasks but also sometimes require dedicated group time, effort, and skills (Becker, Israel, & Allen, 2005; Bradford, 1976). Table 4.2 describes processes that can be practiced to develop a work group that matures to a team capable of producing a better program than any one team member could create alone. The list in Table 4.2 does not include processes for diagnosing and dealing with group problems. Using the skills in Table 4.2 routinely will help the work group avoid many problems, and we encourage the reader to pursue in-depth training in group management and process to attain the skills to manage group problems.

Group management is built on listening to others' ideas with a willingness to review and make transparent for group review one's own assumptions about the health problem and its solutions (Senge, 2006). With this as a starting place, practicing the processes in Table 4.2 can lead

**Table 4.2**    Group Facilitation Processes

| Process | Description |
|---|---|
| **Communication** | |
| Owning a statement | Using first-person singular pronouns (I or me) |
| Completeness and specificity | Clearly stating all necessary information, including the context or frame of reference, intention or goal, and assumptions |
| Congruence | Making verbal and nonverbal communication congruent |
| Redundancy | Using more than one channel of communication (written, oral, or graphic) to clarify meaning |
| Requesting feedback | Asking for information about how a communication is being understood |
| Frame of reference | Making the communication appropriate to the receiver's frame of reference |
| Feelings | Describing feelings by name |
| Describing behavior | Describing behavior of another person without evaluating or interpreting |
| **Task Functions** | |
| Developing the agenda | Enabling the group to list activities, set priorities, and budget time |
| Initiating | Beginning a discussion that includes both substantive offerings (such as the background of an issue) and methodological offerings (such as the suggestion to begin by brainstorming) |
| Information seeking | Eliciting pertinent information by asking for information, keeping issues from closing prematurely, encouraging members to speak, accepting both people and ideas |
| Opinion giving | Allowing opinions to be freely given and valued by the group as coming from the members' experience |
| Elaboration | Asking for elaboration on a partially stated idea |
| Coordination | Joining together ideas from two or more members (ideas that might seem disparate at first) |
| Partializing | Pointing out the fine differences between two ideas that might seem the same at first glance |
| Evaluating | Evaluating ideas but not people |
| Structuring | Deciding and facilitating the ways in which a group can work, such as by using subgroups |
| Energizing | Moving a group through a "stuck" point by restructuring the work or process. For example, introducing a process such as brainstorming, using humor, expressing feeling, or giving or getting feedback |
| Summarizing | Summing up the points, progress, and needs of the group orally in the meeting and in meeting notes, summaries, and action items after the meeting |
| Synthesizing | Making meaning of various ideas expressed in the group |
| **Maintenance and Team-Building Functions** | |
| Gatekeeping | Making opportunities for participation by the less talkative members of the group |
| Encouraging | Encouraging members to participate in the group |
| Harmonizing | Seeking common goals or common ground in a conflict |
| Consensus seeking | Modifying group decisions and plans until group members are relatively comfortable and supportive |
| Giving feedback | Sharing with the whole group a direct, specific, immediate description of the impact of group or individual communication |
| Standard setting | Setting and revisiting group norms regarding efficiency, fairness, power, and communication |
| Processing | Setting aside the final minutes of a meeting for reviewing how the work progressed and how it can be improved |

to a productive work group. The set of individual communication behaviors in the table is from Johnson and Johnson (2012), whereas the group management behaviors are from Bradford (1976), Sampson and Marthas (1990), and Toseland and Rivas (2008).

Other important considerations for working in participatory groups are the facilitation of power equity and inclusive decision making (Johnson and Johnson, 2012). Effective participatory groups are more likely than less effective groups to base power and influence on ability and information rather than position. The groups learn how to equalize influence by explicitly setting group norms and using facilitation processes. Group decision-making procedures should be handled predominantly by consensus and should match the various task situations the work group encounters. A note on evidence: One dilemma that arises in part from the focus on scientific evidence in the work that health promotors do is the tendency to inadvertently devalue contributions from nonacademics in work groups. In this context, some people may feel less confident or less empowered than others to make contributions. As mentioned in Chapter 1, potential answers for every question come from several types of information: theoretical and empirical evidence, practice, and lived experience. Group members can use group processes to allow and encourage ideas and information from many sources.

The types of groups that we are talking about will move back and forth between three types of work group functions within each step of Intervention Mapping: idea generation, decision making, and product development. A hallmark of productive work groups is the ability to generate many ideas from both the most accessible information and experience available to members and from less used and less available experience. Using all of the ideas and data available, groups also have to make decisions and choose goals and direction. Finally, based on decisions, groups produce programs, their components, and an evaluation plan. All of these types of work are crucial to a project's success, and moving between them is a hallmark of effective group function.

The time required for both idea generation and decision-making processes can vary from a few minutes to a few months. A work group needs structure and guidance to produce the end products for each Intervention Mapping step. The tools for keeping the group on track throughout the development, implementation, and evaluation process include participatory meeting agendas, detailed time lines, processes for goal setting, and time in each meeting for debriefing on how the group is progressing.

**Processes for Idea Generation**    Although all work groups will have times when they conduct semistructured meetings and "do work," they also have times, in each Intervention Mapping step, when the important activity is generating ideas. A number of structured processes can help facilitate smooth group functioning. Some of these techniques are structured to avoid judging the merit of ideas so that many ideas are generated. They also help stimulate all group members to participate.

- **Brainstorming or Free Association** encourages group members to generate and record unedited ideas in response to a question. Seeing group members' ideas recorded on a large pad or board serves to prime individual member's idea generation (Buunk & Van Vugt, 2013; Nijstad & Stroebe, 2006; Preskill & Jones, 2009).

- **Nominal Group Technique** is also enacted in response to a posed question, but the ideas are generated independently by each member and then shared one at a time (Delbecq, 1983; Moon, 1999). This prevents group members taking turns (production blocking), which interferes with idea-generation processes (Nijstad & Stroebe, 2006). For the needs assessment, the question might be, "In this neighborhood, what health threat concerns you the most?" Following individual brainstorming, members give answers to the question one at a time, round-robin style. The facilitator records the answers, using a board or large pad. After the list of answers is clarified, group members make preliminary rankings, which they record and discuss. Group members then vote a second time, yielding a final prioritization (Baheiraei, Mirghafourvand, Mohammadi, Charandabi, & Nedjat, 2013; Gilmore & Campbell, 2005). A more formal approach to this process—concept mapping—uses multidimensional scaling and cluster analysis to develop a visual display of themes or categories (Anderson, Day, & Vandenberg, 2011; McFall et al., 2009; Trochim & Kane, 2005). In a less formal approach to categorization, referred to as off-the-wall thinking, individuals write their answers to a single question on Postit notes, and—one at a time—post their notes on a wall or whiteboard in emergent theme categories. Those members who post later offer category modifications to the group based on additions that change the content and meaning of categories and their boundaries. These techniques not only equalize participation but also enable the planner to leave the meeting with lists of answers to the posed question rather than the voluminous transcripts that result from focus groups.

- **Responding to a Paper or Presentation of Evidence** is an efficient way for a planning group to move between steps of Intervention Mapping. For example, data and information from the needs assessment can be presented to the group to enable decisions about what should change and the development of matrices (See Chapter 5). This process was effective in a project to develop an intervention to enable Hispanic and African American men to make informed decisions regarding prostate cancer screening. Team members collected and analyzed data to assess needs in two geographically distant sites. Group members met face to face, shared the findings from the assessments, and, based on presentations from multiple working groups, moved rapidly through Intervention Mapping Step 2, designing a logic model of change (Bartholomew et al., 2010; Chan et al., 2011).

**Processes for Consensus**    Consensus is the process of choice for most decisions made by a health promotion planning team. Most decisions require group members to weigh and understand evidence regarding a certain course of action and to argue the various group decisions based on that evidence. Voting and majority rule are not usually effective for health promotion planning, because they do not encourage full discussion or use minority opinion in the decision-making process. A desire to put a question to a vote in a work group usually indicates a premature closure of deliberation on an issue. To work to consensus, group members need to listen—to seek differences of opinion among the members; help each interested person clearly, fully, and persuasively present a position; critically consider all positions presented; encourage members' willingness to change their minds when they have been logically persuaded of the merit of someone else's argument; tolerate and even encourage intellectual conflict and avoid premature closure of arguments; and focus on the goal of reaching the best possible decision (Johnson & Johnson, 2012). Consensus is not unanimity—group members must be willing to support a decision about an approach, but they do not necessarily need to be enthusiastic about every group decision.

Well-functioning groups make the best decisions possible by embracing conflict in ways that build on and extend the consensus process. Group members proceed through the following process: gathering and organizing information to clarify a problem or a need for a decision; presenting various positions, answers, or alternatives; hearing from members with opposing views; actively acknowledging conceptual conflict and uncertainty; seeking more information to understand the situation from opposing perspectives; and synthesizing ideas presented in the conflict to state a new proposition or answer (Johnson & Johnson, 2012).

### Considering Culture in the Work of the Group

In Chapter 1 we briefly touched on a goal for practice: developing a perspective of cultural humility (Tervalon & Murray-Garcia, 1998). Now we will suggest some ways of preparing oneself to work interculturally (Wilson & Miller, 2003). The thread of discussion regarding the inextricable tie between understanding cultural influences and developing culturally appropriate programs and materials will be picked up again in Chapter 7, where we discuss cultural representations in program development.

The first process in beginning health promotion practice in general, and any one project in particular, is to consider the community and its cultural groups and subgroups, and to make sure that these groups are represented on the planning team. In order to address priority health issues effectively, health educators must develop culturally appropriate programs. Furthermore, culture is not an issue of race and ethnicity alone. Ethnicity is but one of several group designations that act to define enduring aspects of a group culture.

**Exploring Personal Ethnocentricity**   Becoming involved in planning with the potential program participants or beneficiaries is only a beginning; a second aspect is continuing personal development to be able to work both across and within cultures. This personal work involves listening deeply to the people with whom one is working as well as actively exploring one's personal ethnocentrism (Sue, 2003). Locke (1986, 1992) offers the following set of questions as a guide to first steps in developing cultural self-awareness:

- What is my cultural heritage? What was the culture of my parents and grandparents? With what cultural group do I identify?

- What is the cultural relevance of my name?

- What values, beliefs, opinions, and attitudes do I hold that are consistent with the dominant culture? Which are inconsistent? How did I learn these? For example, for someone in the United States, these cultural beliefs might include beliefs in success, the inherent value of work, moral orientation, material comfort, personality and individuality, science and rationality, efficiency, and democracy (Williams, 1970).

- How did I decide to be a [health] educator? What cultural standards were involved in the process? What do I understand to be the relationship between culture and [health] education?

- What unique abilities, aspirations, expectations, and limitations do I have that might influence my relations with culturally diverse individuals?

Through a process of suspending and then observing one's habitual ways of relating to other groups and then observing one's typical ways of seeing and relating to others, a person can move through stages to attain greater cultural awareness, sensitivity, or even humility. The stages may include:

1. feelings of fear, hostility, defensiveness, and superiority

2. denial of cultural differences

3. cultural acceptance and respect

4. empathy

5. integration, multiculturalism, and social justice (Bennett, 1993; Borkan & Neher, 1991; Brown & Mazza, 1997; Rios, McDaniel, & Stowell, 1998).

As next steps, one might structure opportunities in the working group to disclose personal backgrounds, including those related to privilege and power (Tervalon & Murray-Garcia, 1998; Wallerstein & Duran, 2006).

**Exploring and Working in Another Culture**   Only the person who becomes more aware of his or her ethnocentric lens can effectively explore and work in another culture. Another absolute prerequisite is the ability to identify and embrace the positive aspects of that culture (Airhihenbuwa & Liburd, 2006). One way of clearly identifying the positive aspects of a culture as they are related to health is the PEN-3 model (Airhihenbuwa, 1995, 1999; Kannan et al., 2009). In this model, the planner considers three domains of culture. The first domain, cultural identity, defines the priority population through a consideration of extended families and communities as well as individuals. The second domain, relations and expectations, considers aspects of the culture that can affect health and behavior, including perceptions, enablers (community, societal, and structural factors), and nurturers (social support networks such as family, friends, and community members). The third dimension, cultural empowerment, suggests the valence of the relations and perceptions as either positive, negative, or existential (neither positive nor negative) in relation to health (Airhihenbuwa & Webster, 2004; Fitzgibbon & Beech, 2009).

Triandis (1994) presents a different structure for looking at cultures. He describes the cultural syndromes of individualism versus collectivism, complexity versus simplicity, and tightness versus looseness. In an individualist culture, the wishes of the individual are highly prioritized, whereas in a collectivist culture, the group and its needs are paramount. In a tight culture, there is considerable agreement about norms of correct behavior. Understanding elements of these syndromes may be very helpful for health educators. For example, the role of the group may influence the content of health education messages. If a culture focuses on group wants, the message may be directed differently than it would be in a culture in which the individual is emphasized. The strong influence of norms and role-relevant goals in collectivist cultures makes for greater interdependence and embeddedness of social behavior. It may be much more difficult and basically ineffective for someone of a collectivist culture to participate in a program that is solely oriented toward the individual.

Ford and Airhihenbuwa (2010) propose the explicit consideration of racism in health promotion—both in explaining disparities and in intervention development. They propose the analytic framework of critical race theory (Bonilla-Silva, 2006; L. Graham, Brown-Jeffy, Aronson, & Stephen 2011; Thomas, Quinn, Butler, Fryer, & Garza, 2011) as a lens through which to consider racism as a determinant of disparities in health. Key concepts in the theory are race consciousness, or the explicit consideration of the possible influence of race and racism as determinants of behavior and health at the individual, interpersonal, community, and societal levels; centering in the margins, which is the focus of discourse from within the perspective of the marginalized group rather than from the majority viewpoint; and contemporary mechanisms of racism as pervasive and ordinary rather than aberrational (Ford and Airhihenbuwa, 2010).

## BOX 4.1. MAYOR'S PROJECT

Looking in on the health department director and the health promoter, we see the two are struggling with how to keep the planning group moving. The health promoter worries that although the mayor handpicked the planning group, it is not representative enough of the diverse neighborhoods in the city. The planning group may not include some of the project's important stakeholders. She wants permission to add interested community members to the planning group during the needs assessment.

*Health promoter:* Adding more community people will be good for the group and good for planning. We need many diverse perspectives to work effectively on the problem of obesity.

*Health department director:* Yes, but too large a committee is too hard to handle.

*Health promoter:* These will be the people who understand the problem firsthand. And they will also be the people who will ensure successful implementation of whatever program we come up with. Besides, sometimes when people don't feel included, they can sabotage our efforts.

*Health department director:* Okay, I'll get the mayor's approval, but I trust you to really manage this group. Better make sure your group leadership skills are not rusty. I don't have to tell you how anxious the mayor is to see something happening. I know, I know! You say we have to do a needs assessment. I'm convinced, but is the needs-assessment process going to give us the visibility we need? Can we just think of how to do this assessment so that it is clear to everyone that we are actually making progress?

*Health promoter:* Yes, since we talked the last time, I've been thinking about this. We need both qualitative and quantitative evidence about this problem. We also need information from our own community as well as from studies conducted elsewhere. We need information about obesity and its context, but we also need a real feel for the strengths of these communities. What if we could make the complexity work for us in two ways? Maybe the group can function as several smaller teams. Some people will go after the scientific literature. We have some talented library researchers on the team. Another group will get out into the community and talk to people. That will keep us visible. It also will help us balance our examination of needs and strengths. We could structure short interim reports based on our needs-assessment model and present them across the teams and to the mayor as we go along.

*Health department director:* That sounds good. Now that we have that settled, let's get started.

## Conducting a Needs Assessment

The second task in Intervention Mapping Step 1 is to plan and conduct the needs assessment using the PRECEDE model (Green & Kreuter, 2005) to analyze health and quality-of-life problems and their causes.

Before delving into assessment, the planner and the work group will need to plan how to assess the health problem or need (Altschuld & Kumar, 2010). To help us guide the assessment, we use a modified PRECEDE model (Figure 4.1; Green & Kreuter, 2005). A population-based epidemiologic planning framework that is also ecological in perspective, the model can help the planning group figure out what it already knows about the problem and the community along with what further information is needed. Planners conduct needs assessments by using the core processes introduced in Chapter 1. At each part of the needs assessment logic model, the planner will pose questions; brainstorm or figure out what the planning group already knows in relation to the posed question; search the literature for empirical evidence and evaluate the strength of the evidence; access and use theory when appropriate, such as when questions concern determinants; conduct new research; and develop a final summary of answers to the posed questions. PRECEDE is a very useful framework for organizing these questions and the resulting data.

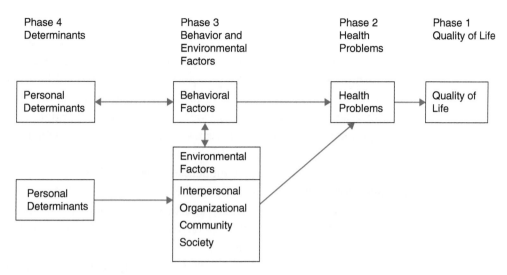

| Phase 4 Determinants | Phase 3 Behavior and Environmental Factors | Phase 2 Health Problems | Phase 1 Quality of Life |

**Figure 4.1**  Logic Model of the Problem

## Understanding PRECEDE as a Logic Model

The model can help the group define the problem, the ecological levels that affect the problem, and the stakeholders who will have opinions and information about both the problem and its solution (Foster-Fishman, Nowell, & Yang, 2007). The lived experience of stakeholders (e.g., community members, program implementers) is as important as the knowledge of experts in assessment of the problem (Foster-Fishman et al., 2007; Midgley, 2006).

The PRECEDE model prescribes an analysis of causation of health problems at multiple ecological levels and the consideration of multiple determinants of health-related behavior and environment. For example, such health problems as coronary artery disease have both behavioral risk factors, such as eating high-cholesterol foods, and environmental causes, such as the unavailability of exercise facilities. The editions of the PRECEDE model, of which there are several, clarify and amplify the important role of both social and physical environment in the causation of health problems (Green & Kreuter, 1991, 1999, 2005). The model has been used as the basis for health education planning in hundreds of programs (see Aboumatar et al., 2012; Buta et al., 2011; Cole & Horacek, 2009; Hazavei, Sabzmakan, Hasanzadeh, Rabiei, & Roohafza, 2012; Li, et al., 2009; Wasilewski, Mateo, & Sidorovsky, 2007; Wright, McGorry, Harris, Jorm, & Pennell, 2006).

The logic model of the problem is developed from right to left, usually beginning with social and epidemiological descriptions of quality-of-life and health problems. When completed, the model is read from left to right as a causal model of the health problem and quality of life. Reducing or eliminating the health problems addressed in the model should be the intention of a health education or promotion intervention. For example, if a planning group wants to address premature mortality and morbidity from cardiovascular disease, the group may also be interested in related quality-of-life issues, such as loss of productive years and the burden of heart disease. Next, the planners would support the description of the health problem and quality-of-life issues with data and would begin finding evidence of behavioral and environmental causes.

Moving to the left in the model, the behavioral analysis typically includes what people do that increases their risk of experiencing the health problem. In the case of secondary and tertiary prevention, the analysis investigates what people do that increases the risk of disability or death from an existing health problem.

The environmental analysis includes conditions in the social and physical environments that influence the health problem directly or through its behavioral causes. In most health problems, the environment plays a significant and modifiable role in causing the problem, either directly, such as air pollution in lung disease, or indirectly through behavior, such as availability of correct medication to prevent and manage an asthma attack and the social norms to consistently use preventive medications for chronic disease.

The next analysis should be of the personal determinants of behavior of the at-risk population and individuals who can influence environmental conditions (i.e., environmental agents). Personal determinants reside at the individual level and include factors such as knowledge, attitudes, beliefs, values, perceptions, and skills that influence behavior (see Chapter 2; Bartholomew & Mullen, 2011; Green & Kreuter, 2005).

A consideration in completing the needs assessment is where to begin in the logic model development: On the far-right side, with assessing the quality of life in the community? With health problems or risks? With behavioral or environmental causes? Although the PRECEDE logic develops the model from right to left, health promotion planners are often unable to enter the model by performing a quality-of-life assessment for a community because their assignment or focus is on a health problem or risk behavior or environmental condition. The agencies that employ the planners are often funded, at least in part, with categorical funds designated for one disease or risk (e.g., cardiovascular disease or smoking). We are often directed to look at needs and problems in terms of the funding or employer's specific focus. The health educator who works for a cancer agency focuses on cancer. The health educator who works for an AIDS agency focuses on HIV. These are health problems, and health educators have entered the assessment model at the health analysis phase. Perhaps, though, the health educator works for the American Cancer Society or the American Lung Association on a tobacco project. The health educator in these instances has entered the assessment model at the behavioral-analysis phase. It is perfectly legitimate to begin in the middle of the assessment model with a behavioral or environmental risk so long as there is strong epidemiologic evidence for the causal relation between the risk and one or more health problems. No matter where a health educator begins the needs assessment, he or she will need to cover all the model's phases, including the relation of health to quality of life. The emphasis on covering all phases of the model, regardless of where health educators begin, is based on the assumption that health is related to quality of life, and that behavior and environment are related to health.

### Describing the Priority Population

The first question in a needs assessment may be "What is the health problem?" but it also may be "Who is the priority population?" Often the needs assessment moves back and forth between these two questions to determine the population at risk (or population in need) and to fully describe problems and causes. The need to define the population at risk requires an epidemiologically and demographically defined population. Precisely defining whom an intervention is meant to affect—who will benefit from the program—enables the planner to know the numerator, or the people who actually participate in the program, and the denominator, or the population for whom the program is intended (Glasgow, Vogt, & Boles, 1999).

The designation "population at risk" refers to a group with a definable boundary and shared characteristics that has or is at risk for having certain health and quality-of-life problems; has health problems and is at risk for the sequelae; or has an identified need for an intervention that will enable individuals to prevent disease or promote their health. The boundaries of the priority population will help define the scope of the needs assessment.

To lay the foundation for intervention, planners will also be concerned with the environmental context of the at-risk group. The environment may contribute directly to the health problem, as in the case of drinking contaminated water causing diarrhea. The influence can also be more indirect, such as the contribution of social networks to the continuation of smoking. We suggest four levels of analysis of the environmental context:

- Interpersonal
- Organizational
- Community
- Societal

The interpersonal level refers to individuals or groups that have close connections to members of the priority population and are likely to have an influence on their health-related behavior. Examples include family members, peers, teachers, and health care providers. At this level, important factors that may influence behavior are role models, norms, reinforcement, and social support.

Organizations are systems with specific objectives and with formal multilevel decision-making processes. Schools, stores, clinics, hospitals, professional associations, and companies are examples (Richard, Potvin, Kishchuk, Prlic, & Green, 1996). Communities in Richard's description require a geographical area comprising people and organizations. Locus is the most commonly cited characteristic of community (MacQueen et al., 2001; Mattessich, Murray-Close, & Monsey, 2001). A geographic community is more than a physical space. It is a social place shared by individuals in units such as families, neighborhoods, and clubs and by organizations such as civic groups, churches, local media, and local government (McKnight, 2012). Groups within a geographic boundary—such as a city, village, or town—usually share a sense of living or working in a location as well as some common elements of values, culture, norms, language, and problems of health and quality of life (Institute of Medicine, 2002). Members of these geographic communities will have perceptions of boundaries, appropriate representatives, and concerns or problems (Sullivan et al., 2003). Communities are systems in which people link together in social networks that can contribute both to causes and cures for health problems. Further, communities—including environmental elements, such as the built environment—are garnering attention for their role in both the cause and maintenance of health risks and their role in potential solutions (Economos, 2007).

We include within communities other groups that exhibit relationships and experience a sense of community among the members of a group whose members may or may not share physical boundaries (Chavis & Wandersman, 1990; Fellin, 1995; Kraft, Beeker, Stokes, & Peterson, 2000; McMillan & Chavis, 1986). In addition to geopolitical boundaries, there are demographic boundaries (e.g., socioeconomic status, gender, age, and family structure) and demographic-ethnic boundaries (e.g., Latino, European American, African American, and Dutch of Surinamese origin). The PEN-3 model offers a set of constructs for moving beyond the labeling of priority groups by race or ethnicity and can help health educators understand cultural factors that can influence both the causes and solutions of health problems (Fitzgibbon & Beech, 2009; Kannan et al., 2009; Scarinci, Bandura, Hidalgo, & Cherrington, 2012).

There are also groups with other shared characteristics, such as people with a certain disease or those served by the same agency. Kraft and colleagues (2000) described community in terms of being with people you identify with and feel similar to because they have the same values, beliefs, and habits. A community may also be a group coming together for a cause or political agenda (Eng & Parker, 1994). Also, people with shared characteristics link together in Internet communities without regard to geographic proximity (Batenburg & Das, 2014; Frost & Massagli, 2008; Hospers, Kok, Harterink, & de Zwart, 2005; Oh & Lee, 2012; Richards & Tangney, 2006; Rier, 2007). Of course, the population may be defined by a combination of variables, such as adults with cystic fibrosis who speak English and live in North America or adolescents ages 13 to 16 who live in the inner city and are at risk for HIV and other sexually transmitted infections (STIs). The important issue is that the populations and their communities are well defined during the assessment process (Altschuld & Kumar, 2010; Gilmore & Campbell, 2005).

Societies are larger systems possessing the means to control several aspects of the lives and development of their constituent systems. Examples of societies are provinces, states, and countries (Richard et al., 1996). We also include in this environmental level multinational structures, such as the European Union, and even global corporations, which certainly have characteristics of community and have even been called living institutions (Senge, 2006).

The broad scope of the environmental context of health problems suggests not only complex causation of health and illness but also the need for health education and promotion interventions on a variety of levels and at a variety of venues (e.g., work sites, schools, communities, and health care organizations). A focal task in performing a needs assessment is to describe the individuals who have the health problem or are at risk of developing the health problem and who, consequently, are the potential beneficiaries of the health-promotion intervention. The at-risk population always is the intended recipient of program benefits such as risk reduction or improvements in health status or quality of life. Therefore, when conducting the needs assessment, the health and quality-of-life analysis is always focused on the population at risk. However, it does not follow that an intervention is always focused on this group. For example, the priority population for behavior could be parents in promoting participation in a national immunization scheme or environmental agents, such as the health care provider in a case of chronic disease management, or organizations and government in a case of primary prevention policy. Also, there may be several targeted groups in a comprehensive, multilevel program, some of whom are populations at risk whereas others are agents that influence the environment.

## Describing Health Problems and Quality of Life

Most health educators begin a needs assessment with some idea of both a health risk or problem and the population groups that have it. They use concepts from epidemiology—the study of the occurrence and distribution of diseases and their risk factors in populations—to further define both the nature of the health problem and the population focused on in the needs assessment in a somewhat interactive process. The basic questions for this process are the following:

- What is the problem?

- Who has it?

- What are the incidence, prevalence, and distribution of the problem?

- What are the demographic characteristics of the population that faces the problem or is at risk for the problem?

- Is there a community? What are its characteristics, including its resources and strengths?

- What segments of the population have an excess burden from the health problem?

- Where can the groups at risk, especially groups at excess risk or excess burden, be reached by a program?

The health educator needs to understand not only the health problem but also how it is exhibited in the particular population of interest and what the health problem or risk means to those who have it. In the process of needs assessment, the health educator will constantly work to understand the groups for whom the program should be a priority. Dimensions of health problems include disability, discomfort, fertility, fitness, morbidity, mortality, and physiological risk factors (Green & Kreuter, 2005). To discover dimensions of the health problem, mostly quantitative data sources are used; whereas to understand the problem's meaning and its quality-of-life effects, qualitative methods may be the most revealing. Dimensions of quality of life include effects of illness on both individual and societal indicators, such as cost of health care, absenteeism, work or school performance, activities of daily living, stigma, isolation and alienation, discrimination, happiness and adjustment, self-esteem, and employment.

The first step is describing demographically who has the health problem and for whom it represents an excess burden. However, the health educator will also need to fully explore the cultural group or groups represented in the priority population beyond a simple description by race or ethnicity (Kreuter, Lukwago, Bucholtz, Clark, & Sanders-Thompson, 2003).

**Rates and Risk**   Risk and rate concepts and statistics are helpful in the process of describing the health problem, and we refer the reader to texts in epidemiology (Friis & Sellers, 2013; Gordis, 2009). The extent of the health problem is usually described as a rate, making possible comparisons among groups and geographic areas as well as judgments of the importance or seriousness of the problem. A rate is the number of events (people with a problem) over a period of time per population of 1,000 or 100,000. A rate can be incidence, the new cases of a problem in a certain time period, or prevalence, the number of existing cases. Usually, both types of rates are needed to fully understand a problem. The number of new cases divided by the number of persons at risk per unit time is the crude incidence rate (Friis & Sellers, 2013; Gordis, 2009).

The importance of rates is that they can be compared across group characteristics and geographic areas to answer questions such as: Is this an important problem in a specific community? Is it more or less prevalent in this community than in other communities? Is it more prevalent than in communities that are demographically similar? Many factors influence rates of a problem. In order to sort out the true extent of a problem in a population, rates may need to be adjusted by demographic variables such as age and gender. Rates are often reported as age-specific and can be weighted to match the age distribution in the population of interest (Gordis, 2009).

Another important concept is that of the probability or risk of developing a disease over time. The term risk is often used to refer to the average risk for a group of people. Because it is a probability, risk is sensitive to the period of time over which observations are made. For example, the risk of developing lung cancer for a smoker increases as the observation period lengthens.

**An Epilepsy Example**   Developers of the clinic-based Management Information Decision-Support Epilepsy Tool (MINDSET) began working on the needs assessment for epilepsy in the Houston metropolitan area, entering the PRECEDE model with the health problem of epilepsy and then exploring related quality-of-life issues (see Figure 4.2.). For more information on MINDSET, see the case study at www.wiley.com/go/bartholomew4e. They partnered with three epilepsy specialty clinics in Houston that provided heterogeneity of clinic type, patient population, and clinician experience. They worked in conjunction with existing epilepsy research programs at these clinics and with the national Managing Epilepsy Well network (Shegog et al., 2013). The developers established a planning group comprising a behavioral scientist, a health economist,

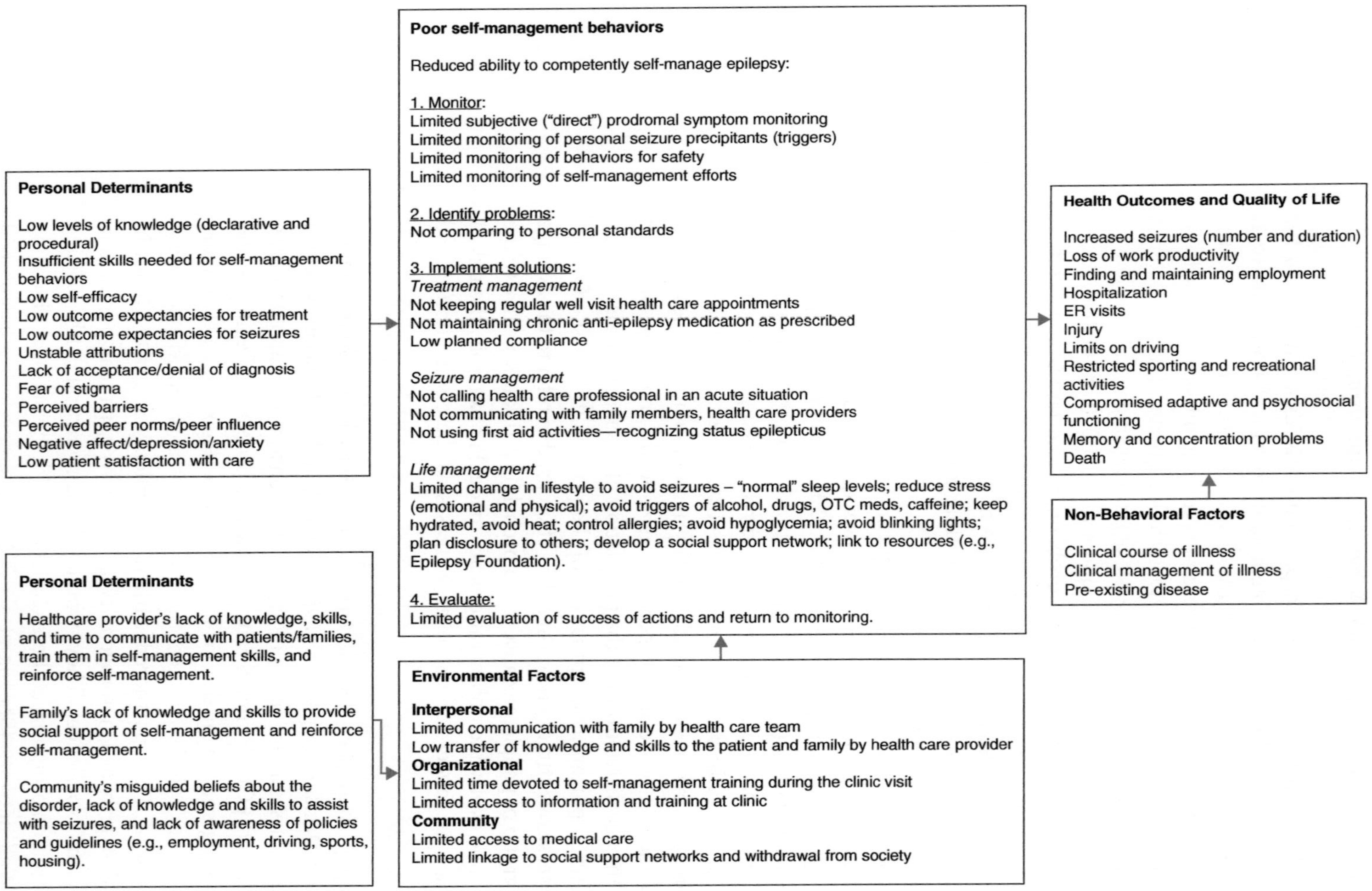

**Poor self-management behaviors**

Reduced ability to competently self-manage epilepsy:

1. Monitor:
Limited subjective ("direct") prodromal symptom monitoring
Limited monitoring of personal seizure precipitants (triggers)
Limited monitoring of behaviors for safety
Limited monitoring of self-management efforts

2. Identify problems:
Not comparing to personal standards

3. Implement solutions:
*Treatment management*
Not keeping regular well visit health care appointments
Not maintaining chronic anti-epilepsy medication as prescribed
Low planned compliance

*Seizure management*
Not calling health care professional in an acute situation
Not communicating with family members, health care providers
Not using first aid activities—recognizing status epilepticus

*Life management*
Limited change in lifestyle to avoid seizures – "normal" sleep levels; reduce stress (emotional and physical); avoid triggers of alcohol, drugs, OTC meds, caffeine; keep hydrated, avoid heat; control allergies; avoid hypoglycemia; avoid blinking lights; plan disclosure to others; develop a social support network; link to resources (e.g., Epilepsy Foundation).

4. Evaluate:
Limited evaluation of success of actions and return to monitoring.

**Health Outcomes and Quality of Life**

Increased seizures (number and duration)
Loss of work productivity
Finding and maintaining employment
Hospitalization
ER visits
Injury
Limits on driving
Restricted sporting and recreational activities
Compromised adaptive and psychosocial functioning
Memory and concentration problems
Death

**Non-Behavioral Factors**

Clinical course of illness
Clinical management of illness
Pre-existing disease

**Personal Determinants**

Low levels of knowledge (declarative and procedural)
Insufficient skills needed for self-management behaviors
Low self-efficacy
Low outcome expectancies for treatment
Low outcome expectancies for seizures
Unstable attributions
Lack of acceptance/denial of diagnosis
Fear of stigma
Perceived barriers
Perceived peer norms/peer influence
Negative affect/depression/anxiety
Low patient satisfaction with care

**Environmental Factors**

**Interpersonal**
Limited communication with family by health care team
Low transfer of knowledge and skills to the patient and family by health care provider
**Organizational**
Limited time devoted to self-management training during the clinic visit
Limited access to information and training at clinic
**Community**
Limited access to medical care
Limited linkage to social support networks and withdrawal from society

**Personal Determinants**

Healthcare provider's lack of knowledge, skills, and time to communicate with patients/families, train them in self-management skills, and reinforce self-management.

Family's lack of knowledge and skills to provide social support of self-management and reinforce self-management.

Community's misguided beliefs about the disorder, lack of knowledge and skills to assist with seizures, and lack of awareness of policies and guidelines (e.g., employment, driving, sports, housing).

**Figure 4.2** Epilepsy PRECEDE Model

neurologists, and specialists in epilepsy care (program developers) as well as nurse educators and health care providers (potential implementers) and epilepsy patients from the participating clinics (end users). Following the core processes regarding the health problem, they asked: What is the prevalence of epilepsy in the United States and in our local community? Does the prevalence or severity vary between individuals of various ages, genders, race or ethnic groups, or socioeconomic statuses? They also wanted to know whether any groups had an excess burden from the disease.

First, they reviewed the literature and found that epilepsy is an important public health problem in the United States. Epilepsy is a neurological condition characterized by recurrent unprovoked seizures. It is the fourth most common neurological disorder in the United States, following migraine, stroke, and Alzheimer's disease (Hirtz et al., 2007). An estimated 2.2 million people in the United States are affected by epilepsy, and approximately 150,000 new cases of epilepsy are diagnosed each year. One in 26 individuals will develop epilepsy at some point in their lifetimes (Institute of Medicine, 2012). Epilepsy is associated with substantially higher rates of mortality than in the general population (Institute of Medicine, 2012). They found that the prevalence of epilepsy was comparable by geographic region—4.0/1000 in the West, 4.4/1000 in the Northeast, 4.9/1000 in the Midwest, and 5.0/1000 in the South (Centers for Disease Control and Prevention, 1994; Theodore et al., 2006). Although epilepsy may start at any age, incidence rates peak before the ages of 5 and after 60. They found that absolute differences in the prevalence of epilepsy by gender were minimal (Banerjee, Filippi, Allen, & Hauser, 2009). A previous study conducted in Houston among health maintenance organization (HMO) enrollees and their families found minimal statistically significant differences in epilepsy incidence by racial/ethnic group. The ethnicity-specific odds ratios for initial unprovoked seizure, using non-Hispanic white as the referent, were 1.04 (0.73–1.49) for African-Americans, 0.97 (0.64–1.48) for Hispanics, and 0.25 (0.08–0.84) for Asian-Americans (Annegers, Dubinsky, Coan, Newmark, & Roht, 1999).

Next, the program planners wanted to understand the impact of epilepsy on quality of life. They asked: How does epilepsy affect the quality of life of individuals living with the condition? How does it impact their activities of daily living, for instance, such as work attendance, risk of injury, utilization of emergency health care services, and hospitalization rates? They also wanted to know how epilepsy contributes to societal indicators such as cost of health care. They found that epilepsy prevalence rates do not fully illustrate the burden of epilepsy on individuals, families, and communities. Epilepsy impacts a wide range of social, physical, and psychological aspects of life and may have a devastating impact on a person's economic and social future, including loss of work productivity, lowered ability to find and maintain employment, high rates of hospitalization, emergency room visits, injuries sustained, limits on driving, restricted sporting and recreational activities, and such types of cognitive dysfunction as memory and concentration problems (Dodson & Trimble, 1994; Institute of Medicine, 2012; Smeets, van Lierop, Vanhoutvin, Aldenkamp, & Nijhuis, 2007). The estimated annual direct medical cost of epilepsy is estimated at $9.6 billion (Institute of Medicine, 2012).

### Describing Possible Causes of Health Problems

Risk factors are those behaviors or environmental conditions that affect the health of populations. The most commonly used measure of the association between exposure to a risk factor and development of a related health problem is relative risk or rate ratio (Gordis, 2009; Kelsey, Whittemore, Evans, & Thompson, 1996). Relative risk is the incidence of the problem in those exposed to the risk factor divided by the incidence of the problem in those not exposed to the risk factor. Another useful statistic is the risk ratio or comparison of probabilities of developing the disease when one is not exposed to the risk factor and when one is exposed (the probability of disease when not exposed divided by the probability of disease when exposed). The risk ratio is particularly applicable when the period of time over which a health problem might develop is fixed, such as the risk of the birth of a low-weight infant.

Another frequently used measure of association is the odds ratio, which is defined in terms of exposure rather than in terms of disease (probability of exposure in the presence of disease divided by the probability of exposure without the presence of disease over the probability of exposure with lack of disease divided by the probability of lack of exposure with lack of disease) (Gordis, 2009; Kelsey et al., 1996).

**Describing Behavior of the At-Risk Group**    Some behaviors of the at-risk group may be causally related to the health problem. For example, a huge body of epidemiologic evidence shows smoking to be associated with both cardiovascular disease and a variety of cancers. Furthermore, as the number of cigarettes smoked increases, the association with cancer increases. This is a dose-response relationship, and is a higher level of epidemiologic evidence. In another example, behavioral risks for HIV transmission include intravenous drug use and unprotected sexual intercourse. When the prevalence of the health problem (or of death from the health problem) and the prevalence of risk factors and the relative risk of acquiring the health problem (or of experiencing mortality from the health problem) are known for a population group, estimates can be made of the proportion of the health problem (or mortality from the health problem) that is attributable to each risk, that is, the attributable fraction (the risk for the exposed minus the risk for the unexposed divided by the risk for the exposed; Kelsey et al., 1996).

**Describing Environmental Risk**   It is helpful to think of environmental factors that influence health directly through disease-causing exposures or indirectly by influencing health-related behavior. These factors can be understood further by ecologic levels, as we have depicted in the PRECEDE-based logic model in Figure 4.1.

Each level of the environment (interpersonal, organizational, community, and societal) can influence both individual behavior and any (lower) level of environment. For example, at the organizational level, health care providers could lack incentives for preventive care. This organizational characteristic could influence providers to omit discussing prevention in the interpersonal interactions with patients (a lower level of environment). In an example of teen alcohol use, peers' reinforcement of teenagers' alcohol use would fall in the interpersonal level of the environment; lack of policy concerning alcohol use at high school parties in the organizational level; social norms for teen drinking in the community level; and laws restricting sales to and possession by minors in the societal level. Individuals with control or authority over social or physical conditions at a given environmental level are referred to as environmental agents. As we shall discuss in Chapter 5, environmental agents may differ from program implementers, and are often themselves the focus of change in a health promotion intervention.

Even though it may be intuitive to think first in terms of the behavior of the at-risk group, the physical and social environment should be a major focus in a needs-assessment study. For example, many authors are studying the effects of environment on physical activity. Growing evidence documents associations between physical environmental factors in a community (e.g., access to trails, parks, and sidewalks) and engagement in physical activity (Ferdinand, Sen, Rahurkar, Engler, & Menachemi, 2012; Taylor et al., 2014). Laws and policies are part of the social environment. Slater and colleagues (2012) found that public elementary schools in the United States were more likely to provide recommended minutes of physical education and recess when states or school districts had a law or policy mandating physical education and recess (Slater, Nicholson, Chriqui, Turner, & Chaloupka, 2012). Fourth-grade students living on the Texas-Mexico border whose families had household rules about limiting the amount of time spent watching television (i.e., family rules) were more likely to meet the American Academy of Pediatrics' recommendation of less than 1–2 hours of TV viewing per day compared to households that did not have TV viewing rules (Springer et al., 2010).

**Behavior and Environment in the Epilepsy Example**     The planners in the epilepsy example (Figure 4.2) next asked: What are the behavioral and environmental contributors to epilepsy morbidity among adults living with the condition? They continued reviewing the literature to understand the behavioral and environmental factors related to epilepsy seizure control and disability. In the behavioral category, lack of adherence to antiseizure medications was a problem, as were failure to monitor and protect against seizure triggers, lack of safety management to minimize the adverse consequences of seizures, and failure to adhere to clinical visit regimens (Buelow, 2001; Institute of Medicine, 2012; Shope, 1988).

At this point the developers used self-management theory to define what individuals might be doing to better care for epilepsy and discovered that researchers and theorists had proposed that self-management steps include monitoring, problem identification, treatment management (e.g., adhering to antiseizure and antidepressant medication regimens), seizure management (e.g., preparation for, and response to, seizure episodes), lifestyle management (e.g., altering behaviors to avoid seizure onset), and evaluation (Buelow, 2001; DiIorio et al., 2004; Institute of Medicine, 2012; Shope, 1988). Many individuals with epilepsy were not following these self-management steps.

However, as they moved to the analysis of environmental factors, they discovered that individuals often did not follow these self-management steps as they had not received guidance from their health care providers. An important aspect of patient self-management is an active partnership between the health care provider, the patient, and the patient's family or significant others to aid in adherence to treatment. Discrepancy between the patient and health care provider regarding the patient's attitudes about epilepsy and their self-management abilities and/or poor communication between the two can undermine the adoption of self-management behavior (Bensing, Roter, & Hulsman, 2003; Clark, 2003; Gilliam et al., 2009). Clinic task analyses and environmental assessment indicated that clinics varied widely in the resources (information, training, educational support) provided as well as the time devoted to patient and provider discussion of self-management issues. Time constraints within the clinic visit often limited the breadth and depth of discussion leading to a focus on epilepsy seziures and medication compliance over other lifestyle self-management domains.

The developers wanted to explore some of these factors in their local area. They conducted surveys with epilepsy patients attending two of the three partnering clinics to assess epilepsy self-management behaviors. The two clinics served socioeconomically diverse populations. About half of participants had experienced an epileptic seizure in the past three months. The developers found that all patients, regardless of socioeconomic status or clinic attended, scored relatively high on individual self-management behaviors related to medication adherence, seizure management, and safety domains, but relatively lower on information and lifestyle domains. Participants also scored relatively low on satisfaction with their health care (Begley et al., 2010).

## Describing Determinants of Behavioral and Environmental Risks

The next part of the needs assessment is asking questions about what factors cause or in some way modify the behavior of the at-risk group or the environmental risks. Here, the planner asks why. Why do members of the at-risk group behave in ways to increase their risk of a health problem? Why do agents in the environment create or maintain unhealthy environmental conditions? We refer to these factors as personal "determinants" because, from an intervention-development perspective, causation is implied. We would not intervene on a factor that was not causing either behavior of the at-risk group or environmental agents. On the other hand, the reality is that the evidence for causation is usually not clear, and planners must weigh the strength and pattern of association between determinants and behavior to judge whether a case for causation can be argued.

Determinants of behavior are factors that rest within the individual (people at risk or environmental agents). These determinants can be changed or modified by interventions that involve influencing how people think about or have the capacity to change a behavior or an environment. In Chapter 2, we described behavior-oriented theories that primarily focus on understanding (and changing) behavior of the at-risk group or environmental agents. In Chapter 3, we described environmental theories that focus on understanding (and changing) environmental conditions to enhance health outcomes. As mentioned in Chapter 1, we agree with Kurt Lewin's adage that nothing is as useful as a good theory (Hochbaum, Sorenson, & Lorig, 1992). The use of theory is necessary in evidence-informed health promotion programs to ensure that we can describe and address the factors that cause health problems and the methods to achieve change.

In an example of asking questions about determinants in a needs assessment, McEachan, Lawton, Jackson, Conner, & Lunt (2008) sought to uncover key barriers to engaging in physical activity in the workplace among employees at worksites in the United Kingdom. Based on focus groups with employees from different types of worksites, the most common barriers to activity in the workplace were:

- Lack of time

- Competing demands on time

- Lack of motivation

- Lack of control (e.g., lack of facilities)

- Negative consequences associated with exercising (e.g., being sweaty, or the manager frowning on you taking breaks)

**Determinants in the Epilepsy Example**   The developers asked the question: Why do individuals with epilepsy often not manage their condition? Using data from their literature review, surveys with patients with epilepsy in partnering clinics, and discussions with the planning group, the developers identified determinants for poor epilepsy self-management behavior. These included the patient's low level of knowledge (declarative and procedural) and limited skill regarding his or her epilepsy self-management, low self-efficacy or confidence that he or she can perform self-management behaviors, low outcome expectations (both in terms of causality of seizure onset as well as causality of treatment), the patient's attributions regarding self-management (particularly in terms of control), limited ability to set goals, acceptance or denial of the diagnosis of epilepsy and perceived stigma related to epilepsy, perceived barriers to managing his or her epilepsy, and the perceived influence of peers (Begley et al., 2010; Buelow, 2001; DiIorio & Faherty, 1994; DiIorio, Faherty, & Manteuffel, 1992; DiIorio et al., 2004; Institute of Medicine, 2012; Levine, Rudy, & Kerns, 1994; May & Pfafflin, 2002; Sabaz, et al., 2003; Shope, 1988; Tedman, Thornton, & Baker, 1995). Stigma includes not only discrimination but also disapproval and rejection by others (Goffman, 1963; Pryor, Reeder, & Monroe, 2012; van der Sanden, Bos, Stutterheim, Pryor, & Kok, 2013). Perceived experience of stigma is associated with epilepsy through poor psychosocial health outcomes, such as low self-esteem, worry, negative feelings about life, and depression (Cramer et al., 1999; Jones et al., 2005; MacLeod & Austin, 2003; Westbrook, Bauman, & Shinnar, 1992). Further, epileptic seizures have been known to be precipitated by psychological triggers (internal precipitants) such as stress, anxiety, anger, and emotions (Ramaratnam, Baker, & Goldstein, 2005); thus, lack of coping skills may contribute to more frequent seizures. Lack of reinforcement from health care providers and lack of social support from family and friends can also lead to poorer self-management. Determinants of environmental factors involve health care providers, families, and the community (Institute of Medicine, 2012). Families lack knowledge and skills for providing support for self-management, and health care providers require greater skills for effectively communicating with patients and families to train them on, and reinforce for them, epilepsy management behaviors (Institute of Medicine, 2012; Rothert, 1991). This is compounded by the general community's misguided beliefs about epilepsy, lack of knowledge and skills to assist with seizures and support management, and lack of awareness of policies and guidelines regarding supporting people with epilepsy in important life functions including employment, driving, sports, and housing (Institute of Medicine, 2012).

### Acquiring Needs Assessment Data

Most needs assessments require multiple data sources, including both qualitative and quantitative measures, because they are answering multiple questions and often seeking various perspectives on the answers. There are many examples of needs assessments and formative research that use multiple methods research. For example, Wright et al. (2006) utilized multiple qualitative and quantitative methods to inform a youth mental-health community awareness campaign intervention in Victoria, Australia. They conducted qualitative focus groups with youth and parents affected by mental health problems, and held consultation forums and presentations with workers from key service organizations. They also conducted a quantitative cross-sectional telephone survey with 600 youth ages 12–25 in the intervention region to assess recognition of mental health disorders, perceived outcomes related to treatment, and exposure to mental health disorders.

Before beginning a needs assessment, we address questions to each phase of our logic model and consider sources of data to answer the questions. Planners should consider the data available from other researchers; cost, time, and other constraints for collecting data; degree of interaction desired with respondents; and which stakeholders should be involved. In general, planners will look for archival data such as organizational records, demographic data, census data, disease registries, medical records, and public-use databases; noninteractive primary data collection such as written, Internet-based, or mailed surveys along with critical incident technique and mailed or Internet-based Delphi technique and observations; and interactive primary data collection such as focus groups, key informant interviews, individual interviews, community forums or public hearings, nominal group technique, and virtual, Web-based applications of any of these processes (Atschuld & Kumar, 2010; see Harmsen et al., 2013, for an example of online focus groups).

In conducting the epilepsy-management needs assessment, the team found that the scientific literature contained considerable information about health and quality-of-life issues. Other questions, such as those regarding local impact, required data collection through surveys, observations, focus groups, and interviews. Some environmental factors, such as the actions of health care providers, could be estimated from reports in the literature, but local data would have required a survey of providers.

We briefly present some of the more common data collection methods but also refer the reader to texts that present needs-assessment techniques in detail (Aday, 1996; Altschuld & Kumar, 2010; Dillman, Smyth, & Christian, 2008; Fowler, 2008; Gilmore & Campbell, 2005).

### *Combining Qualitative and Quantitative Data*

As suggested in Chapter 1, a skill the program planner should bring to bear in Intervention Mapping, including the needs assessment step, is conducting practical, multimethod research (Creswell, Klassen, Plano Clark, & Clegg Smith, 2011; Elliott et al., 2014; Teddlie, & Yu, 2007). A research design using a combination of the qualitative and quantitative research paradigms is described by Creswell as an approach often more focused on the problem at hand or on the research question than on the method itself (Creswell et al., 2011). The benefits from using a practical, combination approach has been described as providing corroboration, confirmation, or triangulation of data (Creswell et al., 2011). Others have suggested the complementarity of the methods such that using more than one method combines the strengths of the two and produces a more nuanced understanding of the topic, allowing planners to increase the validity of their findings (Creswell et al., 2011; Morgan, 2006).

Quantitative methods, such as surveys and disease registries, enable the planner to estimate the incidence and prevalence of health problems and related behaviors in the at-risk population. Quantitative methods also enable estimates of the strength of the correlation of determinants with risk behaviors. On the other hand, qualitative methods can help health educators more fully understand the dynamics of communities, health problems, behavioral and environmental causes, and determinants from the perspectives of the people involved (Farquhar, Parker, Schulz, & Israel, 2006). These methods include ethnographic interviews (Denzin & Lincoln, 2007; Ngo et al., 2007; Small, Kerr, Charette, Schecter, & Spittal, 2006), focus groups (Gilmore & Campbell, 2005; Krueger & Casey, 2009), the problem-posing methods from Freire's education for critical consciousness (Kelso et al., 2014), critical incident technique (Altschuld & Kumar, 2010; Baheiraei et al., 2013; FitzGerald, Seale, Kerins, & McElvaney, 2008), nominal group technique (Baheiraei et al. 2013; Delbecq, Van de Ven, & Gustafson, 1975), photovoice (Catalani & Minkler, 2010; Wang, 2003), and appreciative inquiry (Farrell, Wallis, & Evans, 2007; Fryer-Edwards et al., 2007).

Fernández and colleagues (2005a) combined qualitative and quantitative methods during their formative work to develop a breast- and cervical-screening program for Hispanic farmworkers. First they conducted an extensive literature review and focus groups with farm-working women aged 50 years and older. These methods provided information about quality-of-life issues related to breast and cervical cancer, screening behaviors, and personal and environmental factors influencing screening. From these data, they developed a quantitative face-to-face survey, which was administered to 200 women living in colonias in the Texas Lower Rio Grande Valley to assess the prevalence of screening behaviors in the at-risk group and to assess personal determinants related to screening (Palmer, Fernández, Tortolero-Luna, Gonzales, & Mullen, 2005).

Qualitative and quantitative approaches to problem analysis are not simply two different techniques of arriving at the same answer. They are essentially different in their philosophical origins and approaches to knowledge. The two approaches used together produce a more usable, comprehensive, and accurate assessment product based on better information about and from members of the intended community throughout Intervention Mapping. However, each approach must be used under its own assumptions, and the reader is referred to other texts for instruction in quantitative and qualitative methods.

The methods in each tradition differ in the research object and in design, data collection, and analysis. Patton (1990, 2001) describes qualitative approaches as:

- Inductive
- Discovery oriented
- Iterative
- Question and theory generating
- Subjective and valid with the self as the instrument
- Not usually amenable to counting
- Case oriented
- Not generalizable

Quantitative methods are:

- Deductive
- Theory verification oriented
- Question answering
- Objective and reliable, subject to reliable counting

- Population oriented

- Generalizable

Morgan (2006) suggests that when a researcher uses both types of methods, there are two dimensions of use: sequence and priority. Methods can be used with equal weighting and/or at the same time, but as Morgan (2006) points out, the data analysis can be more difficult when there is no prioritization or sequence. Steckler and colleagues (1992) present a useful diagram of four ways that qualitative and quantitative methods can be used in program evaluation (Figure 4.3). The models are equally appropriate in other steps of Intervention Mapping. In Model l, the planner uses qualitative data-gathering methods—such as focus groups, nominal group technique, observation, ethnographic interviews, or semistructured interviews—to begin hearing perceptions of health problems, related behavioral and environmental causes, determinants, and quality of life in the community.

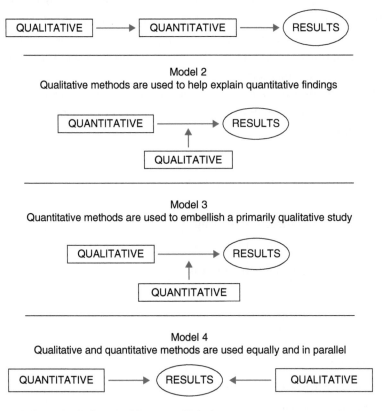

**Model 1**
Qualitative methods are used to help develop quantitative measures and instruments

QUALITATIVE ⟶ QUANTITATIVE ⟶ RESULTS

**Model 2**
Qualitative methods are used to help explain quantitative findings

QUANTITATIVE ⟶ RESULTS
↑
QUALITATIVE

**Model 3**
Quantitative methods are used to embellish a primarily qualitative study

QUALITATIVE ⟶ RESULTS
↑
QUANTITATIVE

**Model 4**
Qualitative and quantitative methods are used equally and in parallel

QUANTITATIVE ⟶ RESULTS ⟵ QUALITATIVE

**Figure 4.3** Integrating Qualitative and Quantitative Methods
Reprinted with permission from Steckler et al. (1992)

After the qualitative phase, surveys can be used to document the prevalence of the issues that emerged from a qualitative study (Fernández et al., 2005a). Beginning with qualitative methods, in this case, gives the planner a better chance of asking pertinent and intelligible questions during a survey phase. This sequence of using qualitative methods to inform survey design may also enable the researcher to develop new hypotheses or to refine existing ones before the quantitative phase of the research. For example, Lehmann, Ruiter, Wicker, van Dam, and Kok (2015) performed focus groups to obtain insight into the determinants influencing health care providers' intentions to get vaccinated against influenza in Belgium, German, and Dutch hospital settings. They then developed a questionnaire to quantify the results of the focus groups and to gain insight into the relative importance of the determinants that influenced intentions to vaccinate (Lehmann, Ruiter, van Dam, Wicker, & Kok, 2015).

In Model 2, planners use qualitative techniques to better understand the meaning of their quantitative findings. In a needs assessment, health educators might use census or epidemiologic data to describe the health problem, behavioral or environmental risk, or determinants, and then conduct qualitative research to better understand the perceptions of the at-risk group (Wingood, Hunter-Gamble, & DiClemente, 1993). For example, Wingood and colleagues (1993) used the focus group technique to better understand the determinants of HIV-associated risk behaviors in African American women. They found that the women they spoke with could bring up with their partners the conversational topic of safer sex, but they could not effectively negotiate condom use. A woman demanding that a partner use condoms could imply lack of trust in a relationship, violate a woman's conflict-avoiding stance, and prove difficult or even dangerous.

In Model 3, the health educator conducts a qualitative study to document the problems or needs in a community and then uses quantitative data to verify and establish the magnitude of the primarily qualitative needs assessment. For example, Fernández and colleagues used focus groups to identify factors associated with colorectal cancer screening among Hispanic men and women living along the Texas-Mexico border and then conducted a survey in three cities (Fernández et al., 2008). The survey data showed that fatalistic beliefs were associated with lower colorectal cancer screening (Fernández et al., 2008). Follow-up qualitative studies that sought to better understand these beliefs revealed that while people were somewhat pessimistic about the ability to survive cancer (perceived survivability), they did not subscribe to the notion that if they were meant to have cancer, they would get it and there was nothing they could do to protect themselves (predeterminism) (Fernández et al., 2015).

These findings helped identify limitations in the quantitative measure of fatalism the researchers had used, and shed light on the specific beliefs that could be addressed through an intervention.

In the final model, qualitative and quantitative methods are used in parallel to shed light on an issue or a problem (Saint-Germain, Bassford, & Montano, 1993). For example, Wittink, Barg, and Gallo (2006) used qualitative and quantitate data concurrently to examine the concordance and discordance between physicians and patients regarding depression status of the latter. Qualitative data were collected using semistructured interviews with patients; quantitative data comprised self-reported patient and physicians' ratings of depression. Among patients who self-rated as depressed, the quantitative data did not differentiate between those whose physicians rated them as depressed and those whose physicians did not rate them as depressed. However, the qualitative data indicated that the patients' perception of their relationship with the physician may have influenced what they were willing to share with their physician.

## Finding and Using Archival Data

Archival or secondary data are data that have been collected for a purpose other than the needs assessment. Many governmental, health, social service, and education agencies collect data describing health problems and demographics that can be useful to the needs assessor. These can be census-type data, in which the goal is to describe every event or person—for example, birth and death records—or they can be survey-type data, in which an attempt is made to capture a representative sample of the population of interest.

Archival sources can be local, regional, national, or international. They can be obtained directly from the agency responsible for collection and analysis or from a library. For example, local health departments collect census data and other data such as birth and death records. National agencies such as the Centers for Disease Control and Prevention in the United States collect a variety of data on disease incidence and prevalence as well as survey data regarding disease risk. The Internet makes acquiring data from agencies at all levels easy. Table 4.3 presents examples of sources of secondary data and their Web addresses.

## Collecting Primary Data

We provide a general description of several data collection methods from individuals and refer the reader to primary sources on survey research (Dillman et al., 2008).

**Table 4.3**    Examples of Secondary Data Sources for Health, Behavior, Environment, and Quality-of-Life Description

| Type of Data | Example Sources | Web Address: |
|---|---|---|
| Demographic | U.S. Census | http://www.census.gov/ |
| | European census information | http://www.hist.umn.edu/&sim;rmccaa/ipums-europe/enumeration_forms.shtml.htm |
| | Statistical abstracts of the U.S. | http://www.census.gov/compendia/statab/ |
| Health and Vital Statistics | National Vital Statistics Report (NVSR) was called MVSR | http://www.cdc.gov/nchs/products/nvsr.htm |
| | Morbidity and Mortality Weekly Report (MMWR) | http://www.cdc.gov/mmwr/ |
| | National Center for Health Statistics | http://www.cdc.gov/nchs/ |
| | Guide to Federal Statistics | http://fedstats.sites.usa.gov |
| | Centers for Disease Control and Prevention (CDC) | http://www.cdc.gov/DataStatistics/ |
| | European Community Health Indicators Monitoring (ECHIM) | http://www.healthindicators.eu/healthindicators/object_document/o4963n28314.html |
| | Health EU: The Public Health Portal of the European Union | http://ec.europa.eu/health/index_en.htm |
| | Canadian Health Statistics | http://www.statcan.gc.ca/eng/health/index |
| | WHO World Health Statistics | http://www.who.int/research/en/ |
| | WHO Weekly Epidemiological Record | http://www.who.int/wer/en/ |
| | Behavioral Risk Factor Surveillance Survey (BRFSS) | http://www.cdc.gov/brfss/ |
| Risk Factors | Youth Risk Behavior Surveillance System | http://www.cdc.gov/HealthyYouth/yrbs/index.htm |
| | National Longitudinal Study of Adolescent Health | http://www.cpc.unc.edu/projects/addhealth |
| | CDC Pregnancy Risk Assessment Monitoring System | http://www.cdc.gov/PRAMS/ |
| | Data Resource Center for Child & Adolescent Health | http://www.childhealthdata.org/content/Default.aspx |
| | Health Information National Trends Survey | http://hints.cancer.gov/ |
| Health Information Access | Environmental Protection Agency | http://www.epa.gov/epahome/data.html |
| Environmental | Air data: Access to Air Pollution Data | http://www.epa.gov/airdata/ |
| | Health Departments, e.g., Texas, Harris County | http://www.dshs.state.tx.us/chs/datalist.shtm http://www.hcphes.org/ |
| Local and Regional Health Data | Texas Department of State Health Services Center for Health Statistics | http://www.dshs.state.tx.us/chs/default.shtml |
| | Texas Cancer Registry, provides access to Cancer Incidence and Mortality Rates in Texas from 1997–2001 | http://www.dshs.state.tx.us/tcr/data.shtm |

(continued)

**Table 4.3**    *(Continued)*

| Type of Data | Example Sources | Web Address: |
|---|---|---|
| Cancer as an example of disease-specific sources | National Cancer Institute | http://seer.cancer.gov/ http://seer.cancer.gov/about/activities.html |
| | American Cancer Society Cancer Facts and Figures | http://www.cancer.org/research/ cancerfactsstatistics/index |
| The Netherlands as an example of country-specific sources | Demographics, the Netherlands | http://www.nidi.nl/nl |
| | Statistics and health, the Netherlands | http://www.cbs.nl |
| | Integrated information, the Netherlands | https://www.volksgezondheidenzorg.info/ |

**Surveys**    Written (including computer-assisted) and telephone surveys are the most often used, with Internet, mobile, and smartphone surveys, and ecological momentary assessment (Runyan et al., 2013; Shiffman, 2009), gaining rapidly in popularity. These use structured forms or protocols that employ a variety of scales and response modes and are relatively easy to administer. As with all data collection activities, questions on surveys should be carefully linked to the purpose of the needs assessment. Key issues are the validity and reliability of items and scales, appropriate sampling to represent the population of interest, and the ability to achieve high response rates (Aday, 1996; Altschuld & Kumar, 2010; Dillman et al., 2008).

**Interviews**    Interviews can be highly structured (much like a survey) or moderately unstructured, using a general guide outlining the set of issues to be addressed. Interviews based on elicitation rather than a rigid protocol of questions have the advantage of allowing the respondent opportunities for free expression, with attitudes more likely to be revealed, but the method requires skilled interviewers and qualitative data analysts. As with surveys, it is important to determine the purpose of the interview and select the sample. Mall intercept interviews, in which potential respondents are approached in public places, are frequently used for structured interviews with convenience samples. Key informants can supply information about needs, barriers, and previous programs (Altschuld & Kumar, 2010; Gilmore & Campbell, 2005).

**Ethnographic Methods**    Ethnographic methods from anthropology provide a key role in describing marginalized settings and hard-to-reach populations, such as commercial sex workers, drug users, people engaging in HIV-risk behaviors, or homeless people (Lankenau, Clatts, Welle, Goldsamt, & Gwadz, 2005; Ngo et al., 2007; Small et al., 2006). Ethnographic methods include participant observation, in-depth interviews, focus groups, and analysis of written textual materials, and they are focused on the description of a culture through the experiences and perspectives of individuals in their own language and on their own terms. Scrimshaw and colleagues have developed rapid-assessment techniques based on anthropological methods, which have been applied in the planning and evaluation of a variety of international programs in such areas as nutrition and primary health care, reproductive health, AIDS, epilepsy, hunger, water and sanitation, and emergency relief (Cifuentes, Alamo, Kendall, Brunkard, & Scrimshaw, 2006; Scrimshaw & Hurtado, 1987, 1992).

**Appreciative Inquiry (AI)**    This approach involves interviews focused on positive experiences related to a topic. Unlike traditional problem-solving approaches, AI focuses on strengths within an organization; it seeks root causes for success instead of root causes for failure (Ludema, Whitney, Mohr, & Griffin, 2003). The key task is to identify and leverage strengths. The use of AI in health care settings has been used successfully in both nursing (Farrell et al., 2007) and medical school settings (Fryer-Edwards et al., 2007). The main inquiry process in this method involves asking a main question with a series of tightly focused subquestions or probes regarding high-point experiences in an organization or community and then eliciting scenarios regarding what the entity would be like if the high points occurred more routinely. Fernández and colleagues (2012) used this method to better understand practice change in primary care settings. They conducted focus groups and in-depth interviews with leaders of federally qualified health centers (FQHCs) to identify factors associated with adopting and implementing evidence-based cancer control programs and practices. They asked leaders to describe a time when clinic staff were energized and satisfied with how things were going and when everything flowed well in response to a particular practice change. This type of inquiry yielded interesting data that would not necessarily have surfaced if they had approached the study with a focus on identifying barriers.

**Planning Groups**    One of the first places to look for information is from the group or groups planners have developed for the program development work. This is usually some combination of a work group and various advisory groups. Both types can contribute to defining the problem and understanding the community if they include a variety of types of community members, including those with the problem. Levy and colleagues (2004) describe a needs-assessment process in two Chicago communities affected disproportionately by diabetes and heart disease. The needs assessment began with providing structure for the planning activities by creating four work groups, each concerned with a different subject: risk factors and programs, quality of clinical care, policy and advocacy, and data and evaluation. The planning group included individuals from different racial and ethnic backgrounds. Members had expertise in public health, medicine, nursing, community organizing, and evaluation. Representatives from voluntary health associations and from the community were also included. (Levy et al., 2004). The work groups reviewed data from all components of the needs assessment and provided critical information and analysis.

**Focus Groups**    Focus groups, a technique borrowed from the field of marketing, are led by a moderator who refers to an interview guide with 5 to 10 questions. They are often used in health promotion as part of a multimethod approach to needs assessment or program development (Fernández, Palmer, & Leong-Wu, 2005b; Fernández et al., 2008; Gilmore & Campbell, 2005; Krueger & Casey, 2009; Morales-Campos, Markham, Peskin, & Fernández, 2013; Santa Maria et al., 2014). The goal of a focus group is to stimulate discussion among 6 to 12 fairly homogenous people to ascertain opinions and attitudes related to the topic of interest. Krueger and Casey (2009) describe processes in planning and conducting focus groups:

- Development of a focus group guide
- Recruitment of participants
- Discussion including introductions, facilitation, and recording
- Transcription
- Analysis

The number of focus groups that should be conducted is based on a variety of considerations: determining whether saturation has been reached and no additional themes are forthcoming, ensuring that different segments of the community are represented, and allowing the opportunity to ask new questions that emerge during earlier focus groups. For example, Fernández and colleagues (2008) stratified their groups on colon cancer screening on the Texas-Mexico border by gender and location. They also conducted separate key informant groups of *promotores* by both age and gender.

**Delphi Technique**    This method is a group survey technique that uses an iterative process to build consensus in a group. There are usually 10–15 respondents with significant knowledge about an issue. The first round of mailed or Internet surveys solicits responses to a limited number of focused questions; the second round follows first-round analysis and asks clarifying questions; a third round often asks for ranking of preferences. Like the nominal group process, this method results in focused information. It also has the advantage of crossing geographic boundaries and of not requiring the scheduling of real-time meetings (De Vet, Brug, De Nooijer, Dijkstra, &

de Vries, 2005; Gilmore & Campbell, 2005; Hsu & Sandford, 2007; Keeney, Hasson, & McKenna, 2011; van Stralen et al., 2008).

**Geographic Methods** Geographic information systems (GIS) are a commonly used tool to geocode, map, and analyze health data in relation to place (S. R. Graham, Carolton, Gaede, & Jamison, 2011). Recent advances in GIS technology have expanded its use beyond the field to a more general audience through online GIS platforms (Highfield, Arthasarnprasit, Ottenweller, & Dasprez, 2011). Online GIS systems— easily accessed and queried—allow users with and without specialized skill sets to access public health data (e.g., incidence, and mortality) and statistics through online maps, both of which are critical for supporting data-driven community needs assessment. In addition, public participation GIS (PPGIS) focuses on the inclusion of the community in the collection, analysis, and use of spatial data for assessing and addressing health needs (Brown, Schebella, & Weber, 2014; Gwede et al., 2010). For example, Friedman et al. (2014) used PPGIS to show practitioners and stakeholders the density of FQHCs in relation to four different types of cancer to facilitate the assessment of where to locate new FQHCs. They used visually appealing maps (made in GIS) to convey complex statistical information to providers and stakeholders about the relationship between FQHC density and cancer rates in the local community (Friedman et al., 2014). The Environmental Systems Research Institute (ESRI) recently developed story maps, which combine traditional GIS data with images, audio, and text (Environmental Systems Research Institute, 2014). Story maps can be used to tell a more comprehensive story about health and are particularly useful for mixed-methods community assessments and for conveying information to a lay audience. Sample story maps can be found on the ESRI website at: http://storymaps.arcgis.com/en/.

> The third task in Intervention Mapping Step 1 is to develop an understanding of the context for the intervention, including the population, community, and setting.

## Describing the Context for the Intervention

### *Balancing the Needs Assessment With an Asset Assessment*

In developing health promotion programs, it is important to balance the needs assessment with an assessment of the community's assets, capacities, and abilities (McKnight & Kretzman, 2012). As described above, by community, we mean the geographic, social, or organizational groups of individuals who may participate in, or benefit from, the program we are developing. An asset approach to program planning seeks to identify the assets and capacities of individuals and their surrounding environments that may be leveraged and incorporated into program planning. In asset mapping, the planning group explores the problems as well as the assets in their community to develop strategies to solve the problems together.

An asset-based approach builds from the strengths of individuals, communities, and environments and is supported by theoretical and practice-based perspectives (Bradley et al., 2009; Ludema et al., 2003; McKnight & Kretzmann, 2012). Incorporating existing assets and capacities into program planning may also enhance the implementation and sustainability of the proposed program (Hebert, Brandt, Armstead, Adams, & Steck, 2009; Tapp & Dulin, 2010). For example, during the needs-assessment phase for the development of Cultivando La Salud, a breast- and cervical-cancer screening intervention for Hispanic farm-working women, Fernández and colleagues (2005a; 2009) identified several strengths and resources within border communities. These included many familial ties in the community, a system of lay health workers available through community clinics, and the acceptability of door-to-door outreach. This information was key for the development of program implementation strategies.

## Conducting an Asset Assessment

Ecological models in health promotion recognize multiple environments that may influence the behavior of the priority population and environmental agents, including social, information, policy, and physical environments (Sallis et al., 2006). By mapping assets and capacities at each of these environmental levels, the planning group may identify existing factors in the community that could be incorporated or leveraged to support a new health promotion program (see Table 4.4).

**Table 4.4**    Community Asset Assessment

| Social Environment Asset Assessment | Information Environment Asset Assessment | Policy/Practice Environment Asset Assessment | Physical Environment Asset Assessment |
|---|---|---|---|
| What are existing social environmental factors that could support the program (e.g., individual capacities, personal income, high school social cohesion and identity)? | What are existing communication channels that could be activated for the program (e.g., community newspapers, local television channels and radio stations, school bulletins, and social media)? | What are existing policies and practices that could be leveraged to support the program? Consider policies and practices at different levels, including national, state, community, organizational, and home (e.g., | What are aspects of the natural or built environment that could be harnessed to support the program (e.g., parks, unused land and buildings)? |
| What are the existing organizations/groups that could help support the intervention (e.g., faith-based organizations, local businesses, community coalitions, and online discussion groups)? | a.<br>b.<br>c.<br>d. | city ordinances, worksite bans on smoking; school policies on required minutes of physical education or recess, and family practices around family meals). | a.<br>b.<br>c.<br>d. |
| a.<br>b.<br>c.<br>d. | | a.<br>b.<br>c.<br>d. | |

Adapted from Springer, n.d.

**Measuring the Social Environment**    Goodman and colleagues' (1998) seminal work defined multiple dimensions of community capacity in the social environment, such as citizen participation, leadership, skills, social and interorganizational networks, social capital, and an understanding of community history, community values, and community power. Validated measures can be used to assess these factors. For example, McKnight & Kretzman (2012) used a "capacity inventory" to identify the skills, talents, knowledge, and experience of individuals living in low-income neighborhoods that could support new approaches or enterprises. Murayama, Wakui, Arami, Sugawara, and Yoshie (2012) assessed indicators of social capital (trust in neighbors, institutional trust in the national social security system, participation in groups with egalitarian relationships, and participation in groups with hierarchical relationships) to assess associations with self-rated health and risk behaviors among adults in Tokyo, Japan.

**Measuring the Information Environment**    The information environment may include local television and radio stations, community newspapers, organizational newsletters, social media, local associations, and outdoor venues, such as public transportation, markets, and shopping malls. Key informant interviews and household surveys can be used to identify relevant communication channels for a new health promotion program. For example, Ramachandran, Jaggarajamma, Muniyandi, and Baluasubraamanian (2006) interviewed key informants and conducted household surveys in rural areas in southern India to identify potential communication channels for a new tuberculosis control program.

**Measuring the Policy Environment**    Several instruments have been developed to examine policies and practices in different community sectors. For example, the School Health Policies and Practices Study is a national survey conducted to assess school health policies and practices at the state, district, school, and classroom levels (Centers for Disease Control and Prevention, 2012b).

**Measuring the Physical Environment**    Environmental audits, such as the Checklist of Health Promotion Environments at Worksites (CHEW), provide observational measures to assess physical features that may affect health behaviors, for example, nutrition, physical activity, and breast feeding (Centers for Disease Control and Prevention, 2010; Oldenburg, Sallis, Harris, & Owen, 2002). Audit tools have also been used to assess the friendliness toward physical activity of neighborhoods and parks (Taylor, Franzini, Olvera, Poston, & Lin, 2012; Taylor et al., 2008; Taylor et al., 2014).

## *Identifying the Intervention Setting*

Developing an asset assessment also assists the planning group in identifying an appropriate setting for the intervention. Ideally, the intervention setting provides widespread access to the priority population and has the capacity to implement the intervention with fidelity. For example, in the It's Your Game...Keep It Real project, the planning group decided to implement the program in middle schools because the schools provided extensive access to early adolescents, and the school district and community had the capacity and support to implement a school-based sexual-health education program.

# Stating Program Goals

The final task for Intervention Mapping Step 1 is to link the needs assessment to program and evaluation planning by specifying desired program goals.

Setting priorities in a needs assessment is an iterative process, occurring throughout the assessment as well as after data analysis at the assessment's end. As health planners ask questions and gather information during the assessment, they make various decisions about the continuing focus. For example, the epilepsy needs assessment came to be focused on adults 18 years and older, as this age group experienced greater prevalence of comorbidities and accidents related to epilepsy than younger age groups. In the It's Your Game example at the end of this chapter (and continuing through the chapters that describe Intervention Mapping steps), planners made a decision to focus both on delaying sexual initiation among middle school students and on promoting condom and contraceptive use among students who were sexually active. On what basis should these health planners make such priority decisions?

Many factors influence priorities. One is the magnitude between what is and what could be (Altschuld & Kumar, 2010). A related criterion is the difference in burden from a problem among groups. Once a problem becomes a focus, priorities may narrow to certain groups due to a heavier burden or to a health inequality or inequity.

A set of practical issues also influences the decision. These are the potential difficulty in ameliorating the needs, the consequences of ignoring the needs, and the possible costs of implementing a solution. Political and other social factors also affect the ultimate priorities and the decision-making process. These include community values, the context of priorities (the local, regional, national, and international priorities), public and leader expectations, available interest and expertise, momentum, and availability of funding and human resources.

Once the health planner has decided on the health problem(s) and population(s) and completed the analysis of behavioral and environmental causes, further decisions are made. We begin to think about what factors need to change, and we move further with this analysis in Chapter 5. Green and Kreuter (2005) recommend rating the importance (that is, relevance) and changeability of behaviors and environmental conditions using findings from the needs assessment. Behaviors and environmental conditions that are both more relevant and more changeable will be a high priority for program focus; factors that are more relevant and less changeable may be a priority for innovative programs for which evaluation is crucial. Factors that are less relevant but more changeable may be deemed as lower priorities except to demonstrate initial change to encourage community support and program participation. Behaviors that are both less relevant and less changeable should not be a focus for intervention. This analysis should be carefully conducted so factors that are very relevant but hard to change are not neglected.

For use in the Intervention Mapping framework, we define program goals as changes in health, quality-of-life, behavioral, or environmental factors from the needs assessment. Looking back at the PRECEDE model, planners target how much change can be expected in indicators over a specified time frame for the priority population. These goals also become the main targets in terms of program evaluation. The major outcome evaluation questions will pertain to whether the intervention developed accomplished the program goals.

The ultimate goals are usually related to health or quality of life. If change in health and quality-of-life outcomes can be accomplished in the program and evaluation time frame, then those become the specified goals. If the time frame is too long for program effects on health and quality of life to be measurable within the program time frame (as, for example, in a program concerned with HIV or cancer), then the planning group can make a decision to define the program goals in terms of behavior or environment. Health indicators include morbidity, mortality, incidence, prevalence, disability, and physiological risk factors. These include a statement (with a strong verb) of what will change in a specified population, by how much, and by what period of time. The amount of expected change and the time frame must be empirically justifiable. For example:

- At the end of three years of intervention, the annual incidence of HIV infection in Austin, Texas, will be reduced by 5 percent.

- Patients with epilepsy who use the MINDSET self-management decision-support system in the context of their usual clinic visit for three consecutive clinic visits over a nine-month period will report at least three fewer "at-risk" self-management behaviors (assessed by the Epilepsy Self-Management scale) compared to patients who do not use MINDSET.

- Following five years of programs to increase physical activity and reduce total caloric consumption, the percentage of obese children in grades five through eight in El Paso, Texas, will be reduced from 35 percent to 30 percent.

The stated program goal that includes *what* will change, for *whom* by *how much* over what *time* is then used in IM Step 2 to guide the statement of expected program outcomes and objectives.

### BOX 4.2. IT'S YOUR GAME . . . KEEP IT REAL

It's Your Game . . . Keep It Real is an example of an application of Intervention Mapping to develop a successful intervention (Tortolero et al., 2010; Markham et al., 2012; Peskin et al., 2014). We present this example step by step at the end of each Intervention Mapping step (Chapters 4 through 9). We organize the example by the tasks that we present in each chapter.

#### Task 1. Establish and Work with a Planning Group

It's Your Game . . . Keep It Real is a sexual-health education program for middle school students, which was developed and evaluated in a large urban school district in the south-central United States. The original project was funded by the National Institute for Mental Health at the National Institutes of Health (Tortolero et al, 2010). The planning team included health educators; behavioral scientists, epidemiologists; a pediatrician; an expert in human sexuality (program developers); representatives from the school district's health and physical education; health and medical services departments; school principals; a school nurse; representatives from local medical, religious, and community organizations (potential implementers and dissemination partners); and parents (end users). A teen advisory group, comprising youth ages 12–15 years from the priority population, also met quarterly during intervention development to review program materials to ensure that they were relevant and engaging for youth.

#### Task 2. Conduct a Needs Assessment to Create a Logic Model of the Problem

The behavioral scientists on the team helped the group choose the PRECEDE model (Green & Kreuter, 2005) as the organizing framework for their needs assessment, and they began immediately putting everything they already knew about adolescent sexual health in the community into the model. They began with the project assumption that they were entering the model at the health problem. They defined the health problem as excess burden of teen pregnancy, STI, and HIV infection among racial/ethnic minority youth.

**Needs Assessment Methods**

In order to flesh out the needs assessment model, they reviewed the literature and secondary surveillance data sources, held focus groups with youth and parents from the priority population, conducted interviews with school district personnel, attended school district meetings, and led discussions with the planning group. They addressed two primary questions: What is the prevalence of teen pregnancy, STIs, and HIV infection? And what behavioral and environmental factors are associated with increased risk of teen pregnancy, STIs, and HIV infection?

They conducted 10 focus groups with seventh- and eighth-grade students from the priority population, and seven focus groups with parents of seventh and eighth graders. The purpose of the qualitative data collection was to explore students' and parents' knowledge, attitudes, and beliefs about dating and relationships, sexual behavior, condom and contraceptive use, and program implementation issues.

*Describing Health Problems, Quality of Life, and the Population at Risk*

The priority population for It's Your Game comprised predominantly African American and Hispanic middle school students attending a large, urban school district in the south-central United States. At the time when the intervention was developed, the school district had 38 middle schools with a seventh-grade population of 13,699 students. Of these students, 36 percent were African American, 52 percent were Hispanic, and 79 percent participated in the school free or reduced-cost lunch program, which is an indicator of low socioeconomic status.

Using the PRECEDE model to guide their needs assessment, they used secondary data sources, empirical literature reviews, and community input to describe health problems and quality-of-life issues related to sexual risk behaviors that may begin in middle school. Minority youth are disproportionately affected both by teen births and STIs, including HIV infection. For instance, nationally, Hispanics experience higher teen birth rates than other racial/ethnic groups, and African Americans represent almost two-thirds of HIV diagnoses among youth (Centers for Disease Control and Prevention, 2014; Hamilton & Ventura, 2012). Many communities in the school district had teen birth rates higher than 100 per 1,000 girls ages 15–19 years, exceeding the state and national rates (63 and 43 per 1,000, respectively; Texas Department of State Health Services, 2007). Chlamydia and gonorrhea cases by age group were highest among 15–19 year old females (Houston Department of Health and Human Services, 2007), and the state ranked fourth among U.S. states for the estimated number of AIDS cases among youth ages 13–19 (Bureau of Epidemiology, 2008). Seventy-five percent of new HIV cases among those 13–19 years old in the target area were among African American youth, and 15 percent were among Hispanics (Bureau of Epidemiology, 2008). In terms of quality of life, teen pregnancy is a major factor in high school dropout, welfare dependency, and negative outcomes for children of teens (Bronte-Tinkew, Burkhauser, & Metz, 2008; Hoffman, 2006; Shuger, 2012). STIs increase the risk of other reproductive health problems, including pelvic inflammatory disease, ectopic pregnancy, infertility, and cancers related to the human papillomavirus (HPV; National Institute of Allergy and Infectious Diseases, 2014). Sexually transmitted infections and HIV infection can lead to issues related to stigma and disclosure (Cunningham, Tschann, Gurvey, Fortenberry, & Ellen, 2002; Tanney, Naar-King, & MacDonnel, 2012).

### Describing Behavior of At-Risk Individuals

Moving to the left in the PRECEDE model (Figure 4.4), they asked the question: What is the behavior of the adolescent at risk that contributes to excess burden of teen pregnancy, STIs, and HIV? African American and Hispanic youth are more likely to initiate sex at a younger age than white youth (Kann et al., 2014). The literature review indicated that youth who initiate sex at or before age 14 are more likely than youth who initiate sex at an older age to have multiple lifetime sexual partners, engage in greater frequency of sex, use alcohol or drugs before sex, and have sex without a condom (Flanigan, 2003; O'Donnell, O'Donnell, & Stueve, 2001; Santelli, Brener, Lowry, Bhatt, & Zabin, 1998). Dating older partners (Marin, Kirby, Hudes, Gomez, & Coyle, 2003) and experience of dating violence (Reed, Miller, Raj, Decker, & Silverman, 2014) are also associated with increased risk of teen pregnancy and STIs. Many youth do not get tested for STIs and HIV, which may delay access to treatment and increase the risk of transmission (Centers for Disease Control and Prevention, 2012a; Centers for Disease Control and Prevention, 2014). The focus groups and discussions with school district personnel and planning group members confirmed these were risk behaviors for the priority population.

### Describing Determinants of Adolescent Sexual Risk Behaviors

Moving again to the left in the PRECEDE model (Figure 4.4), they concentrated on the determinants of adolescent sexual risk behavior by asking, "Why do adolescents engage in sexual risk behaviors?" The literature suggested that many psychosocial determinants—such as knowledge, skills, self-efficacy, beliefs, perceived norms, and low perceived susceptibility—influence adolescent behavior (Buhi & Goodson, 2007; Kirby, Lepore, & Ryan, 2005). The student focus groups corroborated that the majority of seventh- and eighth-grade students was not sexually experienced and lacked basic knowledge regarding STIs, use of contraceptive methods, STI testing, and what types of behaviors are considered sex (e.g., oral sex). The students expressed the belief that people their age needed information about the types and use of contraceptive methods. Students did have some knowledge regarding the consequences of getting pregnant, as well as the characteristics of being in a healthy or unhealthy relationship.

### Describing Environmental Factors Related to Adolescent Sexual Risk Behaviors

At the interpersonal level, family factors, such as low parent-child communication about sexual health and low parental monitoring, influence adolescent sexual behavior

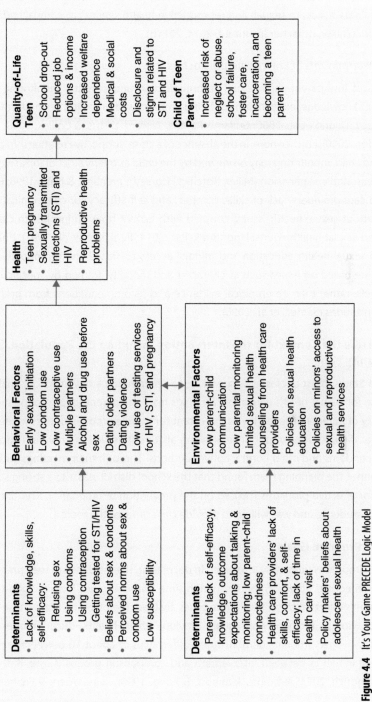

**Determinants**
- Lack of knowledge, skills, self-efficacy:
  - Refusing sex
  - Using condoms
  - Using contraception
  - Getting tested for STI/HIV
- Beliefs about sex & condoms
- Perceived norms about sex & condom use
- Low susceptibility

**Behavioral Factors**
- Early sexual initiation
- Low condom use
- Low contraceptive use
- Multiple partners
- Alcohol and drug use before sex
- Dating older partners
- Dating violence
- Low use of testing services for HIV, STI, and pregnancy

**Health**
- Teen pregnancy
- Sexually transmitted infections (STI) and HIV
- Reproductive health problems

**Quality-of-Life**
**Teen**
- School drop-out
- Reduced job options & income
- Increased welfare dependence
- Medical & social costs
- Disclosure and stigma related to STI and HIV

**Child of Teen Parent**
- Increased risk of neglect or abuse, school failure, foster care, incarceration, and becoming a teen parent

**Determinants**
- Parents' lack of self-efficacy, knowledge, outcome expectations about talking & monitoring; low parent-child connectedness
- Health care providers' lack of skills, comfort, & self-efficacy; lack of time in health care visit
- Policy makers' beliefs about adolescent sexual health

**Environmental Factors**
- Low parent-child communication
- Low parental monitoring
- Limited sexual health counseling from health care providers
- Policies on sexual health education
- Policies on minors' access to sexual and reproductive health services

**Figure 4.4**  It's Your Game PRECEDE Logic Model

(Markham et al., 2010). Health care providers rarely discuss sexual-health issues during adolescent clinic visits (Alexander et al., 2014). Local and state policies on sexual-health education in schools and minors' access to sexual- and reproductive-health services also impact adolescent sexual behavior (The Guttmacher Instititute, 2014, 2014b).

### Describing Determinants of Environmental Factors

Determinants of low parent-child sexual communication and parental monitoring include parents' lack of knowledge, expectations of being embarrassed or feeling uncomfortable, and low self-efficacy (Dilorio et al., 2000; Guilamo-Ramos, Jaccard, Dittus, & Collins, 2008; Jaccard, Dittus, & Gordon, 2000). Furthermore, in the absence of a close, supportive relationship between the parent and child, monitoring may be viewed by the child as overly strict or intrusive control rather than reasonable supervision (Miller, Kotchick, Dorsey, Forehand, & Ham, 1998; Rodgers, 1999). Health care providers' lack of skills, comfort, and self-efficacy for communicating with adolescents about sexual-health issues, coupled with lack of time during health care visits, lead to limited sexual-health counselling (Boekeloo, 2014; Boekeloo et al., 1991). Policies on school-based sexual-health education and minors' access to sexual and reproductive health services may be based on issues such as character and morality, framed by specific religious or moral beliefs, rather than on empirical evidence and recommendations from professional medical organizations (Santelli et al., 2006).

### Task 3. Describe the Context for the Intervention including the Population, Setting, and Community

In the United States, most adolescents spend six to seven hours a day at school, making it a logical setting for sexual-health education. Findings from the parent focus groups suggested that a majority of parents believed it was important for middle school students to receive sex education that discussed the importance of being abstinent as well as providing information about using condoms and other contraceptive methods. Through their meetings with school district personnel, the planning team found that the school district was also a strong supporter of the need for effective programs focused on the prevention of pregnancy, STIs, and HIV for middle school students, and was willing to provide class time for the topic.

### Task 4. State Program Goals

The planning group was ultimately interested in decreasing the incidence of teen pregnancies, STIs, and HIV infection. However, the evaluation time frame was not long enough to assess the intervention's effect on these health outcomes. Instead, the planning team chose to focus on sexual behaviors as proxy program goals. Previous sexual-health education interventions for middle school-aged students demonstrated differences of about 10 percentage points in delayed sexual initiation between intervention and comparison groups (Coyle, Kirby, Marin, Gómez, & Gregorich, 2004; Jemmott, Jemmott, & Fong, 1998; Siegel, Aten, & Enaharo, 2001) and 9 to 30 percent difference in consistent use of condoms or birth control (Jemmott et al., 1998; Mitchell-DiCenso et al., 1997). Using the needs assessment model, the planning team determined that primary program goals for health behavior should include the following:

- After two years of the intervention, the percentage of students in the intervention group who have not initiated sexual intercourse by ninth grade will be 10 percent higher compared to students in the nonintervention group.

- After two years of the intervention, the percentage of sexually active students in the intervention group who used a condom at last sexual intercourse will be 10 percent higher compared to students in the nonintervention group.

## Summary

Chapter 4 describes the process of needs assessment, which is accomplished before beginning work focused on the proposed solutions to identified health problems. The needs assessment begins with involving stakeholders and establishing a participatory planning group. This chapter provides a detailed description of the processes useful in facilitating such a planning group and in carrying out the work of the needs assessment.

Using the PRECEDE model (Green & Kreuter, 2005) as a conceptual framework, the planner conducts an inquiry with a population-based epidemiologic perspective to determine health problem characteristics—such as morbidity and mortality, disease risk, and burden of disease—in various population groups. The inquiry includes an analysis of causation of health problems at multiple levels and the consideration of multiple determinants of health-related behavior and environment.

When conducting the needs assessment, the health and quality-of-life analysis is always focused on the population at risk—that is, the individuals who have the health problem or who are at risk of the health problem. They are the potential beneficiaries of the health promotion intervention. However, it does not follow that an intervention is always focused on this group. There may be several groups in a comprehensive, multilevel program.

Chapter 4 suggests multimethod approaches to needs assessment. The authors describe several data-collection methods including surveys, interviews, ethnographic methods, focus groups, nominal group process, Delphi technique, appreciative inquiry, and geographic techniques. They also describe how to conduct an asset assessment to complete the planning process.

## Discussion Questions and Learning Activities

1. Discuss why a needs assessment is so critical to planning a health promotion program.

2. Explain why it is important for health promotion program planners to balance a needs assessment with an assessment of community capacity and needs. Give examples of measures of community capacity.

3. To develop a health promotion program to address the health problem or related behavior and environmental condition you selected in Chapter 1, describe how you would establish a planning group and who you would include. Briefly describe a process for how you would use the planning group to help conduct the needs assessment.

4. Describe the population at risk for the problem you selected in terms of demographic variables. Provide a rationale for why this population was chosen. Briefly describe the setting for the potential program.

5. Using the problem you selected in Chapter 1, indicate the phase of needs assessment at which you are entering the needs assessment model (e.g., quality of life, health, behavior, or environment). First describe the factor with which you are beginning your model and then describe each of the other factors and their relation to each other.

6. Describe two indicators of quality of life of the selected population. Describe two methods you would use to determine whether these indicators are important to this population. Explain why you selected these methods.

7. Describe health problem(s) that could affect the quality of life for the population. Select at least one of these problems to be addressed by a health promotion program and explain the epidemiologic bases for giving the selected problem(s) priority. Describe the health problem and the incidence/prevalence of the problem in this population. Is it higher compared to other populations? Is there greater burden of disease? If you cannot find data for your chosen population, construct estimates based on comparable populations.

8. Describe behaviors and environmental conditions that are likely causal factors for the health problem selected above. Document and provide references to support the possibility of a causal relationship.

9. From the list generated in Question 8, select the most important behaviors(s) and environmental condition(s) for programmatic focus based on a rating process where you determine the importance (in terms of relation to the health problem) and the changeability of each factor. Present a rationale and evidence.

10. State program goals that would serve as an indicator for the program achieving measurable improvements in health outcomes, quality-of-life outcomes, or behavioral and environmental impact. Consider the time period and use the research literature to justify the amount of change you expect to occur.

11. Specify determinants of the risk behavior and environmental conditions using selected behavioral or social science theories and available empirical evidence.

12. Diagram a logic model that illustrates the casual pathways for how different factors influence increased risk for health problems that have an impact on quality of life for a specified population.

## References

Aboumatar, H., Ristaino, P., Davis, R. O., Thompson, C. B., Maragakis, L., Cosgrove, S., . . . Perl, T. M. (2012). Infection prevention promotion program based on the PRECEDE model: Improving hand hygiene behaviors among healthcare personnel. *Infection, 33*(2), 144–151.

Aday, L. A. (1996). *Designing and conducting health surveys* (2nd ed.). San Francisco, CA: Jossey-Bass.

Airhihenbuwa, C. O. (1995). *Health and culture: Beyond the western paradigm.* Thousand Oaks, CA: Sage.

Airhihenbuwa, C. O. (1999). Of culture and multiverse: Renouncing "the universal truth" in health. *Journal of Health Education, 30*(5), 267–273.

Airhihenbuwa, C. O., & Liburd, L. (2006). Eliminating health disparities in the African American population: The interface of culture, gender, and power. *Health Education & Behavior, 33*(4), 488–501.

Airhihenbuwa, C. O., & Webster, J. D. (2004). Culture and African contexts of HIV/AIDS prevention, care and support. *SAHARA J: Journal of Social Aspects of HIV/AIDS Research Alliance, 1*(1), 4–13.

Alexander, S. C., Fortenberry, J. D., Pollak, K. I., Bravender, T., Davis, J. K., Østbye, T., . . . Shields, C. G. (2014). Sexuality talk during adolescent health maintenance visits. *JAMA Pediatrics, 168*(2), 163–169.

Allegrante, J. P., & Sleet, D. A. (2004). *Derryberry's educating for health: A foundation for contemporary health education practice.* San Francisco, CA: Jossey-Bass.

Altschuld, J. W., & Kumar, D. D. (2010). *Needs assessment: An overview.* Thousand Oaks, CA: Sage.

Anderson, L. A., Day, K. L., & Vandenberg, A. E. (2011). Using a concept map as a tool for strategic planning: The healthy brain initiative. *Preventing Chronic Disease, 8*(5), A116.

Annegers, J. F., Dubinsky, S., Coan, S. P., Newmark, M. E., & Roht, L. (1999). The incidence of epilepsy and unprovoked seizures in multiethnic, urban health maintenance organizations. *Epilepsia, 40*(4), 502–506.

Baheiraei, A., Mirghafourvand, M., Mohammadi, E., Charandabi, S. M., & Nedjat, S. (2013). Determining appropriate strategies for improving women's health promoting behaviours: Using the nominal group technique. *Eastern Mediterranean Health Journal, 19*(5), 409–416.

Banerjee, P. N., Filippi, D., & Allen Hauser, W. (2009). The descriptive epidemiology of epilepsy—A review. *Epilepsy Research, 85*(1), 31–45.

Bartholomew, L. K., & Mullen, P. D. (2011). Five roles for using theory and evidence in the design and testing of behavior change interventions. *Journal of Public Health Dentistry, 71*(s1), S20–S33.

Bartholomew, L. K., Mullen, P. D., Byrd, T., Ureda, J., Volk, R., & Chan, E. (2010). *Developing informed decision making tools for prostate cancer screening: An intervention mapping approach.* Unpublished manuscript.

Batenburg, A., & Das, E. (2014). Emotional coping differences among breast cancer patients from an online support group: A cross-sectional study. *Journal of Medical Internet Research, 16*(2), e28.

Becker, A. B., Israel, B. A., & Allen, A. (2005). Strategies and techniques for effective group process in community-based participatory research partnerships. In B. A. Israel, E. Eng, A. J. Schultz, & E. Parker (Eds.), *Methods in community-based participatory research for health* (pp. 52–72). San Francisco, CA: Jossey-Bass.

Begley, C. E., Shegog, R., Iyagba, B., Chen, V., Talluri, K., Dubinsky, S., . . . Friedman, D. (2010). Socioeconomic status and self-management in epilepsy: Comparison of diverse clinical populations in Houston, Texas. *Epilepsy & Behavior, 19*(3), 232–238.

Belansky, E. S., Cutforth, N., Chavez, R. A., Waters, E., & Bartlett-Horch, K. (2011). An adapted version of intervention mapping (AIM) is a tool for conducting community-based participatory research. *Health Promotion Practice, 12*(3), 440–455.

Bellows, L., Anderson, J., Gould, S. M., & Auld, G. (2008). Formative research and strategic development of a physical activity component to a social marketing campaign for obesity prevention in preschoolers. *Journal of Community Health, 33*(3), 169–178.

Bennett, M. J. (1993). Towards ethnorelativism: A developmental model of intercultural sensitivity. In R. M. Paige (Ed.), *Education for the intercultural experience* (pp. 21–71). Yarmouth, ME: Intercultural Press.

Bensing, J. M., Roter, D. L., & Hulsman, R. L. (2003). Communication patterns of primary care physicians in the United States and the Netherlands. *Journal of General Internal Medicine, 18*(5), 335–342.

Blair, T., & Minkler, M. (2009). Participatory action research with older adults: Key principles in practice. *The Gerontologist, 49*(5), 651–662.

Boekeloo, B. O. (2014). Will you ask? Will they tell you? Are you ready to hear and respond? Barriers to physician-adolescent discussion about sexuality. *JAMA Pediatrics, 168*(2), 111–113.

Boekeloo, B. O., Marx, E. S., Kral, A. H., Coughlin, S. C., Bowman, M., & Rabin, D. L. (1991). Frequency and thoroughness of STD/HIV risk assessment by physicians in a high-risk metropolitan area. *American Journal of Public Health, 81*(12), 1645–1648.

Bonham, C. A., Sommerfeld, D., Willging, C., & Aarons, G. A. (2014). Organizational factors influencing implementation of evidence-based practices for integrated treatment in behavioral health agencies. *Psychiatry Journal, 2014*(4).

Bonilla-Silva, E. (2006). *Racism without racists: Color-blind racism and the persistence of racial inequality in the United States.* Lanham, MD: Rowman & Littlefield.

Borkan, J. M., & Neher, J. O. (1991). A developmental model of ethnosensitivity in family practice training. *Family Medicine, 23*(3), 212–217.

Bradford, L. P. (1976). *Making meetings work: A guide for leaders and group members.* San Diego, CA: University Associates.

Bradley, E. H., Curry, L. A., Ramanadhan, S., Rowe, L., Nembhard, I. M., & Krumholz, H. M. (2009). Research in action: Using positive deviance to improve quality of health care. *Implementation Science, 4,* 1–11.

Bronte-Tinkew, J., Burkhauser, M., & Metz, A. (2008). *Elements of promising practice in teen fatherhood programs: Evidence-based and evidence-informed research findings on what works.* Gaithersburg, MD: National Responsible Fatherhood Clearinghouse.

Brown, C., & Mazza, G. (1997). *Healing into action: A leadership guide for creating diverse communities.* Washington, DC: National Coalition Building Institute.

Brown, G., Schebella, M. F., & Weber, D. (2014). Using participatory GIS to measure physical activity and urban park benefits. *Landscape and Urban Planning, 121,* 34–44.

Bryant, L. L., Altpeter, M., & Whitelaw, N. A. (2006). Evaluation of health promotion programs for older adults: An introduction. *Journal of Applied Gerontology, 25*(3), 197–213.

Buelow, J. M. (2001). Epilepsy management issues and techniques. *Journal of Neuroscience Nursing, 33*(5), 260–269.

Buhi, E. R., & Goodson, P. (2007). Predictors of adolescent sexual behavior and intention: A theory-guided systematic review. *Journal of Adolescent Health, 40*(1), 4–21.

Bureau of Epidemiology Houston Department of Health and Human Services. (2008). AIDS: Summary of Houston/Harris county cases cumulative—Reported 1981 through 121/31/2008. Retrieved from http://www.houstontx.gov/health/HIV-STD/4thQRT2008.pdf

Buta, B., Brewer, L., Hamlin, D. L., Palmer, M. W., Bowie, J., & Gielen, A. (2011). An innovative faith-based healthy eating program: From class assignment to real-world application of PRECEDE/PROCEED. *Health Promotion Practice, 12*(6), 867–875.

Buunk, A. P., & Van Vugt, M. (2013). *Applying social psychology: From problems to solutions* (2nd ed.). London: Sage.

Cargo, M., & Mercer, S. L. (2008). The value and challenges of participatory research: Strengthening its practice. *Annual Review of Public Health, 29,* 325–350.

Catalani, C., & Minkler, M. (2010). Photovoice: A review of the literature in health and public health. *Health Education & Behavior, 37*(3), 424–451.

Centers for Disease Control and Prevention. (1994). Current trends: Prevalence of self reported epilepsy: United States 1986–1990. *Morbidity and Mortality Weekly Report, 43*, 810–811.

Centers for Disease Control and Prevention. (2010). Environmental audits. Retrieved from http://www.cdc.gov/nccdphp/dnpao/hwi/programdesign/environmental_audits.htm

Centers for Disease Control and Prevention. (2012a). *HIV among youth in the US.* CDC Vitalsigns. Retrieved from http://www.cdc.gov/vitalsigns/HIVAmongYouth/index.html

Centers for Disease Control and Prevention. (2012b). SHPPS 2012. School health policies and practices study. Retrieved from http://www.cdc.gov/healthyyouth/shpps/2012/factsheets/pdf/FS_Overview_SHPPS2012.pdf

Centers for Disease Control and Prevention. (2014). Diagnoses of HIV infection and population among young adults aged 20–24 years, by race/ethnicity 2011—United States. Retrieved from http://www.cdc.gov/hiv/pdf/statistics_surveillance_Adolescents.pdf

Centers for Disease Control and Prevention & Oak Ridge Institute for Science and Education. (2003). Cdcynergy: Your guide to effective health communication (version 3.0) [computer software]. Retrieved from http://www.cdc.gov/healthmarketing/cdcynergy/

Centers for Disease Control and Prevention Program Performance and Evaluation Office. (2012). A framework for program evaluation. Retrieved from www.cdc.gov/EVAL/framework

Chan, E. C., McFall, S. L., Byrd, T. L., Mullen, P. D., Volk, R. J., Ureda, J., . . . Kay Bartholomew, L. (2011). A community-based intervention to promote informed decision making for prostate cancer screening among Hispanic American men changed knowledge and role preferences: A cluster RCT. *Patient Education and Counseling, 84*(2), e44–e51.

Chavis, D. M., & Wandersman, A. (1990). Sense of community in the urban environment: A catalyst for participation and community development. *American Journal of Community Psychology, 18*(1), 55–81.

Christopher, S., Watts, V., McCormick, A. K., & Young, S. (2008). Building and maintaining trust in a community-based participatory research partnership. *American Journal of Public Health, 98*(8), 1398–1406.

Cifuentes, E., Alamo, U., Kendall, T., Brunkard, J., & Scrimshaw, S. (2006). Rapid assessment procedures in environmental sanitation research: A case study from the northern border of Mexico. *Canadian Journal of Public Health/Revue Canadienne De Sante'e Publique, 97*(1), 24–28.

Clark, N. M. (2003). Management of chronic disease by patients. *Annual Review of Public Health, 24*(1), 289–313.

Cole, R. E., & Horacek, T. (2009). Applying precede-proceed to develop an intuitive eating nondieting approach to weight management pilot program. *Journal of Nutrition Education and Behavior, 41*(2), 120–126.

Coyle, K. K., Kirby, D. B., Marin, B. V., Gómez, C. A., & Gregorich, S. E. (2004). Draw the line/respect the line: A randomized trial of a middle school intervention to reduce sexual risk behaviors. *American Journal of Public Health, 94*(5), 843–851.

Cramer, J. A., Westbrook, L. E., Devinsky, O., Perrine, K., Glassman, M. B., & Camfield, C. (1999). Development of the quality of life in epilepsy inventory for adolescents: The QOLIE-AD-48. *Epilepsia, 40*(8), 1114–1121.

Creswell, J. W., Klassen, A. C., Plano Clark, V. L. & Clegg Smith, K. (2011). Best practices for mixed methods research in the health sciences. *Report commissioned by the office of behavioral and social sciences research (OBSSR).* Retrieved from http://obssr.od.nih.gov/scientific_areas/methodology/mixed_ methods_research/section2.aspx

Cunningham, S. D., Tschann, J., Gurvey, J. E., Fortenberry, J. D., & Ellen, J. M. (2002). Attitudes about sexual disclosure and perceptions of stigma and shame. *Sexually Transmitted Infections, 78*(5), 334–338.

Damschroder, L. J., Aron, D. C., Keith, R. E., Kirsh, S. R., Alexander, J. A., & Lowery, J. C. (2009). Fostering implementation of health services research findings into practice: A consolidated framework for advancing implementation science. *Implementation Science, 4*(1), 50.

De Vet, E., Brug, J., De Nooijer, J., Dijkstra, A., & De Vries, N. K. (2005). Determinants of forward stage transitions: A Delphi study. *Health Education Research, 20*(2), 195–205.

Delbecq, A. (1983). The nominal group as a technique for understanding the qualitative dimensions of client needs. In R. A. Bell (Ed.), *Assessing health and human service needs* (pp. 191–209). New York, NY: Human Sciences Press.

Delbecq, A. L., Van de Ven, Andrew H, & Gustafson, D. H. (1975). *Group techniques for program planning: A guide to nominal group and Delphi processes.* Glenview, IL: Scott, Foresman.

Denzin, N. K., & Lincoln, Y. S. (Eds.). (2007). *Collecting and interpreting qualitative materials* (3rd ed.). Thousand Oaks, CA: Sage.

DiIorio, C., & Faherty, B. (1994). Epilepsy self management: Partial replication and extension. *Research in Nursing & Health, 17*(3), 167–174.

DiIorio, C., Faherty, B., & Manteuffel, B. (1992). Self-efficacy and social support in self-management of epilepsy. *Western Journal of Nursing Research, 14*(3), 292–307.

DiIorio, C., Resnicow, K., Dudley, W. N., Thomas, S., Wang, D. T., Van Marter, D. F., . . . Lipana, J. (2000). Social cognitive factors associated with mother-adolescent communication about sex. *Journal of Health Communication, 5*(1), 41–51.

DiIorio, C., Shafer, P. O., Letz, R., Henry, T. R., Schomer, D. L., Yeager, K., & Project EASE Study Group. (2004). Project EASE: A study to test a psychosocial model of epilepsy medication management. *Epilepsy & Behavior, 5*(6), 926–936.

Dillman, D. A., Smyth, J. D., & Christian, L. M. (2008). *Internet, mail and mixed-mode surveys: The tailored design method* (3rd ed.). Hoboken, NJ: John Wiley & Sons.

Dodson, W. E., & Trimble, M. R. (1994). Epilogue: Quality of life in epilepsy. In M. R. Trimble, & W. E. Dodson (Eds.), *Epilepsy and quality of life*. New York, NY: Raven Press Ltd.

Economos, C. D. (2007). Community interventions: A brief overview and their application to the obesity epidemic. *The Journal of Law, Medicine & Ethics*, *35*(1), 131–137.

Edgren, K. K., Parker, E. A., Israel, B. A., Lewis, T. C., Salinas, M. A., Robins, T. G., & Hill, Y. R. (2005). Community involvement in the conduct of a health education intervention and research project: Community action against asthma. *Health Promotion Practice*, *6*(3), 263–269.

Elliott, L., McBride, T. D., Allen, P., Jacob, R. R., Jones, E., Kerner, J., & Brownson, R. (2014). Health care system collaboration to address chronic diseases: A nationwide snapshot from state public health practitioners. *Preventing Chronic Disease*, *11*, E152.

Eng, E., & Parker, E. (1994). Measuring community competence in the Mississippi Delta: The interface between program evaluation and empowerment. *Health Education & Behavior*, *21*(2), 199–220.

Environmental Systems Research Institute. Story maps. Retrieved from http://storymaps.arcgis.com/en/

Farquhar, S. A., Parker, E. A., Schulz, A. J., & Israel, B. A. (2006). Application of qualitative methods in program planning for health promotion interventions. *Health Promotion Practice*, *7*(2), 234–242.

Farrell, M., Wallis, N. C., & Evans, M. T. (2007). A replication study of priorities and attitudes of two nursing programs' communities of interest: An appreciative inquiry. *Journal of Professional Nursing*, *23*(5), 267–277.

Fawcett, S. B., Francisco, V. T., Schultz, J. A., Berkowitz, B., Wolff, T. J., & Nagy, G. (2000). The community tool box: A web-based resource for building healthier communities. *Public Health Reports (Washington, D.C.: 1974)*, *115*(2–3), 274–278.

Fellin, P. (1995). Understanding American communities. In J. Rothman, J. L. Erlich, & J. E. Tropman (Eds.), *Strategies of community intervention: Macro practice* (5th ed.). Itasca, IL: F.E. Peacock.

Ferdinand, A. O., Sen, B., Rahurkar, S., Engler, S., & Menachemi, N. (2012). The relationship between built environments and physical activity: A systematic review. *American Journal of Public Health*, *102*(10), e7–e13.

Fernández, M. (2012, Aug 21). Factors influencing implementation of evidence-based cancer prevention and control practices in FQHCs: A qualitative study. Oral presentation at the center for disease control national cancer conference. Washington, DC.

Fernández, M. E., Gonzales, A., Tortolero-Luna, G., Partida, S., & Bartholomew, L. K. (2005a). Using intervention mapping to develop a breast and cervical cancer screening program for Hispanic farmworkers: Cultivando La Salud. *Health Promotion Practice*, *6*(4), 394–404.

Fernández, M. E., Gonzales, A., Tortolero-Luna, G., Williams, J., Saavedra-Embesi, M., & Vernon, S. (2009). Effectiveness of Cultivando La Salud: A breast and cervical cancer screening education program for low income Hispanic women living in farmworker communities. *Cancer Causes & Control, 99*(5), 936–943.

Fernández, M. E., Palmer, R. C., & Leong-Wu, C. A. (2005b). Repeat mammography screening among low-income and minority women: A qualitative study. *Cancer Control, 12*(Suppl 2), 77–83.

Fernández, M. E., Savas, L. S., Wilson, K. M., Byrd, T. L., Atkinson, J., Torres-Vigil, I., & Vernon, S. W. (2015). Colorectal cancer screening among Latinos in three communities on the Texas-Mexico border. *Health Education & Behavior, 42*(1), 16–25.

Fernández, M. E., Wippold, R., Torres-Vigil, I., Byrd, T., Freeberg, D., Bains, Y., . . . Vernon, S. W. (2008). Colorectal cancer screening among Latinos from US cities along the Texas–Mexico border. *Cancer Causes & Control, 19*(2), 195–206.

Fishbein, M., & Ajzen, I. (2010). *Predicting and changing behaviour: The Reasoned Action Approach*. New York, NY: Taylor & Francis.

Fisher, E. B., Sussman, L. K., Arfken, C., Harrison, D., Munro, J., Sykes, R. K., . . . Strunk, R. C. (1994). Targeting high risk groups: Neighborhood organization for pediatric asthma management in the neighborhood asthma coalition. *CHEST Journal, 106*(4_Supplement), 248S–259S.

FitzGerald, K., Seale, N. S., Kerins, C. A., & McElvaney, R. (2008). The critical incident technique: A useful tool for conducting qualitative research. *Journal of Dental Education, 72*(3), 299–304.

Fitzgibbon, M. L., & Beech, B. M. (2009). The role of culture in the context of school-based BMI screening. *Pediatrics, 124* Suppl 1, S50–62.

Flanigan, C. M. (2003). Sexual activity among girls under age 15: Findings from the national survey of family growth. In B. Albert, S. Brown & C. M. Flanigan (Eds.), *14 and younger: The sexual behavior of young adolescents* (pp. 57–64). Washington, DC: The National Campaign to Prevent Teen Pregnancy.

Ford, C. L., & Airhihenbuwa, C. O. (2010). Critical race theory, race equity, and public health: Toward antiracism praxis. *American Journal of Public Health, 100*(S1), S30–S35.

Foster-Fishman, P. G., Nowell, B., & Yang, H. (2007). Putting the system back into systems change: A framework for understanding and changing organizational and community systems. *American Journal of Community Psychology, 39*(3–4), 197–215.

Fowler, F. J. (2008). *Survey research methods* (4th ed.). Thousand Oaks, CA: Sage.

Friedman, D. B., Brandt, H. M., Freedman, D. A., Adams, S. A., Young, V. M., Ureda, J. R., . . . Hebert, J. R. (2014). Innovative and community-driven communication practices of the South Carolina cancer prevention and control research network. *Preventing Chronic Disease, 11*, E127.

Friis, R. H., & Sellers, T. (2013). *Epidemiology for public health practice*. Burlington, MA: Jones & Bartlett Publishing.

Frost, J. H., & Massagli, M. P. (2008). Social uses of personal health information within PatientsLikeMe, an online patient community: What can happen when patients have access to one another's data. *Journal of Medical Internet Research*, *10*(3), e15.

Fryer-Edwards, K., Van Eaton, E., Goldstein, E. A., Kimball, H. R., Veith, R. C., Pellegrini, C. A., & Ramsey, P. G. (2007). Overcoming institutional challenges through continuous professionalism improvement: The University of Washington experience. *Academic Medicine, 82*(11), 1073–1078.

Gilliam, F., Penovich, P. E., Eagan, C. A., Stern, J. M., Labiner, D. M., Onofrey, M., . . . Cramer, J. (2009). Conversations between community-based neurologists and patients with epilepsy: Results of an observational linguistic study. *Epilepsy & Behavior, 16*(2), 315–320.

Gilmore, G. D., & Campbell, M. D. (2005). *Needs and capacity assessment strategies for health education and health promotion* (3rd ed.). Sudbury, MA: Jones and Bartlett.

Gittelsohn, J., Steckler, A., Johnson, C. C., Pratt, C., Grieser, M., Pickrel, J., . . . Staten, L. K. (2006). Formative research in school and community-based health programs and studies: "State of the art" and the TAAG approach. *Health Education & Behavior, 33*(1), 25–39.

Glasgow, R. E., Marcus, A. C., Bull, S. S., & Wilson, K. M. (2004). Disseminating effective cancer screening interventions. *Cancer, 101*(S5), 1239–1250.

Glasgow, R. E., Vogt, T. M., & Boles, S. M. (1999). Evaluating the public health impact of health promotion interventions: The RE-AIM framework. *American Journal of Public Health, 89*(9), 1322–1327.

Goffman, E. (1963). *Stigma*. Englewood Cliffs, NJ: Prentice Hall.

Goodman, R. M., Speers, M. A., McLeroy, K., Fawcett, S., Kegler, M., Parker, E., . . . Wallerstein, N. (1998). Identifying and defining the dimensions of community capacity to provide a basis for measurement. *Health Education & Behavior, 25*(3), 258–278.

Goodman, R. M., & Steckler, A. (1989). A model for the institutionalization of health promotion programs. *Family & Community Health, 11*(4), 63–78.

Gordis, L. (2009). *Epidemiology* (3rd ed.). Philadelphia, PA: Saunders.

Graham, L., Brown-Jeffy, S., Aronson, R., & Stephens, C. (2011). Critical race theory as theoretical framework and analysis tool for population health research. *Critical Public Health, 21*(1), 81–93.

Graham, S. R., Carlton, C., Gaede, D., & Jamison, B. (2011). The benefits of using geographic information systems as a community assessment tool. *Public Health Reports (Washington, D.C.: 1974), 126*(2), 298–303.

Green, L. W., & Kreuter, M. W. (1991). *Health promotion planning: An educational and environmental approach* (2nd ed.). Mountain View, CA: Mayfield.

Green, L. W., & Kreuter, M. W. (1999). *Health program planning: An educational and ecological approach* (3rd ed.). Mountain View, CA: Mayfield.

Green, L. W., & Kreuter, M. W. (2005). *Health program planning: An educational and ecological approach* (4th ed.). New York, NY: McGraw Hill Professional.

Guilamo-Ramos, V., Jaccard, J., Dittus, P., & Collins, S. (2008). Parent-adolescent communication about sexual intercourse: An analysis of maternal reluctance to communicate. *Health Psychology, 27*(6), 760–769.

The Guttmacher Institute. (2014a). State policies in brief: An overview of minors' consent law. Retrieved from http://www.guttmacher.org/statecenter/spibs/ spib_OMCL.pdf

The Guttmacher Institute. (2014b). State policies in brief: Sex and HIV education. Retrieved from http://www.guttmacher.org/statecenter/spibs/spib_SE.pdf

Gwede, C. K., Menard, J. M., Martinez-Tyson, D., Lee, J. H., Vadaparampil, S. T., Padhya, T. A., ... Tampa Bay Community Cancer Network Community Partners. (2010). Strategies for assessing community challenges and strengths for cancer disparities participatory research and outreach. *Health Promotion Practice, 11*(6), 876–887.

Hamilton, B. E., & Ventura, S. J. (2012). *Birth rates for US teenagers reach historic lows for all age and ethnic groups. (Data brief number 89).* US Department of Health and Human Services, Centers for Disease Control and Prevention, National Center for Health Statistics.

Harmsen, I. A., Mollema, L., Ruiter, R. A. C., Paulussen, T. G., de Melker, H. E., & Kok, G. (2013). Why parents refuse childhood vaccination: A qualitative study using online focus groups. *BMC Public Health, 13*(1), 1183.

Hawe, P., King, L., Noort, M., Gifford, S. M., & Lloyd, B. (1998). Working invisibly: Health workers talk about capacity-building in health promotion. *Health Promotion International, 13*(4), 285–295.

Hazavei, S. M. M., Sabzmakan, L., Hasanzadeh, A., Rabiei, K., & Roohafza, H. (2012). The effects of an educational program based on PRECEDE model on depression levels in patients with coronary artery bypass grafting. *ARYA Atherosclerosis, 8*(1), 36.

Hebert, J. R., Brandt, H. M., Armstead, C. A., Adams, S. A., & Steck, S. E. (2009). Interdisciplinary, translational, and community-based participatory research: Finding a common language to improve cancer research. *Cancer Epidemiology, Biomarkers & Prevention, 18*(4), 1213–1217.

Highfield, L., Arthasarnprasit, J., Ottenweller, C. A., & Dasprez, A. (2011). Interactive web-based mapping: Bridging technology and data for health. *International Journal of Health Geographics, 10,* 69.

Hirtz, D., Thurman, D. J., Gwinn-Hardy, K., Mohamed, M., Chaudhuri, A. R., & Zalutsky, R. (2007). How common are the "common" neurologic disorders? *Neurology, 68*(5), 326–337.

Hochbaum, G. M., Sorenson, J. R., & Lorig, K. (1992). Theory in health education practice. *Health Education & Behavior, 19*(3), 295–313.

Hoffman, S. D. (2006). *By the numbers: The public costs of teen childbearing.* Washington, DC: National Campaign to Prevent Teen Pregnancy.

Horn, K., McCracken, L., Dino, G., & Brayboy, M. (2008). Applying community-based participatory research principles to the development of a smoking-cessation program for American Indian teens: "Telling our story". *Health Education & Behavior, 35*(1), 44–69.

Hospers, H. J., Kok, G., Harterink, P., & de Zwart, O. (2005). A new meeting place: Chatting on the internet, e-dating and sexual risk behaviour among Dutch men who have sex with men. *AIDS, 19*(10), 1097–1101.

Houston Department of Health and Human Services. (2007). Statistical information on chlamydia, gonorrhea, and syphilis. Retrieved from http://www.houstontx .gov/health/HIV-STD/statistics.html

Hsu, C., & Sandford, B. A. (2007). The Delphi technique: Making sense of consensus. *Practical Assessment, Research & Evaluation, 12*(10), 1–8.

Hugentobler, M. K., Israel, B. A., & Schurman, S. J. (1992). An action research approach to workplace health: Integrating methods. *Health Education & Behavior, 19*(1), 55–76.

Institute of Medicine. (2002). *Speaking of health: Assessing health communication strategies for diverse populations.* Washington, DC: National Academies Press.

Institute of Medicine. (2012). *Epilepsy across the spectrum: Promoting health and understanding.* Washington, DC: The National Academies Press.

Israel, B. A., Schulz, A. J., Parker, E. A., Becker, A. B., Allen, A. J. I., & Guzman, J. R. (2003). Critical issues in developing and following community based participatory research principles. In M. Minkler & N. Wallerstein (Eds.), *Community-based participatory research for health* (pp. 53–76). San Francisco, CA: Jossey-Bass.

Jaccard, J., Dittus, P. J., & Gordon, V. V. (2000). Parent-teen communication about premarital sex factors associated with the extent of communication. *Journal of Adolescent Research, 15*(2), 187–208.

Jemmott, J. B., III, Jemmott, L. S., & Fong, G. T. (1998). Abstinence and safer sex HIV risk-reduction interventions for African American adolescents: A randomized controlled trial. *Journal of the American Medical Association, 279*(19), 1529–1536.

Johnson, D. R., & Johnson, F. P. (2012). *Joining together: Group theory and group skills* (11th ed.). Upper Saddle River, NJ: Pearson.

Jones, J. E., Hermann, B. P., Woodard, J. L., Barry, J. J., Gilliam, F., Kanner, A. M., & Meador, K. J. (2005). Screening for major depression in epilepsy with common self-report depression inventories. *Epilepsia, 46*(5), 731–735.

Kann, L., Kinchen, S., Shanklin, S. L., Flint, K. H., Kawkins, J., Harris, W. A.,... Chyen, D. (2014). Youth risk behavior surveillance—United States, 2013. *MMWR Surveillance Summaries, 63*(Suppl 4), 1–168.

Kannan, S., Schulz, A., Israel, B., Ayra, I., Weir, S., Dvonch, T. J.,... Benjamin, A. (2008). A community-based participatory approach to personalized, computer-generated nutrition feedback reports: The healthy environments partnership. *Progress in Community Health Partnerships: Research, Education, and Action, 2*(1), 41–53.

Kannan, S., Webster, D., Sparks, A., Acker, C. M., Greene-Moton, E., Tropiano, E., & Turner, T. (2009). Using a cultural framework to assess the nutrition influences in relation to birth outcomes among African American women of childbearing age: Application of the PEN-3 theoretical model. *Health Promotion Practice, 10*(3), 349–358.

Keeney, S., Hasson, F., & McKenna, H. (2011). *The Delphi technique in nursing and health research*. Oxford, UK: Wiley Online Library.

Kelsey, J. L., Whittemore, A. S., Evans, A. S., & Thompson, W. D. (1996). *Methods in observational epidemiology*. Oxford, UK: Oxford University Press.

Kelso, G. A., Cohen, M. H., Weber, K. M., Dale, S. K., Cruise, R. C., & Brody, L. R. (2014). Critical consciousness, racial and gender discrimination, and HIV disease markers in African American women with HIV. *AIDS and Behavior*, *18*(7), 1237–1246.

Kirby, D., Lepore, G., & Ryan, J. (2005). *Sexual risk and protective factors: Factors affecting teen sexual behavior, pregnancy, childbearing, and sexually transmitted disease: Which are important? Which can you change?* Washington, DC: National Campaign to Prevent Teen Pregnancy.

Kraft, J. M., Beeker, C., Stokes, J. P., & Peterson, J. L. (2000). Finding the "community" in community-level HIV/AIDS interventions: Formative research with young African American men who have sex with men. *Health Education & Behavior*, *27*(4), 430–441.

Kreuter, M. W., Lukwago, S. N., Bucholtz, R. D., Clark, E. M., & Sanders-Thompson, V. (2003). Achieving cultural appropriateness in health promotion programs: Targeted and tailored approaches. *Health Education & Behavior*, *30*(2), 133–146.

Krieger, J., Allen, C., Cheadle, A., Ciske, S., Schier, J. K., Senturia, K., & Sullivan, M. (2002). Using community-based participatory research to address social determinants of health: Lessons learned from Seattle partners for healthy communities. *Health Education & Behavior*, *29*(3), 361–382.

Krueger, R. A., & Casey, M. A. (2009). *Focus groups: A practical guide for applied research* (4th ed.). Thousand Oaks, CA: Sage.

Lankenau, S. E., Clatts, M. C., Welle, D., Goldsamt, L. A., & Gwadz, M. V. (2005). Street careers: Homelessness, drug use, and sex work among young men who have sex with men (YMSM). *International Journal of Drug Policy*, *16*(1), 10–18.

Lehmann, B., Ruiter, R. A. C., van Dam, D., Wicker, S., & Kok, G. (2015). Sociocognitive predictors of the intention of healthcare workers to receive the influenza vaccine in Belgian, Dutch and German hospital settings. *Journal of Hospital Infection*, *89*(3), 202–209.

Lehmann, B. A., Ruiter, R. A. C., Wicker, S., Van Dam, D., & Kok, G. (2014). "I don't see an added value for myself": A qualitative study exploring the social cognitive variables associated with influenza vaccination of Belgian, Dutch and German healthcare personnel. *BMC Public Health*, *14*, 407.

Levine, J., Rudy, T., & Kerns, R. (1994). A two factor model of denial of illness: A confirmatory factor analysis. *Journal of Psychosomatic Research*, *38*(2), 99–110.

Levy, S. R., Anderson, E. E., Issel, L. M., Willis, M. A., Dancy, B. L., Jacobson, K. M., . . . Hebert-Beirne, J. (2004). Using multilevel, multisource needs assessment data for planning community interventions. *Health Promotion Practice*, *5*(1), 59–68.

Lewin, S., Munabi-Babigumira, S., Glenton, C., Daniels, K., Bosch-Capblanch, X., van Wyk, B. E., . . . Zwarenstein, M. (2010). Lay health workers in primary and community health care for maternal and child health and the management of infectious diseases. *Cochrane Database of Systematic Reviews, 3.*

Li, Y., Cao, J., Lin, H., Li, D., Wang, Y., & He, J. (2009). Community health needs assessment with precede-proceed model: A mixed methods study. *BMC Health Services Research, 9,* 181.

Locke, D. C. (1986). Cross-cultural counseling issues. In W. J. Weikel & A. J. Palmo (Eds.), *Foundation of mental health counseling.* Springfield, IL: Charles C. Thomas.

Locke, D. C. (1992). *Increasing multicultural understanding: A comprehensive model.* Thousand Oaks, CA: Sage.

Ludema, J. D., Whitney, D., Mohr, B. J., & Griffin, T. J. (2003). *The appreciative inquiry summit: A practitioner's guide for leading large-group change.* San Francisco, CA: Berrett-Koehler.

MacLeod, J. S., & Austin, J. K. (2003). Stigma in the lives of adolescents with epilepsy: A review of the literature. *Epilepsy & Behavior, 4*(2), 112–117.

MacQueen, K. M., McLellan, E., Metzger, D. S., Kegeles, S., Strauss, R. P., Scotti, R., . . . Trotter, R. T. (2001). What is community? An evidence-based definition for participatory public health. *American Journal of Public Health, 91*(12), 1929–1938.

Marin, B., Kirby, D., Hudes, E., Gomez, C., & Coyle, K. (2003). Youth with older boyfriends and girlfriends: Associations with sexual risk. In B. Albert, S. Brown, & C. Flanigan (Eds.), *Too much, too soon: The sex lives of young teens* (pp. 83–90). Washington, DC: The National Campaign to Prevent Teen Pregnancy.

Markham, C. M., Lormand, D., Gloppen, K. M., Peskin, M. F., Flores, B., Low, B., & House, L. D. (2010). Connectedness as a predictor of sexual and reproductive health outcomes for youth. *Journal of Adolescent Health, 46*(3), S23–S41.

Markham, C. M., Tortolero, S. R., Peskin, M. F., Shegog, R., Thiel, M., Baumler, E. R., . . . Robin, L. (2012). Sexual risk avoidance and sexual risk reduction interventions for middle school youth: A randomized controlled trial. *Journal of Adolescent Health, 50*(3), 279–288.

Mattessich, P. W., Murray-Close, M., & Monsey, B. R. (2001). *Collaboration: What makes it work? A review of factors influencing successful community building.* St. Paul, MN: Amherst H. Wilder Foundation.

May, T. W., & Pfäfflin, M. (2002). The efficacy of an educational treatment program for patients with epilepsy (MOSES): Results of a controlled, randomized study. *Epilepsia, 43*(5), 539–549.

McEachan, R. R., Lawton, R. J., Jackson, C., Conner, M., & Lunt, J. (2008). Evidence, theory and context: Using intervention mapping to develop a worksite physical activity intervention. *BMC Public Health, 8,* 326.

McFall, S. L., Ureda, J., Byrd, T. L., Valdes, A., Morales, P., Scott, D. B., . . . Chan, E. C. (2009). What is needed for informed decisions about prostate cancer screening: Perspectives of African-American and Hispanic men. *Health Education Research, 24*(2), 280–291.

McKnight, J. (2012). *The abundant community: Awakening the power of families and neighborhoods.* San Francisco, CA: Berrett-Koehler Publishers, Inc.

McKnight, J. L., & Kretzmann, J. P. (2012). Mapping community capacity. In M. Minkler (Ed.), *Community organizing and community building for health* (pp. 171–186). New Brunswick, NJ: Rutgers University Press.

McMillan, D. W., & Chavis, D. M. (1986). Sense of community: A definition and theory. *Journal of Community Psychology, 14*(1), 6–23.

Merzel, C., & D'Afflitti, J. (2003). Reconsidering community-based health promotion: Promise, performance, and potential. *American Journal of Public Health, 93*(4), 557–574.

Midgley, G. (2006). Systemic intervention for public health. *American Journal of Public Health, 96*(3), 466–472.

Miller, K. S., Kotchick, B. A., Dorsey, S., Forehand, R., & Ham, A. Y. (1998). Family communication about sex: What are parents saying and are their adolescents listening? *Family Planning Perspectives, 30*(5), 218–235.

Minkler, M. (1997). Community organizing among the elderly poor in San Francisco's Tenderloin District. In M. Minkler (Ed.), *Community organizing and community building* (pp. 244–258). New Brunswick, NJ: Rutgers University Press.

Minkler, M. (Ed.). (2012). *Community organizing and community building for health and welfare* (3rd ed.). New Brunswick, NJ: Rutgers University Press.

Minkler, M. (2005). Community-based research partnerships: Challenges and opportunities. *Journal of Urban Health, 82*, ii3–ii12.

Minkler, M., Wallerstein, N., & Wilson, N. (2008). Improving health through community organization and community building. In K. Glanz, F. M. Lewis, & B. K. Rimer (Eds.), *Health behavior and health education: Theory, research, and practice* (4th ed., pp. 287–312). San Francisco, CA: Jossey-Bass.

Mitchell-DiCenso, A., Thomas, B. H., Devlin, M. C., Goldsmith, C. H., Willan, A., Singer, J.,…Hewson, S. (1997). Evaluation of an educational program to prevent adolescent pregnancy. *Health Education & Behavior, 24*(3), 300–312.

Moon, R. H. (1999). Finding diamonds in the trenches with the nominal group process. *Family Practice Management, 6*(5), 49–50.

Morales-Campos, D. Y., Markham, C. M., Peskin, M. F., & Fernández, M. E. (2013). Hispanic mothers' and high school girls' perceptions of cervical cancer, human papilloma virus, and the human papilloma virus vaccine. *Journal of Adolescent Health, 52*(5), S69–S75.

Morgan, D. L. (2006). Practical strategies for combining qualitative and quantitative methods: Applications to health research. In C. N. Hesse-Biber & P. Leavy (Eds.), *Emergent methods in social research* (pp. 165–182). Thousand Oaks, CA: Sage.

Murayama, H., Wakui, T., Arami, R., Sugawara, I., & Yoshie, S. (2012). Contextual effect of different components of social capital on health in a suburban city of the greater Tokyo area: A multilevel analysis. *Social Science & Medicine, 75*(12), 2472–2480.

National Institute of Allergy and Infectious Diseases. (2014). Sexually transmitted diseases (STDs). Retrieved from http://www.niaid.nih.gov/topics/std/Pages/default.aspx

Ngo, A. D., McCurdy, S. A., Ross, M. W., Markham, C., Ratliff, E. A., & Pham, H. T. (2007). The lives of female sex workers in Vietnam: Findings from a qualitative study. *Culture, Health & Sexuality*, 9(6), 555–570.

Nijstad, B. A., & Stroebe, W. (2006). How the group affects the mind: A cognitive model of idea generation in groups. *Personality and Social Psychology Review*, 10(3), 186–213.

O'Donnell, L., O'Donnell, C. R., & Stueve, A. (2001). Early sexual initiation and subsequent sex-related risks among urban minority youth: The reach for health study. *Family Planning Perspectives*, 33(6), 268–275.

Oh, H. J., & Lee, B. (2012). The effect of computer-mediated social support in online communities on patient empowerment and doctor–patient communication. *Health Communication*, 27(1), 30–41.

Oldenburg, B., Sallis, J. F., Harris, D., & Owen, N. (2002). Checklist of health promotion environments at work (CHEW): Development and measurement characteristics. *American Journal of Health Promotion*, 16(5), 288–299.

Orlandi, M. A. (1986). The diffusion and adoption of worksite health promotion innovations: An analysis of barriers. *Preventive Medicine*, 15(5), 522–536.

Orlandi, M. A. (1987). Promoting health and preventing disease in health care settings: An analysis of barriers. *Preventive Medicine*, 16(1), 119–130.

Orlandi, M. A., Landers, C., Weston, R., & Haley, N. (1990). Diffusion of health promotion innovations. In K. Glanz, F. M. Lewis, & B. K. Rimer (Eds.), *Health behavior and health education: Theory, research, and practice* (1st ed., pp. 288–313). San Francisco, CA: Jossey-Bass.

Palmer, R. C., Fernández, M. E., Tortolero-Luna, G., Gonzales, A., & Mullen, P. D. (2005). Correlates of mammography screening among Hispanic women living in lower Rio Grande Valley farmworker communities. *Health Education and Behavior*, 32(4), 488–503.

Patton, M. Q. (1990). *Qualitative evaluation and research methods* (2nd ed.). Thousand Oaks, CA: Sage.

Patton, M. Q. (2001). *Qualitative evaluation and research methods* (3rd ed.). Thousand Oaks, CA: Sage.

Peskin, M. F., Markham, C. M., Shegog, R., Baumler, E. R., Addy, R. C., & Tortolero, S. R. (2014). Effects of the *It's Your Game . . . Keep It Real* program on dating violence in ethnic-minority middle school youths: A group randomized trial. *American Journal of Public Health*, 104(8), 1471–1477.

Preskill, H., & Jones, N. (2009). *A practical guide for engaging stakeholders in developing evaluation questions*. Princeton, NJ: Robert Wood Johnson Foundation.

Pryor, J. B., Reeder, G. D., & Monroe, A. E. (2012). The infection of bad company: Stigma by association. *Journal of Personality and Social Psychology*, 102(2), 224.

Ramachandran, R., Jaggarajamma, K., Muniyandi, M., & Balasubramanian, R. (2006). Identifying effective communication channels in a rural community: A field report from south India. *Indian Journal of Tuberculosis*, 53, 206–211.

Ramaratnam, S., Baker, G., & Goldstein, L. (2005). Psychological treatments for epilepsy. *The Cochrane Library*, 2.

Reed, E., Miller, E., Raj, A., Decker, M. R., & Silverman, J. G. (2014). Teen dating violence perpetration and relation to STI and sexual risk behaviours among adolescent males. *Sexually Transmitted Infections, 90*(4), 322–324.

Richard, L., Potvin, L., Kishchuk, N., Prlic, H., & Green, L. W. (1996). Assessment of the integration of the ecological approach in health promotion programs. *American Journal of Health Promotion, 10*(4), 318–328.

Richards, D., & Tangney, B. (2006). Towards an informal online learning community for student mental health at university. In P. Isaias, M. McPherson, & F. Bannister (Eds.), *IADIS international conference on e-society* (pp. 197–201). IADIS.

Rier, D. A. (2007). Internet social support groups as moral agents: The ethical dynamics of HIV status disclosure. *Sociology of Health & Illness, 29*(7), 1043–1058.

Rios, R. A., McDaniel, J. E., & Stowell, J. P. (1998). Pursuing the possibilities of passion: The affective domain of multicultural education. In M. Dillworth (Ed.), *Being responsive to cultural differences: How teachers learn* (pp. 160–181). Thousand Oaks, CA: Corwin Press.

Rodgers, K. B. (1999). Parenting processes related to sexual risk-taking behaviors of adolescent males and females. *Journal of Marriage and the Family, 61*(1), 99–109.

Rothert, M. L. (1991). Perspectives and issues in studying patients' decision-making. In H. Hibbard, P. A. Nutting, & M. L. Grady (Eds.), *Primary care and research: Theory and methods* (pp. 175–179). Washington, DC: U.S. Department of Health and Human Services.

Rubenstein, L. V., & Pugh, J. (2006). Strategies for promoting organizational and practice change by advancing implementation research. *Journal of General Internal Medicine, 21*(S2), S58–S64.

Runyan, J. D., Steenbergh, T. A., Bainbridge, C., Daugherty, D. A., Oke, L., & Fry, B. N. (2013). A smartphone ecological momentary assessment/intervention "app" for collecting real-time data and promoting self-awareness. *PLoS ONE, 8*(8), e71325.

Sabaz, M., Lawson, J. A., Cairns, D. R., Duchowny, M. S., Resnick, T. J., Dean, P. M., & Bye, A. M. (2003). Validation of the quality of life in childhood epilepsy questionnaire in American epilepsy patients. *Epilepsy & Behavior, 4*(6), 680–691.

Saint-Germain, M. A., Bassford, T. L., & Montano, G. (1993). Surveys and focus groups in health research with older Hispanic women. *Qualitative Health Research, 3*(3), 341–367.

Sallis, J. F., Cervero, R. B., Ascher, W., Henderson, K. A., Kraft, M. K., & Kerr, J. (2006). An ecological approach to creating active living communities. *Annual Review of Public Health, 27*, 297–322.

Sampson, E. E., & Marthas, M. (1990). *Group process for the health professions* (3rd ed.). Albany, NY: Delmar Thomson Learning.

Santa Maria, D., Swartz, M. C., Markham, C., Chandra, J., McCurdy, S., & Basen-Engquist, K. (2014). Exploring parental factors related to weight management in survivors of childhood central nervous system tumors. *Journal of Pediatric Oncology Nursing*, *31*(2), 84–94.

Santelli, J. S., Brener, N. D., Lowry, R., Bhatt, A., & Zabin, L. S. (1998). Multiple sexual partners among US adolescents and young adults. *Family Planning Perspectives*, *20*(6), 271–275.

Santelli, J., Ott, M. A., Lyon, M., Rogers, J., Summers, D., & Schleifer, R. (2006). Abstinence and abstinence-only education: A review of US policies and programs. *Journal of Adolescent Health*, *38*(1), 72–81.

Scarinci, I. C., Bandura, L., Hidalgo, B., & Cherrington, A. (2012). Development of a theory-based (PEN-3 and Health Belief Model), culturally relevant intervention on cervical cancer prevention among Latina immigrants using Intervention Mapping. *Health Promotion Practice*, *13*(1), 29–40.

Scrimshaw, S. C. M., & Hurtado, E. (1987). *Rapid assessment procedures for nutrition and primary health care*. Los Angeles, CA: UCLA Latin American Center Publications.

Scrimshaw, S. C. M., & Hurtado, E. (1992). *Rapid assessment procedures: Qualitative methodology for planning and evaluation of health related programmes*. Boston, MA: International Nutrition Foundation for Developing Countries.

Senge, P. M. (2006). *The fifth discipline: The art and practice of the learning organization*. New York, NY: Doubleday.

Shegog, R., Bamps, Y. A., Patel, A., Kakacek, J., Escoffery, C., Johnson, E. K., & Ilozumba, U. O. (2013). Managing epilepsy well: Emerging e-tools for epilepsy self-management. *Epilepsy & Behavior*, *29*(1), 133–140.

Shiffman, S. (2009). Ecological momentary assessment (EMA) in studies of substance use. *Psychological Assessment*, *21*, 486–497.

Shope, J. T. (1988). Compliance in children and adults: Review of studies. *Epilepsy Research, Supplement*, *1*, 23–47.

Shuger, L. (2012). *Teen pregnancy and high school dropout: What communities can do to address these issues*. Washington, DC: The National Campaign to Prevent Teen and Unplanned Pregnancy.

Siegel, D. M., Aten, M. J., & Enaharo, M. (2001). Long-term effects of a middle school- and high school–based human immunodeficiency virus sexual risk prevention intervention. *Archives of Pediatrics & Adolescent Medicine*, *155*(10), 1117–1126.

Slater, S. J., Nicholson, L., Chriqui, J., Turner, L., & Chaloupka, F. (2012). The impact of state laws and district policies on physical education and recess practices in a nationally representative sample of US public elementary schools. *Archives of Pediatrics & Adolescent Medicine*, *166*(4), 311–316.

Small, W., Kerr, T., Charette, J., Schechter, M. T., & Spittal, P. M. (2006). Impacts of intensified police activity on injection drug users: Evidence from an ethnographic investigation. *International Journal of Drug Policy*, *17*(2), 85–95.

Smeets, V. M., van Lierop, B. A., Vanhoutvin, J. P., Aldenkamp, A. P., & Nijhuis, F. J. (2007). Epilepsy and employment: Literature review. *Epilepsy & Behavior*, *10*(3), 354–362.

Springer, A. (n.d.). *Assessing environmental assets for health promotion program planning: A practical framework for health promotion practitioners.* Unpublished manuscript.

Springer, A. E., Kelder, S. H., Barroso, C. S., Drenner, K. L., Shegog, R., Ranjit, N., & Hoelscher, D. M. (2010). Parental influences on television watching among children living on the Texas–Mexico border. *Preventive Medicine, 51*(2), 112–117.

Steckler, A., McLeroy, K. R., Goodman, R. M., Bird, S. T., & McCormick, L. (1992). Toward integrating qualitative and quantitative methods: An introduction. *Health Education Quarterly, 19*(1), 1–8.

Sue, D. W. (2003). *Overcoming our racism.* San Francisco, CA: Jossey-Bass.

Sullivan, M., Chao, S. S., Allen, C. A., Kone, A., Pierre-Louise, M., & Krieger, J. (2003). Community-research partnerships: Perspectives from the field. In M. Minkler & N. Wallerstein (Eds.), *Community-based participatory research for health* (pp. 113–130). San Francisco, CA: Jossey-Bass.

Tanney, M. R., Naar-King, S., & MacDonnel, K. (2012). Depression and stigma in high-risk youth living with HIV: A multi-site study. *Journal of Pediatric Health Care, 26*(4), 300–305.

Tapp, H., & Dulin, M. (2010). The science of primary health-care improvement: Potential and use of community-based participatory research by practice-based research networks for translation of research into practice. *Experimental Biology and Medicine (Maywood, N.J.), 235*(3), 290–299.

Taylor, W. C., Franzini, L., Olvera, N., Poston, W. S. C., & Lin, G. (2012). Environmental audits of friendliness toward physical activity in three income levels. *Journal of Urban Health, 89*(2), 296–307.

Taylor, W. C., Hepworth, J. T., Lees, E., Feliz, K., Ahsan, S., Cassells, A., . . . Tobin, J. N. (2008). Obesity, physical activity, and the environment: Is there a legal basis for environmental injustices? *Environmental Justice, 1*(1), 45–48.

Taylor, W. C., Upchurch, S. L., Brosnan, C. A., Selwyn, B. J., Nguyen, T. Q., Villagomez, E. T., & Meininger, J. C. (2014). Features of the built environment related to physical activity friendliness and children's obesity and other risk factors. *Public Health Nursing, 31*(6), 545–555.

Teddlie, C., & Yu, F. (2007). Mixed methods sampling a typology with examples. *Journal of Mixed Methods Research, 1*(1), 77–100.

Tedman, S., Thornton, E., & Baker, G. (1995). Development of a scale to measure core beliefs and perceived self efficacy in adults with epilepsy. *Seizure, 4*(3), 221–231.

Tervalon, M., & Murray-Garcia, J. (1998). Cultural humility versus cultural competence: A critical distinction in defining physician training outcomes in multicultural education. *Journal of Health Care for the Poor and Underserved, 9*(2), 117–125.

Teufel-Shone, N. I., Siyuja, T., Watahomigie, H. J., & Irwin, S. (2006). Community-based participatory research: Conducting a formative assessment of factors that influence youth wellness in the Hualapai community. *American Journal of Public Health, 96*, 1623–1628.

Texas Department of State Health Services. (2007). *Bureau of vital statistics.*

Theodore, W. H., Spencer, S. S., Wiebe, S., Langfitt, J. T., Ali, A., Shafer, P. O., ... Vickrey, B. G. (2006). Epilepsy in North America: A report prepared under the auspices of the Global Campaign Against Epilepsy, the International Bureau for Epilepsy, the International League Against Epilepsy, and the World Health Organization. *Epilepsia, 47*(10), 1700–1722.

Thomas, S. B., Quinn, S. C., Butler, J., Fryer, C. S., & Garza, M. A. (2011). Toward a fourth generation of disparities research to achieve health equity. *Annual Review of Public Health, 32,* 399–416.

Tortolero, S. R., Markham, C. M., Peskin, M. F., Shegog, R., Addy, R. C., Escobar-Chaves, S. L., & Baumler, E. R. (2010). It's your game: Keep it real: Delaying sexual behavior with an effective middle school program. *Journal of Adolescent Health, 46*(2), 169–179.

Toseland, R. W., & Rivas, R. F. (2008). *An introduction to group work practice* (6th ed.). Boston, MA: Allyn & Bacon.

Triandis, H. C. (1994). *Culture and social behavior.* New York, NY: McGraw-Hill.

Trochim, W., & Kane, M. (2005). Concept mapping: An introduction to structured conceptualization in health care. *International Journal for Quality in Health Care, 17*(3), 187–191.

van der Sanden, Remko L. M., Bos, A. E., Stutterheim, S. E., Pryor, J. B., & Kok, G. (2013). Experiences of stigma by association among family members of people with mental illness. *Rehabilitation Psychology, 58*(1), 73–80.

van Stralen, M. M., Kok, G., de Vries, H., Mudde, A. N., Bolman, C., & Lechner, L. (2008). The active plus protocol: Systematic development of two theory- and evidence-based tailored physical activity interventions for the over-fifties. *BMC Public Health, 8,* 399.

Vu, M. B., Murrie, D., Gonzalez, V., & Jobe, J. B. (2006). Listening to girls and boys talk about girls' physical activity behaviors. *Health Education & Behavior, 33*(1), 81–96.

Wallerstein, N. B., & Duran, B. (2006). Using community-based participatory research to address health disparities. *Health Promotion Practice, 7*(3), 312–323.

Wang, C. C. (2003). Using Photovoice as a participatory assessment and issue select tool. In M. Minkler & N. Wallerstein (Eds.), *Community-based participatory research for health* (p. 196). San Francisco, CA: Jossey-Bass.

Wasilewski, R. M., Mateo, P., & Sidorovsky, P. (2007). Preventing work-related musculoskeletal disorders within supermarket cashiers: An ergonomic training program based on the theoretical framework of the PRECEDE-PROCEED model. *Work: A Journal of Prevention, Assessment and Rehabilitation, 28*(1), 23–31.

Westbrook, L. E., Bauman, L. J., & Shinnar, S. (1992). Applying stigma theory to epilepsy: A test of a conceptual model. *Journal of Pediatric Psychology, 17*(5), 633–649.

Williams, R. M. J. (1970). *American society: A sociological interpretation.* New York, NY: Knopf.

Wilson, B. D., & Miller, R. L. (2003). Examining strategies for culturally grounded HIV prevention: A review. *AIDS Education and Prevention, 15*(2), 184–202.

Wingood, G. M., Hunter-Gamble, D., & DiClemente, R. J. (1993). A pilot study of sexual communication and negotiation among young African American women: Implications for HIV prevention. *Journal of Black Psychology, 19*(2), 190–203.

Wittink, M. N., Barg, F. K., & Gallo, J. J. (2006). Unwritten rules of talking to doctors about depression: Integrating qualitative and quantitative methods. *Annals of Family Medicine, 4*(4), 302–309.

Wright, A., McGorry, P. D., Harris, M. G., Jorm, A. F., & Pennell, K. (2006). Development and evaluation of a youth mental health community awareness campaign—the compass strategy. *BMC Public Health, 6*, 215.

Yoo, S., Butler, J., Elias, T. I., & Goodman, R. M. (2009). The 6-step model for community empowerment: Revisited in public housing communities for low-income senior citizens. *Health Promotion Practice, 10*(2), 262–275.

Young, D. R., Johnson, C. C., Steckler, A., Gittelsohn, J., Saunders, R. P., Saksvig, B. I., ... McKenzie, T. L. (2006). Data to action: Using formative research to develop intervention programs to increase physical activity in adolescent girls. *Health Education & Behavior, 33*(1), 97–111.

Zapka, J., Lemon, S. C., Estabrook, B. B., & Jolicoeur, D. G. (2007). Keeping a step ahead: Formative phase of a workplace intervention trial to prevent obesity. *Obesity, 15*(S1), 27S–36S.

# CHAPTER 5

# INTERVENTION MAPPING STEP 2

*Program Outcomes and Objectives – Logic Model of Change*

## Competency

- Develop matrices of change objectives that specify what needs to change in behavior and the environment to improve health and quality of life.

The basic tool for Intervention Mapping is the matrix of change objectives. Change objectives state what needs to be achieved to accomplish performance objectives that will lead to changes in behavior or environmental conditions that will, in turn, accomplish the health and quality-of-life program goals. In this chapter we explain how program planners use the findings from the needs assessment and other information to state intended change in individual health-related behaviors and environmental outcomes at the interpersonal, organizational, community, and societal levels. Once the intended change is specified, the planner writes performance objectives for behaviors and for environmental outcomes at each ecological level. These performance objectives describe exactly what the at-risk population members and the agents or influential people at each environmental level need to do to accomplish improvements in health outcomes.

Matrices—created by the intersection of the performance objectives and determinants for the at-risk group—along with the performance objectives and determinants of environmental agents, are the foundation for completing program development, steps that we explain in Chapters 6 and 7. The matrices contain the change objectives that the program will target to influence change in determinants and the accomplishment of performance objectives. This chapter describes the principle components of matrices in detail and guides the reader to use the core processes and information from the needs assessment to create sound matrices. The final product of Step 2 of the Intervention Mapping process is a set of matrices that specifies the immediate objectives for a health promotion program.

---

**BOX 5.1. MAYOR'S PROJECT**

The mayor's planning group did a great job on the needs assessment. Many of the members commented that they had no idea that the problem of obesity was so complex. Looking at the theories helped them to delve into some of the causes of obesity among the youth in their neighborhoods. They were practically bubbling over with enthusiasm, and they were sure that they were ready to talk about intervention.

> *Health Care Provider:* Now that we know what some of the factors that are related to obesity, let's go after them.

> *School Superintendent:* I could call all my associate superintendents at the district tomorrow for a big meeting, because surely we will want to intervene in the schools.

> *Business Community Rep:* Yeah, and what about that Communities in Schools Group?

> *Parent:* We could . . .

The health educator sat quietly for a moment, getting up the courage to tell them the truth. They had completed only the first phase of their planning. Things were likely to get more complex before a coherent planning framework could emerge. Finally, the health educator said, "Let's back up for just a minute. There are some other things we need to do before we can talk about intervention."

Amid the moans and groans, she told the group about the building blocks of matrices. She reminded the group, "Before we design an intervention, we need to know exactly what needs to change or be accomplished to prevent obesity."

---

## Perspectives

In this section we highlight the importance of continuing with the ecological perspective for program development and building the program logic model.

### Continuing With the Ecological Framework

One perspective in this chapter is the continued use of an ecological framework for planning health promotion programs. Most health problems are caused by a web of factors that occur at multiple levels. Some external influences work through the behavior of at-risk individuals, as regarding the effects of advertising on the smoking behavior of adolescents (Audrain-McGovern et al., 2006; Gilpin, White, Messer, & Pierce, 2007; Hanewinkel, Isensee, Sargent, & Morgenstern, 2011; Shadel, Tharp-Taylor, & Fryer, 2009), whereas others, such as air quality, work directly on health (Chuang, Chan, Su, Lee, & Tang, 2007; Loomis et al., 2013; Pope & Dockery, 2006). These levels of causation are represented in this chapter's matrix products. However, in this step, the focus is on changing behavior and the environment instead of on explaining the causes of health problems as addressed in the needs assessment in Step 1.

## The Logic Model of Change

The logic model in this step (see Figure 5.1) is similar to the logic model for the needs assessment, except the logic model of change represents pathways of program effects rather than pathways of problem causation. It begins, on the right side, with the program goals for health and quality-of-life outcomes to be achieved by the health promotion program. This was the last task in Step 1 and forms the basis for continued planning in Step 2. Working from right to left in the logic model of change, the program planner states the behavioral and environmental changes necessary to achieve the health and quality-of-life outcomes. The process for creating a matrix of change objectives is based on the assumption that behaviors or environmental conditions that cause health or quality-of-life problems were identified in the needs assessment. The next assumption is that development of certain more-favorable behavioral or environmental outcomes will lead to better health and improved quality of life. Thus, the first task in creating a causal pathway for influencing change is to state the behavioral and environmental outcomes that the health promotion program seeks to accomplish.

The next link in the model is the specification of performance objectives for obtaining the behavioral and environmental outcomes. Performance objectives are statements of what a program participant will do or how the

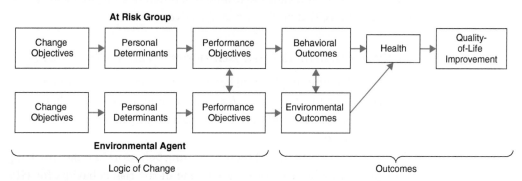

**Figure 5.1** Logic Model of Change

individual will modify the environment. Performance objectives can comprise a somewhat complex list of processes or actions required to perform the health behavior or environmental change. Performance objectives are then examined in light of the determinants of behavior and environmental modifications to generate change objectives. Change objectives specify what needs to change in the determinants of behavioral or environmental outcomes to accomplish the performance objectives, further delineating the logic of change. In Step 1, the needs assessment can be considered a "risk model" that defines the causes of the health problem. In Step 2, working from the risk model, the planner shifts to a "change model" that defines what the intervention needs to change to reduce risk for the problem or to promote, protect, and improve health.

## Tasks for Step 2

### Stating Behavioral and Environmental Outcomes

The first task in Step 2 of Intervention Mapping is to state expected program outcomes for health behaviors and environmental conditions to improve health and quality of life.

The needs assessment (see Chapter 4) should provide a clear statement of behaviors and environmental conditions linked to a health problem. To create a logic model of change, the planner will look at these conditions in the logic model of the problem and state what needs to change—in other words, what the health promotion program is intended to accomplish. Thus, starting in Step 2, the planning shifts to focus on health-promoting behaviors and healthy environmental outcomes. For example, a behavioral cause of lung cancer is smoking, but the behavioral outcome for an intervention could be either not starting to smoke or quitting smoking (U.S. Department of Health and Human Services, 2012). Likewise, the environment can stimulate or support smoking, but an intervention would have to address a specific part of environmental change, such as eliminating advertising campaigns by tobacco product manufacturers (Brownson, Haire-Joshu, & Luke, 2006; Hanewinkel et al., 2011; Yong et al., 2008). Well-defined behavioral and environmental outcomes will, in the next task, lead to better specified performance objectives.

#### *Identifying Health-Related Behaviors of the At-Risk Group*

One of the difficulties in planning health promotion programs is confusion over what is meant by the term *behavior*. Examples of types of behavior are risk reduction, health promotion, screening and early detection, adherence, and self-management actions.

Intervention development requires stating behaviors as either reducing risk or promoting health. For example, one of the risk behaviors for HIV infection is having unprotected sexual intercourse. This risk behavior can be restated into two health-promoting behaviors: (a) using condoms when having sexual intercourse and (b) choosing not to have sexual intercourse. In this case the objectives of the Intervention Mapping process would be directed at obtaining and improving the performance of these two behaviors (Schaalma, Abraham, Gillmore, & Kok, 2004; Tortolero et al., 2002; Tortolero et al., 2008; van Empelen & Kok, 2008).

**Risk-Reduction Behaviors**   Some behaviors are causally related to morbidity and mortality. For example, heart disease is associated with hyperlipidemia (a physiological risk), which is strongly influenced by diet (a behavioral risk) (Appel et al., 2005; Bayne-Smith et al., 2004; Smalley, Wittler, & Oliverson, 2004). Thus, risk behaviors are defined as actions, such as eating certain foods that have been demonstrated to directly increase the risk of disease or disability. Even when an intervention is designed from a population perspective with the goal of reducing the prevalence of a risk behavior within a defined population, it is still helpful to consider the behavior that an individual will (or will not) perform. Because of the addictive nature of some behaviors, such as smoking, the goal is the elimination, not just a reduction, of the behavior. For other behaviors—for example, fat intake—the goal is for a reduction. For example, 2010 dietary guidelines recommend consuming less than 10 percent of calories from saturated fats (U.S. Department of Agriculture & U.S. Department of Health and Human Services, 2010). The desired impact of a health promotion program on risk behaviors is to reduce or eliminate the practice and prevalence of these behaviors.

**Health-Promoting Behaviors**   Health-promoting behavior is action taken to protect or enhance health. For example, getting immunizations, wearing a bicycle helmet, and wearing a seat belt are health-promoting behaviors, because they protect against a potential risk (Eluru & Bhat, 2007; Kelly, Zito, & Weber, 2003). Other health-promoting behaviors are more specific to certain risks, diseases, or conditions. For example, the practice of yoga among breast cancer survivors has been shown to enhance health and quality of life by reducing fatigue, anxiety, and depression (Stan, Collins, Olsen, Croghan, & Pruthi, 2012).

Some health promotion programs are directed to primary prevention (preventing a health problem before it occurs); others are directed toward secondary prevention (reducing the consequences of a disease or slowing its progress). Secondary prevention is especially important for diseases in which early signs or symptoms are not apparent. When symptoms are not present or not easily detected by laypeople, screening is necessary to identify individuals at high risk for the disease or to detect the disease process early so that appropriate medical treatment can be started to prevent more severe illnesses or mortality (U.S. Preventive Services Task Force, 2014). For example, mammography is used to screen for changes in the breast to detect breast cancer in the early stages, when treatment has the best chance of effectiveness (D. W. Smith, Steckler, McCormick, & McLeroy, 1995; R. A. Smith et al., 2003; U.S. Preventive Services Task Force, 2014). Tests for blood pressure and blood cholesterol levels screen for elevated risk for cardiovascular disease (Abel, Darby, & Ramachandran, 1994; Chobanian et al., 2003; Labarthe, 1998; Ohkubo et al., 1997; F. E. Thompson & Byers, 1994; S. G. Thompson, Pyke, & Wood, 1996). Screening tests are also used to detect infectious diseases such as sexually transmitted infections (STIs) and HIV (U.S. Preventive Services Task Force, 2014; Workowski & Berman, 2006) and genetic diseases such as Tay-Sachs disease (Natowicz & Prence, 1996) and cystic fibrosis (Brock, 1990; Livingstone, Axton, Mennie, Gilfillan, & Brock, 1993).

Screening and early detection range from self-administered tests to complicated medical procedures, but almost all require some behavior by the person at risk. Generally speaking, interventions are designed to motivate individuals to participate in self-administered screening or to seek out and attend screening procedures by health professionals in accordance with current screening guidelines (Craun & Deffenbacher, 1987; Fernández et al., 2009; R. A. Smith, Cokkinides, & Brawley, 2009; U.S. Preventive Services Task Force, 2014). The exact nature of the behavior is specific to the screening method and the purpose of the screening. Some screening involves a one-time or infrequently repeated behavior (that is, going to a health care facility and having blood or other specimens taken to be examined by a laboratory or health care professional); others may require more frequent screening (e.g., blood sugar levels or blood pressure).

**Adherence and Self-Management Behaviors**    Patient education—a specific type of health education—can help individuals who are receiving health care for a diagnosed problem to not only adhere to the prescribed therapy but also understand the disease and treatment better, and to use the information effectively (Alewijnse, Mesters, Metsemakers, & van den Borne, 2002; Coulter et al., 2015; Grover & Joshi, 2014). With medical therapy, the patient is expected to follow through with the recommendations of the health care provider, and the extent to which the patient follows through with the recommended action is referred to as a level of adherence (Brawley & Culos-Reed, 2000; DiMatteo, 2004). There has been a movement in the field from the term *compliance* to *adherence* to avoid the implication that the patient is being told what to do without having any involvement in the decision. For example, if a patient were instructed to take antibiotic medication three times a day for 10 days, full adherence would mean taking the right dose at the right time each day for 10 days. Studies have shown that, for most medical recommendations, adherence is incomplete (DiMatteo 2004; Leffler et al., 2011; Zullig et al., 2015). Thus, the goal of health promotion interventions in this case is to improve adherence behavior.

Often the behavior required for follow-up to medical care is much more complex than simply adhering to a set of instructions, especially in the case of chronic illnesses for which management of the condition requires the patients or their families to take continuing action at home or somewhere else that also falls outside of health care facilities (Brug, Schols, & Mesters, 2004; E. B. Fisher et al., 2005; Glasgow, Fisher, Skaff, Mullan, & Toobert, 2007; Harrington & Valerio, 2014; Heijmans, Waverijn, Rademakers, van der Vaart, & Rijken, 2015; Rust, Davis & Moore, 2015; Shegog et al., 2013a; Shegog, Markham, Leonard, Bui, & Paul, 2012). Self-management and self-regulation refer to the same phenomenon: an active, iterative process of goal setting, choosing strategies, self-observation, making judgments based on observation (as opposed to ones based on habit, fear, or tradition), reacting appropriately in the light of one's goal, and revising one's strategy accordingly (Clark, 2003; Clark, Gong, & Kaciroti, 2014; Clark & Zimmerman, 2014; Shegog et al., 2013b). The process is iterative, because feedback loops, through which one sees discrepancies between goals and outcomes, play an essential part in self-regulation (Clark, Valerio, & Gong, 2008; Scheier & Carver, 2003). Good disease management depends on making judgments to take action based on changing physiological conditions and life situations (Nutbeam, 2008). For example, people with epilepsy must manage the disease by adhering to antiseizure medication regimens and altering their lifestyle to avoid seizure onset (DiIorio et al., 2004; Institute of Medicine, 2012; Nutbeam, 2008; Shegog et al., 2013b). This type of behavior is referred to as self-management because monitoring, decision making, and action must occur independently of the health care provider (Clark et al., 2014; Clark & Zimmerman, 2004). The goals for self-management may include increasing the performance of the behavior as well as improving the quality of the behavior—for example, helping the patient become better at decision making and problem solving (Cameron & Leventhal, 2003; Kruse, Bolton, & Freriks, 2015; Lorig, Ritter, Moreland, & Laurent, 2015; Shegog et al., 2013b).

### Stating Behavioral Outcomes

Behavioral outcomes should be stated in terms of the behaviors to be accomplished as a result of the health promotion program. The following statements are examples of health-related behavioral outcomes:

- Consume less than 10 percent of calories from saturated fats.
- Use condoms correctly and consistently when having sexual inter-course.

- Engage in moderate to vigorous physical activity at least 150 minutes a week.

- Take antiseizure medications as prescribed by a health care provider.

- Women ages 50–74 years obtain a mammogram every two years.

The description of It's Your Game...Keep It Real, introduced in Chapter 4, is continued in this chapter and presented in Box 5.2 at the end of the chapter to provide examples of tasks completed for Step 2. Recall from the needs assessment that the primary behavior that increased the risk of poor sexual health outcomes for teens was sexual initiation at an early age. In Step 2, the program planners agreed that the health-promoting behavior for the at-risk population (middle school students) was to delay the age of sexual initiation. Thus, the primary behavioral outcome for the intervention was stated as, "Middle school students choose not to have sex." However, they also recognized that students may become sexually active during their middle or high school years, and that some students were already having sex. Thus, they additionally included the following behavioral outcomes: to have healthy dating relationships, to use condoms correctly and consistently, to use an effective birth control method along with condoms, and to obtain regular testing for pregnancy, HIV, and STIs for sexually active students.

In a project that used Intervention Mapping to create a program to address physical activity in adults over 50, planners identified two health promoting behaviors (van Stralen, de Vries, Mudde, Bolman, & Lechner, 2009; van Stralen et al., 2008) (see publisher's website for the case study; www.wiley.com/go/bartholomew4e) The first was to increase recreational physical activity, such as by playing sports, walking, and cycling. The second was to increase physical activity in people's daily routines, such as by walking and cycling for transport, taking the stairs instead of the lift (elevator), and going for a walk during lunch breaks at work, along with doing gardening, chores, and other household activities at home. The strength of this example is that specific ways of achieving increased physical activity are stated. However, the behaviors could be made even stronger by stating a target for the size of the increase or setting a minimum standard. For example, a worksite program designed to increase physical activity recognized that individuals would be at different baseline levels of physical activity and may not be able to immediately reach the recommended goal of 30 minutes of moderate physical activity at least five days a week. The planners approached adding specificity to the expected behavior by having participants set graded goals for themselves and show cumulative increases throughout the intervention (McEachan, Lawton, Jackson, Conner, & Lunt, 2008).There are many ways to state behaviors, and to the extent possible, the statements should clearly express what participants in the program will be expected to do as a result of the intervention.

## *Identifying and Stating Environmental Outcomes*

In the needs assessment (Chapter 4), we referred to those aspects of the environment identified as causes of a health problem as environmental conditions. However, when stating how the environment needs to change as a result of an intervention, we refer to them as environmental outcomes—at the interpersonal, organizational, community, and societal levels. Stating environmental outcomes communicates to the planners and the recipients of an intervention the expected outcome if the intervention is successful.

**Interpersonal Environment**    The first place to consider environmental outcomes is in the behavior of individuals in the interpersonal environment of the at-risk group. Humans are embedded in social systems that change as people develop. Families are the primary influence for socialization of children and continue to have an effect on behavior throughout life. As children grow older, peer groups become more important, beginning with playmates and continuing with friends, neighbors, coworkers, and members of organizations with which they affiliate (such as churches, social clubs, and service groups). Certain individuals may hold special influence in accordance with the roles they play, such as teachers, coaches, religious leaders, or health care providers.

Interpersonal environmental outcomes can also be considered as social constructs, such as social support. Researchers have extensively studied social support as a protective factor for many health outcomes (Abbott & Freeth, 2008; Beets, Cardinal & Alderman, 2010; Bond et al., 2007; Heaney & Israel, 2002; Hogan, Linden, & Najarian, 2002; Reblin & Uchino, 2008; Tomaka, Thompson, & Palacios, 2006). The types of support that individuals may receive from their social networks include emotional support, information or advice, material support, maintenance of social identity, and social outreach (Abbott & Freeth, 2008; Barrera, Toobert, Angell, Glasgow, & Mackinnon, 2006; Canary, 2008; Heaney & Israel, 2002; Valente, 2015; van Dam et al., 2005). There is considerable evidence that social support buffers the effects of stress through the processes of cognitive appraisal of stress and coping (Berkman, 1984; Berkman & Glass, 2000; Fujishiro & Heaney, 2009; Heaney & Israel, 2002; Rhodes, Contreras, & Mangelsdorf, 1994; Taylor & Stanton, 2007). The social environment may provide modeling and reinforcement for the practice of specific health behaviors (Bandura, 1986; Bandura, 2004a; Bandura, 2006), and it may directly influence physiological health, including immune function and blood pressure (Kiecolt-Glaser, McGuire, Robles, & Glaser, 2002; Reblin & Uchino, 2008; Seeman, 2000; Uchino, 2006). The presence or absence of supports from important others within the individuals' immediate interpersonal environment may have an influence on the performance of the health behavior as well as on the health outcomes.

The ToyBox-Study, a kindergarten-based, family-involved intervention to increase physical activity and decrease sedentary behavior among preschoolers in six European countries, is an example of how program planning can focus on instrumental support of children's health behaviors by parents and teachers (De Craemer et al., 2014; De Decker et al., 2014; Duvinage et al., 2014). Because preschoolers spend much of their time at home or at kindergarten, the program planners intended the ToyBox intervention to enhance physical activity levels and decrease sedentary behavior in both environments. The program goals for their at-risk population (preschoolers) were: "Children between 4 and 6 years old increase their total physical activity throughout the entire day by 10 percent at the end of the intervention," and "Children between 4 and 6 years old decrease their sitting time (screen viewing activities and other sedentary activities) by 10 percent at home and during their time at kindergarten at the end of the intervention." At the interpersonal level, they developed two outcomes for parents/caregivers to support the children's behavior change:

- Parents/caregivers support preschoolers to be more physically active.
- Parents/caregivers support preschoolers to decrease sitting time.

They developed similar organizational level outcomes for teachers to promote physical activity and decrease sedentary behavior among preschoolers in kindergarten.

**Organizational Environment**    Organizational environments include elements such as norms, policies, practices, and facilities (Sallis et al., 2006; Sallis & Glanz, 2009; Steenhuis, Van Assema, & Glanz, 2001; Stetler, McQueen, Demakis, & Mittman, 2008). For example, policies can exert strong control over behavior, as in worksite bans on smoking, which have been shown to reduce the prevalence among workers (Bauer, Hyland, Li, Steger, & Cummings, 2005; Helakorpi et al., 2008; Hopkins et al., 2010). Similarly, combinations of preventive health care policies and health care facility characteristics such as service hours can determine whether workers obtain care. For example, in Cultivando La Salud, Fernández and colleagues (2005) targeted change at the clinic level to make mammography and Pap tests more available to Hispanic farm-working women.

In the T.L.L. Temple Foundation Stroke Project, the planning team developed an intervention to improve the rapid treatment of ischemic stroke victims in rural communities in East Texas (Morgenstern et al.,

2002; Morgenstern et al., 2003). (See publisher's website for the case study; www.wiley.com/go/bartholomew4e) At the time, intravenous recombinant tissue plasminogen activator (rtPA) had been approved for use by the U.S. Food and Drug Administration. However, only a small minority of patients were receiving the treatment, and even fewer in rural areas. To be effective, treatment must begin within 3 hours of symptom onset. During their needs assessment, the planning group identified three organizations—the hospital emergency department, the emergency medical services, and community primary care physicians—as the key organizations with agents who were able to make a change in stroke treatment. Thus, in Step 2, they developed organizational outcomes for each entity:

- Emergency department personnel provide acute stroke therapy for all eligible patients within 3 hours of symptom onset.

- Emergency services personnel transport possible stroke victims to the emergency department at the highest priority.

- Community primary care physicians facilitate rapid treatment of patients who experience possible stroke.

**Community Environment**   The community environment contains conditions that affect the health of populations, either directly or through behavior. Examples of these conditions include availability of work and income, the quality and quantity of housing, health care, availability of recreational resources, smoking and other health ordinances, law enforcement, judicial practices, and treatment resources for social problems such as child abuse, violence, and drug addiction. Further, community environment issues deal with social capital and community capacity for forming and maintaining problem-solving relationships (Lempa, Goodman, Rice, & Becker, 2008; Norton, McLeroy, Burdine, Felix, & Dorsey, 2002; Springer et al., 2012; Springer, Parcel, Baumler, & Ross, 2006). Examples of supportive environments that communities have achieved through health promotion projects include increasing physical activity options and healthful food availability (Coffield, Nihiser, Sherry, & Economos, 2015; Economos et al., 2007), protecting communities against diesel fuel particulates (Kinney, Aggarwal, Northridge, Janssen, & Shepard, 2000; Northridge et al., 1999), and protecting children from the hazard of high unbarred windows from which they could fall (Schulz & Northridge, 2004). Flewelling and colleagues (2013) developed a community-based intervention to reduce underage access to alcohol in Oregon through greater enforcement of underage drinking laws. Two examples of health-related community level outcomes were:

- Community members support laws targeting underage drinking.

- Off-premise alcohol outlets comply with underage drinking laws.

**Societal Environment**   The societal level focuses on legislation, enforcement, regulation, and resource allocation as well as policies, programs, and facilities of large political and geographic groups. Societal influences often function through governments—at the local, state, province, national, or international level. For example, legislation that influences tobacco use includes minors' access laws, clean air acts, and tobacco excise taxes. These laws, along with lawsuits against tobacco companies by states and individuals, have been pivotal to the success of the tobacco control movement (De Leeuw, Townsend, Martin, Jones, & Clavier, 2013; Douglas, Davis, & Beasley, 2006; Helakorpi et al., 2008; Hopkins et al., 2010; Levy, Chaloupka, & Gitchell, 2004; Levy & Friend, 2003; McMullen, Brownson, Luke, & Chriqui, 2005; Sweda, 2004; Wisotzky, Albuquerque, Pechacek, & Park, 2004). State and federal agencies—including those for health, human services, education, agriculture, transportation, and food and drugs—originate regulations, policies, and programs that affect health status. The following statements are examples of health-related societal-level outcomes:

- State legislators prohibit smoking in all enclosed public places in the state.

- The federal government requires food labeling for most prepared foods.

## Specifying Performance Objectives

The second task in Intervention Mapping Step 2 is to subdivide behavioral and environmental outcomes into performance objectives.

Once the program planners have defined the program's behavioral and environmental outcomes, they write performance objectives for each of them. The use of performance objectives is not new, nor is it unique to health promotion. For example, therapeutic outcomes are sometimes stated in performance terms at the individual client level. On an organizational level, quality assurance defines a standard of performance to maintain certain levels of service or production. In education, performance objectives usually reflect academic performance (Armstrong, 2015; Bloom, 1956). In the area of training, participants must perform at a criterion level for a program to be successful. Although the term *performance objective* may not be applied exactly the same way in each of these examples, they are all used to further delineate behavioral and environmental program outcomes.

### Specifying Performance Objectives for Behaviors

As described above, when we first state behavioral outcomes, they are broad conceptualizations: Exercise aerobically 30 minutes per day. As we continue toward intervention development, we use performance objectives to clarify the exact performance it would take to achieve the behavioral outcome. To determine the performance objectives, planners ask: What do the participants in this program or the environmental agents need to do to perform the behavior or to make the environmental change stated in the behavioral or environmental outcomes? Performance objectives enable planners to make a transition from a behavior or environmental condition to a detailed description of its components. For example, eliminating trans-fats from the diet is a health-promoting behavior, but many sub-behaviors or components make up that broader behavior. To perform the behavior, an individual would need to take many actions, including the following: read food labels, select foods without transfats, and inquire about ingredients at restaurants.

These sub-behaviors, specified by action words, become the performance objectives. They refine, focus, and make more specific what the program participants must do as a result of the intervention. For the It's Your Game project presented in Box 5.2 at the end of the chapter, four performance objectives for the behavioral outcome "Middle school students choose not to have sex" provide what a student needs to do to choose to wait until he or she is older before having sex.

The performance objectives also help ensure the appropriateness of the program's behavioral expectations. For example, managing a chronic disease, such as diabetes, would have different performance objectives for schoolchildren than for an adult, because the two groups have different maturity levels and cognitive skills. The performance objectives must also be practical in terms of what the priority population is both able and willing to do.

Intervention Mapping makes a clear distinction between performance objectives and change objectives. Most cognitive and affective performance represents determinants of behavior rather than the behavior itself. Determinants (why people do, or would do, the behavior) are, along with performance objectives, the parts that make up change objectives. Change objectives are described later in this chapter. Planners can distinguish performance objectives from change objectives by thinking of the performance objective as an observable subset of the behavior and a change objective as what the program participants must learn or change to meet or maintain the performance objective.

Changing health-related behaviors and environmental conditions usually requires complex multistep processes. The specification of performance objectives helps program planners to sequence the behavioral learning process when the learner needs to learn one part before another and to

**Table 5.1**    Performance Objectives for Consistently and Correctly Using Condoms During Sexual Intercourse

The adolescent will:

1.  Make the decision to use condoms.

    1.1.    Locate condom displays in drug or grocery store.

    1.2.    Choose condoms that are product tested.

2.  Carry condoms or have condoms easily available.

    2.1.    Carry condoms in wallet or purse for no longer than a month.

    2.2.    Carry or store condoms in place that is not susceptible to extreme temperatures.

3.  Negotiate the use of a condom with a partner.*

    3.1.    State mutual goals, such as pregnancy or HIV prevention.

    3.2.    State clearly intention of using a condom as a prerequisite for intercourse.

    3.3.    Listen to partner's concerns.

    3.4.    Pose solutions to partner's concerns that reference mutual goals and personal requirements.

4.  Correctly apply condoms during use.

    4.1.    Use a water-soluble rather than petroleum-based lubricant.

    4.2.    Use a new condom for each occurrence of intercourse.

    4.3.    Follow instructions on package insert for use.

    4.4.    Follow instructions on package insert for disposal.

5.  Maintain use over time.

*Example of using theory to specify performance objectives. This uses negotiation theory as described by R. Fisher and Ury (1991).

include all necessary supports for the behavior. For example, Table 5.1 illustrates how the behavior of using condoms correctly and consistently when having sexual intercourse can be broken down into subcomponents, which are the performance objectives.

In another example, the following performance objectives were stated for the management of the daily antiretroviral treatment (ART) for people living with HIV (Côté, Godin, Garcia, Gagnon, & Rouleau, 2008). Notice that the performance objectives are stated in a general way and could be made more specific with subobjectives, as illustrated in Table 5.1. Another option would be for the planners to make each performance objective a separate behavior with each having its own performance objectives. Either approach can work depending on what is most useful for the planners.

PO.1. Follow and integrate the treatment plan properly in the daily routine

PO.2. Handle situations in which ART is difficult to take

PO.3. Cope with side effects

PO.4. Interact and deal with health professionals

PO.5. Maintain relationships with resources person and immediate social circle

## Specifying Performance Objectives for Environmental Outcomes

The process for writing performance objectives for environmental outcomes parallels the process for writing performance objectives for health behaviors. An environmental outcome to increase plant-based components of school meals (Dietary Guidelines Advisory Committee, 2015) must be broken down into its component parts. For example, at the organizational level, the following might be performance objectives for the change agents at school:

- Food service directors will modify menus so that all meals contain three choices of fruits and vegetables with no added sugar.

- Food service directors will modify purchase order specifications to reduce the fat content of vendor-prepared foods and to increase fresh fruits and vegetables.

- Nutritionists will modify recipes to find appetizing/attractive presentations of fruits and vegetables.

- Nutritionists will replace most desserts with fruits and grains.

- Cooks will modify cooking practices to follow new recipes.

- Food service directors will involve school children in pilot testing new menus.

The basic question when stating performance objectives for environmental outcomes is: What does someone in the environment need to do to accomplish the environmental outcome? This general question addresses who is doing the action to accomplish the objective, because the agent may be different for each of the performance objectives. This question is somewhat different from the question asked about performance objectives for the health-related behavior, because the health behavior question assumes a reference to the behavior of the at-risk population. Environmental change usually requires people outside the at-risk population to take action to modify the environmental conditions.

Exactly who will be taking the action to accomplish the performance objectives will depend on the agent in the environment who has control over or can influence a modification in the environmental factor. This agent might be, for example, a family member, policy maker, lawmaker, resource controller, or service provider. In the beginning of the planning process, it may be difficult to identify specific people to include in the performance objectives for modifying an environmental condition. We suggest starting with whatever information may be available about the agent and stating the "who" in terms of general groups of people or appropriate positions of responsibility—that is, roles or agents that may be able to accomplish the performance objective. As work on the intervention progresses, the health educator can figure out specifically who, in terms of either roles or individuals, will perform the modification in the environment.

The ToyBox-Study provides a good example. The performance objectives listed in Table 5.2 were constructed to enable modification of the preschoolers' environment. At the interpersonal level of the environment, the focus was on action to be taken by the parents/caregivers. At the organizational level, the focus was on action to be taken by teachers to increase the children's physical activity levels in the kindergarten setting. The environmental outcomes for parents and teachers were fairly simple (to increase preschoolers' physical activity levels and decrease their sedentary behavior). However, the stated performance objectives added specificity that enabled the program planners to more effectively communicate the essential components the intervention should address. Note that each performance objective states who will perform the action.

The T.L.L. Temple Foundation Stroke Project provides additional examples of performance objectives for environmental outcomes. Recall that the environmental outcome was to provide acute stroke therapy for all eligible patients. To accomplish this outcome, performance objectives were stated for three different groups of agents in the organizational environment of the health care system: emergency department of the hospital, the emergency medical service, and the community primary care physicians. The performance objectives listed in Table 5.3 provide a clear statement of *who* needs to do *what*. The *who* varies with each performance objective depending on who has responsibility for performing the action that will contribute to a change in the environment.

Our last example concerns performance objectives for HIV-related stigma reduction (see sections on Stigma and Discrimination in Chapters 2 and 6) to illustrate how performance objectives can be stated across all levels to address the environmental outcome of HIV-related stigma reduction. See Table 5.4. One of the environmental factors hindering HIV prevention, and especially promoting HIV testing, is stigma (Bos, Dijker, & Koomen, 2007; Stutterheim et al., 2009). People who are afraid of being stigmatized hesitate to go for HIV testing. To reduce stigmatization and promote HIV testing, we distinguish performance objectives at various environmental levels. Stigmatizing behavior involves people at all levels, starting with public stigma at the interpersonal level. In addition to the environmental levels, the people who are being stigmatized because of HIV can also behave in ways that will decrease stigmatizing behavior by others. They can do the following: Seek and secure social support (Stutterheim et al., 2010); disclose HIV status, when prepared to do so (Paxton, 2002b); express distress to others who are most likely to be empathetic, such as female

**Table 5.2**   Environmental Performance Objectives for the ToyBox-Study

### Interpersonal Environment

Environmental outcome 1: Parents/caregivers support preschoolers in becoming more physically active.

Parents and caregivers will:

1.1.   Facilitate children to be more physically active.

1.2.   Use active transport to move from place to place together with their child.

1.3.   Participate in sports activities and/or unstructured physical activities inside, together with their children.

1.4.   Participate in sports activities and/or unstructured physical activities outside, together with their children.

1.5.   Motivate (verbally) their children to play outside.

1.6.   Be physically active themselves to provide a role model for their children.

Environmental outcome 2: Parents/caregivers support preschoolers to decrease sitting time.

Parents and caregivers will:

2.1.   Limit preschoolers' screen-viewing activities to 1 hour per day.

2.2.   Motivate (verbally) their children to do other activities instead of screen-viewing activities.

2.3.   Do activities with their child instead of screen-viewing activities.

2.4.   Limit their own sitting time to provide a role model for their children.

### Organizational Environment

Environmental outcome 3: Kindergarten teachers support preschoolers to be more physically active.

Kindergarten teachers will:

3.1.   Every day, organize movement breaks that last between 1 and 5 minutes in the kindergarten classroom (2 in the morning and 2 in the afternoon).

3.2.   Encourage the children's parents to use active transport.

3.3.   Use active ways to teach (e.g., counting while jumping, movement stories).

Environmental outcome 4: Kindergarten teachers support preschoolers to decrease sitting time.

Kindergarten teachers will:

4.1.   Use different strategies (e.g., classroom environmental changes) to decrease preschoolers' total sitting time per day at kindergarten.

4.2.   Give assignments that the preschoolers need to fulfill standing up.

4.3.   Encourage the preschoolers to stand up when they are sitting down at the playground.

4.4.   Act as a role model for the preschoolers and limit sitting down themselves.

4.5.   Encourage preschoolers to switch from sitting down to standing up.

Source: De Craemer et al., 2014; De Decker et al., 2014.

friends (Bos et al., 2007); and actively cope with the stigma using downward comparison, external attribution, or shift in comparison level (Crocker, Major, & Steele, 1998).

## *Using the Core Processes to Write Performance Objectives*

How to break down a health-related behavior or an environmental condition into subparts is not always apparent and may require additional thinking and information. The core processes presented in Chapter 1 serve as

**Table 5.3**    Environmental Performance Objectives for T.L.L. Temple Foundation Stroke Project

## Organizational Environment

Environmental outcome 1: Emergency department personnel provide acute stroke therapy for all eligible patients within three hours of symptom onset.

| | |
|---|---|
| 1.1. | ED physicians and teams complete stroke evaluation in 10 minutes. |
| 1.1.a. | Triage nurses have patient seen by the physician in 10 minutes. |
| 1.1.b. | ED physicians notify the designated ED stroke team within 15 minutes. |
| 1.2. | ED stroke teams send lab work STAT (HCT, platelets, glucose, PT, PTT) and get it back. |
| 1.3. | ED physicians and stroke teams make rapid differential diagnosis of stroke (use modified NIH scale and protocol). |
| 1.4 | ED stroke teams perform pulse oximetry, attach cardiac monitor, and perform EKG. |
| 1.5. | ED stroke teams obtain accurate onset of time of stroke symptoms. |
| 1.6. | ED stroke teams ensure patient receives CT scan within 25 minutes and notify on-call radiologist. |
| 1.7. | Radiologists and stroke teams read the CT scan immediately (within 45 minutes of arrival). |
| 1.8. | ED stroke teams rule out contraindications. |
| 1.9. | ED stroke teams manage diagnosed stroke. |
| 1.9.a. | ED staff members insert an IV in each arm if not done by EMS. |
| 1.9.b. | ED physicians administer rtPA within 60 minutes. |
| 1.9.c. | ED physicians treat blood pressure appropriately. |
| 1.9.c. | ED physicians give appropriate dose of rtPA; infuse properly; document time (do not give heparin or coumadin). |

Environmental outcome 2: Emergency services personnel transport possible stroke victims to the emergency department at the highest priority.

| | |
|---|---|
| 2.1. | Dispatchers triage to highest priority of transport. |
| 2.2. | Dispatchers convey stroke possibility and urgency to responders. |
| 2.3. | Responders perform "load and go." |
| 2.4. | Responders call ahead to the hospital. |
| 2.5. | Responders encourage a family member or witness to accompany the individual to the hospital. |
| 2.6. | Responders interview patient and witness to determine symptom onset. |
| 2.7. | Responders deliver patient with IV in both arms (perform in ambulance). |

Environmental outcome 3: Primary care physicians facilitate rapid treatment of patients who experience possible stroke.

| | |
|---|---|
| 3.1. | Receptionists and nurses tell the person with the possible stroke to call 911. |
| 3.2. | Primary care providers identify high-risk patients for stroke and tell patients about their stroke risk, possible symptoms, and instructions for calling 911. |
| 3.3. | Primary care providers educate office staff regarding how to recognize stroke and what to tell patients (such as to call 911 immediately). |

ED = Emergency Department; EMS = Emergency Medical Services

**Table 5.4**    Performance Objectives to Reduce Stigma and Promote HIV Testing

**Interpersonal Level**

Relatives and friends

PO1. Replace blaming and stereotyping by expressing empathy when interacting with persons with HIV (Dijker & Koomen, 2007).

PO2. Give social support (Stutterheim et al., 2010).

PO3. Support stigmatized person if disclosing (Paxton, 2002a).

**Organizational Level**

PO4. Coworkers replace blaming and stereotyping by expressing empathy when interacting with persons with HIV (Dijker & Koomen, 2007).

PO5. Health care providers protect confidential information about people with HIV.

PO6. Hospital managers and company managers develop policies against discrimination and stigmatization, instead endorsing providing information, training, and interventions (Link & Phelan, 2001; Parker & Aggleton, 2003).

**Community Level**

PO7. Opinion leaders communicate norms for treating every community member with respect regardless of HIV status.

PO8. Community members give social support to people with HIV (Stutterheim et al., 2010).

PO9. Community members replace blaming and stereotyping by expressing empathy when interacting with persons with HIV (Dijker & Koomen, 2007).

**Societal Level**

PO10. Elected officials develop policies and laws that support programs that provide information, education, procedures, and enforcement for nondiscrimination of people with HIV (Parker & Aggleton, 2003).

PO11. Elected official support programs and efforts to reduce power inequalities in society (Link & Phelan, 2001).

guides for writing performance objectives, as applied in the following steps. Formulating a question is the starting place. For health-related behavior, the question is: What do the participants of this program need to do to perform the health-related behavior? For environmental conditions, the question is: What does someone in the environment need to do to accomplish the environmental outcome? The answers to these questions form a logical sequence of smaller steps that are necessary to perform the behavior or achieve the environmental outcome. Sometimes planners begin with this provisional list. An initial list can also come from the literature. For example, many countries have guidelines for approaches to treat various illnesses, which can be helpful in constructing illness management performance objectives (guidelines.gov). Searching the research and practice literature by topic can also be helpful in creating or refining an initial list. Finally, the planner will review the list of performance objectives and reduce the list to objectives essential for performing the behavior or achieving the environmental outcome. This step is important because each performance objective is the basis for further work. Each will be linked with determinants to form change objectives. Nonessential (interesting but not necessary) performance objectives will expand the subsequent planning and potentially diffuse the intervention's focus.

**Using Theory as a Basis for Performance Objectives**    Sometimes theory provides a rationale for performance objectives. For example, a self-management or self-regulation approach to behavior change can help the planner develop performance objectives, especially for complex behavior. In that case, the self-management processes of goal setting, making plans or implementation intentions, self-monitoring, comparison to a personal standard, self-evaluation, self-control, and reward would become performance objectives as they relate to a specific behavior (Abraham, Sheeran, & Johnston, 1998; Gollwitzer, in press; Gollwitzer, Martiny-Huenger, & Oettingen, 2014; Gollwitzer & Oettingen, 2015; Shegog et al., 2012, 2013a). Behavior change for establishing a healthier diet, for instance, might be approached with specific dietary advice, such as choosing low-fat cheese or abstaining from snacks, but such a list of specific behaviors might be long and unmanageable. A self-regulatory approach would look quite different from a list of specific dos and don'ts, and it may include the following performance objectives (the specific actions needed would vary by person and setting):

- Monitor one's own food intake
- Compare intake to personal goals based on guidelines for a healthy diet
- Decide if discrepancies exist
- Make a detailed plan of implementation intentions and take action to improve dietary behavior
- Evaluate the action's effects
- Recycle to self-monitoring

Health educators may find it useful to consider the self-regulatory process when designating health-promoting behaviors for the self-management of chronic disease. For example, in the Partners in School Asthma Management program, Kay Bartholomew and colleagues (2006) conceptualized both asthma-specific behaviors (e.g., taking control medications) and self-regulatory behaviors (e.g., for symptoms of asthma) in their performance objectives. For the Familias project, Fernández, Bartholomew, Lopez, and colleagues (2000) described specific performance objectives using self-regulatory constructs for parents' management of their child's asthma. Another example of the application of a self-regulatory approach to health behaviors can be found in HIV-prevention programs. Table 5.5 presents performance objectives for condom use among HIV-positive gay men using a self-regulatory approach, and focusing on safe sex in a broader framework of sexual health, which is a more complex behavior (Van Kesteren, Hospers, Kok, & van Empelen, 2005).

**Validating Performance Objectives** Once planners have a set of performance objectives, they will need to collect new data to determine their validity. What do potential participants in the program actually do, or say they do, when performing the behavior? Data may also be collected from service providers, key informants, or people who may implement the program. Surveys and interviews are good methods for this purpose. Through focus groups or interviews, potential program participants can be asked whether the performance objectives fit with their views of how they would go about performing the health-related behaviors. Feedback from individuals who have had both successful and unsuccessful experience with the health behavior or the environmental outcome can be very helpful.

An often overlooked, but in some cases essential, source of information about performance objectives is direct observation of the health behavior or environmental outcomes. For some health problems, there may be a limited amount of information, experience, or documentation of how the related health behavior is performed or how environmental outcomes break down into component parts. Observation of performance in natural settings as well as in simulated settings can be very helpful. For example, program planners developing a nutrition improvement program for schoolchildren can spend time in the school cafeteria observing how children select, trade, modify, and eat or do not eat food.

Performance objectives may also be validated by using quantitative methods to predict health-related behaviors from the performance objectives specified within the priority population. This approach is illustrated

**Table 5.5** Performance Objectives for Condom Use Among HIV+ Men Who Have Sex With Men (MSM) Using a Self-Regulatory Approach (Van Kesteren, Hospers, Kok, & van Empelen, 2005)

| | |
|---|---|
| 1. | Self-observe sexual behavior and compare sexual behavior to standard of safer sex |
| 2. | Identify when a problem exists |
| 3. | Implement solutions |
| 3.1. | Decide to use nonpenetrative sexual techniques |
| 3.2. | Decide to use condoms for anal sex |
| 3.2.1. | Purchase condoms |
| 3.2.2. | Carry condoms or have condoms easily available |
| 3.2.3. | Negotiate condoms for anal sex |
| 3.2.4. | Use condoms correctly and consistently |
| 3.2.5. | Maintain use over time |
| 4. | Implement selected coping strategies |
| 5. | Evaluate actions and return to monitoring |

by a study conducted by van Empelen and Kok (2008) that examined the role of preparatory performance in explaining condom use among adolescents. In writing the performance objectives, they relied on experts along with theoretical and empirical evidence. From the evidence available, van Empelen and Kok (2008) derived young people's performance objectives and then conducted a prospective study among 400 secondary school students to validate them. Among sexually active students, condom use with steady sex partners could be explained by the decision to use condoms with steady sex partners (operationalized as intention) and the relationship was mediated by buying and carrying condoms and by communicating about condom use (performance objectives) (van Empelen & Kok, 2008). When focusing on condom use with casual sex partners, van Empelen and Kok (2008) did not find the predicted sequence of performance objectives. Actual condom use with casual sex partners was predicted only by the decision to use condoms, not by the additional performance objectives. Does this mean that they are not important? Not at all. First of all, the data showed that adolescents simply do not prepare themselves for casual sexual encounters and that young people are more willing to engage in unsafe sex. Thus, although the researchers were not able to validate the sequence of performance objectives in the case of casual sex, they were able to show that the lack of such performance objectives enhances risk-taking behavior (that is, not using condoms). This study might suggest the need to consider additional or different performance objectives for casual sex.

## Selecting Personal Determinants

The third task in Step 2 is to select important and changeable determinants of the health behavioral and environmental outcomes.

Those factors that rest within individuals (people at risk or agents in the environment) and are subject to their direct control or influence are referred to as personal determinants. These factors can be changed or influenced by interventions that involve influencing how people think about or have the capacity to change a behavior or the environment. Personal determinants usually include cognitive factors (such as knowledge, attitudes, beliefs, values, self-efficacy, and expectations) and capabilities, such as skills. In this text, when referring to determinants, in most cases this will mean personal determinants.

Those factors that rest outside the individual and influence behavior are considered environmental conditions and are addressed in Intervention Mapping as environmental outcomes, as discussed in the previous section. These environmental conditions may include such factors as social influences (such as norms, social support, and reinforcement) or structural influences (such as access to resources, policies, and organizational climate). The individuals at risk for a health problem are not usually able to control these conditions directly; therefore, change is not likely to be accomplished unless action is taken by agents or groups within the various levels of the environment. Therefore, personal determinants can be identified as important influences for changing health behavior of the at-risk population as well as action to be taken by agents who can exert change in environmental outcomes.

### Using Core Processes to Select Determinants

Coming up with an appropriate set of evidence- and theory-informed determinants for the performance objectives for behavior and environment require the use of the core processes (see Chapter 1). Briefly, core processes mean asking a question, generating a provisional list of answers, and validating the answers against the literature and new data.

In the needs assessment (see Chapter 4), the planner will have already asked and answered questions about determinants regarding the risk behavior(s) and environmental conditions. The needs assessment should provide a good starting list of personal determinants in answer to these questions:

* Why would a person perform a particular risky behavior?

* Why do certain environmental conditions exist?

In Step 2, planners are posing questions about the determinants of the health-promoting behavior and environmental outcomes that will support the health behavior or affect health directly.

* Why would people perform the health-promoting behavior or performance objectives?

* Why would a certain environmental agent make an environmental modification?

To answer these questions, the planning group first creates a provisional list of answers. To refine or add to this provisional list, the planner undertakes a review of the literature to find empirical studies, theoretical constructs associated with the topic at hand, and general theories that include some of the identified determinants as constructs within those theories (Kok et al., 1992; Kok, Schaalma, Ruiter, van Empelen, & Brug, 2004; Murphy & Bennett, 2004). For example, if self-efficacy was defined in the literature review as a possible determinant of the behavior, then going to the literature on Social Cognitive Theory (SCT) for which self-efficacy is a central construct would be useful (Bandura, 1986; Bandura, 2004a, 2004b; Kelder, Hoelscher, & Perry, 2015; McAlister, Perry, & Parcel, 2008). A review of the general theory may suggest other constructs that might be considered as important determinants of behavior.

The needs assessment and the literature reviews provide the planner with informed or hypothesized relationships of personal determinants to the health behavior or behavior of the environmental agents. Determinants on the provisional list should be well supported by the literature, and the planner should retain only those with the strongest relation to the behaviors.

Planners often need to collect data from the at-risk group and environmental agents to identify additional determinants and to understand how determinants manifest in a particular group. Qualitative methods, such as focus groups or interviews, can be helpful in generating new ideas for determinants or in verifying some of the findings from the research literature (Peters, 2014). Quantitative data collection, using questionnaires that measure the determinants and the behavior of interest, can be especially helpful in judging the strength of the association between potential determinants and behavior. With both types of data collection, planners can estimate the presence or absence of the determinant, as well as its importance for influencing change. For example, in designing an AIDS-prevention program for adolescents, knowledge about the seriousness of AIDS may at first be viewed as an important determinant of risk-reduction behavior. However, formative research may show that adolescents already know about AIDS and consider it a serious condition. Therefore, it is unlikely that an intervention to increase knowledge about AIDS will have much of an effect on the group's behavior to prevent AIDS. Another way to judge whether a determinant is important is to measure the determinant in population subgroups: those who practice the behavior and those who do not. For example, if children who eat five servings of fruits and vegetables daily have a high self-efficacy for the behavior and those who eat only two servings have a low self-efficacy for the behavior, then self-efficacy is likely to be an important determinant.

### Rating Importance of Determinants

Eventually, the planner must refine the list of determinants. A long list of determinants is not practical for program development. Determinants that have weak evidence of association to the performance objectives or no logical or theoretical basis for their causal relation to the performance are unlikely to be important targets for an intervention. Therefore, careful analysis of the determinants at this stage improves planning results at later stages. To conduct this analysis, planners can start by using evidence to rate each determinant in terms of relevance (that is, strength of association with the behavior) and changeability (that is, how likely it is that health education or promotion intervention is going to influence a change in the determinant). Table 5.6 shows an example of a table used to access

**Table 5.6**    Judging Importance of Determinants of Performance Objectives

| Determinants | Importance | Changeability | Evidence for Importance |
|---|---|---|---|
| Knowledge | + | +++ | Precondition for personal attitude. |
| Risk perception | + | + | Precondition for personal relevance. |
| Attitude | ++ | + | r = .52, p< .01 (with intention to always use condoms). |
| Anticipated regret | ++ | + | r = .70, p <.01. |
| Personal norm | +++ | + | r = .78, p <.01. |
| Subjective norm | + | + | r = .29, p <.01. |
| Self-efficacy | +++ | + | r = .71, p <.01. |
| Skills | ++ | + | Precondition for self-efficacy improvement. |
| Habit | ++ | + | Making the healthy behavior automatic behavior. |

*Note*: Importance = the strength of the evidence for the causal relationship between the determinant and the behavior we want to change; changeability = the strength of the evidence that the proposed change can be realized by a program; + means: not very important, not easy to change; ++ means: important, changeable; +++ means: very important.

relevance and changeability of determinants provided by an Intervention Mapping project to develop an Internet HIV-prevention program for men having sex with men (Kok, Harterink, Vriens, de Zwart, & Hospers, 2006). In this example the term *importance* is used to represent relevance.

As much as possible, the basis for rating relevance and changeability should be based on evidence from the research literature. Sometimes, the literature will not adequately discuss a proposed determinant, and the planner will need to collect data from the at-risk group and from others in the field. Alternatively, decisions to retain or delete determinants may be based entirely on a theoretical or conceptual basis when data are not available. For example, the evidence may be strong for one determinant (such as self-efficacy), but the literature may provide little evidence to support the relevance of a related factor (such as outcome expectations). However, the theoretical literature suggests that these two constructs are interrelated, and for some behaviors, it may be important to address both with methods to promote change (Bandura, 1986; Bandura, 1997). There may be situations in which the literature provides little evidence for a hypothetical determinant, but planners may find literature that supports the importance of a determinant for a similar behavior. For example, evidence may not be available to support the relationship between perceived risk and use of clinical breast examination, but there may be literature that supports the importance of this determinant for mammography screening.

The process of using findings from empirical studies of the specific health problem, the theoretical literature, and new research is illustrated in the development of MINDSET, a clinic-based information management decision-support epilepsy tool (Begley et al., 2010; Shegog et al., 2013a; Shegog et al., 2013b). (See the case study at www.wiley.com/

go/bartholomew4e.) After reviewing findings from the empirical literature, Social Cognitive Theory, and self-regulation models, motivational enhancement therapy, and their own formative research, the program planners identified knowledge, self-efficacy, skills, and perceived importance as important and changeable determinants of epilepsy self-management.

Some personal determinants and environmental conditions have a reciprocal relationship. For example, subjective norms are considered personal determinants because they derive from an individual's perception of the norms for behavior and are subject to his or her control. The actual norms for behavior are considered environmental conditions because they are external to the individual and outside her or his control. Both subjective norms and the actual norms may influence health behavior; however, the processes for change may be very different. On the one hand, actual norms are very difficult to change and require environmental change methods. Subjective norms, on the other hand, may be influenced by intervention methods that focus on how individuals think about and perceive norms. If subjective norms and actual norms are both considered influences of behavioral outcomes for a health promotion program, the program planners can approach change by selecting subjective norms as a determinant of behavior and linking it to performance objectives and stating change objectives in the matrix for behavior of the at-risk population. On the other hand, the planners may decide that it is important and possible to change the actual norms and address them as an environmental outcome for one or more of the environmental levels.

In some situations the actual norms are supportive of the health behavior but the perception of the norms by the priority population is not consistent with the actual norms. For example, in the United States, young adolescents tend to overestimate the proportion of youth smokers, thinking that many adolescents smoke, when in reality less than 5 percent of middle school students and 14 percent of high school students smoke (Centers for Disease Control and Prevention, 2013). The focus of many smoking prevention programs is to correct the perception of what is normative for youth smoking. In other situations, it is difficult to modify an environmental condition; program planners must decide whether to plan for an intervention for an environmental outcome or to prepare the at-risk population to deal with the environmental condition. For example, financial resources may be an important environmental condition and skills in coping with resource limitations may be a personal determinant.

## Constructing Matrices of Change Objectives

Matrices of change objectives are constructed by crossing performance objectives with determinants and writing change objectives. These matrices are simple tables formed by entering the performance objectives in the left column and the determinants along the top (see the matrices for the It's Your Game project in Box 5.2 at end of chapter, Tables 5.15, 5.16, and 5.17). The planner then writes change objectives in the cells formed at the intersection of each performance objective and determinant. Conceptually, a matrix of change objectives represents the pathways for the most immediate changes in motivation and capability to influence health behavior and actions taken by environmental agents.

*The fourth task in Step 2 is to create a matrix of change objectives for each ecological level to be included in the intervention (individual, interpersonal, organizational, community, and societal).*

## Selecting Intervention Levels

Planners will construct separate matrices for each level of intervention for which program planners have written performance objectives. The final number of matrices of program objectives is different for each program and is influenced by the problem's complexity, the span of the program across levels, and the population's diversity. To select intervention levels, program planners ask: At what levels of intervention is it necessary to attain the performance objectives? For example, the ToyBox-Study was developed for the home and kindergarten settings (interpersonal and organizational levels), and the project team identified performance objectives for children at the individual level. However, most of the emphasis was on parents and kindergarten teachers, who were to create environmental changes to support the children's physical activity efforts. Therefore, the intervention also addressed interpersonal and organizational levels; and planners created matrices for the individual (Table 5.7), interpersonal, and organizational (Table 5.8) levels. Had the needs assessment identified important community or governmental factors influencing young children's physical activity and sedentary behavior, then these levels would have also been reflected in the performance objectives.

For the Partners in School Asthma Management Program, the focus was on the child's behavior as well as the child's interpersonal environment, including parents and providers and the organizational environmental of the school (see Web-based Case Study at www.wiley.com/go/bartholomew4e.). The program planners developed performance objectives and matrices for the children and parents, health care providers, and school organization. Additional examples of matrices developed for the individual level and the organizational level are illustrated in the T.L.L. Temple Foundation Stroke Project, another Web-based Case Study (see www.wiley.com/go/bartholomew4e.).

## Differentiating the Intervention Population

Planners may also need to create separate matrices for subgroups at any level of intervention (most often at the individual or at-risk group

**Table 5.7**   Sample Matrix for Children in the ToyBox-Study (De Decker et al., 2014)

| Behavior: Preschoolers decrease their sitting time at home and at kindergarten | | | | |
|---|---|---|---|---|
| | **Personal Determinants** | | | |
| **Performance Objectives (Preschoolers)** | **Attitudes** | **Self-Efficacy** | **Preference** | **Behavioral Capability** |
| PO.1. Decrease total sitting time per day at kindergarten | A.1. Express positive feelings toward devoting less time sitting down at kindergarten | SE.1. Express confidence about decreasing total sitting time per day at kindergarten, even when other children want to sit down/are sitting down | P.1. Prefer to stand up instead of sitting down in the classroom at kindergarten | BC.1. Demonstrates ability to decrease total sitting time per day at kindergarten |
| PO.2. Decrease total sitting time per day at home or during leisure time | A.2. Express positive feelings toward being less sedentary, at home and during leisure time | SE.2. Express confidence about decreasing total sitting time per day at home and during leisure time, even when their siblings are sitting down | P.2. Prefer to stand up instead of sitting down at home and during leisure time | BC.2. Demonstrates ability to decrease total sitting time per day at home and during leisure time |
| PO.3. Limit screen viewing time (e.g., TV viewing, computer time) to 1 hour per day at kindergarten | A.3. Express positive feelings toward limiting screen viewing time by doing other nonsedentary activities at kindergarten | SE.3. Express confidence about limiting screen viewing to less than 1 hour per day at kindergarten, even when other children are watching TV, playing on the computer, or doing other screen viewing activities | P.3. Prefer to limit screen viewing to less than 1 hour per day at kindergarten | BC.3. Demonstrates ability to limit screen viewing time to less than one hour per day at kindergarten |
| PO.4. Limit screen viewing time (e.g., TV viewing, computer time) to 1 hour per day or less at home (with help from their parents/caregivers) | A.4. Express positive feelings toward limiting screen viewing time (with help from their parents/caregivers) by doing other activities at home | SE.4. Express confidence about limiting screen viewing time to 1 hour per day or less (with help from their parents/caregivers), even when their siblings are watching TV, playing on the computer, or doing other screen viewing activities | P.4. Prefer to limit screen viewing to 1 hour per day or less at home (with help from their parents/caregivers) | BC.4. Demonstrates ability to limit screen viewing time to one hour per day or less at home (with help from their parents/caregivers) |
| PO.5. Switch from sitting down to standing up for some activities | A.5. Express positive feelings toward switching from sitting down to standing up for some activities | SE.5.a. Express confidence about switching from sitting down to standing up, even when other children do these activities sitting down<br><br>SE.5.b. Express confidence about switching from sitting down to standing up, even when the teacher does not give prompts to do this | P.5. Prefer to switch from sitting down to standing up for some activities | BC.5. Demonstrates ability to switch from sitting down to standing up for some activities |

**Table 5.8**    Sample of Rows From Matrices for Interpersonal and Organizational Environmental Change in the ToyBox-Study (De Decker et al., 2014)

| Interpersonal Outcome: Parents/Caregivers Support Preschoolers to Decrease Sitting Time | | | | |
|---|---|---|---|---|
| **Personal Determinants** | | | | |
| **Performance Objectives (Parents/Caregivers)** | **Attitudes** | **Self-Efficacy** | **Knowledge** | **Social Influence** |
| PO.1. Parents/caregivers limit preschoolers' screen viewing activities to 1 hour per day | A.1. Express positive feelings about the benefits that limiting screen viewing activities to 1 hour per day by using different strategies has for their child | SE.1. Express confidence that they can use different strategies to limit screen viewing activities even when their child wants to continue doing screen viewing activities | K.1.a. State that it is recommended to limit screen activities of their child to 1 hour per day <br> K.1.b. List different strategies to limit screen viewing activities | |
| PO.2. Parents/caregivers motivate (verbally) their children to do other activities instead of screen viewing activities | A.2. Express positive feelings about the benefits that doing other activities instead of screen viewing activities has for their child | SE.2. Express confidence that they can motivate their child to do other activities instead of screen viewing activities even when their child is nagging | K.2. Describe how to motivate their child to do other activities instead of screen viewing activities (e.g., tips, tricks) | SI.2. Indicate that they are able to motivate their child to do other activities instead of screen viewing activities even when their friends/neigbors do not motivate their own children |
| PO.3. Parents/caregivers do other activities with their child instead of screen viewing activities | A.3. Express positive feelings about the benefits about doing other activities together with their child instead of screen viewing activities has for their child | SE.3. Express confidence that they can do activities with their child that are not screen viewing activities even when their child only wants to do screen viewing activities | K.3. List activities that can be done instead of screen viewing activities (e.g., tips, tricks) | |
| PO.4. Parents/caregivers are role models for their children and limit their own time sitting down | A.4. Express positive feelings about being a role model for their child because the child will copy their behavior | SE.4. Express confidence that they can be a role model for their child even when they had a rough day | K.4. Describe how being a role model for their child by limiting their own sitting down time encourages their child to do the same | |

*(continued)*

**Table 5.8** *(Continued)*

| Organizational Outcome: Kindergarten Teachers Support Preschoolers to Decrease Sitting Time | | | | |
| --- | --- | --- | --- | --- |
| | **Personal Determinants** | | | |
| **Performance Objectives (Teachers)** | **Attitudes** | **Self-Efficacy** | **Knowledge** | **Social Influence** |
| PO.1. Teachers use different strategies to decrease preschoolers' total sitting time per day in kindergarten (e.g., performing standing classroom activities) | A.1. Express positive feelings about the benefits of using different strategies to decrease preschoolers' total sitting time | SE.1. Express confidence that they can use different strategies to decrease preschoolers' total sitting time in kindergarten even when they have a tight schedule to follow | K.1.a. List different strategies to decrease preschoolers' total sitting time a day | SI.1. Indicate that they use different strategies to decrease preschoolers' total sitting time per day in kindergarten even when other teachers stick to sedentary activities |
| PO.2. Teachers give assignments that the preschoolers need to fulfil standing up | A.2. Express positive feelings about the benefits of giving assignments that the preschoolers need to fulfil standing up | SE.2. Express confidence that they can give assignments that the preschoolers need to fulfil standing up even when they need to rearrange their classroom | K.2. Describe assignments that the preschoolers need to fulfil standing up | SI.2. Indicate that they plan to give assignments that the preschoolers need to fulfil standing up even when other teachers stick to assignments sitting down |
| PO.3. Teachers encourage the preschoolers to stand up when they are sitting down at the playground | A.3. Express positive feelings about the benefits that encouraging preschoolers to stand up when they are sitting down at the playground has for the preschoolers | SE.3. Express confidence that they can encourage preschoolers to stand up when they are sitting down at the playground even when there is already a lot of noise and commotion | | SI.3. Encourage the preschoolers to stand up when they are sitting down at the playground even when other teachers do not do this |
| PO.4. Teachers are a role models for the preschoolers and limit sitting down themselves | A.4. Express positive feelings about being role models for the preschoolers by limiting their own time sitting down | SE.4. Express confidence that they are role models for the preschoolers in limiting sitting down even when they are tired | K.4. Describe how being a role model for the preschoolers encourages the preschoolers to sit down less | |

level). To differentiate a population means to make a distinction between two or more subgroups because they differ in either the performance objectives or determinants of the health-related behavior or environmental outcomes. Differentiating a population often occurs simultaneously with writing performance objectives or exploring determinants because of the question that guides differentiation: Are either performance objectives or determinants substantially different for subgroups?

The rationale for differentiating a population is the basic understanding that populations are made up of individuals and groups with different characteristics and needs, all of which must be considered in relation to a health problem and to a health promotion program. The greater these differences, the less likely that a single intervention focus will fit everyone in the intervention population. If a subgroup has different behaviors or environmental conditions, the program planner may need to develop separate matrices for that subgroup and conduct a parallel planning process. If subgroups differ only on a few performance objectives and/or determinants the planner may be able to use the same matrices but make a note that certain performance objectives or change objectives pertain to a specific subgroup. The decision to differentiate the population should be very carefully considered, because each differentiation into two or more subgroups will expand the details of the planning process and potentially increase the program's complexity and costs. If identified differences in the subpopulations are not great, planners can often accommodate them within the program with a few variations of the intervention applications to address differences.

Some of the variables that may be important to consider in the differentiation of a population are the ones that were mentioned in the needs assessment. They include age and gender, geographic location, socioeconomic status, education, and cultural group. In addition, using stage theories and models such as child development, adult development, stages of change models (C. C. DiClemente & Prochaska, 1998; Nidecker, DiClemente, Bennett, & Bellack, 2008; Werch, Ames, Moore, Thombs, & Hart, 2009), and stages of organizational change (Cooperrider & Sekerka, 2006; Cummings & Worley, 2014) to differentiate populations will in many cases enhance a planner's ability to develop change objectives that successfully define what needs to change.

In summary, differentiating the population leads to separate matrices of program objectives for each group. The matrices are used to guide program planning to design interventions appropriate for each subgroup. The result may be a separate program for each group or a single program with multiple components, methods, or practical applications that can accommodate differences between groups. Careful consideration should be given to decisions to differentiate the priority population to ensure that the differences in the subgroups are significant enough to warrant the detailed planning involved in the creation of separate matrices for each subgroup. Modest differences between the subgroups can often be dealt with by adding designated performance objectives or change objectives for the subgroups within matrices for the priority population. This avoids the potential of overlapping matrices and a duplication of change objectives, which leads to the unnecessary expansion of work needed to plan the program.

## Constructing Matrices and Writing Change Objectives

At this point, the planner has made a preliminary decision about the number of matrices for the project, based on population differentiation and levels of environmental change. For each behavioral outcome and environmental outcome, the planner enters the performance objectives down the left side of a matrix and the determinants across the top. The next task is to assess each cell of the matrix to judge whether the determinant is likely to influence accomplishment of the performance objective. It is unlikely that each of the determinants will be an important influence for every performance objective. Because change objectives are needed for those cells in which the determinant is likely to influence accomplishment of the performance objective, this task can be a process of review and elimination. One way that the planner accomplishes this task is to look at each cell, decide whether change in a particular determinant is necessary for the performance objective, put an X through unimportant cells, and then write change objectives for the cells that remain. The planner then writes change objectives for the personal determinants.

The question that leads to formation of a change objective for personal determinants is: What needs to change related to the determinant for the program participants to do the performance objective? For example, Table 5.9 shows a matrix from the It's Your Game project in which the performance objective "Buy or obtain free condoms" is paired with the determinant of "knowledge." The question used to address this cell can be worded this way: What needs to change related to knowledge for the participants to be able to buy or obtain a condom? Answers to this question lead to the following change objectives (Table 5.9):

- List places to buy or obtain condoms for free
- Identify the different types of condoms and the relative advantages and disadvantages of each type

In Step 3, these change objectives will become the targets for program change methods and practical applications to increase knowledge. In another example that uses the same performance objective (buy or obtain condoms), a focus on the cell connected with the determinant of skills and self-efficacy leads to the question: What needs to change regarding skills and self-efficacy for program participants to purchase condoms? This question yields the following change objectives:

- Express confidence in ability to buy or obtain a free condom
- Express confidence in ability to deal with embarrassment when buying a condom

**Table 5.9**     Examples of Cells From a Behavior Matrix: Consistently and Correctly Using Condoms During Sexual Intercourse

| | Personal Determinants | | | |
| Performance Objectives | Knowledge | Skills and Self-Efficacy | Outcome Expectations | Perceived Norms |
| --- | --- | --- | --- | --- |
| PO.1. Make the decision to use condoms | K.1.a. State the consequences of not using a condom if you have sex <br> K.1.b. Recognize that using condoms when having sex will reduce your risk of getting HIV, STDs, or becoming pregnant | SSE.1. Feel confident in being able to make the decision to use condoms | OE.1.Recognize that making the decision to use condoms reduces the risk of getting pregnant, STDs, and HIV | PN.1.a. Recognize that most sexually active teens feel it is important to use condoms <br> PN.1.b. Recognize that most sexually active teens who decide to use condoms are more likely to use condoms |
| PO.2. Buy or obtain free condoms | K.2.a. List places to buy or obtain condoms for free <br> K.2.b. Identify the different types of condoms and the relative advantages and disadvantages of each type | SSE.2.a. Express confidence in the ability to buy or obtain a free condom <br> SSE.2.b. Express confidence in ability to deal with embarrassment when buying a condom | OE.2. Expect that buying or obtaining a condom will increase the likelihood of using a condom | PN.2. Explain that peers go into stores and buy condoms |
| PO.3. Carry condoms or have condoms easily available | K.3.a. List private, effective places to keep condoms <br> K.3.b. Describe how long condoms can be kept without increasing risk of breakage | SSE.3.a. Demonstrate the ability to carry condom discretely <br> SSE.3.b. Express confidence that can find a private, safe, accessible place for condoms | OE.3. Describe how having condoms easily available will result in more routine condom use | PN.3. State that peers have condoms easily available |
| PO.4. Negotiate the use of a condom with a partner | K.4. List the steps of successful negotiation | SSE.4.a. Demonstrate the ability to negotiate the use of condoms. <br> SSE.4.b.Express confidence in ability to not have sex if negotiation fails | OE.4.Describe personal beliefs that negotiation will lead to positive experience where both partners are satisfied and result in condom use | PN.4. Explain that peers talk to their partners about condom use |
| PO.4.1. Communicate your intentions to use a condom | K.4.1.a. Describe ways to communicate your intentions to use condoms to partner <br> K.4.1.b. State your personal rule to use condoms | SSE.4.1.a. Demonstrate ability to communicate intention to use a condom to partner <br> SSE. 4.1.b. Express confidence in ability to communicate intention to use a condom to partner | OE.4.1.a. Expect that communicating your intention will result in condom use | PN.4.1. Recognize that sexually active teens communicate their intentions to use condoms with their partners |

*(continued)*

**Table 5.9**    (Continued)

| | | Personal Determinants | | |
| --- | --- | --- | --- | --- |
| Performance Objectives | Knowledge | Skills and Self-Efficacy | Outcome Expectations | Perceived Norms |
| PO.4.2. Elicit partner's intentions to use a condom | K.4.2. Describe ways to elicit partner's intentions to use a condom | SSE. 4.2.a. Demonstrate ability to elicit partner's intention to use a condom<br>SSE.4.2b. Express confidence in ability to elicit partner's intention to use a condom | OE.4.2.Expect that eliciting partner's intention will lead to more effective negotiation not to have sex without a condom | PN.4.2. Recognize that sexually active teens elicit their partner's intentions to use a condom |
| PO.4.3. Actively listen to partner's concerns | K.4.3. Describe components of active listening | SSE.4.3.a. Demonstrate actively listening to partner's concerns<br>SSE.4.3.b. Express confidence in ability to actively listen to partner's concerns | OE.4.3. Expect that actively listening to partner's concerns will result in a mutual decision to use a condom or not have sex without one | PN.4.3. Recognize that sexually active teens actively listen to their partner's concerns |
| PO.4.4. Make an agreement to use condoms or not have sex | K.4.4. Describe steps to make an agreement | SSE.4.4.a. Demonstrate ability to come to an agreement to use condoms<br>SSE.4.4.b. Express confidence in ability to come to an agreement to use condoms or not have sex | OE.4.4. Expect that having an agreement about using condoms or not having sex will increase the chances of this agreement being successful | PN.4.4. Recognize that sexually active teens make an agreement to use condoms or not have sex |
| PO.5. Use a condom correctly | K.5.a. Explain how to evaluate the condition of a condom<br>K.5.b. Describe how to correctly apply a condom<br>K.5.c. Describe how to safely remove and dispose of a condom | SSE.5.a. Demonstrate ability to use a condom correctly<br>SSE.5.b. Express confidence in ability to use a condom correctly | OE.5. Expect that using a condom correctly will reduce the risk of getting HIV or STDs or becoming pregnant | PN.5. Recognize that sexually active teens use condoms correctly |
| PO.6. Maintain condom use with every partner every time you have sex | K.6. Explain why condom use is important with regular partners as well as with casual partners for all types of sex (oral, vaginal, and anal) | SSE.6. Express confidence to use a condom with regular partners as well as with casual partners every time you have sex | OE.6.a. Recognize that using condoms every time you have sex reduces the risk of getting HIV or STDs or becoming pregnancy<br>OE.6.b. Expect that using a condom with every partner will reduce the risk of getting HIV or STDs or becoming pregnant | PN.6.a. Recognize that teens use condoms with regular and casual partners<br>PN.6.b. Recognize that teens feel it is important to use condoms for all types of sex |

**Table 5.10**    List of Action Words for Writing Change Objectives: Organized by Levels of Complexity of Learning Tasks

| Knowledge | Understand | Applications | Analysis | Synthesis | Evaluation |
|-----------|-----------|--------------|----------|-----------|------------|
| define | describe | apply | analyze | arrange | appraise |
| label | discuss | demonstrate | appraise | assemble | assess |
| list | explain | dramatize | calculate | collect | choose |
| name | express | execute | categorize | compose | compare |
| recall | identify | illustrate | compare | construct | conclude |
| record | interpret | illustrate | contrast | create | critique |
| repeat | locate | implement | debate | design | estimate |
| state | recognize | interpret | diagram | formulate | evaluate |
| tell | report | modify | differentiate | manage | judge |
| | restate | operate | distinguish | organize | justify |
| | review | practice | examine | plan | measure |
| | summarize | predict | experiment | prepare | rate |
| | translate | schedule | inspect | propose | revise |
| | | sketch | inventory | relate | score |
| | | use | question | set up | select |
| | | | relate | | value |
| | | | solve | | |
| | | | test | | |

These examples show that change objectives are stated with action verbs. Table 5.10 includes words to help with this task (Caffarella, 1985). Notice in Table 5.10 that the action verbs are organized by complexity of learning or change process. For example, "comprehension" is more complex that just "knowing," and "application" is more complex than "comprehension" (Krathwohl, 2002). The selection of the action verb enables the planners to determine the level of complexity required for a performance objective to be accomplished. Change objectives begin with a verb that defines the action and are followed by a statement of the expected result of the intervention. The purpose of stating a change objective in this manner is to make as specific as possible what change in the determinant needs to be achieved to accomplish the performance objective. Planners who write change objectives with an action verb and specified change in the determinants have a clear direction to the next steps in the Intervention Mapping process: selecting intervention methods and translating methods into practical applications.

**Dealing With Automaticity in the Matrix of Change Objectives**    As discussed in Chapter 2, automaticity (impulsivity, habits, or prejudice) is not a standard determinant but a characteristic of the behavior and mostly outside of an individual's awareness. Theory predicts that automatic reactions can be overcome by reflective reactions, coping skills, and control motivation. Habits may be changed by cue altering, counterconditioning, and stimulus control. However, most of these change methods refer to performance objectives in combination with change objectives. For example:

- Teach people to change a stimulus that elicits or signals a behavior.

- Encourage removing cues for unhealthy habits and adding prompts for healthier alternatives (Wood & Neal, 2007).

- Get the person to identify potential barriers and ways to overcome these (Marlatt & Donovan, 2005).

- Have people choose a (larger) delayed reward far in advance (Robbins, Schwartz, & Wasserman, 2001).

- Stimulate pledging, promising, or engaging oneself to perform the healthful behavior, and announce that decision to others (Ajzen, Czasch, & Flood, 2009).

It is not advisable to place Automaticity or Habit in the matrix as a determinant; it is very difficult to formulate clear change objectives. For the matrix, automaticity may best be handled in terms of specific performance objectives derived from methods to change Habitual, Automatic, and Impulsive Behaviors (see Chapter 6, Table 6.6) in combination with awareness, attitudes, social norms, and (social) coping skills and (control) self-efficacy. Those performance objectives may, for example, be derived applying a self-management approach: monitoring, evaluating, planning coping responses, implementing, and recycling (Clark, 2003; Rothman, Baldwin, & Hertel, 2004). Changing a habitual chain by moving the cookie jar from its normal place is a (sub) performance objective; being confident and able to find and implement that coping response are change objectives. Table 5.11 provides a simulated matrix of change objectives for worksite employees to establish a healthy diet.

### Identifying Environmental Agents and Program Implementers

A common source of confusion for program planners is the distinction between using agents in the environment to make environmental changes and using them to implement components of an intervention program. For example, in a school-based program such as Coordinated Approach to Child Health (CATCH), a cardiovascular disease prevention program for children, teachers may be both agents to change the environmental conditions and program implementers (Coleman et al., 2005; Hoelscher et al., 2010). A component of the intervention in the CATCH program has been directed at performance and change objectives for ensuring that children have scheduled time during the school day to engage in moderate

**Table 5.11**     Examples of Cells From a Simulated Matrix to Address a Habitual Behavior

| Behavior: Establish a Healthy Diet | | | |
| --- | --- | --- | --- |
| **Performance Objectives** | **Awareness** | **Attitudes** | **Self-Efficacy and Skills** |
| PO.1. Monitor food intake | A.1. Acknowledge the habitual character of eating high fat food, especially snacks | ATT.1. Feel positive about monitoring food intake | SSE.1. Express confidence in ability to correctly monitor one's own food intake |
| PO.2. Decide if discrepancies exist | | | SSE.2. Demonstrate the ability to evaluate fat content of food intake |
| PO.3. Make plan, e.g., change a stimulus that elicits or signals a behavior | A.3. Acknowledge the need to change environmental cues | ATT.3. Recognize the advantages of changing behavior | SSE.3. Express confidence in ability to generate coping strategies to deal with habitual behaviors |
| PO.4. Take action, e.g., moving the cookie jar from its normal place | | | SSE.4. Demonstrate the ability to recognize automaticity in behavior chains and identify points for cue altering |
| PO.5. Evaluate (and Recycle to Monitoring) | A.5. Explain the importance of self-evaluation skills | ATT.5. Feel positive about evaluating and returning to self-monitoring if necessary | SSE.5. Express confidence in ability to evaluate implemented coping strategies and return to self-monitoring if necessary |

physical activity. This was part of the school's environmental change program. They were thus important agents at the organizational level. In addition, the teachers implemented the physical education program that enabled the children to be physically active at school. A training program helped prepare the teachers to implement the physical education program. Program implementation is not part of planning done in Step 2 but is addressed in Step 5, following a similar set of tasks focused on implementation outcomes rather than health behavior or environmental change outcomes.

## Creating a Logic Model of Change

In contrast to the PRECEDE model developed in Step 1, which depicts pathways of problem causation, the logic model of change created in Step 2 illustrates pathways of program effects. Program planners use information from Step 1 regarding desired health and quality-of-life outcomes and information from the previous tasks in Step 2 (behavior and environmental outcomes, performance objectives, determinants, and change objectives) to begin populating a logic model of change, which is read from left to right. Figure 5.2 presents the initial logic model of change for the It's Your Game project. Subsequent information from Steps 3, 4, and 5 will be added to the model to complete the logic of change and to guide evaluation planning.

The final task in Step 2 is for program planners to begin creating a logic model of change for their health promotion program.

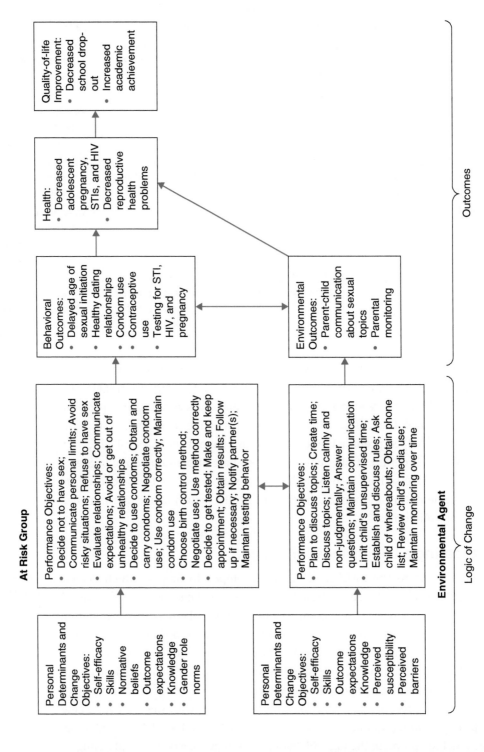

**Figure 5.2** IYG Logic Model of Change

# Using Matrices of Change Objectives for Program Evaluation

Each task in Step 2 produces information that is used to guide the program evaluation (see Chapter 9). In the first task, the planners specified the behavioral and environmental outcomes that the program would address. For program evaluation these outcomes are measured to determine the impact of the program on behavior and environmental conditions (Abbema, van Assema, Kok, Leew, & de Vries, 2004; Hou, Fernández, Baumler, & Parcel, 2002).

In the second task, the planners further delineated the behavioral and environmental conditions by writing performance objectives. These performance objectives help define the critical components and necessary prerequisites for the performance of the behavior and environmental outcomes. As part of the program evaluation, questions can be asked to determine whether program participants achieved the performance objective, which provides valuable information to better understand a program's effectiveness. For example, if the behavior was performed, then responses to questions about the performance objectives help the evaluators to know the relative importance of the objectives to the performance of the behavior. If the behavior was not performed, then the responses to questions about the performance objectives may help explain why the program did not have an effect on behavior and may provide important information to guide revisions of the program. In some cases the performance objectives help in defining behavioral or environmental outcome and can be used to construct evaluation questions to measure the behavior. For example, eating a low-fat diet so that less than 30 percent of calories are from fat cannot be effectively measured without more specific questions about what and how much was eaten, which can be guided by performance objectives such as "drink low-fat milk instead of whole milk."

In the final task in Step 2, the planners create matrices for change objectives that the intervention program will address. These matrices can also be used to guide the development of measures to evaluate the most immediate impact of the program. The program design is intended to address the change objectives, as the first effect in the logic model of change (see Figure 5.1). Accomplishment of the change objectives is intended to influence changes in the personal determinants of the performance objectives. For impact evaluation the evaluator will want to know whether the program was successful in influencing changes in the determinants. The change objectives in the cells of the matrices can be used to help guide the development of instruments to measure the determinants. For example, to develop a knowledge instrument, the change objectives for knowledge constitute the critical knowledge needed to accomplish the performance objectives. Planners can thus use the change objectives for knowledge to construct questions to measure participants' knowledge before and after participating in the intervention program. This same principle can be applied to the construction of items to measure other determinants, such as self-efficacy, subjective norms, attitudes, and beliefs.

It is most difficult to evaluate the effectiveness of a health promotion program if the planners have not clearly stated the program's objectives and outcomes. Step 2 of Intervention Mapping provides the program evaluators with clearly stated behavioral and environmental outcomes, performance objectives, and change objectives that can guide the program evaluation (Markham et al., 2012; Tortolero et al., 2010).

---

### BOX 5.2. IT'S YOUR GAME . . . KEEP IT REAL PROJECT

**The first task in Step 2 is to state what health behaviors and environmental conditions need to change.**

Following from the needs assessment for the It's Your Game . . . Keep It Real Project introduced in Chapter 4, the program planners identified the primary health-related behavior outcome for the at-risk group (middle school students) as "choose not to have sex." However, they identified the need for additional behavior outcomes related to having healthy friendships and dating relationships, using condoms correctly and consistently when having sex, using an effective method of birth control along with condoms, and obtaining regular testing for pregnancy, HIV, and STIs if a student was sexually active. In the environment, the planners identified two interpersonal outcomes for parents:

- Parents communicate with their child about dating, intimate/healthy relationships, and sexual behavior.

- Parents monitor their child's time, friendships, and dating activities.

**The second task is to subdivide behavioral and environmental outcomes into performance objectives.**

The performance objectives for the at-risk group (middle school students) and for parents are listed in Table 5.12.

**The third task in Step 2 is to select important and changeable determinants of the health behavior and environmental outcomes.**

Based on the needs assessment (Chapter 4, It's Your Game), the planning group brainstormed possible determinants for the health-promoting behaviors and environmental outcomes. The planners worked first on student performance objectives and then on the parent objectives. The brainstormed preliminary list included ideas from the focus groups and literature review. The planners modified the preliminary list using theoretical constructs

**Table 5.12**    Behavioral Outcomes, Environmental Outcomes, and Performance Objectives for It's Your Game . . . Keep It Real

| Behavioral Outcomes (BO) Students will: | Associated Performance Objectives |
|---|---|
| BO.1. Choose not to have sex | Decide to not have sex |
| | Communicate personal limits regarding sex |
| | Avoid situations which could lead to sex |
| | Refuse to have sex |
| BO.2. Use condoms correctly and consistently if having sex | Make the decision to use condoms |
| | Buy or obtain a free condom |
| | Carry condoms |
| | Negotiate the use of condom with every partner |
| | Use a condom correctly |
| | Maintain condom use with every partner every time you have sex |
| BO.3. Use effective method of contraception along with condoms if having sex | Make decision to use birth control |
| | Choose appropriate birth control method |
| | Negotiate use of birth control method each time you engage in sex |
| | Use chosen birth control method effectively and consistently |
| BO.4. Get tested and counseled for HIV, STIs, and pregnancy if having sex | Make the decision to get tested |
| | Make appointment to get tested by health care provider |
| | Keep appointment to get tested |
| | Obtain test results |
| | Obtain and follow through with health care if necessary |
| | Notify partner(s) of test results |
| | Maintain testing behavior over time |
| BO.5. Have healthy relationships with friends, girlfriends, or boyfriends | Evaluate past, current, and potential relationships |
| | Communicate expectations about healthy relationships |
| | Avoid relationships with friends, boyfriends/girlfriends that are not healthy |
| | Get out of relationships with friends, boyfriends/girlfriends that are not healthy |
| **Environmental Outcomes (EO) Parents will:** | **Associated Performance Objectives** |
| EO.1. Communicate with child about dating and sexual health topics | Plan to discuss dating, healthy relationships, and sexual behaviors with child |
| | Create appropriate time and location to talk to child |
| | Discuss healthy dating relationships |
| | Discuss advantages of abstinence |
| | Discuss refusal skills |
| | Discuss avoidance of risky situations |
| | Discuss alternatives to having sex |
| | Discuss use of condoms and other contraceptive methods |
| | Listen to child's feelings and opinions calmly and nonjudgmentally |
| | Answer child's questions or concerns |
| | Maintain open channel of communication with child over time |

*(continued)*

**Table 5.12**    (Continued)

| Environmental Outcomes (EO) Parents will: | Associated Performance Objectives |
|---|---|
| EO.2. Monitor child's time, friendships, and dating activities | Limit child's unsupervised time |
| | Establish rules on how child spends time, friendships, & dating |
| | Discuss rules with child |
| | Ask child where he is going, with whom, and what they will be doing |
| | Discuss with child and other parents about the potential exposure to risk at the location where the child will be |
| | Obtain and update list of names and phone numbers of child's friends, boyfriends, and girlfriends |
| | Review child's Internet & other media use |
| | Evaluate if activity is appropriate |
| | If activity is inappropriate, negotiate an alternative activity with child |
| | Maintain monitoring behaviors over time |

from Social Cognitive Theory (SCT) and the Theory of Planned Behavior (TPB), the two theories that matched most closely the preliminary ideas from the needs assessment. For the healthy relationships outcome, the planners added perceived gender role norms as an important determinant, as this has been targeted in previous effective dating violence prevention programs (Cornelius & Resseguie, 2007; Foshee et al., 2005). For parent outcomes, the planner added perceived susceptibility and perceived barriers from the Health Belief Model (HBM) as these emerged as determinants in the parent focus groups. Examples of work on determinants are presented in Tables 5.13 and 5.14.

**Table 5.13**    Work on Determinants of Middle School Students' Choosing Not to Have Sex

| Preliminary List | Final List |
|---|---|
| Confidence about avoiding situations that make it hard to say no to sex | Self-efficacy (effective communication and refusal) |
| Ability to refuse unwanted sexual advances | Skills (effective communication and refusal) |
| Thinking that friends and parents support waiting until you are older to have sex | Normative beliefs |
| Knowing a teen parent | Outcome expectations |
| Knowing how to say no | Knowledge (effective communication and refusal) |
| Not being embarrassed to talk with their partner | Self-efficacy (effective communication) |

**The fourth task in Step 2 is to create the matrices.**

The planners created five separate matrices for the at-risk group, that is, middle school students, and two matrices for parents at the interpersonal level. Sample matrices are shown in Tables 5.15, 5.16, and 5.17.

**Table 5.14**    Work on Determinants of Parents' Communication With Child

| Preliminary List | Final List |
|---|---|
| Understanding the positive influence that parents can have on child's dating and sexual behavior | Outcome expectations |
| Confidence about talking with child about sexual topics | Self-efficacy |
| Choosing the right time and place to start a conversation about sexual topics | Skills |
| Having current information about condoms and contraceptive methods | Knowledge |
| Recognizing that child will eventually start to date and have sex | Perceived susceptibility |
| Anticipating negative responses from child | Perceived barriers |
| Confidence in answering difficult questions | |
| Not believing that talking to children about sexual topics will encourage them to become sexually active | |
| Overcoming embarrassment or anxiety to talk with child about sexual topics | |
| Knowing current rates of teen dating violence, teen pregnancy, and STIs | |

**Table 5.15**    Matrix for Behavioral Outcome: Student Chooses Not to Have Sex

| Performance Objectives The middle school student will: | Personal Determinants | | | | |
|---|---|---|---|---|---|
| | Knowledge | Skills | Self-Efficacy | Normative Beliefs | Outcome Expectations |
| PO.1. Decide to not have sex | K.1.a. Define the different types of sex (oral, vaginal, and anal sex) K.1.b. State the physical, emotional, and social consequences of having sex K.1.c. Recognize that the only 100% effective way of avoiding HIV, STI, or getting pregnant is to not have sex | S.1. Demonstrate ability to make the decision to not have sex | SE.1. Express confidence in ability to make the decision to not have sex | NB.1.a. State that significant others approve and respect your decision to not have sex NB.1.b. Recognize that most parents feel it is important for teens to not to have sex | OE.1. State that abstaining from sex will help in achieving life goals, self-respect, and respect for others |
| PO.2. Communicate personal limits regarding sex | K.2.a. Describe what a personal limit is K.2.b. List your personal limits regarding sex K.2.c. List ways to communicate personal limits to friends/ boyfriend/ girlfriend | S.2. Demonstrate ability to communicate to friends or boyfriend/girlfriend your personal limit to wait to have sex | SE.2. Express confidence in ability to communicate to friends or boyfriend/girlfriend your personal limit to wait to have sex | NB.2.a. Recognize that friends and partners approve of you communicating your personal limits NB.2.b. Recognize that parents want you to communicate your intention to not have sex to friends and partners | OE.2.a. State that communicating your personal limits will decrease risk of HIV, STIs, & pregnancy OE.2.b. State that communicating your personal limits will lead to better relationship with boyfriend/girlfriend |

*(continued)*

**Table 5.15**    *(Continued)*

| Performance Objectives The middle school student will: | Personal Determinants | | | | |
|---|---|---|---|---|---|
| | **Knowledge** | **Skills** | **Self-Efficacy** | **Normative Beliefs** | **Outcome Expectations** |
| PO.3. Avoid situations that might lead to sex | K.3.a. List situations (places, peers, times) that may make it hard to say no to sex<br><br>K.3.b. Identify signs (feeling pressure to do something, lack of adult supervision, alcohol and drugs) and situations (places, peers, times) that make it hard to say no<br><br>K.3.c. Identify useful strategies for avoiding these types of situations | S.3.a. Demonstrate ability to identify signs and situations that may make it hard to say no to sex<br><br>S.3.b. Demonstrate ability to avoid these situations | SE.3.a. Express confidence in ability to identify signs and situations that may make it hard to say no to sex<br><br>SE.3.b. Express confidence in ability to avoid these situations | NB.3. State that significant others approve and respect your decision to avoid situations that may make it hard to say no to sex | OE.3. State that avoiding a high risk situation will help you to not have sex |
| PO.4. Refuse to have sex | K.4.a. Identify the signs of being in a situation where it may be hard to say no to sex<br><br>K.4.b. Recognize these signs as cues to use refusal strategies<br><br>K.4.c. Describe characteristics of clear refusal skills | S.4. Demonstrate the ability to use refusal skills in multiple situations (e.g., peer pressure, social situations, when you really like the person) | SE.4.a. State a high degree of confidence in being able to use refusal skills in a variety of situations (nonsex related)<br><br>SE.4.b. State a high degree of confidence in being able to refuse sex in a variety of situations | NB.4.a. State that significant others approve and respect you refusing to do things that you choose not to do (nonsex related behaviors)<br><br>NB.4.b. State that significant others approve and respect your refusing to have sex | OE.4.a. State that use of appropriate refusal skills will keep you from doing things you do not want to do (nonsex related) without jeopardizing friendships<br><br>OE.4.b. State that use of appropriate refusal skills will lead to successful abstinence without jeopardizing interpersonal relationships<br><br>OE.4.c. State that use of refusal skills will reduce the risk of HIV, STIs, or becoming pregnant |

**Table 5.16**    Matrix for Behavioral Outcome: Student Has Healthy Relationships With Friends, Girlfriends, or Boyfriends

| Performance Objectives *The middle school student will:* | Personal Determinants | | | | |
|---|---|---|---|---|---|
| | **Knowledge** | **Skills** | **Self-Efficacy** | **Normative Beliefs** | **Gender Role Norms** |
| PO.1. Decide to have healthy relationships with friends, boyfriends, or girlfriends | K.1.a. List characteristics of healthy/unhealthy relationships K.1.b. State the physical, emotional, and social consequences of unhealthy relationships | | SE.1. Express confidence in ability to make the decision to have only healthy relationships with friends, boyfriends, or girlfriends | NB.1. State that significant others approve and respect your decision to have healthy relationships with friends, boyfriends, or girlfriends | GRN.1. List ways gender role norms can influence a relationship |
| PO.2. Evaluate past, current, and potential relationships | K.2. List characteristics of past & current relationships | S.2. Demonstrate ability to evaluate relationships | SE.2. Express confidence in ability to evaluate relationships | | GRN.2. State ways that gender roles have influenced your past & current relationships |
| PO.3. Communicate expectations about healthy relationships | K.3.a. List your own expectations about healthy relationships K.3.b. List verbal & nonverbal communication strategies | S.3. Demonstrate the ability to communicate your own expectation | SE.3.a. Express confidence in ability to communicate your expectations SE.3.b. Express confidence in ability to listen to your partner's expectations | | GRN.3.a. State ways that gender roles influence your ability to communicate your expectations GRN.3.b. State ways that gender roles influence your ability to listen to your partner's expectations. |
| PO.4. Avoid relationships with friends, boyfriends/ girlfriends that are not healthy | K.4.a. Identify current & potential relationships with friends, boyfriends, or girlfriends that are not healthy K.4.b. List ways/strategies to avoid friends, boyfriends, or girlfriends that are not healthy | S.4.a. Demonstrate the ability to avoid unhealthy relationships S.4.b. Demonstrate the ability to be comfortable by yourself | SE.4.a. Express confidence in ability to avoid unhealthy relationships SE.4.b. Express confidence in ability to be comfortable by yourself | | GRN.4. Recognize how gender roles influence ability to avoid unhealthy relationships |
| PO.5. Get out of relationships with friends, boyfriends, or girlfriends that are not healthy | K.5.a. List ways to end an unhealthy relationship (be clear, consider location, be respectful, set boundaries) K.5.a. Identify situations where you need help getting out of an unhealthy relationship | S.5. Demonstrate ability to get out of unhealthy relationship | SE.5. Express confidence in ability to get out of an unhealthy relationship | NB.5. State that significant others believe it is important to end unhealthy relationships | GRN.5. Recognize how gender roles influence ability to get out of unhealthy relationships |

**Table 5.17**   Sample Cells for Matrix for Interpersonal Environmental Outcome: Parent Communicates With Child About Dating and Sexual Health Topics

| Performance Objectives Parents will: | Personal Determinants | | | | |
|---|---|---|---|---|---|
| | Knowledge | Skills and Self-Efficacy | Perceived Susceptibility | Perceived Barriers | Outcome Expectations |
| PO.1. Plan to discuss dating, healthy relationships, and sexual behavior with child | K.1.a. Describe the importance of talking to child about dating, healthy relationships, and sexual behavior K.1.b. State that parents can influence child's dating & sexual behavior K.1.c. State that talking about dating and sexual behavior does not lead to child's participation in these behaviors | SSE.1. Express confidence in ability to plan a discussion about dating, healthy relationships, and sexual behavior with child | PS.1.a. Recognize that their child may be starting to date or engage in sexual behavior PS.1.b. Describe the risks in their community (STIs, HIV, pregnancy, and dating violence rates) | PB.1.a. Anticipate negative responses of child PB.1.b. Recognize their own barriers to discussing dating & sexual behaviors with their child | OE.1. Expect to be better prepared to discuss dating, healthy relationships, and sexual behavior with child if they plan ahead |
| PO.2. Create appropriate time and location to talk to child | K.2.a. State potential times and locations to talk with child K.2.b. Recognize characteristics of a teachable moment | SSE.2.a Demonstrate ability to approach child to discuss these topics SSE.2.b. Express confidence in ability to approach child to discuss these topics SSE.2.c. Express confidence in ability to identify and act on teachable moments | | PB.2. Anticipate barriers to finding appropriate time and location to discuss these topics | OE.2. Expect that identifying an appropriate time/location will ensure that the discussion is better received by child |
| PO.3. Discuss healthy dating relationships | K.3.a. Describe characteristics of healthy/unhealthy relationships K.3.b. List expectations for child's dating (e.g., acceptable age for group/solo dates) | SSE.3. Express confidence in ability to communicate expectations about healthy dating relationships | PS.3. Recognize that middle school students are at risk for being victims and perpetrators of dating violence | | OE.3. Expect that sharing your expectations about dating will help child to avoid unhealthy relationships |

**Table 5.17**    (*Continued*)

| Performance Objectives *Parents will:* | Personal Determinants | | | | |
|---|---|---|---|---|---|
| | **Knowledge** | **Skills and Self-Efficacy** | **Perceived Susceptibility** | **Perceived Barriers** | **Outcome Expectations** |
| PO.4. Discuss advantages of abstinence (choosing to wait until child is older to have sex) | K.4.a. State the advantages of sexual abstinence (e.g., time to focus on goals, avoid potential negative consequences) | SSE.4.a. Demonstrate the ability to discuss advantages of abstinence SSE.4.b. Express confidence in ability to discuss advantages of abstinence | PS.4.Recognize that some middle school students are having sex | PB.4. Anticipate negative responses of child | OE.4. Expect that discussing advantages of abstinence with child will reduce likelihood of him/her engaging in risky sexual behavior |
| PO.5. Discuss avoidance of risky situations (e.g., being home alone, going to a party with alcohol) | K.5.a. State characteristics of risky situations (i.e., situations that could lead to unwanted sex) K.5.b. Identify strategies to avoid risky situations | SSE.5.a. Demonstrate ability to discuss avoidance of risky situations SSE.5.b. Express confidence in ability to discuss avoidance of risky situations | PS.5. Recognize that child may be pressured or put themselves in risky situations | PB.5.a. Recognize own discomfort in discussing avoidance of risky situations PB.5.b. Anticipate child's negative response to discussing avoidance of risky situations | OE.5. Expect that discussing ways to avoid risky situations will reduce likelihood that child will be pressured to have sex |
| PO.6. Discuss use of condoms and other contraceptive methods | K.6.a. Describe steps for correct condom use to child K.6.b. List available contraceptive methods and their effectiveness K.6.c. Direct their child to where they can obtain condoms and contraceptive methods | SSE.6.a. Demonstrate how to use a condom correctly SSE.6.b. Express confidence in ability to demonstrate correct condom use SSE.6.c. Express confidence in ability to discuss contraceptive methods | PS.6. Recognize that middle school students who have sex are at risk for unintended pregnancy, HIV, and STIs | PB.6. Recognize that discussing about condoms and contraception will not encourage child to become sexually active sooner | OE.6. Expect that discussing about condoms and contraception will reduce the likelihood that child has unprotected sex when they become sexually active |
| PO.7. Listen to child's feelings and opinions calmly and nonjudgmentally | K.7.a. State characteristics of active listening K.7.b. State importance of listening to child's feelings and opinions actively and nonjudgmentally (e.g., will elicit more honest answers, child will feel supported) | SSE.7.a. Demonstrate ability to listen calmly and nonjudgmentally SSE.7.b. Express confidence in ability to listen calmly and nonjudgmentally | | PB.7.a. Anticipate increased need for patience and self-control to actively listen to child PB.7.b. Recognize that distractions can make it difficult to actively listen to child | OE.7. Expect that effective active listening will reduce likelihood of child failing to communicate or miscommunicating important information |

(*continued*)

**Table 5.17**    (Continued)

| Performance Objectives Parents will: | Personal Determinants | | | | |
|---|---|---|---|---|---|
| | Knowledge | Skills and Self-Efficacy | Perceived Susceptibility | Perceived Barriers | Outcome Expectations |
| PO.8. Answer child's questions or concerns | K.8.a. Describe ways to respond to questions for which you have an answer, as well as questions for which you do not have an answer K.8.b. List possible motives behind the questions asked (e.g., Am I normal? Permission seeking?) K.8.c.Recognize that parent does not need to share their personal sexual experiences with child | SSE.8.a. Demonstrate ability to effectively answer child's questions SSE.8.b. Demonstrate ability to provide an appropriate delayed response SSE.8.c. Express confidence in ability to identify motive behind question and answer appropriately | | PB.8.a. Anticipate questions child may have about dating and sexual behavior | OE.8. Expect that answering child's questions or concerns will reduce likelihood of engaging in unhealthy relationships or risky sexual behaviors |
| PO.9. Maintain open channel of communication with child over time | K.9.a. Recognize that the information you discuss with child about dating and sexual behavior will change as the child matures K.9.b. Identify ways to keep an open channel of communication with child | SSE.9.a. Demonstrate ability to keep an open channel of communication with child SSE.9.b. Express confidence in ability to keep an open channel of communication with child | PS.9. Recognize that child's likelihood of being in an unhealthy dating relationship or engaging in risky sexual behavior may increase with age | PB.9. Identify barriers to maintaining open communication with child (e.g., time availability, child's resistance, difficulty accepting/giving feedback) | OE.9. Expect that maintaining open communication will reduce child's likelihood of engaging in unhealthy relationships or risky sexual behaviors |

**The fifth task in Step 2 is to create a logic model of change.**

The planners created a logic model of change for It's Your Game based on the matrices of change objectives developed in Step 2 and the health and quality-of-life outcomes identified in Step 1 (Figure 5.2).

## Summary

In Step 2 of Intervention Mapping, a transition is made from the needs assessment conducted in Step 1 to assessing what should change to prevent a health problem or improve health and quality-of-life outcomes. This transition is a shift from a logic model for causes of a health problem to a logic model for what changes will be addressed by an intervention. The starting points for this assessment are the program goals for health and quality of life stated at the end of Step 1. The first task in this step is to state the behavior and environmental outcomes that need to be achieved to reach the program goals for improved health and quality of life. The second task of Step 2 is to subdivide each behavior and environmental outcome into performance objectives that specify exactly what needs to change by whom so that the overall behavior or environmental outcome is accomplished.

The third task in Step 2 is to select potential important and changeable determinants for each behavior and environmental outcome. Determinants are factors derived from behavioral science theory and evidence from empirical studies that suggest a change in the factors may influence a change in the behavior of the at-risk group or of environmental agents capable of changing environmental conditions. The final task is to create a matrix of change objectives for each behavior and environmental outcome by linking the selected determinants to the performance objectives and forming cells to write change objectives. These change objectives represent what needs to be modified as a result of the intervention to influence performance objectives to achieve the behavior and environmental outcomes. Thus, the matrix of change objectives describes the most immediate change to be addressed by the intervention and provides the detail for the selection of intervention methods and practical applications for the health promotion program. In addition, the matrix of change objectives provides a basis for formulating questions and measurement instruments for the evaluation of the health promotion program.

Most program planning will require multiple matrices to address the behavior of the at-risk population as well as describe each level of the environment to be addressed by the intervention. In some cases it is necessary to break down the population into subpopulations due to important differences in behavior, performance objectives, or determinants and to create separate matrices of change objectives for each group. The final product of Step 2 of the Intervention Mapping process is a set of matrices that specifies the immediate objectives of a health promotion program.

## Discussion Questions and Learning Activities

1. In Step 2 of Intervention Mapping, the program planners make the transition from a risk model created in Step 1 to a change model that describes what the intervention will change to achieve the health outcome goal. Construct a logic model that illustrates the causal

pathways for influencing achievement of the health outcome goal and impact on quality of life.

2. Explain why it is important to be very specific when stating behavioral and environmental outcomes.

3. Give examples of the questions planners can use to: (a) state the behavioral and environmental outcomes to be achieved by a health promotion program; (b) subdivide behavioral and environmental outcomes into performance objectives; and (c) write change objectives for the cells of the matrices.

4. For the health problem and population you selected for the needs assessment in Step 1 (Chapter 4), state the behavioral and environmental outcomes to be accomplished by the intervention. What will your intervention try to change? Justify your decisions using evidence from the literature.

5. Priority population differentiation: Whom is this intervention meant to affect? Are there important subgroups? On what variables should the population be grouped? Explain the rationale for differentiation or nondifferentiation into subgroup for planning the program.

6. Performance objectives: Specify performance objectives for the health behavior and environmental outcomes for at least one of the priority groups you have differentiated. Briefly describe the process you would use to validate these performance objectives.

7. Specify determinants of the health behaviors and environmental outcomes. Specify and justify, using theory and empirical findings, the most important personal determinants for each behavioral outcome and environmental outcome (that is, those most important to address in your program). Describe any new research you would plan to supplement what you are able to ascertain from the literature.

8. Change objectives: For each health behavior and environmental outcome, create matrices to write change objectives and give at least one example in each relevant cell of the matrix.

## References

Abbema, E. A., van Assema, P., Kok, G. J., De Leeuw, E., & de Vries, N. K. (2004). Effect evaluation of a comprehensive community intervention aimed at reducing socioeconomic health inequalities in the Netherlands. *Health Promotion International*, *19*(2), 141–156.

Abbott, S., & Freeth, D. (2008). Social capital and health. *Journal of Health Psychology*, *13*(7), 874–883.

Abel, E., Darby, A. L., & Ramachandran, R. (1994). Managing hypertension among veterans in an outpatient screening program. *Journal of the American Academy of Nurse Practitioners, 6*(9), 413–419.

Abraham, C., Sheeran, P., & Johnston, M. (Jul 1998). From health beliefs to self-regulation: Theoretical advances in the psychology of action control. *Psychology & Health, 13*(4), 569–591.

Ajzen, I., Czasch, C., & Flood, M. G. (2009). From intentions to behavior: Implementation intention, commitment, and conscientiousness. *Journal of Applied Social Psychology, 39*(6), 1356–1372.

Alewijnse, D., Mesters, I. E., Metsemakers, J. F., & van den Borne, B. H. (2002). Program development for promoting adherence during and after exercise therapy for urinary incontinence. *Patient Education & Counseling, 48*(2), 147–160.

Appel, L. J., Sacks, F. M., Carey, V. J., Obarzanek, E., Swain, J. F., Miller, E. R., 3rd,...Bishop, L. M. (2005). Effects of protein, monounsaturated fat, and carbohydrate intake on blood pressure and serum lipids: Results of the OmniHeart randomized trial. *JAMA, 294*(19), 2455–2464.

Armstrong, P. (2015). *Bloom's taxonomy*. Retrieved from http://cft.vanderbilt.edu/guides-sub-pages/blooms-taxonomy/

Audrain-McGovern, J., Rodriguez, D., Patel, V., Faith, M. S., Rodgers, K., & Cuevas, J. (2006). How do psychological factors influence adolescent smoking progression? The evidence for indirect effects through tobacco advertising receptivity. *Pediatrics, 117*(4), 1216–1225.

Bandura, A. (1986). *Social foundations of thought and action: A Social Cognitive Theory*. Englewood Cliffs, NJ: Prentice-Hall.

Bandura, A. (1997). *Self-efficacy: The exercise of control*. New York, NY: W.H. Freeman.

Bandura, A. (2004a). Health promotion by social cognitive means. *Health Education & Behavior, 31*(2), 143–164.

Bandura, A. (2004b). Swimming against the mainstream: The early years from chilly tributary to transformative mainstream. *Behaviour Research & Therapy, 42*(6), 613–630.

Bandura, A. (2006). On integrating social cognitive and social diffusion theories. In A. Singhal & J. Dearing (Eds.), *Communication of innovations: A journey with Ev Rogers* (pp. 111–134). Thousand Oaks, CA: Sage.

Barrera, M., Jr., Toobert, D. J., Angell, K. L., Glasgow, R. E., & Mackinnon, D. P. (2006). Social support and social-ecological resources as mediators of lifestyle intervention effects for type 2 diabetes. *Journal of Health Psychology, 11*(3), 483–495.

Bauer, J. E., Hyland, A., Li, Q., Steger, C., & Cummings, K. M. (2005). A longitudinal assessment of the impact of smoke-free worksite policies on tobacco use. *American Journal of Public Health, 95*(6), 1024.

Bayne-Smith, M., Fardy, P. S., Azzollini, A., Magel, J., Schmitz, K. H., & Agin, D. (2004). Improvements in heart health behaviors and reduction in coronary artery disease risk factors in urban teenaged girls through a school-based intervention: The PATH program. *American Journal of Public Health*, *94*(9), 1538–1543.

Beets, M. W., Cardinal, B. J., & Alderman, B. L. (2010). Parental social support and the physical activity-related behaviors of youth: A review. *Health Education & Behavior*, *37*(5), 621–644.

Begley, C. E., Shegog, R., Iyagba, B., Chen, V., Talluri, K., Dubinsky, S., . . . Friedman, D. (2010). Socioeconomic status and self-management in epilepsy: Comparison of diverse clinical populations in Houston, Texas. *Epilepsy & Behavior*, *19*(3), 232–238.

Berkman, L. F. (1984). Assessing the physical health effects of social networks and social support. *Annual Review of Public Health*, *5*, 413–432.

Berkman, L. F., & Glass, T. (2000). Social integration, social networks, social support, and health. In L. F. Berkman (Ed.), *Social epidemiology* (pp. 137–173). New York, NY: Oxford University Press.

Bloom, S. S. (1956). *Taxonomy of education objectives: Handbook I: Cognitive domain*. New York: NY: McKay.

Bond, L., Butler, H., Thomas, L., Carlin, J., Glover, S., Bowes, G., & Patton, G. (2007). Social and school connectedness in early secondary school as predictors of late teenage substance use, mental health, and academic outcomes. *Journal of Adolescent Health*, *40*(4), 357. e9–e18.

Bos, A. E., Dijker, A. J., & Koomen, W. (2007). Sex differences in emotional and behavioral responses to HIV individuals' expression of distress. *Psychology and Health*, *22*(4), 493–511.

Brawley, L. R., & Culos-Reed, S. N. (2000). Studying adherence to therapeutic regimens: Overview, theories, recommendations. *Controlled Clinical Trials*, *21*(5), S156–S163.

Brock, D. (1990). Population screening for cystic fibrosis. *American Journal of Human Genetics*, *47*(1), 164–165.

Brownson, R. C., Haire-Joshu, D., & Luke, D. A. (2006). Shaping the context of health: A review of environmental and policy approaches in the prevention of chronic diseases. *Annual Review of Public Health*, *27*, 341–370.

Brug, J., Schols, A., & Mesters, I. (2004). Dietary change, nutrition education and chronic obstructive pulmonary disease. *Patient Education and Counseling*, *52*(3), 249–257.

Caffarella, R. (1985). *Planning programs for adult learners: A practical guide for educators, trainees, and staff developers*. San Francisco, CA: Jossey-Bass.

Cameron, L. D., & Leventhal, H. (Eds.). (2003). *The self-regulation of health and illness behaviour*. New York, NY: Routeledge.

Canary, H. E. (2008). Creating supportive connections: A decade of research on support for families of children with disabilities. *Health Communication*, *23*(5), 413–426.

Centers for Disease Control and Prevention. (2013). Tobacco product use among middle and high school students—United States, 2011 and 2012. *MMWR. Morbidity and Mortality Weekly Report*, *62*(45), 893–897.

Chobanian, A. V., Bakris, G. L., Black, H. R., Cushman, W. C., Green, L. A., Izzo, J. L., Jr.,. . . National High Blood Pressure Education Program Coordinating Committee. (2003). Seventh report of the joint national committee on prevention, detection, evaluation, and treatment of high blood pressure. *Hypertension, 42*(6), 1206–1252.

Chuang, K., Chan, C., Su, T., Lee, C., & Tang, C. (2007). The effect of urban air pollution on inflammation, oxidative stress, coagulation, and autonomic dysfunction in young adults. *American Journal of Respiratory and Critical Care Medicine, 176*(4), 370–376.

Clark, N. M. (2003). Management of chronic disease by patients. *Annual Review of Public Health, 24*(1), 289–313.

Clark, N. M., Gong, M., & Kaciroti, N. (2014). A model of self-regulation for control of chronic disease. *Health Education & Behavior, 41*(5), 499–508.

Clark, N. M., Valerio, M. A., & Gong, Z. M. (2008). Self-regulation and women with asthma. *Current Opinion in Allergy and Clinical Immunology, 8*(3), 222–227.

Clark, N. M., & Zimmerman, B. J. (2014). A social cognitive view of self-regulated learning about health. *Health Education & Behavior, 41*(5), 485–491.

Coffield, E., Nihiser, A. J., Sherry, B., & Economos, C. D. (2015). Shape up Somerville: Change in parent body mass indexes during a child-targeted, community-based environmental change intervention. *American Journal of Public Health, 105*(2), e83–e89.

Coleman, K. J., Tiller, C. L., Sanchez, J., Heath, E. M., Sy, O., Milliken, G., & Dzewaltowski, D. A. (2005). Prevention of the epidemic increase in child risk of overweight in low-income schools: The El Paso coordinated approach to child health. *Archives of Pediatrics & Adolescent Medicine, 159*(3), 217–224.

Cooperrider, D. L., & Sekerka, L. E. (2006). Toward a theory of positive organizational change. In J. V. Gallos (Ed.), *Organization development* (pp. 223–238). San Francisco, CA: Jossey-Bass.

Cornelius, T. L., & Resseguie, N. (2007). Primary and secondary prevention programs for dating violence: A review of the literature. *Aggression and Violent Behavior, 12*(3), 364–375.

Côté, J., Godin, G., Garcia, P. R., Gagnon, M., & Rouleau, G. (2008). Program development for enhancing adherence to antiretroviral therapy among persons living with HIV. *AIDS Patient Care and STDs, 22*(12), 965–975.

Coulter, A., Entwistle, V. A., Eccles, A., Ryan, S., Shepperd, S., & Perera, R. (2015). Personalised care planning for adults with chronic or long-term health conditions. *Cochrane Database of Systematic Reviews,* (3).

Craun, A. M., & Deffenbacher, J. L. (1987). The effects of information, behavioral rehearsal, and prompting on breast self-exams. *Journal of Behavioral Medicine, 10*(4), 351–365.

Crocker, J., Major, B., & Steele, C. (1998). Social stigma. In D. T. Gilbert, S. T. Fiske, & G. Lindzey (Eds.), *The handbook of social psychology* (Vol. 2; 4th ed., pp. 504–553). Boston, MA: McGraw Hill.

Cummings, T. G., & Worley, C. G. (2014). *Organization development and change* (10th ed.). Mason, OH: South-Western Cengage Learning.

De Craemer, M., De Decker, E., De Bourdeaudhuij, I., Verloigne, M., Duvinage, K., Koletzko, B.,...Cardon, G. (2014). Applying the intervention mapping protocol to develop a kindergarten-based, family-involved intervention to increase European preschool children's physical activity levels: The ToyBox-Study. *Obesity Reviews, 15*, 14–26.

De Decker, E., De Craemer, M., De Bourdeaudhuij, I., Verbestel, V., Duvinage, K., Iotova, V.,...Cardon, G. (2014). Using the intervention mapping protocol to reduce European preschoolers' sedentary behavior, an application to the ToyBox-Study. *International Journal of Behavioral Nutrition & Physical Activity, 11*(1), 1–35.

de Leeuw, E., Townsend, B., Martin, E., Jones, C. M., & Clavier, C. (2013). Emerging theoretical frameworks for global health governance. In C. Clavier & E. de Leew (Eds.), *Health promotion and the policy process* (pp. 104–130). Oxford, United Kingdom: Oxford University Press.

DiClemente, C. C., & Prochaska, J. O. (1998). Toward a comprehensive transtheoretical model of change. In W. Miller, & N. Heather (Eds.), *Treating addictive behaviors* (pp. 3–24). New York, NY: Plenum Press.

Dietary Guidelines Advisory Committee. (2015). Scientific report of the 2015 dietary guidelines advisory committee. Part B. Chapter 2: 2015 DGAC themes and recommendations: Integrating the evidence. Retrieved from http://www .health.gov/dietaryguidelines/2015-scientific-report/04-integration.asp

DiIorio, C., Shafer, P. O., Letz, R., Henry, T. R., Schomer, D. L., Yeager, K., & Project EASE Study Group. (2004). Project EASE: A study to test a psychosocial model of epilepsy medication management. *Epilepsy & Behavior, 5*(6), 926–936.

Dijker, A., & Koomen, W. (2007). *Stigmatization, tolerance and repair: An integrative psychological analysis of responses to deviance.* Cambridge, United Kingdom: Cambridge University Press.

DiMatteo, M. R. (2004). Variations in patients' adherence to medical recommendations: A quantitative review of 50 years of research. *Medical Care, 42*(3), 200–209.

Douglas, C. E., Davis, R. M., & Beasley, J. K. (2006). Epidemiology of the third wave of tobacco litigation in the United States, 1994–2005. *Tobacco Control, 15* Suppl 4, iv9–16.

Duvinage, K., Ibrügger, S., Kreichauf, S., Wildgruber, A., De Craemer, M., De Decker, E.,...Socha, P. (2014). Developing the intervention material to increase physical activity levels of European preschool children: The ToyBoxStudy. *Obesity Reviews, 15*(S3), 27–39.

Economos, C. D., Hyatt, R. R., Goldberg, J. P., Must, A., Naumova, E. N., Collins, J. J., & Nelson, M. E. (2007). A community intervention reduces BMI z-score in children: Shape up Somerville first year results. *Obesity, 15*(5), 1325–1336.

Eluru, N., & Bhat, C. R. (2007). A joint econometric analysis of seat belt use and crash-related injury severity. *Accident Analysis & Prevention, 39*(5), 1037–1049.

Fernández, M. E., Bartholomew, L. K., Lopez, A., Tyrrell, S., Czyzewski, D., & Sockrider, M. M. (2000b). *Using Intervention Mapping in the development of a school-based asthma management intervention for Latino children and families:*

*The FAMILIAS project*. Paper presented at the meeting of the American Public Health Association, Boston, MA.

Fernández, M. E., Gonzales, A., Tortolero-Luna, G., Williams, J., Saavedra-Embesi, M., Chan, W., & Vernon, S. W. (2009). Effectiveness of Cultivando La Salud: A breast and cervical cancer screening promotion program for low-income Hispanic women. *American Journal of Public Health*, 99(5), 936–943.

Fernández, M. E., Gonzales, A., Tortolero-Luna, G., Partida, S., & Bartholomew, L. K. (2005a). Using Intervention Mapping to develop a breast and cervical cancer screening program for Hispanic farmworkers: Cultivando La Salud. *Health Promotion Practice*, 6(4), 394–404.

Fisher, E. B., Brownson, C. A., O'Toole, M. L., Shetty, G., Anwuri, V. V., & Glasgow, R. E. (2005). Ecological approaches to self-management: The case of diabetes. *American Journal of Public Health*, 95(9), 1523–1535.

Fisher, R., & Ury, W. (1991). *Getting to yes: Negotiating agreement without giving in* (2nd ed.). New York, NY: Penguin Books.

Flewelling, R. L., Grube, J. W., Paschall, M., Biglan, A., Kraft, A., Black, C., . . . Ruscoe, J. (2013). Reducing youth access to alcohol: Findings from a community-based randomized trial. *American Journal of Community Psychology*, 51(1–2), 264–277.

Foshee, V. A., Bauman, K. E., Ennett, S. T., Suchindran, C., Benefield, T., & Linder, G. F. (2005). Assessing the effects of the dating violence prevention program "Safe dates" using random coefficient regression modeling. *Prevention Science*, 6(3), 245–258.

Fujishiro, K., & Heaney, C. A. (2009). Justice at work, job stress, and employee health. *Health Education & Behavior*, 36(3), 487–504.

Gilpin, E. A., White, M. M., Messer, K., & Pierce, J. P. (2007). Receptivity to tobacco advertising and promotions among young adolescents as a predictor of established smoking in young adulthood. *American Journal of Public Health*, 97(8), 1489–1495.

Glasgow, R. E., Fisher, L., Skaff, M., Mullan, J., & Toobert, D. J. (2007). Problem solving and diabetes self-management: Investigation in a large, multiracial sample. *Diabetes Care*, 30(1), 33–37.

Gollwitzer, P. M. (in press). Setting one's mind on action: Planning out goal striving in advance. In R. Scott & S. Kosslyn (Eds.), *Emerging trends in the social and behavioral sciences*. Thousand Oaks, CA: Sage.

Gollwitzer, P. M., Martiny-Huenger, T., & Oettingen, G. (2014). Affective consequences of intentional action control. In A. J. Elliot (Ed.), *Advances in motivation science* (Vol. 1; pp. 49–84). San Diego, CA: Academic Press.

Gollwitzer, P. M., & Oettingen, G. (2015). From studying the determinants of action to analysing its regulation: A commentary on Sniehotta, Presseau and Araújo-Soares. *Health Psychology Review*, 9(2), 146–150.

Grover, A., & Joshi, A. (2014). An overview of chronic disease models: A systematic literature review. *Global Journal of Health Science*, 7(2), 210.

Hanewinkel, R., Isensee, B., Sargent, J. D., & Morgenstern, M. (2011). Cigarette advertising and teen smoking initiation. *Pediatrics*, 127(2), e271–e278.

Harrington, K. F., & Valerio, M. A. (2014). A conceptual model of verbal exchange health literacy. *Patient Education and Counseling, 94*(3), 403–410.

Heaney, C. A., & Israel, B. A. (2002). Social networks and social support. In K. Glanz, B. K. Rimer, & F. M. Lewis (Eds.), *Health behavior and health education: Theory, research and practice* (3rd ed., pp. 185–209). San Francisco, CA: Jossey-Bass.

Heijmans, M., Waverijn, G., Rademakers, J., van der Vaart, R., & Rijken, M. (2015). Functional, communicative and critical health literacy of chronic disease patients and their importance for self-management. *Patient Education and Counseling, 98*(1), 41–48.

Helakorpi, S. A., Martelin, T. P., Torppa, J. O., Patja, K. M., Kiiskinen, U. A., Vartiainen, E. A., & Uutela, A. K. (2008). Did the tobacco control act amendment in 1995 affect daily smoking in Finland? Effects of a restrictive workplace smoking policy. *Journal of Public Health (Oxford, England), 30*(4), 407–414.

Hoelscher, D. M., Springer, A. E., Ranjit, N., Perry, C. L., Evans, A. E., Stigler, M., & Kelder, S. H. (2010). Reductions in child obesity among disadvantaged school children with community involvement: The Travis County CATCH trial. *Obesity, 18*(S1), S36–S44.

Hogan, B. E., Linden, W., & Najarian, B. (2002). Social support interventions: Do they work? *Clinical Psychology Review, 22*(3), 381–440.

Hopkins, D. P., Razi, S., Leeks, K. D., Kalra, G. P., Chattopadhyay, S. K., Soler, R. E., & Task Force on Community Preventive Services. (2010). Smokefree policies to reduce tobacco use: A systematic review. *American Journal of Preventive Medicine, 38*(2), S275–S289.

Hou, S., Fernández, M. E., Baumler, E., & Parcel, G. S. (2002). Effectiveness of an intervention to increase Pap test screening among Chinese women in Taiwan. *Journal of Community Health, 27*(4), 277.

Institute of Medicine. (2012). *Epilepsy across the spectrum: Promoting health and understanding*. Washington, DC: The National Academies Press.

Kay Bartholomew, L., Sockrider, M. M., Abramson, S. L., Swank, P. R., Czyzewski, D. I., Tortolero, S. R., ... Tyrrell, S. (2006). Partners in school asthma management: Evaluation of a Self-Management program for children with asthma. *Journal of School Health, 76*(6), 283–290.

Kelder, S., Hoelscher, D., & Perry, C. L. (2015). How individuals, environments, and health behaviour interact: Social Cognitive Theory. In K. Glanz, B. K. Rimer, & K. Viswanath (Eds.), *Health behavior and health education: Theory, research, and practice* (5th ed., pp. 285–325). San Francisco, CA: Jossey-Bass.

Kelly, D. L., Zito, M. A., & Weber, D. (2003). Using a stage model of behavior change to prompt action in an immunization project. *Joint Commission Journal on Quality and Safety, 29*(6), 321–323.

Kiecolt-Glaser, J. K., McGuire, L., Robles, T. F., & Glaser, R. (2002). Psychoneuroimmunology and psychosomatic medicine: Back to the future. *Psychosomatic Medicine, 64*(1), 15–28.

Kinney, P. L., Aggarwal, M., Northridge, M. E., Janssen, N. A., & Shepard, P. (2000). Airborne concentrations of PM(2.5) and diesel exhaust particles on Harlem sidewalks: A community-based pilot study. *Environmental Health Perspectives, 108*(3), 213–218.

Kok, G., Den Boer, D. J., de Vries, H., Gerards, F., Hospers, H. J., & Mudde, A. N. (1992). Self efficacy and attribution theory in health education. In R. Schwarzer (Ed.), *Self-efficacy: Thought control of action* (pp. 245–262). Washington, DC: Hemisphere.

Kok, G., Harterink, P., Vriens, P., de Zwart, O., & Hospers, H. J. (2006). The gay cruise: Developing a theory-and evidence-based internet HIV-prevention intervention. *Sexuality Research & Social Policy, 3*(2), 52–67.

Kok, G., Schaalma, H., Ruiter, R. A. C., van Empelen, P., & Brug, J. (2004). Intervention mapping: Protocol for applying health psychology theory to prevention programmes. *Journal of Health Psychology, 9*(1), 85–98.

Krathwohl, D. R. (2002). A revision of Bloom's taxonomy: An overview. *Theory into Practice, 41*(4), 212–218.

Kruse, C. S., Bolton, K., & Freriks, G. (2015). The effect of patient portals on quality outcomes and its implications to meaningful use: A systematic review. *Journal of Medical Internet Research, 17*(2), e44.

Labarthe, D. R. (1998). *Epidemiology and prevention of cardiovascular diseases: A global challenge.* Gaithersburg, MD: Aspen.

Leffler, D. A., Neeman, N., Rabb, J. M., Shin, J. Y., Landon, B. E., Pallav, K., . . . Aronson, M. D. (2011). An alerting system improves adherence to follow-up recommendations from colonoscopy examinations. *Gastroenterology, 140*(4), 1166–1173.

Lempa, M., Goodman, R. M., Rice, J., & Becker, A. B. (2008). Development of scales measuring the capacity of community-based initiatives. *Health Education & Behavior, 35*(3), 298–315.

Levy, D. T., Chaloupka, F., & Gitchell, J. (2004). The effects of tobacco control policies on smoking rates: A tobacco control scorecard. *Journal of Public Health Management and Practice, 10*, 338–353.

Levy, D. T. & Friend, K. B. (2003). The effects of clean indoor air laws: What do we know and what do we need to know? *Health Education Research, 18*, 592–609.

Link, B. G., & Phelan, J. C. (2001). Conceptualizing stigma. *Annual Review of Sociology, 17*, 363–385.

Livingstone, J., Axton, R., Mennie, M., Gilfillan, A., & Brock, D. (1993). A preliminary trial of couple screening for cystic fibrosis: Designing an appropriate information leaflet. *Clinical Genetics, 43*(2), 57–62.

Loomis, D., Grosse, Y., Lauby-Secretan, B., Ghissassi, F. E., Bouvard, V., Benbrahim-Tallaa, L., . . . Straif, K. (2013). The carcinogenicity of outdoor air pollution. *The Lancet Oncology, 14*(13), 1262–1263.

Lorig, K., Ritter, P. L., Moreland, C., & Laurent, D. D. (2015). Can a box of mailed materials achieve the triple aims of health care? The mailed chronic disease self-management tool kit study. *Health Promotion Practice*, doi:1524839915571633

Markham, C. M., Tortolero, S. R., Peskin, M. F., Shegog, R., Thiel, M., Baumler, E. R., . . . Robin, L. (2012). Sexual risk avoidance and sexual risk reduction interventions for middle school youth: A randomized controlled trial. *Journal of Adolescent Health, 50*(3), 279–288.

Marlatt, G. A., & Donovan, D. M. (Eds.). (2005). *Relapse prevention: Maintenance strategies in the treatment of addictive behaviors* (2nd ed.). New York, NY: Guilford.

McAlister, A. L., Perry, C. L., & Parcel, G. S. (2008). How individuals, environments, and health behaviors interact: Social Cognitive Theory. In K. Glanz, B. K. Rimer, & K. Viswanath (Eds.), *Health behavior and health education* (4th ed., pp. 169–188). San Francisco, CA: Jossey-Bass.

McEachan, R. R., Lawton, R. J., Jackson, C., Conner, M., & Lunt, J. (2008). Evidence, theory and context: Using intervention mapping to develop a worksite physical activity intervention. *BMC Public Health, 8,* 326.

McMullen, K. M., Brownson, R. C., Luke, D., & Chriqui, J. (2005). Strength of clean indoor air laws and smoking-related outcomes in the USA. *Tobacco Control, 14,* 43–48.

Morgenstern, L. B., Bartholomew, L. K., Grotta, J. C., Staub, L., King, M., & Chan, W. (2003). Sustained benefit of a community and professional intervention to increase acute stroke therapy. *Archives of Internal Medicine, 163*(18), 2198–2202.

Morgenstern, L. B., Staub, L., Chan, W., Wein, T. H., Bartholomew, L. K., King, M., . . . Grotta, J. C. (2002). Improving delivery of acute stroke therapy: The TLL Temple Foundation stroke project. *Stroke; a Journal of Cerebral Circulation, 33*(1), 160–166.

Murphy, S., & Bennett, P. (2004). Health psychology and public health: Theoretical possibilities. *Journal of Health Psychology, 9*(1), 13–27.

Natowicz, M. R., & Prence, E. M. (1996). Heterozygote screening for Tay-Sachs disease: Past successes and future challenges. *Current Opinion in Pediatrics, 8*(6), 625–629.

Nidecker, M., DiClemente, C. C., Bennett, M. E., & Bellack, A. S. (2008). Application of the Transtheoretical Model of change: Psychometric properties of leading measures in patients with co-occurring drug abuse and severe mental illness. *Addictive Behaviors, 33*(8), 1021–1030.

Northridge, M. E., Yankura, J., Kinney, P. L., Santella, R. M., Shepard, P., Riojas, Y., . . . Strickland, P. (1999). Diesel exhaust exposure among adolescents in Harlem: A community-driven study. *American Journal of Public Health, 89*(7), 998–1002.

Norton, B. L., McLeory, K. R., Burdine, J. N., Felix, M. R. J., & Dorsey, A. M. (2002). Community capacity: Concept, theory and methods. In R. J. DiClemente, R. A. Crosby, & M. C. Kegler (Eds.), *Emerging theories in health promotion practice and research: Strategies for improving public health* (pp. 197–227). San Francisco, CA: Jossey-Bass.

Nutbeam, D. (2008). The evolving concept of health literacy. *Social Science & Medicine, 67*(12), 2072–2078.

Ohkubo, T., Imai, Y., Tsuji, I., Nagai, K., Watanabe, N., Minami, N., . . . Fukao, A. (1997). Prediction of mortality by ambulatory blood pressure monitoring versus screening blood pressure measurements: A pilot study in Ohasama. *Journal of Hypertension, 15*(4), 357–364.

Parker, R., & Aggleton, P. (2003). HIV and AIDS-related stigma and discrimination: A conceptual framework and implications for action. *Social Science & Medicine, 57*(1), 13–24.

Paxton, S. (2002a). The impact of utilizing HIV-positive speakers in AIDS education. *AIDS Education and Prevention, 14*(4), 282–294.

Paxton, S. (2002b). The paradox of public HIV disclosure. *AIDS Care, 14*(4), 559–567.

Peters, G. Y. (2014). A practical guide to effective behavior change: How to identify what to change in the first place. *European Health Psychologist, 16*(5), 142–155.

Pope, C. A., III, & Dockery, D. W. (2006). Health effects of fine particulate air pollution: Lines that connect. *Journal of the Air & Waste Management Association, 56*(6), 709–742.

Reblin, M., & Uchino, B. N. (2008). Social and emotional support and its implication for health. *Current Opinion in Psychiatry, 21*(2), 201–205.

Rhodes, J. E., Contreras, J. M., & Mangelsdorf, S. C. (1994). Natural mentor relationships among Latina adolescent mothers: Psychological adjustment, moderating processes, and the role of early parental acceptance. *American Journal of Community Psychology, 22*(2), 211–227.

Robbins, S. J., Schwartz, B., & Wasserman, E. A. (2001). *Psychology of learning and behavior* (5th ed.). New York, NY: Norton.

Rothman, A. J., Baldwin, A. S., & Hertel, A. W. (2004). Self-regulation and behavior change. In R. F. Baumeister & K. D. Vohs (Eds.), *Handbook of self-regulation: Research, theory, and applications* (pp. 130–148). New York, NY: Guilford Press.

Rust, C. F., Davis, C., & Moore, M. R. (2015). Medication adherence skills training for African-American breast cancer survivors: The effects on health literacy, medication adherence, and self-efficacy. *Social Work in Health Care, 54*(1), 33–46.

Sallis, J. F., Cervero, R. B., Ascher, W., Henderson, K. A., Kraft, M. K., & Kerr, J. (2006). An ecological approach to creating active living communities. *Annual Review of Public Health, 27*, 297–322.

Sallis, J. F., & Glanz, K. (2009). Physical activity and food environments: Solutions to the obesity epidemic. *Milbank Quarterly, 87*(1), 123–154.

Schaalma, H. P., Abraham, C., Gillmore, M. R., & Kok, G. (2004). Sex education as health promotion: What does it take? *Archives of Sexual Behavior, 33*(3), 259–269.

Scheier, M. F., & Carver, C. S. (2003). Goals and confidence as self-regulatory elements underlying health and illness behavior. In L. D. Cameron & H. Leventhal (Eds.), *The self-regulation of health and illness behavior* (pp. 17–41). New York, NY: Routledge.

Schulz, A., & Northridge, M. E. (2004). Social determinants of health: Implications for environmental health promotion. *Health Education & Behavior, 31*(4), 455–471.

Seeman, T. E. (2000). Health promoting effects of friends and family on health outcomes in older adults. *American Journal of Health Promotion, 14*(6), 362–370.

Shadel, W. G., Tharp-Taylor, S., & Fryer, C. S. (2009). How does exposure to cigarette advertising contribute to smoking in adolescents? The role of the developing self-concept and identification with advertising models. *Addictive Behaviors, 34*(11), 932–937.

Shegog, R., Bamps, Y. A., Patel, A., Kakacek, J., Escoffery, C., Johnson, E. K., & Ilozumba, U. O. (2013a). Managing epilepsy well: Emerging e-tools for epilepsy self-management. *Epilepsy & Behavior, 29*(1), 133–140.

Shegog, R., Begley, C. E., Harding, A., Dubinsky, S., Goldsmith, C., Hope, O., & Newmark, M. (2013b). Description and feasibility of MINDSET: A clinic decision aid for epilepsy self-management. *Epilepsy & Behavior, 29*(3), 527–536.

Shegog, R., Markham, C. M., Leonard, A. D., Bui, T. C., & Paul, M. E. (2012). "CLICK": Pilot of a web-based training program to enhance ART adherence among HIV-positive youth. *AIDS Care, 24*(3), 310–318.

Smalley, S. E., Wittler, R. R., & Oliverson, R. H. (2004). Adolescent assessment of cardiovascular heart disease risk factor attitudes and habits. *Journal of Adolescent Health, 35*(5), 374–379.

Smith, D. W., Steckler, A. B., McCormick, L. K., & McLeroy, K. R. (1995). Lessons learned about disseminating health curricula to schools. *Journal of Health Education, 26*(1), 37–43.

Smith, R. A., Cokkinides, V., & Brawley, O. W. (2009). Cancer screening in the United States, 2009: A review of current American Cancer Society guidelines and issues in cancer screening. *CA: A Cancer Journal for Clinicians, 59*(1), 27–41.

Smith, R. A., Saslow, D., Sawyer, K. A., Burke, W., Costanza, M. E., Evans, W., . . . Sener, S. (2003). American cancer society guidelines for breast cancer screening: Update 2003. *CA: A Cancer Journal for Clinicians, 53*(3), 141–169.

Springer, A. E., Kelder, S. H., Ranjit, N., Hochberg-Garrett, H., Crow, S., & Delk, J. (2012). Promoting physical activity and fruit and vegetable consumption through a community-school partnership: The effects of Marathon Kids® on low-income elementary school children in Texas. *Journal of Physical Activity and Health, 9*(5), 739.

Springer, A., Parcel, G., Baumler, E., & Ross, M. (2006). Supportive social relationships and adolescent health risk behavior among secondary school students in El Salvador. *Social Science & Medicine, 62*(7), 1628–1640.

Stan, D. L., Collins, N. M., Olsen, M. M., Croghan, I., & Pruthi, S. (2012). The evolution of mindfulness-based physical interventions in breast cancer survivors. *Evidence-Based Complementary and Alternative Medicine, 20*(15s), 1–15.

Steenhuis, I. H., Van Assema, P., & Glanz, K. (2001). Strengthening environmental and educational nutrition programmes in worksite cafeterias and supermarkets in the Netherlands. *Health Promotion International, 16*(1), 21–33.

Stetler, C. B., McQueen, L., Demakis, J., & Mittman, B. S. (2008). An organizational framework and strategic implementation for system-level change to enhance research-based practice: QUERI series. *Implementation Science, 3*(1), 1–11.

Stutterheim, S. E., Bos, A. E. R., Pryor, J. B., Brands, R., Liebregts, M., & Schaalma, H. P. (2010). *Does having a choice matter? Psychological and social correlates of HIV status disclosure among those with and without visible symptoms.* Unpublished manuscript.

Stutterheim, S. E., Pryor, J. B., Bos, A. E., Hoogendijk, R., Muris, P., & Schaalma, H. P. (2009). HIV-related stigma and psychological distress: The harmful effects of specific stigma manifestations in various social settings. *AIDS (London, England), 23*(17), 2353–2357.

Sweda, E. L. (2004). Lawsuits and secondhand smoke. *Tobacco Control, 13*(S1), i61–i66.

Taylor, S. E., & Stanton, A. L. (2007). Coping resources, coping processes, and mental health. *Annual Review of Clinical Psychology, 3*, 377–401.

Thompson, F. E., & Byers, T. (1994). Dietary assessment resource manual. *The Journal of Nutrition, 124*(11 Suppl), 2245S–2317S.

Thompson, S. G., Pyke, S. D., & Wood, D. A. (1996). Using a coronary risk score for screening and intervention in general practice. *British family heart study. Journal of Cardiovascular Risk, 3*(301), 306.

Tomaka, J., Thompson, S., & Palacios, R. (2006). The relation of social isolation, loneliness, and social support to disease outcomes among the elderly. *Journal of Aging and Health, 18*(3), 359–384.

Tortolero, S. R., Bartholomew, L. K., Tyrrell, S., Abramson, S. L., Sockrider, M. M., Markham, C. M.,...Parcel, G. S. (2002). Environmental allergens and irritants in schools: A focus on asthma. *Journal of School Health, 72*(1), 33–38.

Tortolero, S. R., Markham, C. M., Addy, R. C., Baumler, E. R., Escobar-Chaves, S. L., Basen-Engquist, K. M.,...Parcel, G. S. (2008). Safer choices 2: Rationale, design issues, and baseline results in evaluating school-based health promotion for alternative school students. *Contemporary Clinical Trials, 29*(1), 70–82.

Tortolero, S. R., Markham, C. M., Peskin, M. F., Shegog, R., Addy, R. C., Escobar-Chaves, S. L., & Baumler, E. R. (2010). It's Your Game: Keep It Real: Delaying sexual behavior with an effective middle school program. *Journal of Adolescent Health, 46*(2), 169–179.

Uchino, B. N. (2006). Social support and health: A review of physiological processes potentially underlying links to disease outcomes. *Journal of Behavioral Medicine, 29*(4), 377–387.

U.S. Department of Agriculture & U.S. Department of Health and Human Services. (2010). *Dietary guidelines for Americans* (7th ed.). Washington, D.C.: Government Printing Office.

U.S. Department of Health and Human Services. (2012). *Preventing tobacco use among youth and young adults: A report of the surgeon general.* Atlanta, GA: U.S. Department of Health and Human Services, Centers for Disease Control and Prevention, National Center for Chronic Disease Prevention and Health Promotion, Office on Smoking and Health.

U.S. Preventive Services Task Force. (2014). *Guide to clinical preventive services.* Rockville, MD: Agency for Healthcare Research and Quality.

Valente, T. (2015). Social networks and health behavior. In K. Glanz., B. Rimer, & K. Viswanath (Eds.), *Health behavior: Theory, research and practice* (5th ed.). San Francisco, CA: Jossey-Bass.

van Dam, H. A., van der Horst, F. G., Knoops, L., Ryckman, R. M., Crebolder, H. F., & van den Borne, B. H. W. (2005). Social support in diabetes: A systematic review of controlled intervention studies. *Patient Education and Counseling, 59*(1), 1–12.

van Empelen, P., & Kok, G. (2008). Action-specific cognitions of planned and preparatory behaviors of condom use among Dutch adolescents. *Archives of Sexual Behavior, 37*(4), 626–640.

van Kesteren, N. M., Hospers, H. J., Kok, G., & van Empelen, P. (2005). Sexuality and sexual risk behavior in HIV-positive men who have sex with men. *Qualitative Health Research, 15*(2), 145–168.

van Stralen, M. M., de Vries, H., Mudde, A. N., Bolman, C., & Lechner, L. (2009). Efficacy of two tailored interventions promoting physical activity in older adults. *American Journal of Preventive Medicine, 37*(5), 405–417.

van Stralen, M. M., Kok, G., de Vries, H., Mudde, A. N., Bolman, C., & Lechner, L. (2008). The active plus protocol: Systematic development of two theory- and evidence-based tailored physical activity interventions for the over-fifties. *BMC Public Health, 8,* 399.

Werch, C. E., Ames, S., Moore, M. J., Thombs, D., & Hart, A. (2009). Health behavior insights: The Transtheoretical/stages of change model: Carlo C. DiClemente, PhD. *Health Promotion Practice, 10*(1), 41–48.

Wisotzky, M., Albuquerque, M., Pechacek, T. F., & Park, B. Z. (2004). The National Tobacco Control Program: Focusing on policy to broaden impact. *Public Health Reports, 119,* 303–310.

Wood, W., & Neal, D. T. (2007). A new look at habits and the habit-goal interface. *Psychological Review, 114*(4), 843.

Workowski, K. A., & Berman, S. M. (2006). *Sexually transmitted diseases treatment guidelines,* 2006. U.S. Department of Health and Human Services, Centers for Disease Control and Prevention.

Zullig, L. L., Shaw, R. J., Shah, B. R., Peterson, E. D., Lindquist, J. H., Crowley, M. J.,...Bosworth, H. B. (2015). Patient–provider communication, self-reported medication adherence, and race in a postmyocardial infarction population. *Patient Preference and Adherence, 9,* 311.

# CHAPTER 6

# INTERVENTION MAPPING STEP 3

*Program Design*

## Competency

- Generate program ideas, including change methods and practical applications.

## Deciding How to Start

In Step 3, planners work from the logic model of change (established in Step 2) to begin to conceptualize and design the intervention. The plan from this step will include intervention themes, components, scope, sequence, theory- and evidence-based methods, and practical applications.

Intervention Mapping guides the planner through steps of conducting the needs assessment, developing the matrices for performance and change objectives, selecting change methods that are translated into practical applications, and then creating the actual intervention program. However, after completing the matrices, most planners already have some ideas about the concrete aspects of their program—how they can best reach their priority populations and the practical applications and program materials that will be culturally congruent and can garner the attention of the participants. People have different work styles; work groups do too. In selecting methods and practical applications, health promoters may take any of several routes based on their experience with theory and practice. Some will begin with the less abstract ideas about their program (delivery, themes, scope, and sequence) and then move to matching methods and their applications to change objectives and embedding the same in the program components. Others will move from change objectives

**LEARNING OBJECTIVES AND TASKS**

- Generate program themes, components, scope, and sequence

- Choose theory- and evidence-based change methods

- Select or design practical applications to deliver change methods to change methods and then to applications. Still others will move from objectives to applications and then back to the underlying methods or will brainstorm change methods and applications simultaneously. For example, a health promoter may think of commitment as a theoretical method for increasing self-efficacy of adolescents to remain nonsmokers and then brainstorm about practical applications to apply that method. Another health promoter may think of a nonsmoking contract as an application for improving self-efficacy, later finding out from the literature that the underlying theoretical method is commitment. While reading about theory, the health promoter might also find alternatives to a nonsmoking contract that may have the same, or even better, results.

Regardless of the work style, it is essential that planners identify methods and link them to the change objectives they are meant to influence. Further, the planners will need to keep in mind the parameters of the methods—the conditions under which the methods are shown to be effective—during the translation from method to application and to program. For example, the health promoter who likes the idea of a nonsmoking contract should be aware that commitment is only effective as a method for increasing self-efficacy when the act of commitment has been made public (parameter). Therefore, contracts that individuals make in private settings may have positive effects as reminders, but they do not have the strong effect of public commitment.

## Program Aspects

A health promotion program based on a systematic theory- and evidence-based planning process such as Intervention Mapping will contain effective change methods. Also, planners will figure out many practical aspects of the program. For example, questions will include: How many different types of target participants will the program have? At what environmental levels? What is the extent of the program and its duration (scope)? In what order will it be delivered (sequence)? Will the program have a theme, more than one theme, and a title? Some planning groups will have ideas about the program aspects as soon as they begin working through Intervention Mapping and will want to begin with them in this step; others will begin with change methods.

## Theory- and Evidence-Based Change Methods

A main idea behind the steps of Intervention Mapping is enabling planners to develop a solid foundation in theory and evidence. Planners must find a balance between preliminary ideas for programs on the one hand and theory- and evidence-informed decisions for change methods, applications, and programs on the other hand. What planners think about the effectiveness of methods is not always congruent with the scientific evidence. For example, mass media campaigns may be useful for changing social norms but probably seldom useful for increasing self-efficacy and skills. Fear-arousing messages may be popular with the representatives of the at-risk population and intermediates, but they often are not effective at influencing behavior (G. Y. Peters, Ruiter, & Kok, 2014; Ten Hoor et al., 2012).

In this chapter we present various methods for different determinants, starting with methods for determinants that are related to change in the individual health behavior of the at-risk group. Then we discuss methods for changing determinants at environmental levels, which are more specifically appropriate for groups, organizations, communities, and public policy. We describe only a sample of methods that can be used to address change objectives, based on frequency in health promotion publications; there are many more. A theory- and evidence-based change method is a general technique for influencing the determinants of behaviors and environmental conditions. Practical applications refer to delivery of the methods in ways that fit the intervention population and the context in which the intervention will be conducted. For example, a change objective for an intervention might be to increase adolescents' self-efficacy to resist social pressure to use drugs. For the change objective of increasing self-efficacy, change might include modeling, skill training, guided practice with feedback, and reinforcement. One application for modeling could be a videotaped step-by-step demonstration by adolescents of how to resist peer pressure in situations they commonly encounter.

In another example, an environmental condition of adolescent drug use could be the availability of drugs for sale in neighborhoods where adolescents live, with a performance objective of the mayor getting police to actively enforce laws against neighborhood drug dealers. A change objective for this might be to increase the mayor's positive outcome expectations—for example, that this enforcement will save children's lives, be popular with constituents, be positively received by powerful groups in the city, and increase tourism to the city. The primary method for this could be advocacy, which includes methods of information, persuasion, negotiation, and coercion. One application might be for influential neighborhood activists to hold a breakfast meeting with the mayor, neighborhood constituents, and key city opinion leaders. The activists might present detailed case histories of neighborhood teens, along with pictures of open drug dealing on the street. If the mayor does not respond to this application, the group might undertake, as additional applications, media advocacy with an exposé story calling for action by the mayor on the local television channel.

As shown in Figure 6.1, planners choose methods and applications to influence change objectives. Change objectives describe the desired changes in the determinants of performance objectives for health behavior

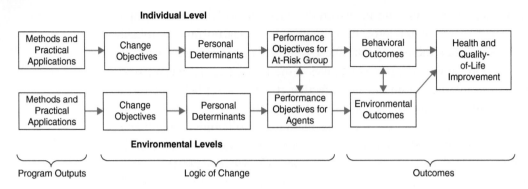

**Figure 6.1** Intervention Logic Model

and environmental conditions, at both individual and higher environmental levels. Modeling may change individual health behavior, but it could also be applied to influence the behavior of decision makers in organizations that are required to make changes in the environment. For example, persuasive communication could be applied to influence the behavior of politicians to take action to enforce laws that would change environmental conditions. In addition, the methods for change objectives can be applied to the change agent, who, in turn, may apply a method to the priority population. For example, an organization manager may provide incentives to influence employee behavior to increase physical activity. A special case is the training of those who deliver the intervention to influence the priority population (see Chapter 8 on program implementation). Note that the decision makers' performance objectives are influenced by environmental conditions as well as personal determinants (see Figure 6.2 for an example).

## Practical Applications

Practical applications are the ways in which the theory-based methods are presented and delivered in an intervention—ways that are culturally appropriate and acceptable to the population as well as the context in which the intervention will be conducted. The planner makes a selection of intervention methods that correspond to the program objectives stated in Step 2. The translation of selected methods into action is completed through the development of applications. In this step and the next (Step 4), designing the program should be fun; creativity and scientific rigor should go hand in hand. Change methods and practical applications form a continuum that extends from abstract theoretical methods through practical applications to organized programs with specified scope, sequence, and support materials. For instance, skills training is a theoretical method; a step-by-step instruction from a videotape with guided practice would be

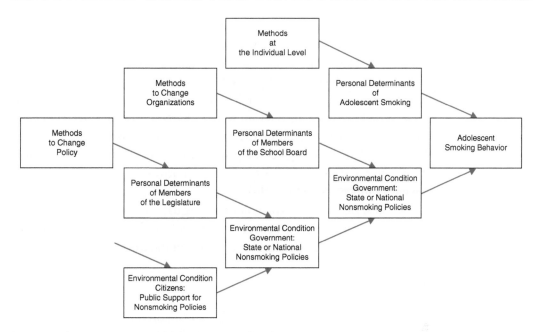

**Figure 6.2**   Schematic Representation of Shift in Environmental Levels

a practical application to deliver the skills training; and a program would include descriptions of when and how the training would be delivered and supported. The difference between theoretical methods and practical applications can be confusing. Modeling is a method; use of role-model stories is an application; and demonstrations are applications. The point is that methods should always be considered, and applications should never be devoid of the effective component—the method. Yet methods are easy to overlook because health promoters often think in terms of concrete program components, such as a videotape or a brochure.

There is no reason why planners cannot start with applications and then think about theoretical methods. However, the essential question here is: Why would the particular application work? For every creative idea, there needs to be a theoretical process describing why the expected effects are going to happen. The central challenge in translating change methods into practical applications is to adhere to parameters within which the methods can be expected to be effective.

In one example, health promoters working with gay men who chat on the Internet to meet others for dating and sex decided to use an Internet application with a virtual guide with the characteristics of an attractive gay man to lead the user through a Web-based program for HIV prevention (Kok, Harterink, Vriens, de Zwart, & Hospers, 2006; Mikolajczak, Kok, & Hospers, 2008). The potential participants had very clear but different preferences for the choice of guides from six options. Most men selected one guide and stayed with him when they returned to the site. Why would this application be expected to work? The guides and the municipal health service that produced the site were both seen as sources of information. Research on persuasive communication (a method for attitude change) suggests that theoretically relevant source characteristics are attractiveness and expertise (parameters for the method). In this case, giving the men the choice of their own guide helped to ensure they would see the guide as attractive and the source as credible to improve the effectiveness of the persuasive messages on the website. Of course, the quality of the arguments in the messages given by the guides was equally important. Guides who were chosen for their attractiveness but lacked good arguments would probably have had little impact on the users of the website.

## Perspectives

Our perspectives in this chapter concern the importance of being creative in generating program ideas while ensuring that programs contain theory- and evidence-based methods that can produce planned change at the planner's desired ecological level (Fishbein & Cappella, 2006; Glanz & Bishop, 2010; G. Y. Peters, de Bruin, & Crutzen, 2015; Schaalma & Kok, 2009).

### Enabling Creativity to Flourish

Planning should allow creativity to flourish. In this step, program planners liberate their creativity based on the objectives they have developed in the previous steps. They may close the books, put the matrices away, and even close their eyes to dream what a program could be like. The planning group should be cohesive by this point, so its members can feel free to come forth with many ideas. Some of the ideas may be farfetched or even ridiculous on further consideration. However, the most exciting and effective programs emerge from a creative, unrestrained process. The foundation is laid in the matrices of Step 2; the design task should be fun and creative, with scientific rigor going hand in hand. Regardless of the work style of the planning team, it is essential that within all program ideas, there are change methods that will be effective to influence the objectives in the matrices. Further, the team will want to keep in mind the parameters of the methods—the conditions under which the methods have been shown effective—so that there is effective translation from method to application to program.

### The Case of the Missing Methods

Unfortunately, articles presenting interventions in the health education literature often do not report the causal chain from determinants to objectives to change methods to applications. Without this description, the reader may not be able to judge the theory and evidence base for what the planners have chosen to include in the intervention. Most publications on health education interventions, often evaluation studies, lack clear information about how the authors expected to cause a change. They often present the application and the program—for example, a tailored letter to encourage mammography or a videotape to discourage tobacco use. However, they may not be explicit about what change methods they used in the letter or how the videotape discouraged the risk behavior. Tailoring can be considered a general method, but the letter must also use specific methods that would, according to theory, "cause" a woman to obtain a mammogram. Did the researchers use persuasion, modeling with vicarious reinforcement, a cue to action, or some other method? In another example, researchers might write that they used nonsmoking contracts to stimulate resistance to smoking, but they do not mention the theoretical method of commitment on which the application was presumably based—a method that would include, to be effective, making a *public* commitment. All program theory- and evidence-based methods should be linked to change objectives as well as practical applications and intervention components suited to reach the priority population.

## Using Methods Correctly

One source of confusion about change methods may be that the same concept, such as modeling or reinforcement, can be used to describe both determinants and methods. The double use of these concepts suggests that the theory explains both behavior and behavior change. The difference for health promoters is that modeling as a determinant refers to what happens in the actual situation, whereas modeling as a method will be part of a well-designed program. For instance, with respect to condom use, modeling that occurs in the television shows and movies that adolescents see may be negative, whereas health promoters may use positive role models in their interventions to compensate for those negative counterparts in the media (Schaalma, Abraham, Gillmore, & Kok, 2004).

Translating methods into applications demands a sufficient understanding of the theory behind the method, especially the theoretical parameters that are necessary for the effectiveness of the theoretical process (de Bruin, Crutzen, & Peters, 2015; Kok, Schaalma, Ruiter, van Empelen, & Brug, 2004; G. Y. Peters et al., 2015). For example, modeling can be a strong method but only when certain parameters are met, such as reinforcement of the modeled behavior (Kelder, Hoelscher, & Perry, 2015). People or environmental decision makers do not usually imitate behavior simply because a model demonstrates that behavior; they behave comparably to the model only when the model exhibits certain characteristics, such as being reinforced for that particular behavior and when they expect to be reinforced in a similar way. Translating the method modeling to a practical application includes taking care that, in the actual program, from the perspective of the program participants, the model is reinforced. As a second example, goal setting can be a very effective method to enhance performance, but only when the goal is challenging as well as acceptable for the actor. People often choose goals outside those parameters. A third classic example is provided by the method implementation intentions. While very effective when properly applied, violation of its parameter for effectiveness (a preexisting intention to perform the behavior) greatly reduces or eliminates this effectiveness. Finally, fear appeals are popular (G. Y. Peters et al., 2014; Ten Hoor et al., 2012) but are only effective when the at-risk population has high self-efficacy, and they may be counterproductive when self-efficacy is low (G. Y. Peters, Ruiter, & Kok, 2013).

## Using Different Methods at Different Levels of Intervention

There are two basic differences between descriptions in the literature of behavioral change methods and those of methods for changing environmental conditions. One difference is that theories that focus on individual behavior change are more likely to focus on processes (that is, closer to what we call methods), whereas theories regarding environmental change are more likely to focus on practice (that is, closer to what we call applications) (Butterfoss, Kegler, & Francisco, 2008; Porras & Robertson, 1987).

The second difference is in the way that knowledge is garnered regarding the application of different types of theories to health education. In individual behavior change, there has been a somewhat deductive approach: Program planners extract behavioral science theoretical change constructs and then apply them to health. On the one hand, this approach to theory application is not theory testing—it is still a theory-of-the-problem approach—but in its philosophy, it resembles theory testing. On the other hand, social change activities—people doing things such as community organization and coalition building—have been reported in the literature as case examples. It sometimes is not possible to determine whether these activities are change methods or applications and whether theoretical constructs are involved in the applications. Possibly this approach to intervention is more inductive, intervening with an application without naming the method. Where possible in this chapter, we label the methods inherent in community-oriented applications.

Change methods at the individual level can be directed toward agents at higher ecological levels. See Figure 6.2. The theoretical process behind the method is the same; however, often the application of the method is somewhat different, depending on the target. For instance, in a study about interventions to change environmental conditions, persuasion was applied at various environmental levels (Kok, Gottlieb, Commers, & Smerecnik, 2008). For example, in a project to decrease carbon dioxide transmission, the health promoter reported a persuasive communication approach that illustrated to businesses the advantages of approaching and dealing with the issue of carbon dioxide emissions. The health promoter showed them how reducing carbon dioxide is profitable and made it clear to companies that being environmentally friendly is good for company image. The potential effect on the image of and profit for the company are typical organizational-level arguments. In another example, the persuasive message was surprisingly similar: A health promoter approached an online condom store to increase the accessibility and availability of condoms. The health promoter persuaded the company by stressing positive influences on their image and explained that cooperating would be in their own commercial and economic interest. Cooperation would mean that more customers would find their way to their online store. The educator also stressed the responsibility of the condom store in HIV and STI prevention.

In another example, smoking by adolescents is influenced by personal determinants but also by a supportive school environment. When the school environment is not supportive enough, the health promoter will want to change this environmental condition by urging the school management to develop and implement a nonsmoking school policy. So the focus of the health promoter will shift, in this instance, to the behavior of agents related to the school. Perhaps the school management, school board, superintendent, or parents could be persuaded to implement a nonsmoking policy. The health promoter might use methods of persuasive communication and modeling to influence the school management's decision making. However, there are environmental influences on the school management's decision making as well, in the form of state and national regulations related to nonsmoking policies in schools. When those regulations are lacking, the health promoter might want to change this environmental condition by urging state, provincial, or national agencies to declare stricter rules banning smoking in schools. The health promoter will use the method of political advocacy to influence this policy-making process. Figure 6.2 offers a schematic representation of this chain of events. Even a government will be influenced by external factors, such as public support. Again, by applying methods from the community level, the health promoter may be able to influence citizens to advocate for school policies that ban smoking.

Planners frequently bundle together methods at the individual level to create a change method at a higher ecological level. This is because environmental agents along with organization and community members are also individuals, and the determinants of their behaviors are similar to determinants of behavior at the individual level. The change target and the overall method, however, are specific to the environmental change level. For example, community organization can include the individual methods of persuasion, modeling, skills training, and public commitment; however, these methods are bundled together to accomplish a change in a community-level problem and to increase community capacity. Organizational development, in fact, has been defined as the transfer of behavioral science knowledge to increase organizational effectiveness, and the process resembles behavioral self-regulation applied to the organizational level (see McLean, 2005).

There may be different approaches for targeting a level or being targeted from a level (Kok, Gottlieb, Panne, & Smerecnik, 2012). On the one hand, organizations may apply methods for improving the health of their employees, such as to increase physical activity (Abraham & Graham-Rowe, 2009). Those methods might include tailoring, goal setting, and modeling. The activities are initiated by the management and are directed at the employees. On the other hand, health promoters and health-promoting organizations may apply methods to get organizations to start health-promoting activities, as in the earlier examples above—reducing carbon dioxide transmissions or increasing the availability of condoms. A national voluntary heart organization may try to encourage companies to facilitate physical activity programs for their employees. Methods that are used include persuasive communication, advocacy and lobbying, and organizational modeling and facilitation. These activities are initiated outside the organization, usually by a health promoter, and are directed at the organization, often the management. An interesting parallel to this process can be found in the research tradition of corporate social responsibility (Maon, Lindgreen, & Swaen, 2009). An example of corporate social responsibility is a community focusing on a company with respect to environmental pollution. In this case, the community initiates an activity focusing on an organization applying a method of coalition formation. These communities may have themselves been the focus of health-promoting organizations applying a method of community organizing.

## A Taxonomy of Change Methods

There is increasing interest in systematic descriptions of health promotion interventions, the theory- and evidence-based change methods they contain, and the determinants that are targeted for change. For instance, Abraham and Michie (2008) and Michie et al. (2011, 2013) provide a theory-linked coding taxonomy generally applicable to health behavior change techniques (BCTs), all directed at individual change. Some of those techniques are linked with determinants of behavior, an approach comparable to what is presented in Intervention Mapping (Michie et al., 2011; Michie et al., 2013). Other authors combine the original taxonomy by Abraham & Michie (2008) with the Intervention Mapping approach to develop a checklist for coding methods in patient education interventions (de Bruin et al., 2010; van Achterberg et al., 2011). Addressing higher environmental levels, Khan and colleagues (2009) identify a set of applications and associated measurements that communities and local governments can use to plan and monitor environmental and policy-level changes for obesity prevention (Khan et al., 2009). For other descriptions of change methods, we refer the reader to behavioral science texts, particularly those with explicit applications to health promotion (DiClemente, Crosby, & Kegler, 2009; Edberg & APA Publications and Communications Board Working Group on Journal Article Reporting Standards, 2007; Glanz, Rimer, & Viswanath, 2015; Goodson, 2009; Hayden, 2008; Kok, Gottlieb, Peters, Mullen, Parcel, Ruiter, Fernández, Markham, & Bartholomew, 2015; Minkler, 2012; Minkler & Wallerstein, 2008).

# Tasks for Step 3

## Generating Program Themes, Components, Scope, and Sequence

The planning group, established in the first step of Intervention Mapping, should include both members of the potential program participants and implementers to make sure the group has a good forum for balancing ideas on applications and programs, theoretical and empirical input on change methods, and limitations and potentials of the program context.

The first task in Step 3 is to generate ideas for program themes, components, scope, and sequence with the planning group.

The product of the first part of this step is an initial plan that describes the program. The program plan should account for the contacts with each group of program participants. For example, in a program for patients, three contacts might be a video presentation followed by a discussion with a nurse and a reminder by a physician. The overall program might also include contacts to train the health care provider. Health promoters will specify both the amount of the program that is expected to be delivered (dosage) and the way the program should look at each interface with participants. They will also outline the extent and length of the program (scope) and the order in which components and materials will be delivered (sequence). The format for the initial program plan will vary from program to program, but it should include at least the following: (1) the program scope and sequence, and (2) a description of each population group and program interface with a list of the program materials and staff required for that interface. Budget for production of materials and a list of other resources are also important, and planners will have an early estimate here, and a more complete idea for production in the next step. See Chapter 7.

### Generating Program Ideas

A central problem plagues planners in every profession—how to have a good idea ... how to "think outside of the box." The key to having a good idea is to have more than one idea—maybe even hundreds (de Bono, 2008; 2015; Gedney & Fultz, 1988). And the key to having a hundred ideas is to generate them without editing and without adhering to strictly logical process. Prior to considering real-world constraints, de Bono suggests a lateral process that creates movement from one idea to another, breaks up current thinking, and disrupts reliance on the status quo (de Bono, 2006). At this point, planners can dismiss all preconceived notions and program constraints. They can ask themselves, "What would we do if we could do anything that comes to mind?" The diversity of the planning group will allow for the generation of unique ideas and innovative concepts.

The core processes (Chapter 1) can also be useful to generate ideas but should not take the place of brainstorming and lateral thinking. A literature review can identify the types of practical applications and programs others have used and the evidence for success using such approaches.

Using behavior change theory will help with generating thoughts about methods and ways to use them. Finally, going to the potential participants (formative research) and continuing to fuel the process with their ideas is imperative. Focus groups can be used for this purpose and are particularly suited, because stimulus materials can be created from the change objectives, change methods, and practical applications and will generate discussion regarding acceptability and potential effectiveness. Sample questions include "If you were trying to figure out how to [change objective X], what would you do?" For example: "If you were going to increase the confidence of teenage girls in negotiating condom use, what would you do?"

### Program Themes

A program theme is a general organizing construct or idea for a program. A program often has a theme as well as several recurring visual and linguistic subthemes or ideas that "brand" the program while delivering a key change objective-related message. Both themes and recurring subthemes can be based on the health topic, such as the themes for the stroke project, "call 911" and "Is there treatment for stroke?" (See publisher's website www .wiley.com/go/bartholomew4e). Heinen and colleagues developed a self-management program to increase physical activity and reduce wound days in leg ulcer patients: the "Lively Legs" program (Heinen, Bartholomew, Wensing, van de Kerkhof, & van Achterbert, 2005, 2006; 2012; Van de Glind, Heinen, Evers, Wensing, & van Achterberg, 2012).

Themes also may be based on the behavioral or community change objectives. For example, the Watch, Discover, Think, and Act theme of an intervention for asthma was based on the self-regulatory processes taught in the computer program, informed by Bandura's theory of self-regulation (see publisher's website www.wiley.com/go/bartholomew4e). This primary message became the program title and a structure in recurring visuals and messaging (Bartholomew et al., 2000c; Bartholomew et al., 2000b; Shegog et al., 1999; Shegog et al., 2006).

Themes may also be unrelated to the program content. The third-grade component of the CATCH program (Perry et al., 1997) used a theme of space creatures that had come to Earth to teach Earth children about diet and physical activity. Themes may also derive from characteristics of the at-risk groups, cultures, or preferred learning styles identified through formative research. For example, in It's Your Game . . . Keep It Real, program planners selected the theme based on input from the target audience and the vernacular language that urban youth used for being healthy and responsible ("keeping it real") (see Box 6.2 It's Your Game). Similarly, in an intervention to increase breast and cervical cancer screening for U.S. Hispanic farm-working women, the program theme was "Cultivando La Salud" ("Cultivating Health"), which expressed a culturally significant message for the at-risk group (Fernández et al., 2005a) (Figure 6.3). The key to the themes is connecting back to appropriate behavioral change messages. The overarching message that a theme can deliver may reach not only the primary target audience, participants, but also a secondary audience—parents, peers, and community members, promoting the adoption of the change behavior or support of the behavior.

## Program Components, Scope, and Sequence

Health education and promotion programs have components (units or modules) with an identifiable scope and sequence. The questions to ask are: Who will get what part of this program? When will they get it? How will they get it? How long will it last overall? How long will each interaction be?

While objectives of typical curriculum planning are cognitive or academic skills, these program components have more diverse change

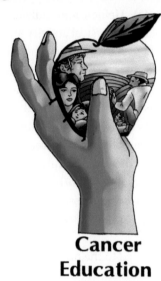

## Cancer Education Program

**Figure 6.3**   Cultivando La Salud
Reprinted with permission from the National Center for Farmworker Health.

objectives. The components might be combinations of change methods, practical applications, and delivery mechanisms aimed at various objectives. For example, a program might comprise messages that neighborhood volunteers deliver one-to-one and mass media messages delivered in public service announcements (PSAs) and billboards, all tied together across time with a theme. Interventions are combinations of components. For example, in the It's Your Game intervention, program components included a classroom curriculum comprising group-based activities facilitated by classroom teachers and individual computer-based activities, along with support materials (newsletters) for parents.

The scope is the breadth and amount of a program (what is included in the program and what is not). The scope reflects the choice of change objectives. The sequence is the order in which programs are delivered across time. For example, in the TLL Temple Foundation Stroke Project (see publisher's website www.wiley.com/go/bartholomew4e), the program had two major components, one that addressed the lay audience—the

**Table 6.1**    Scope and Sequence of the T.L.L. Temple Foundation Stroke Project

| Weeks 1–2 | Weeks 2–8 | Weeks 8–16 | Weeks 16–32 | Weeks 32+ |
|---|---|---|---|---|
| **Professional Module 1:** Change planning meetings with hospital EDs | **Professional Module 2:** Orientation meetings with hospital medical staff | **Professional Module 3:** Training meetings (mock stroke code at a worksite) for ED and EMS teams | **Professional Module 4:** Review training meetings for ED and EMS teams | **Professional Module 5:** Reinforcement for protocol use via newsletters |
| Change planning meetings with local EMS | Guideline and protocol development with med staff and critical care committees | **Community Module 1:** One-to-One train the trainer + Brochure | **Community Module 1:** One-to-One Train the Trainer + Brochure | **Community Module 1:** One-to-One Train the Trainer + Brochure |
| | Guideline and protocol development meetings with EMS directors and medical directors | **Community Module 2:** Placement of billboards and PSAs | | **Community Module 2A:** Change out billboards and PSAs to use real stories |
| | | **Community Module 3A:** Newspaper stories and news releases introducing the program and objectives; coverage of the mock stroke code | **Community Module 3B:** Newspaper stories regarding stroke symptoms, new treatments, and steps to take | **Community Module 3C:** Newspaper stories about stroke treatment successes |

at-risk group—and another that addressed health care providers. See Table 6.1. The overall scope of the project encompassed a year of community directed messages via radio, television, and billboards and an initial organizational change and training period for health care providers. For another example of a scope and sequence, see It's Your Game . . . Keep It Real (Box 6.2 and Table 6.20).

## Channels and Vehicles for Change Methods, Practical Applications, and Messages

Program design demands decisions not only about themes but also about messages and how to deliver them. Modes for delivery of messages are constantly changing—for example, with the adoption of technology via smartphones, short messaging services, and social media. A communication channel can be interpersonal or mediated; a vehicle is how a message is actually packaged and delivered. Before the planners can choose channels and vehicles for delivery of program components, they must ascertain the preferred and most accepted media use by the intended audiences. Keep in mind that the decision to use certain channels and vehicles should serve the program and should not dictate the program. Also, most interventions incorporate multiple channels and vehicles, often having a primary delivery method and a secondary method that may focus on reinforcement of key change behaviors and the intervention theme.

Choosing delivery vehicles is a matter of balancing the needs and preferences of the intended program participants with logistics, budget constraints, team skills, and sustainability. With children, for example, planners often look to school-based education, using teachers and peer leaders; to health care providers and caregivers; to magazines, radio, and television addressed to children; and to computer and video games and instruction.

Techniques that help focus our interventions and identification of vehicles include social-marketing strategies such as audience segmentation, which can help define the various segments of a priority audience in terms of the context in which they will interact with a new behavior, their current behavior, readiness to change, and benefits desired from the new behavior (Cheng, Kotler, & Lee, 2011; Randolph & Viswanath, 2004; Storey, Hess, & Saffitz, 2015). Keep in mind that these vehicles may help reach a secondary audience, caregivers, family or friends, who are influential in motivating and promoting change objectives. See Table 6.2 for examples of communication channels and vehicles and their use.

Many interventions include an interpersonal communication channel; the specific delivery vehicle may be teachers, health care providers, lay health workers, and many different types of community volunteers. These individuals may deliver a variety of methods and practical applications. For example, teachers may use tutorials (one-on-one instruction), group discussions, and lectures, depending on the context and on the content and objectives of the instruction. Tutorials and small-group learning have the advantage over lectures in that learner performance can be elicited and feedback provided with greater individualization. Other interactive vehicles for change, such as community coalitions, have been used to address alcohol, tobacco, and other drug abuse prevention; immunization promotion; oral health promotion; injury prevention; HIV/AIDS prevention; asthma; children's health insurance; and chronic disease prevention (Butterfoss, 2007). Coalitions often draw members from education, law enforcement, local government, health care, human services, business, and other community sectors. Blueprints used by coalitions for accomplishing performance objectives are comparable to the program design documents we discuss later in Chapter 7 and include guidelines for selecting coalition members, meeting agendas, protocols for legislative visits, and sample letters for advocacy. These members are also key to program adoption and sustainability (Chapter 8).

**Table 6.2**   Communication Channels and Vehicles

| Channels and Vehicles | Typical Uses, Methods, and Practical Applications | Advantages | Disadvantages |
|---|---|---|---|
| **Interpersonal** Community volunteers Peer leaders Community health workers (promotoras) | Skill training Social reinforcement Modeling Tutoring Small-group discussion | Powerful source of influence and persuasion Can be inexpensive Involve community and enhance capacity Cultural connectivity | Difficult to train and motivate individuals to deliver one-on-one or small-group messages Expert involvement needed for delivery of specific content and reinforcement |
| **Interpersonal** Teachers | Mastery learning Tutoring Small-group discussion Lecture Modeling | Expert in didactic teaching techniques Fit organizational context of school Sustainable model for school setting and integration for dissemination and implementation | Can be resistant to truly interactive techniques Can be crippled by curriculum and examination time constraints Content may need approval from decision makers |
| **Interpersonal** Health care providers | Skill training Social reinforcement Modeling Counseling Tutoring | Powerful source of influence and persuasion Expert in patient assessment and counseling Captive audiences interested in personal health issues Content expertise and ability to integrate evidence-based messages | Can be difficult to train and motivate Lack of time Have difficulty integrating counseling techniques if they are used to a more directive "medical model" Can be perceived as too dissimilar from the patient Incentives may be needed if certified educator may need continuing education |
| **Circulating Print** Local and online newspapers | Letters to the editor Editorial commentary Role-model stories Information Persuasion Vicarious reinforcement | Inexpensive Wide audience Extends expertise Detailed Very flexible Positive consumer attitudes about vehicle Tailored narratives focused on community needs Can be niche based Ownership of materials by community advisory boards and planning groups Fast and timely dissemination Integrates well into multistrategy approaches | Depends on reading literacy Reaches only certain segments Short life span Clutter (many vehicles on the market compete for attention) Not for demonstration Poor visual quality (if print) Require health educator cultivation of relationship with gatekeepers such as health reporters at the newspaper Require health educator to capitalize on short media attention span for issues |

*(continued)*

**Table 6.2**    (*Continued*)

| Channels and Vehicles | Typical Uses, Methods, and Practical Applications | Advantages | Disadvantages |
|---|---|---|---|
| **Circulating Print or Online**<br>Magazines | Editorial commentary<br>Role-model stories<br>Information<br>Persuasion<br>Vicarious reinforcement | Good audience segmentation<br>High audience receptivity<br>Credibility and prestige<br>Long life span<br>Visual quality<br>Multiple messages with ongoing reach<br>Targeted and tailored by cultural relevance and language | Depends on reading literacy<br>Reaches only certain segments<br>Short life span<br>Clutter (many vehicles on the market compete for attention)<br>Lack of flexibility<br>Lack of control of distribution |
| **Circulating Print and Online**<br>Newsletters and e-mail blasts | Letters to the editor and editorial commentary<br>Role-model stories<br>Information<br>Persuasion<br>Vicarious reinforcement | Good audience segmentation<br>High audience receptivity<br>Strong possibility for tailoring<br>Control of distribution<br>Multiple messages with ongoing reach | Require high degree of novelty<br>Access to subscribers and continued reach to subscriber population |
| **Display Print**<br>Billboards<br>Posters | Attention<br>Awareness<br>Cue to action | Can be very effective in calling attention to a campaign<br>Direct messages<br>Able to tailor to audience and use novel images and language | Can only effect limited learning and change objectives (such as knowledge and awareness)<br>Limited view time<br>Expense can be significant |
| **Display Print**<br>Brochures<br>Flip-charts | Skill Training<br>Modeling<br>Information with extensive detail<br>Persuasion<br>Vicarious reinforcement | Can effect a variety of learning and change objectives<br>Focused on single issue or build as part of multistrategy messages<br>Use for community based learning and entry into households by community health workers<br>Used to reinforce messages and delivery of key messages<br>Lend to multilanguage formatting | No standard distribution routes exist as they do for circulating print.<br>Use for specific project |
| **Radio**<br>News Items<br>Interviews<br>Public service announcements (PSAs) | Information<br>Awareness<br>Role-model stories<br>Persuasion | Good audience segmentation<br>High audience receptivity<br>Language specific reach<br>Novel methods including radio novellas – multiseries spots<br>Messaging with key words and tag lines for branding | Require cultivation of relationship with station gatekeepers<br>Require ability to capitalize on short media attention span for issues; also short life span<br>Require high degree of novelty<br>Role-model stories not supported by visuals |

**Table 6.2** *(Continued)*

| Channels and Vehicles | Typical Uses, Methods, and Practical Applications | Advantages | Disadvantages |
|---|---|---|---|
| **Television**<br>News stories<br>Talk shows<br>Interviews | Skill training<br>Modeling<br>Information with extensive detail<br>Persuasion<br>Vicarious reinforcement | Wide distribution<br>Possibility for segmentation<br>Language specific reach<br>Novel methods including radio novellas – multiseries spots | Lack of control over content<br>Require cultivation of relationship with station gatekeepers<br>Require ability to capitalize on short media attention span for issues; also short life span<br>Require high degree of novelty<br>Competition with broadcast clutter |
| **Television**<br>Entertainment TV | Intense role-model stories | Wide distribution<br>Natural segmentation<br>Norm changing capabilities | Require relationships with producers<br>Can be very long |
| **Television and theatre**<br>PSAs | To stimulate awareness | Wide distribution<br>Natural segmentation<br>Novel methods including novellas – multiseries spots | Channel surfing or theatre attendance cuts down on audience.<br>Must have excellent production qualities<br>Often used at off-peak or not used |
| **Television**<br>Infomercials – novellas | Product awareness and persuasion | Can provide large amounts of detail<br>Multiseries spots | Channel surfing is problematic |
| **Computer- and Internet-based Interventions**<br>Decision-support<br>Curricula<br>Serious games<br>Simulations | Skill training<br>Information with extensive detail<br>Modeling<br>Vicarious reinforcement | Interactive<br>Tailored content to learner/user needs<br>Learner/user-controlled<br>24/7 access<br>High fidelity<br>Wide reach<br>Multimethod strategies | Can be costly to develop and revise<br>Programming skills are rare and in high demand.<br>Production time may be lengthy |
| **Videotape**<br>Training<br>Documentary | Just about anything | Control over content | Can be costly<br>Distribution systems must be planned. |
| **Phones and smartphones (see also computers above)**<br>Text messaging<br>Interactive voice response | Product awareness and persuasion<br>Information with limited detail<br>Vicarious reinforcement | Wide distribution<br>Possibility for segmentation<br>Language specific reach<br>Novel methods– multiseries texts<br>Control over content | Require ability to capitalize on short media attention span for issues; also short life span<br>Require high degree of novelty<br>Skill to design short messaging service with limited characters<br>Concern over data security |

*(continued)*

**Table 6.2**    (*Continued*)

| Channels and Vehicles | Typical Uses, Methods, and Practical Applications | Advantages | Disadvantages |
|---|---|---|---|
| **Social Media** (Facebook, Twitter, and other emerging networks) | Skill training<br>Modeling<br>Information with extensive detail<br>Persuasion<br>Vicarious reinforcement | Multimethod strategies<br>Wide distribution<br>Possibility for segmentation<br>Language specific reach<br>Novel methods including radio novellas – multiseries spots | Lack of control over comments and sharing of information<br>Require cultivation of relationship with association and page gatekeepers<br>Require ability to capitalize on short attention span for issues; also short life span<br>Require high degree of novelty<br>Need to monitor comments and update information – must change messages and keep audience engaged<br>Concern over data security |

## eHealth Interventions

Electronic health (eHealth) is a rapidly growing field that encompasses the application of digital technology in the service of health promotion, disease prevention, and disease management. eHealth includes computer- or Internet-based interventions to provide tailored messaging, decision support, and education and interventions using social media, serious gaming, and interactive voice response. Platforms for these interventions are diverse and include desktop computers, mobile computers such as laptops and tablets, mobile phones, and wearable devices.

**Computer- and Internet-Based Tailored Interventions**    The ubiquity of the Internet and consistently increasing bandwidth has made it the ideal platform to optimize reach for tailored computer-based programs. The ability to access websites and stream or download content on varied mobile platforms has closed the definition gap between computer-based and Internet-based interventions. Advantages include extraordinary reach, user 24/7 accessibility, anonymity, self-pace, low cost, and appealing multimedia educational strategies (Griffiths, Lindenmyer, Powell, Lowe, & Thorogood, 2006; Napolitano & Marcus, 2002). From a health promoter's point of view, the Internet offers improved opportunities for maintenance and updating of interventions (Atkinson & Gold, 2002). Computer-based interventions can be an effective way to deliver health promotion to many diverse groups (Kohl, Crutzen, & de Vries, 2013; Portnoy, Scott-Sheldon, Johnson, & Carey, 2008) and can be designed to be highly responsive to the user, providing feedback on inputted data (healthy or unhealthy choices made), and provide opportunities to practice new skills in a low risk virtual context (de Vries & Brug, 1999).

Individual tailoring through interactivity is a fundamental cornerstone of eHealth. Tailoring refers to strategies and information provided for an individual that are based on "characteristics that are unique to that individual, related to the outcome of interest, and derived from the individual assessment" (Kreuter, Strecher, & Glassman, 1999, p. 277). For the past 20 years, health education researchers have been testing computer-tailored interventions that enable tailoring of communications to certain participant characteristics (Hawkins, Kreuter, Resnicow, Fishbein, & Dijkstra, 2008). Although research is continuing to determine exactly on what demographic, clinical, or cognitive characteristic, tailoring should be based, there is enough evidence of effectiveness to import these practical applications into common practice (Krebs, Prochaska, & Rossi, 2010; Noar, Benac, & Harris, 2007). The characteristics on which to base tailoring in a particular program must be well justified empirically and theoretically (Kreuter et al., 1999).

The most common type of tailored expert decision support in eHealth education is a program that generates behavior-change messages tailored to the receiver's specific characteristics. In other words, the program contains one or more databases of messages based on theoretical constructs that vary as they apply to different characteristics of individuals and algorithms for matching the messages to the individual. The message channel could be anything that facilitates delivery of the message, such as a computer-assisted instruction on a tablet computer or text-message decision support on a mobile phone. All the systems described in the literature are based on similar configurations (see Figure 6.4), with a theoretical framework and specification of relevant hypothesized determinants of the health behavior; use of the determinant model to create a data collection tool and a series of messages; several databases, including at least a data file and a feedback message file; decision rules and a tailoring program; communications; and delivery vehicles (Dijkstra & de Vries, 1999).

In a Web-based computer-tailored intervention aimed to prevent weight gain or achieve modest weight loss by making small changes in dietary intake or physical activity, feedback was given by means of video and text messages (Walthouwer, Oenema, Soetens, Lechner, & de Vries, 2013). Feedback was used not only for increasing individuals' awareness about their body weight, physical activity level, and dietary intake but also to help participants set appropriate goals. Participants who achieved their goals were subsequently complimented, while those who failed to achieve their goals received feedback in which the failure was externally attributed to prevent a decrease in motivation.

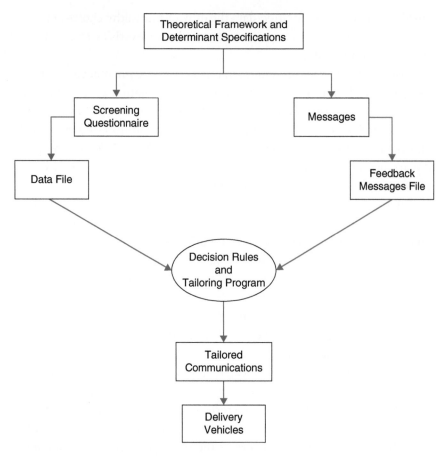

**Figure 6.4** Developing Tailored Feedback
Source: Adapted with permission from Brug, Steenhuis, van Assema, and de Vries, 1996.

Tailored decision support includes systems that offer assistance with just-in-time information, action planning, and social linkage. The Comprehensive Health Enhancement Support System (CHESS) is one of the first programs to explicitly use theoretical methods such as problem solving, decision support, self-monitoring, social support, and action planning in a computer-delivered program. The program is intended for people who have health crises; and the first problem areas to be developed were breast cancer, HIV, sexual assault, adult children of alcoholics, academic crisis, and stress management (Gustafson, Bosworth, Chewning, & Hawkins, 1987; Gustafson et al., 2002; Gustafson et al., 1994; Shaw et al., 2006). The program shell consists of three components: (a) information delivered through an instant library, questions and answers, "ask an expert," and help and support; (b) decision and planning support delivered through decision analysis, action planning, and risk assessment; and (c) social support delivered through personal stories and a discussion group.

The Management Information Decision Support Epilepsy Tool (MINDSET) (See publisher website www.wiley.com/go/bartholomew4e) provides decision support to patients and health care providers in the context of their clinic visit (Begley et al., 2015; Shegog et al., 2013b). Based on patient input on items that assess the patient's self-management (seizure management, medication management, and lifestyle management) MINDSET provides a goal-oriented action plan focused on those behaviors for which the patient is not being adherent, that have the greatest perceived importance for the patient, and for which the patient has the greatest confidence that they can perform. The action plan also cues the health care provider on what behaviors to discuss in the teachable moment of the clinic visit.

Community-based decision support is emerging to guide health promoters to adopt evidence-based programs. For example, iCHAMPSS provides online decision support for schools in adopting and implementing evidence based sexual health education (see publisher's website www.wiley.com/go/bartholomew4e). Based on the CHAMPSS Model (Choosing and Maintaining Programs for Sex Education in Schools), the program assists school health stakeholders (administrators, teachers, parents, nurses, and school health advisory council members) in navigating seven steps to assess their school district's readiness to adopt a program and to prepare for adoption, implementation, and maintenance of the program (Hernandez et al., 2011). The iCHAMPSS staging algorithm allows the user to define their district's readiness to adopt and then provides over 60 decision tools (e.g., form templates, fact sheets, video-based training, testimonials) tailored for each stage in the adoption process.

Entire disease-prevention educational experiences can be tailored on specific user input. For example, ASPIRE (A Smoking Prevention Interactive Experience), an online smoking cessation and prevention curriculum for high school students, provides lessons based on the student's self-reported stage of readiness to quit or to adopt cigarette smoking behavior. The program elicits student information using a validated readiness staging algorithm (Prokhorov et al., 2008). A student in the preparation stage receives lesson content incorporating processes of cognitive change such as consciousness raising, dramatic relief, and environmental reevaluation so as to elicit movement to contemplation. A student who is in the contemplation stage receives content focused on behavioral processes such as stimulus control and counterconditioning to move them to the action stage.

**Social Media Interventions**    Initially, Internet-delivered interventions were websites. With the advent of Web 2.0, interpersonal communication proliferated through chatrooms, blogs, and texts, the users no longer passive recipients of information but creators of it—the era of social networking was born. MySpace and Facebook were the vanguard of what are now hundreds of emerging social apps. The social environment, as a nexus of behavioral influence, has attracted research efforts on social networks and their potential impact. The use of social media as a vehicle to inform and engender social action has been amply demonstrated in contexts involving charitable campaigns, political rallying, and even national regime change. Applications of text messaging for health have been shown impactful in smoking cessation, weight loss, physical activity, and diabetes management (Cole-Lewis & Kershaw, 2010; Fjeldsoe, Marshall, & Miller, 2009; Whittaker et al., 2009). Social media applications range from an inexpensive way to send reminders for health care appointments (Gurol-Urganci, De Jongh, Vodopivec-Jamsek, Atun, & Car, 2013) to promotion of lifestyle changes such as smoking cessation or physical activity (Head, Noar, Iannarino, & Harrington, 2013). In reviews on the use of social media to effectively change health behavior, to date, a few studies have demonstrated significant effects in improving health behaviors or health outcomes (Maher et al., 2014).

Social media is increasingly used to publicize, support, and evaluate health promotion campaigns. A social media campaign requires thoughtful strategic planning to define scope and function. The Heart Truth Campaign triangulated the use of multiple social network platforms, including Twitter, Facebook, Flickr, YouTube, widgets, and badges to raise awareness of heart health among women. Awareness of the campaign and awareness of heart disease as a leading cause of death have risen significantly though it is difficult to factor out the potential influence of extraneous variables and secular trends (Long, Taubenheim, Wayman, Temple, & Ruoff, 2008; Mosca, Mochari-Greenberger, Dolor, Newby, & Robb, 2010). The precise impact of social media adjuncts in health promotion requires more study (Chang, Chopra, Zhang, & Woolford, 2013; Gold et al., 2011).

**Serious Gaming Interventions**    Using games and gaming technology to teach, train, and change behaviors is known as serious gaming (Baranowski, Buday, Thompson, & Baranowski, 2008). Games for health represent a subcategory of serious games that are focused on health promotion and disease prevention. Digital games have been designed to change health-related behaviors by changing determinants of behavior (e.g., self-efficacy, attitudes), by incorporating the behavior into the game design to advance game play (e.g., problem solving), or to influence health by changing health precursors (e.g., relaxation or anxiety reduction before surgery) (Kato, 2010). Effects on behavior have been reported in systematic literature reviews of serious games for health or safety behaviors (Hieftje, Edelman,

Camenga, & Fiellin, 2013), factors associated with traumatic brain injury (Pietrzak, Pullman, & McGuire, 2014), and obesity prevention (Lu, Kharrazi, Gharghabi, & Thompson, 2013). A recent meta-analysis of 64 games promoting healthy lifestyles revealed that games had statistically significant effects on behaviors, stronger effects on behavior determinants, and even effects on health outcomes, though these effects were weaker (DeSmet et al., 2014). Despite this, studies were limited by diverse measures, small samples, variable use of control groups and randomization, and often short duration.

**Telephone and Smartphone Interventions**   The telephone has been used as an instrument for providing health care since its debut (Soet & Basch, 1997). There is a great body of literature on the use of the telephone as an instrument of health education and promotion, ranging from simple information hotlines through a midrange of standardized messages aimed at health behavior, to more complex live coaching and computerized counseling for behavior change (Hawkes et al., 2009; Ramelson, Friedman, & Ockene, 1999). The telephone as a delivery mechanism has many advantages. It is interactive, and messages can be individualized or tailored. Voice or text messaging can be used. Visual privacy can make intervention less stressful and more productive for individuals who are reluctant to discuss a particular issue. The telephone also can reach dispersed (e.g., rural and small villages) or homebound populations and can accommodate limited literacy and language differences. There is some risk of meaning loss with this medium (as there is for print vehicles) because 65 to 95 percent of social meaning comes from visual cues in face-to-face interaction. Huang and colleagues (2011, 2014) recently used a messaging system in combination with self-management education to help adolescents with chronic illness transition to adult care (Huang et al., 2011, 2014).

Earlier programs using telephone delivery have combined expert system technology with interactive (digitized voice) telephone counseling. This technology enables a real-time assessment and contingent delivery of messages and feedback regarding attempts to perform a health behavior. Automated systems are increasingly being used in managed care situations and other health care settings. For example, the telephone linked communication (TLC) system, based on interactive voice recognition (IVR), which can function as an at-home monitor, educator, and counselor for patients and consumers (Friedman, Stollerman, Mahoney, & Rozenblyum, 1997; Migneault, Farzanfar, Wright, & Friedman, 2006; Ramelson et al., 1999). These messages may be programed or delivered by trained health promoters who can tailor self-management messages to the needs of the participant.

More recently, the use of cloud computing has been demonstrated feasible for global applications of IVR (Piette et al., 2011).

**Emerging eHealth Technology**    In the last couple of years, the availability of smartphones and wearable devices has mushroomed, resulting in numerous technical capabilities in addition to text messaging and Internet access in mobile (or mHealth) platforms. The proliferation of smartphone applications ("apps") offers the unprecedented potential to impact behavior change now that individuals have ready access to tools to monitor their physiological, behavioral, and environmental indicators and to access tailored decision support or behavioral intervention in convenient and inexpensive platforms. Apps have been described as technology in search of a theory, lacking grounding in human computer interface design, health behavior, and communication theory (Vollmer Dahlke et al., 2015). Despite this possible criticism, apps have been well received by users and have been found feasible and acceptable for delivering health interventions (Payne, Lister, West, & Bernhardt, 2015). However, this mushrooming technology has outpaced the research community's ability to collectively assess its utility, effectiveness, and safety (Bender, Yue, To, Deacken, & Jadad, 2013).

As real-time monitoring through wearable or embedded devices becomes coupled with the ability to integrate data through machine learning, behavioral interventions will continue to (a) move toward more seamless integration within a person's everyday life, and (b) enable more intelligent and synchronous interventions concordant with immediate health prevention or treatment needs. A reemergence of more versatile virtual reality simulation technology and haptic sensory devices is occurring that will allow the virtual learning environment to more closely approximate reality through more acute and higher fidelity visual, auditory, and tactile sensory input. eHealth technology is rapidly evolving, making this a challenging and exciting field for the development and evaluation of innovative health behavior change solutions.

## Choosing Theory- and Evidence-Based Change Methods to Address Program Objectives

The next task is to choose theory- and evidence-based change methods to address program objectives.

Theory- and evidence-based change methods are general techniques for influencing changes in determinants of behaviors of the at-risk group or environmental agents. To match a method with a change objective, the linking concept is the determinant involved. For example, take the following change objective: adolescents (the population) demonstrate skills (the determinant) in communicating with a partner about condom use (the performance objective). The method to reach this objective can be identified by considering methods for the determinant: skills. Of course, within the various methods for skills training, the planner will need to also consider the population and the performance objectives. Adolescents can be reached through the schools, and teachers may have ideas on what skills training methods they would want to apply with the topic of condom use.

To get from the matrices with change objectives as a result of Step 2 to the selection of methods in Step 3, planners reorganize the change objectives by determinants. They make a list of all change objectives related to increasing knowledge, another list of all change objectives related to changing outcome expectations, and so forth. They then match change methods to the determinants. Often they have multiple change methods for a determinant as well as multiple objectives to be influenced by each method. For example, modeling is often used for skills-related change objectives, but for training some skills, it may also be necessary to use guided practice. In the HIV-prevention program for Dutch adolescents, described in Table 6.3, the awareness and risk perception change objectives were matched with a number of methods. The table shows three change objectives for two performance objectives, as well as four methods for changing awareness and risk perception. The planners of this intervention elected to use personalized risk as a method for all three objectives. They also decided to apply three other methods for the third objective—consciousness raising, scenario-based risk information, and framing (loss frame)—because they found that objective to be especially relevant for this priority group: many adolescents see themselves as monogamous, whereas in fact they are serially monogamous, resulting in multiple sex partners.

**Table 6.3**    Examples of Objectives and Methods for Changing Awareness and Risk Perception

| Determinant: Awareness and Risk Perception | |
|---|---|
| **Change Objectives** | **Methods** |
| *Performance objective: Plan condom use* | |
| Recognize that HIV and sexually transmitted infections are related to behavior, not to risk group | Personalize risk |
| Recognize the possibility of finding oneself in situations in which infection is possible | Personalize risk<br>Scenario-based risk information |
| *Performance objective: Use condoms with regular partner* | |
| Describe own sexual behavior as serial monogamous rather than monogamous | Consciousness raising<br>Scenario-based risk information<br>Personalize risk<br>Framing: Loss frame |

## Roles, Determinants, and Change Methods for Environmental Conditions

Environmental conditions are not likely to be under the direct control of the individuals at risk for the health problem. They are controlled by external agents, such as parents, peers, teachers, managers, decision makers, and other gatekeepers. Therefore, performance objectives for environmental outcomes are formulated by referring to an environmental agent. Moreover, there may be various environmental levels: interpersonal, organizational, community, and societal. For example, in the ToyBox-Study (see Chapter 5), there are matrices for the at-risk individual, interpersonal, and organizational levels: children, parents, and teachers (De Craemer et al., 2014).

The same methods can be applied at any ecological level; however, methods at the higher levels often take a different form than similar methods at the individual level. Persuasive communication with individuals in a counseling context is different from persuasive communication as a part of political advocacy in a meeting between politicians and a lobbying group or in a meeting between company managers and union representatives. The determinant may be the same (i.e., outcome expectations), but the content and the vehicle for delivering a selected method—in this case persuasive communication—are different. Therefore, when addressing the behavior of agents in the environment, planners will most often select methods for individual change by determinant, and then follow up by higher level methods for environmental change that are directed at the same determinants. For example, in the ToyBox-Study, there were two change objectives for attitude change—one at the individual level (child) and one at the interpersonal level (parent) (see Table 6.4). Modeling is a useful method for attitude change and can easily be applied with the children with reinforcement of the model as an essential parameter (a condition under which the method is effective). Modeling can also be applied with the parent, but the content will be different. In this case, the parents are responsible for the healthy development of their child, so self-reevaluation may be another very effective method to change their attitudes. For example, they have to realize how their behavior influences the health of their children. If that method were not effective, planners could move to methods for other determinants, such as resistance to social pressure by providing parents with tip cards (De Decker et al, 2014).

To summarize, to select methods for environmental conditions, the first thing to do is to identify who may be in a position to make the expected change. The planner has to specify the performance objectives for the agent who will actually change the environmental condition. The health promoter then applies methods for influencing the determinants of the

**Table 6.4**    Examples of Objectives and Methods at Various Levels

| Determinant: Attitude Change | |
| --- | --- |
| **Change Objectives** | **Methods** |
| *Individual level performance objective:* | |
| Child limits screen viewing time (e.g., TV viewing, computer time) to one hour per day or less at home | |
| Change objective: Express positive feelings toward limiting screen viewing time at home | Modeling<br>Reinforcement |
| *Interpersonal level performance objective:* | |
| Parents limit preschoolers' screen viewing activities to one hour per day | |
| Change objective: Express positive feelings about the benefits that limiting screen viewing activities to one hour per day has for their child | Modeling<br>Self-reevaluation<br>Resistance to social pressure |

agent's performance objectives. Notice that determinants often have different content at various ecological levels, depending on the environmental agent's role. The adolescent's outcome expectations (e.g., that not smoking will result in more clean-smelling breath and clothes) differ from the school management's outcome expectations about implementing a nonsmoking policy (e.g., that parents will appreciate the school's having a nonsmoking policy), and those are different still from the government's outcome expectations about declaring a national nonsmoking policy for schools (e.g., that constituents will support a stricter policy). Therefore, methods directed at the same type of determinant, such as outcome expectations or skills, will be different for various environmental levels. That is why later in this chapter we describe methods for change organized by environmental level: interpersonal, organization, community, and society.

## Using Core Processes

Two of the core processes presented in Chapter 1 are essential for identifying and selecting change methods: reviewing existing empirical evidence in the literature and reviewing theories of change. With the topic approach to finding and using theory, the health promoter goes back to the literature on the problem. For example, when searching the topic drug abuse, the health promoter will discover what change methods others have used to influence various program objectives including the specific performance objective of resisting social pressure. Unfortunately, many articles are vague about change methods and more forthcoming about practical applications. The health promoter can then use the construct approach to find methods targeted toward specific determinants. For example, if a change objective is stated as "resist social pressure (determinant) to use drugs," a planner will look for methods specifically about resisting social pressure to use drugs, resisting social pressure to other risk behaviors such as smoking, and resisting social pressure in general. The health promoter may find that this literature cites theories on conformity and nonconformity and on social comparison (Cialdini, 2008). The health promoter may also use the general theories approach to explore those theories that address behavior change in general—for example, Social Cognitive Theory (Kelder et al., 2015), and discover what those general theories have to offer about accomplishing this particular objective.

There may be several change methods for one objective as well as one method for multiple objectives. In cases in which available information is extremely sparse, such as reducing fear of social contact with people with AIDS, planners may have to develop more insight on appropriate methods through a third core process: additional research with the intervention group (see Stigma in Chapter 2).

## BOX 6.1.  MAYOR'S PROJECT

When we drop in on the mayor's work group, we hear the group deliberating on what to do next. The one person who had used Intervention Mapping previously is quite comfortable continuing in a somewhat linear process.

*Teacher:* Okay, now we just group the change objectives at each ecological level by determinants. Then we discuss what methods could change that group of objectives. You see, the whole process at this point is driven by the determinants.

*Business Community Rep:* What? I thought we had already dealt with the determinants. Now we are back at the matrices with the change objectives?

*Parent:* Yes, that's right. It's just that the determinant part of the matrix—the determinant grouping—guides this process.

Many in the mayor's group groan.

*Community Agency Rep:* I am so tired of tables. I just cannot think this way anymore. Isn't there any other way of doing this? I have so many ideas about this program, and I've managed to keep up my enthusiasm through this entire Intervention Mapping process to this point. But to tell the truth, if I have to do one more table, I might lose all of my creative program ideas.

*Business Community Rep:* I feel the same way. And on top of that, I don't understand the difference between a change method and a practical application. It seems to me that this is just one more set of unnecessary vocabulary words that get in the way of really being creative about a program. Furthermore, throughout the planning process, I have been asked to hold on to my program ideas. When do I get to stop holding on? Is that now?

The health promoter listens to her colleagues and recommends that they all close their Intervention Mapping notes and put away their matrices. The group structures the next hour as a brainstorming session. Brainstorming had worked well for this group in the past, and they liked generating ideas without censure or correction. The health promoter draws two lines on the board to create three columns which she labels *Program Ideas, Change Methods*, and *Practical Applications*. She then asks the question: Thinking about our determinants and change objectives—How are we going to produce change? What are we thinking about our program? As the group members list ideas, the health promoter lists it where it fits and the group begins to get comfortable with whether each idea is a theory- and evidence-based way to change the determinant (a method), an idea about how to deliver methods (practical application), or a program idea about components, themes, scope, and sequence.

After the brainstorming, the group makes a decision about how to further organize thoughts about the program. Some members want to get the concrete program ideas out on the table: How will we reach our target populations? How long will the program be? What will the theme be? Other members are comfortable with matching change methods to objectives and then translating the methods to practical applications. They decide to discuss concrete ideas first for a set amount of time, then to turn their attention to methods.

After discussing how the program might "look and feel," the group moves on to change methods. They make a list of change objectives grouped by determinants and match the change methods on their preliminary list to each set of objectives. Where they do not have adequate coverage, they generate more change methods. At the end of the afternoon of work, the group looks at their lists and realizes that the pieces of a program are beginning to take shape.

## Methods for Changing Behavior

This section describes theoretical methods for change, summarized in tables. The first part presents basic methods and methods geared to changing certain determinants (e.g., attitude and skills) of the at-risk individuals (Tables 6.5 to 6.12). The second part presents basic method and methods for change in determinants of agents within the various environmental levels (Tables 6.13 to 6.18). For instance, attitude change of an individual could be facilitated by persuasive communication. Interventions at the level of the at-risk group are embedded in social and physical systems. A child with asthma is in an environment with parents, nurses, doctors, and other children. An adolescent in an HIV-prevention

**Table 6.5**   Basic Methods at the Individual Level

| Method (Related Theories and References) | Definition | Parameters | Examples |
|---|---|---|---|
| **Participation** (Diffusion of Innovations Theory; Theories of Power; Organizational Development Theories; Models of Community Organization: Cummings & Worley, 2014; McCullum, Pelletier, Barr, Wilkins, & Habicht, 2004; Roggers, 2003; World Health Organization, 2002) | Assuring high level engagement of the participants' group in problem solving, decision making, and change activities; with highest level being control by the participants' group. | Requires willingness by the health promoter or convener to accept the participants as having a high level of influence; requires participants' group to possess appropriate motivation and skills. | A health promoter includes representatives of students in the project group that is developing a new sex education program for schools. |
| **Belief selection** (Theory of Planned Behavior; Reasoned Action Approach: Fishbein & Ajzen, 2010) | Using messages designed to strengthen positive beliefs, weaken negative beliefs, and introduce new beliefs. | Requires investigation of the current attitudinal, normative, and efficacy beliefs of the individual before choosing the beliefs on which to intervene. | In a program for HIV prevention for Hispanic men, the men's belief that condoms were unclean needed to be changed; the importance of family values needed to be reinforced; and the belief that condoms could prevent HIV infection needed to be introduced. |
| **Persuasive communication** (Communication-Persuasion Matrix; Elaboration Likelihood Model; Diffusion of Innovations Theory: McGuire, 2001; Petty, Barden, & Wheeler, 2009, Rogers, 2003) | Guiding individuals and environmental agents toward the adoption of an idea, attitude, or action by using arguments or other means. | Messages need to be relevant and not too discrepant from the beliefs of the individual; can be stimulated by surprise and repetition; will include arguments. | Viewing a television broadcast on the health consequences to children from environmental tobacco smoke and the benefits of protecting children from smoke may influence a mother to declare her home smoke free. |
| **Active learning** (Elaboration Likelihood Model; Social Cognitive Theory: Petty et al., 2009; Kelder et al., 2015) | Encouraging learning from goal-driven and activity-based experience. | Time, information, and skills. | Getting individuals to search for answers to questions they pose as a result of some stimulus leads to better information processing and learning than passive learning and to increased change in determinants and behavior. |

**Table 6.5**    (*Continued*)

| Method (Related Theories and References) | Definition | Parameters | Examples |
|---|---|---|---|
| **Tailoring** (Trans-Theoretical Model; Precaution Adoption Process Model; Protection Motivation Theory; Communication-Persuasion Matrix: Lustria, Cortese, Noar, & Glueckauf, 2009; Weinstein, Sandman, & Blalock, 2008; Werrij, Ruiter, Riet, & De Vries, 2012; McGuire, 2001) | Matching the intervention or components to previously measured characteristics of the participant. | Tailoring variables or factors related to behavior change (such as stage) or to relevance (such as culture or socioeconomic status). | A patient educator motivates her patients to engage in vigorous physical activity by giving different messages based on the stage of change of each patient, for example providing information that physical activity will reduce their cardiovascular risk and increase their stamina to patients who are precontemplators. |
| **Individualization** (Trans-Theoretical Model: Bartholomew et al., 2000a, 2000b; Prochaska, Redding, & Evers, 2015) | Providing opportunities for learners to have personal questions answered or instructions paced according to their individual progress. | Personal communication that responds to a learner's needs. | An AIDS services organization provides a phone facility for young gay people to ask questions about their sexual identity and coming-out. |
| **Modeling** (Social Cognitive Theory; Theories of Learning: Kelder et al., 2015; Kazdin, 2012) | Providing an appropriate model; being reinforced for the desired action. | Attention, remembrance, self-efficacy and skills, reinforcement of model; identification with model; coping model instead of mastery model. | The health promoter finds a role model from the community or at-risk group who will encourage identification and serve as a coping model: "I tried to quit smoking several times and was not successful, then I tried . . . Now I have been off cigarettes for . . . " |
| **Feedback** (Theories of Learning; Goal-Setting Theory, Social Cognitive Theory: Kazdin, 2012; Kelder et al., 2015; Latham & Locke, 2007) | Giving information to individuals and environmental agents regarding the extent to which they are accomplishing learning or performance, or the extent to which performance is having an impact. | Feedback needs to be individual, follow the behavior in time, and be specific. | A physical activity counselor informs a client that her body mass index has decreased by 4% since she has begun her physical activity program. |
| **Reinforcement** (Theories of Learning; Social Cognitive Theory: Kazdin, 2012; Kelder et al., 2015; McSweeney & Murphy, 2014) | Providing reinforcement: linking a behavior to any consequence that increases the behavior's rate, frequency, or probability. | Reinforcement needs to be tailored to the individual, group, or organization, to follow the behavior in time, and to be seen as a consequence of the behavior. | An elementary school teacher praises a student for selecting a healthful dessert. |

(*continued*)

**Table 6.5** (*Continued*)

| Method (Related Theories and References) | Definition | Parameters | Examples |
|---|---|---|---|
| **Punishment** (Theories of Learning: Kazdin, 2012; McSweeney & Murphy, 2014) | Providing punishment: linking a behavior to any consequence that decreases the behavior's rate, frequency, or probability. | Punishment needs to be tailored to the individual, group, or organization, to follow the behavior in time, and to be seen as a consequence of the behavior. Punishment should be avoided because of negative side effects. If used, emphasis should be on positive reinforcement. | In the framework of behavior modification (e.g., with tantrums or aggression), one method that is applied is the so-called timeout: a period of time in a less reinforcing environment, made contingent on a behavior. |
| **Motivational interviewing, MI** (Self-Determination Theory; Theories of self-regulation: Miller & Rollnick, 2012; Ng et al., 2012; Ryan & Deci, 2000) | Providing a collaborative, goal-oriented style of communication with particular attention to the language of change; designed to strengthen personal motivation for and commitment to a specific goal by eliciting and exploring the person's own reasons for change within an atmosphere of acceptance and compassion. | A supportive relationship between client and professional combined with the evocation of patient change talk. Professionals must recognize that MI involves collaboration not confrontation, evocation not education, autonomy rather than authority, and exploration instead of explanation. | A practitioner supports the autonomy of an adolescent with a chronic medical condition by valuing of the patient's perspective (e.g., reflecting ambivalence about treatment), minimizing pressures and demands (e.g., asking for permission before providing information), and offering choices wherever possible (e.g., providing a menu of self-care options). |
| **Facilitation** (Social Cognitive Theory: Bandura, 1986) | Creating an environment that makes the action easier or reduces barriers to action. | Requires real changes in the environment instead of in the perceptions of the environment. Requires the identification of barriers and facilitators and the power for making the appropriate changes. Facilitating conditions on one environmental level are usually dealt with by intervening on a higher environmental level. | A program that targets improvement in drug users' self-efficacy for using clean needles must also facilitate accessibility of clean needles. |
| **Nudging** (Theories of Automatic, Impulsive and Habitual Behavior: de Ridder, 2014; Thaler & Sunstein, 2008) | Simple changes in the presentation of choice alternatives that make the desired choice the easy, automatic, or default choice. | Requires autonomy: freedom of choice, a sense of awareness, and the healthy choice being default: easy and attractive. | In a university building, orange colored footsteps on the floor stimulate students and faculty to take the stairs instead of the elevator. |

program is in an environment with friends, sexual partners, parents, teachers, and community leaders. Worksite employees participating in a smoking-cessation program are in an environment with colleagues, health professionals, supervisors, and worksite policies. It is important for health promotion planners to consider intervention methods at both the individual and environmental levels.

In each table, for each method there is a definition, description, example of use, and parameter for effectiveness. Parameters for use are the conditions under which the theory-based method will be effective. We developed the tables of behavior change methods in a conceptual analysis that was repeated over time with the four editions of this book (Bartholomew, Parcel, Kok, & Gottlieb, 2001, 2006; Bartholomew, Parcel, Kok, Gottlieb, & Fernández, 2011; Bartholomew et al., 2016). We derived most of the definitions of intervention methods directly from the theories within which they are described from textbooks, reviews, and meta-analysis of theories of (health) behavior and change. Some of the definitions are based on methods summaries and definitions by others (e.g., Abraham & Michie, 2008). In addition, we conducted two studies with colleagues in the field of health promotion and health psychology for consensus building on the definition of change methods (Kok et al., 2012).

**How to Use the Tables**   To effectively use the tables, planners will have created change objectives by clearly stating the behavioral outcomes, identifying who will be expected to perform the behavior, and naming determinants to create change objectives (Chapter 5). To select methods they will do the following:

1.  Check the table for each relevant determinant from the matrices.

2.  For each potential method, inspect the definition and the parameters to determine whether the method is applicable given the situation.

3.  Use the references included in the tables to study the relevant literature for ideas about how the method has been used. Use bibliographic databases, such as Google Scholar, to locate more recent studies.

4.  Repeat these steps for all determinants, until methods have been identified to address all the determinants. Then translate these methods into practical applications.

The tables have some complexities. The various determinants are not independent of each other. For example, knowledge is the basis for many other determinants, such as risk perception, attitude, and skill. Risk perception in turn is a specific part of attitude. Change methods described for one determinant may sometimes be used for other determinants as well. The tables combine comparable determinants when they appear in more than one theory—for example, attitudes, beliefs, and outcome expectations. Further, the planner should always consider change methods that may be applied to almost any determinant, is described in a table of "Basic Methods." See Chapters 2 and 3 for the theoretical foundations of the change methods.

**Basic Methods for Behavior Change**    Some methods for change at the individual level are useful for all determinants and at various levels. The members of the intervention group, for example, must pay attention to the intervention message, understand the content, and process the information carefully. Table 6.5 lists these basic requirements of health education and promotion at the individual level: participation, belief selection, persuasive communication, active learning, tailoring, individualization, modeling, feedback, reinforcement and punishment, motivational interviewing, facilitation, and nudging.

**Methods to Increase Knowledge**    Table 6.6 gives an overview of the methods and parameters for influencing knowledge. Knowledge is a necessary (though not sufficient) prerequisite for most other determinants, such as risk perception, behavioral beliefs, perceived norms, and skills. Many change methods for other determinants will also change knowledge. Conventional wisdom has long held that giving people information could change their behavior and thereby solve health and social problems. However, knowledge does not generally lead directly to behavior change; nor is assuring that the priority population attains knowledge necessarily an easy task. Theories of Information Processing provide several concepts that suggest methods for successfully conveying information.

**Methods to Change Awareness and Risk Perception**    Table 6.7 presents methods that may help people perceive their risk. Before they become motivated to make a health-promoting behavior change, people need to be aware of a risk. Most of these methods are derived from theories on risk perception and risk communication; others come from stages of behavioral change theories that start with an awareness stage.

**Methods to Change Habitual, Automatic, and Impulsive Behaviors**
Table 6.8 summarizes methods for changing habitual and automatic behaviors, as well as methods to promote action control over impulsive behaviors. Many behaviors are automatic and habitual. Even when people make reasoned and planned behavioral intentions, they may fail to follow up on those intentions. The attention of the scientific community to this type of behavior has increased in recent years; however, the evidence for effective methods is still limited.

**Table 6.6**    Methods to Increase Knowledge

| Method (Related Theories and References) | Definition | Parameters | Examples |
|---|---|---|---|
| **Chunking** (Theories of Information Processing: Gobet et al., 2001; Smith, 2008) | Using stimulus patterns that may be made up of parts but that one perceives as a whole. | Labels or acronyms are assigned to material to aid memory. | Children in the asthma self-management program learned a rap song with the words "watch, discover, think, and act" for the stages of self-management. |
| **Advance organizers** (Theories of Information Processing: Kools, 2012; Kools, van de Wiel, Ruiter, Crüts, & Kok, 2006) | Presenting an overview of the material that enables a learner to activate relevant schemas so that new material can be associated. | Schematic representations of the content or guides to what is to be learned. | In a brochure for children with asthma, graphic organizers were placed on the top of every page, with the relevant concepts addressed on that page highlighted by means of thick lines and shadings. |
| **Using imagery** (Theories of Information Processing: Steen, 2007; Wright, 2012) | Using artifacts that have a similar appearance to some subject. | Familiar physical or verbal images as analogies to a less familiar process. | A patient educator helps a learner memorize a long self-care process by attaching the steps in the procedure to landmarks on a familiar daily route. |
| **Discussion** (Elaboration Likelihood Model: Petty et al., 2009) | Encouraging consideration of a topic in open informal debate. | Listening to the learner to ensure that the correct schemas are activated. | A classroom teacher has students discuss what they learned in a video about defusing a bullying situation. |
| **Elaboration** (Theories of Information Processing; Elaboration Likelihood Model: Smith 2008; Petty et al., 2009) | Stimulating the learner to add meaning to the information that is processed. | Individuals with high motivation and high cognitive ability; messages that are personally relevant, surprising, repeated, self-pacing, not distracting, easily understandable, and include direct instructions; messages that are not too discrepant and cause anticipation of interaction. | A classroom teacher has students discuss the safe sex message: "When you want to get pregnant, use a condom"; stimulating adolescents to discover that Chlamydia can cause infertility: "If you want to get pregnant *later*, use a condom *now*." |
| **Providing cues** (Theories of Information Processing: Godden & Baddeley, 1975) | Assuring that the same cues are present at the time of learning and the time of retrieval. | Cues work best when people are allowed to select and provide their own cues. | For teens who are learning to negotiate condom use, the cues present during learning, such as what the partner says, should be as similar as possible to what teens will actually encounter in real life. |

**Table 6.7**    Methods to Change Awareness and Risk Perception

| Method (Related Theories and References) | Definition | Parameters | Examples |
|---|---|---|---|
| **Consciousness raising** (Health Belief Model; Precaution-Adoption Process Model; Trans-Theoretical Model: Skinner, Tiro, & Champion, 2015; Prochaska et al., 2015; Weinstein et al., 2008) | Providing information, feedback, or confrontation about the causes, consequences, and alternatives for a problem or a problem behavior. | Can use feedback and confrontation; however, raising awareness must be quickly followed by increase in problem-solving ability and (collective) self-efficacy. | An HIV counselor reminds a person of recent episodes of failure to use condoms when having sex and the potential consequences of that behavior on significant others. |
| **Personalize risk** (Precaution-Adoption Process Model: Skinner et al., 2015) | Providing information about personal costs or risks of action or inaction with respect to target behavior. | Present messages as individual and undeniable, and compare them with absolute and normative standards. | Individuals receive personal risk feedback on their fat intake, indicating whether it is higher than their self-rated level. |
| **Scenario-based risk information** (Precaution-Adoption Process Model: Mevissen, Meertens, Ruiter, Feenstra, & Schaalma, 2009) | Providing information that may aid the construction of an image of the ways in which a future loss or accident might occur. | Plausible scenario with a cause and an outcome; imagery. Most effective when people generate their own scenario or when multiple scenarios are provided. | Peer models in an HIV-prevention program present a series of scenarios in which they describe how they found themselves in risky situations, e.g., a sexual relationship over the summer holidays. |
| **Framing** (Protection Motivation Theory: Van't Riet et al., 2014; Werrij et al., 2012) | Using gain-framed messages emphasizing the advantages of performing the healthy behavior; or loss-framed messages, emphasizing the disadvantages of not performing the healthy behavior. | Requires high self-efficacy expectations. Gain frames are more readily accepted and prevent defensive reactions. | Missing early detection of cancer by not getting a Pap test every year can cost you your life (loss frame). Getting a Pap test every year may enable you to live to see your grandchildren grow up (gain frame). |
| **Self-reevaluation** (Trans-Theoretical Model: Prochaska et al., 2015) | Encouraging combining both cognitive and affective assessments of one's self-image with and without an unhealthy behavior. | Stimulation of both cognitive and affective appraisal of self-image. Can use feedback and confrontation; however, raising awareness must be quickly followed by increase in problem-solving ability and self-efficacy. | A person can compare his or her image as a sedentary person to a possible image as an active person. |
| **Dramatic relief** (Trans-Theoretical Model: Prochaska et al., 2015) | Encouraging emotional experiences, followed by reduced affect or anticipated relief if appropriate action is taken | Preferably should be done in counseling context so that emotions can be aroused and subsequently relieved. | A counselor encourages a client to role-play a traumatic experience so that the emotion can be experienced and then relieved. |

**Table 6.7** *(Continued)*

| Method (Related Theories and References) | Definition | Parameters | Examples |
|---|---|---|---|
| **Environmental reevaluation** (Trans-Theoretical Model: Prochaska et al., 2015) | Encouraging combining the affective and cognitive assessments of how the presence or absence of a personal behavior affects one's social environment. | May include awareness about serving as a role model for others. | In a smoking cessation class, participants describe how their family members feel about their smoking. |
| **Fear arousal** (Protection Motivation Theory; Extended Parallel Process Model: G. Y. Peters, Ruiter, & Kok, 2013; Ruiter, Kessels, Peters, & Kok, 2014) | Arousing negative emotional reactions in order to promote self-protective motivation and action. | Requires high self-efficacy expectations rather than high outcome expectations alone; is rarely effective. | A health promoter shows in an emotionally moving way how a child is hurt by fireworks before demonstrating techniques for safer firework handling. |
| **Self-affirmation** (Self-Affirmation Theory: Cohen & Sherman, 2014) | Increasing people's self-image by having them elaborate on their relevant values or desirable characteristics. | Must be tailored to individual self-image. | A stress management class includes a writing exercise in which people record as many of their desirable characteristics as they can think of. |

**Table 6.8** Methods to Change Habitual, Automatic, and Impulsive Behaviors

| Method (Related Theories and References) | Definition | Parameters | Examples |
|---|---|---|---|
| **Deconditioning** (Theories of Learning: Robbins, Schwartz, & Wasserman, 2001) | Letting people experience a lack of reinforcement or even negative outcomes of the undesired behavior. | Slow process, especially when reinforcement schedule was intermittent. It may be necessary to create a continuous lack of positive reinforcement. | A health educator advises parents to ignore a child's requests to buy unhealthy foods as they shop in a store. |
| **Counterconditioning** (Theories of Automatic, Impulsive and Habitual Behavior: Wood & Neal, 2007) | Encouraging the learning of healthier behaviors that can substitute for problem behaviors. | Availability of substitute behaviors. | When they feel the urge to smoke, smokers in a cessation program are instructed to do other behaviors than smoking, such as taking a short walk, chewing gum, or making a positive self-statement. |
| **Implementation intentions** (Theories of Goal Directed Behavior; Theories of Automatic, Impulsive and Habitual Behavior: Gollwitzer & Sheeran, 2006; Verplanken & Aarts, 1999) | Prompting making if-then plans that link situational cues with responses that are effective in attaining goals or desired outcomes. | Existing positive intention. | You are more likely to go for a cervical smear if you decide when and where you will go. Please write in below when, where, and how you will make an appointment. |

*(continued)*

**Table 6.8**     (*Continued*)

| Method (Related Theories and References) | Definition | Parameters | Examples |
|---|---|---|---|
| **Cue altering** (Theories of Goal Directed Behavior; Theories of Automatic, Impulsive and Habitual Behavior: Verplanken & Aarts, 1999; Wood & Neal, 2007) | Teaching people to change a stimulus that elicits or signals a behavior. | Existing positive intention. | Dieters change the places they keep snack food in order to prevent taking the snack automatically. |
| **Stimulus control** (Theories of Automatic, Impulsive and Habitual Behavior; Trans-Theoretical Model: Prochaska et al., 2015; Wood & Neal, 2007) | Encouraging removing cues for unhealthy habits and adding prompts for healthier alternatives. | Needs insight in the behavioral chain leading to the automatic response. | Interventions to break habits should be directed at people when they are in new environments. For example, smokers are encouraged to remove all smoking paraphernalia (e.g., ashtrays, matches) from their houses and cars. |
| **Planning coping responses** (Attribution Theory and Relapse Prevention Theory; Theories of Goal Directed Behavior: Hoffman, Friese, & Wiers, 2008; Marlatt & Donovan, 2005) | Getting the person to identify potential barriers and ways to overcome these. | Identification of high-risk situations and practice of coping response. | The HIV nurse and the patient define the causes of nonadherence as caused by habits. Then the HIV nurse and the patient formulate solutions to solve or avoid the causes for nonadherence. |
| **Early commitment** (Theories of Learning: Robbins et al., 2001) | Having people choose a (larger) delayed reward far in advance. | Making the choice may be forced but the choice for the delayed reward needs to be voluntary. | A designated driver who voluntarily refrains from alcohol (immediate reward) during a party to bring friends safely home feels good about his role and will use a friend's service as designated driver at the next party (delayed reward). |
| **Public commitment** (Theories of Automatic, Impulsive and Habitual Behavior: Ajzen, Czasch, & Flood, 2009) | Stimulating pledging, promising or engaging oneself to perform the healthful behavior, and announcing that decision to others. | Most effective when publicly announced; may include contracting. | A patient trying to get more exercise makes a private commitment to self and then announces her decision to others in the social environment. |
| **Training executive function** (Theories of Automatic, Impulsive and Habitual Behavior: Diamond, 2013) | Improving the top-down mental control processes that are used when going on automatic or relying on instinct or intuition would be ill-advised, insufficient, or impossible. | The task has to be challenging and substantial repetition is required to sufficiently train the executive functions. | A child will engage in computerized working memory training, such as Cogmed. |

## Methods to Change Attitudes, Beliefs, and Outcome Expectations

Table 6.9 lists methods that may be used to change people's attitudes toward health. Attitudes are a positive or negative reaction to something; however, they can include the more specific constructs of beliefs, outcome expectations, assessments of advantages and disadvantages, perceptions of benefits and barriers, self-evaluations, and motivations to act. Social psychology has devoted much attention to attitude change, and the table represents a very brief summary of this work here (for a more in-depth review, see Crano & Prislin, 2011; Petty & Cacioppo, 2012).

**Table 6.9**  Methods to Change Attitudes, Beliefs, and Outcome Expectations

| Method (Related Theories and References) | Definition | Parameters | Examples |
|---|---|---|---|
| **Classical conditioning** (Theories of Learning: Kazdin, 2012) | Stimulating the learning of an association between an unconditioned stimulus (UCS) and a conditioned stimulus (CS). | Most effective when the time interval is short and the CS precedes the UCS. | Women with high body concern completed a conditioning procedure in which pictures of their bodies were selectively linked to positive social feedback: smiling faces. |
| **Self-reevaluation** (Trans-Theoretical Model: Prochaska et al., 2015) | Encouraging combining both cognitive and affective assessments of one's self-image with and without an unhealthy behavior. | Stimulation of both cognitive and affective appraisal of self-image. Can use feedback and confrontation; however, raising awareness must be quickly followed by increase in problem-solving ability and self-efficacy. | A person can compare his or her image as a sedentary person to a possible image of themselves as an active person. |
| **Environmental reevaluation** (Trans-Theoretical Model: Prochaska et al., 2015) | Encouraging realizing the negative impact of the unhealthy behavior and the positive impact of the healthful behavior. | Stimulation of both cognitive and affective appraisal to improve appraisal and empathy skills. | Empathy training, viewing of documentaries or testimonials, or family interventions. |
| **Shifting perspective** (Theories of Stigma and Discrimination: Batson, Chang, Orr, & Rowland, 2002) | Encouraging taking the perspective of the other. | Initiation from the perspective of the learner; needs imaginary competence. | Parents instructing small children to cross the street kneel down to see traffic from the child's height. |
| **Arguments** (Communication-Persuasion Matrix; Elaboration Likelihood Model: McGuire, 2001; Petty & Wegener, 1998) | Using a set of one or more meaningful premises and a conclusion. | For central processing of arguments they need to be new to the message receiver. | Hearing for the first time about the benefits of protecting children from smoke may influence a mother to declare her home smoke free. |

*(continued)*

**Table 6.9**    (*Continued*)

| Method (Related Theories and References) | Definition | Parameters | Examples |
|---|---|---|---|
| **Direct experience** (Theories of Learning: Maibach & Cotton, 1995) | Encouraging a process whereby knowledge is created through the interpretation of experience. | Rewarding outcomes from the individual's experience with the behavior or assurance that the individual can cope with and reframe negative outcomes. | Rehabilitation counselors in training try taking a trip while in a wheelchair. This may change their attitudes about what it is like to use a wheelchair. |
| **Elaboration** (Theories of Information Processing; Elaboration Likelihood Model: Smith, 2008; Petty et al., 2009) | Stimulating the learner to add meaning to the information that is processed. | Individuals with high motivation and high cognitive ability; messages that are personally relevant, surprising, repeated, self-pacing, not distracting, easily understandable, and include direct instructions; messages that are not too discrepant and cause anticipation of interaction. | *Sex, Games, and Videotapes*, an HIV-prevention program for homeless mentally ill men in a New York shelter, made messages personally relevant, surprising, and repeated by embedding them in playing competitive games, storytelling, and watching videos, activities that were salient pastimes in the shelter. |
| **Anticipated regret** (Theory of Planned Behavior; Reasoned Action Approach: Richard, Pligt, & de Vries, 1995) | Stimulating people to focus on their feelings after unintended risky behavior, before any losses actually materialize. | Stimulation of imagery; assumes a positive intention to avoid the risky behavior. | A sex educator asks people to imagine how they would feel after risky behavior such as having had unsafe sex. |
| **Repeated exposure** (Theories of Learning: Zajonc, 2001) | Making a stimulus repeatedly accessible to the individual's sensory receptors. | Neutrality of original attitude. | Adolescents may be shown condoms repeatedly in classroom HIV-prevention education. |
| **Cultural similarity** (Communication-Persuasion Matrix: Kreuter & McClure, 2004) | Using characteristics of the target group in source, message, and channel. | Using surface characteristics of the target group enhances receptivity. Using social-cultural characteristics leads to a more positive reception of the message. | Trained members of the Latino community give culturally relevant messages for cancer prevention and screening trials. |

**Methods for Changing Social Influence**    Table 6.10 presents methods for changing social influence. The influence of the social environment is an important determinant of many behaviors and as such occurs frequently in change objectives. The Theory of Planned Behavior (TPB) and its successor the Reasoned Action Approach (Fishbein & Ajzen, 2010; Montaño & Kasprzyk, 2015) explain social influence. In these theories, behavior is determined by intention, and that intention is determined by attitudes, perceived norms, and perceived behavioral control (self-efficacy). Social influence in this theory is described as perceived expectations of "people who are important to me" and perceived behavior of "people like me"

**Table 6.10**    Methods to Change Social Influence

| Method (Related Theories and References) | Definition | Parameters | Examples |
|---|---|---|---|
| **Information about others' approval** (Theory of Planned Behavior; Reasoned Action Approach; Social Comparison Theory: Forsyth, 2014; Mollen, Ruiter, & Kok, 2010 ) | Providing information about what others think about the person's behavior and whether others will approve or disapprove of any proposed behavior change. | Positive expectations are available in the environment. | University students are given data showing the percentage of students who drink on campus, which usually is less than the students predict. |
| **Resistance to social pressure** (Theory of Planned Behavior; Reasoned Action Approach: Evans, Getz, & Raines, 1992) | Stimulating building skills for resistance to social pressure. | Commitment to earlier intention; relating intended behavior to values; psychological inoculation against pressure. | Young women learn effective refusal skills to use when a partner does not want to use a condom. |
| **Shifting focus** (Theory of Planned Behavior; Reasoned Action Approach: Fishbein & Ajzen, 2010) | Prompting hiding of the unpopular behavior or shifting attention away from the behavior. | Preferably shift focus to a new reason for performing the behavior. | Young women tell a partner that they want to use a condom to prevent pregnancy (instead of preventing STI/HIV). |
| **Mobilizing social support** (Diffusion of Innovations Theory; Theories of Social Networks and Social Support: Holt-Lundstad & Uchino, 2015; Valente, 2015) | Prompting communication about behavior change in order to provide instrumental and emotional social support. | Combines caring, trust, openness, and acceptance with support for behavioral change; positive support is available in the environment. | An exercise in a sex education program has students talk about safe sex and using condoms to make the positive expectations for using condoms more visible. |
| **Provide opportunities for social comparison** (Social Comparison Theory: Suls, Martin, & Wheeler, 2002) | Facilitating observation of nonexpert others in order to evaluate one's own opinions and performance abilities. | Upward comparison may help setting better goals; downward comparison may help feeling better or more self-efficacious. | A breast cancer patient may have had a lumpectomy, but sees herself as better off than another patient who lost her breast (downward comparison). |

(comparable to modeling). Social influence through modeling is a central construct in Social Cognitive Theory, which explicates intervention methods that change the social environment as well as perceived social influence (Bandura, 1986; Kelder et al., 2015). Social influence may also occur as upward and downward social comparison: Facilitating the observation of nonexpert others in order to evaluate one's own opinions and performance abilities (Suls et al., 2002).

**Methods to Influence Skills, Capability, and Self-Efficacy and to Overcome Barriers**    Table 6.11 presents change methods to enhance skills and self-efficacy. Constructs addressed in this section are self-efficacy, perceived behavioral control, perceived barriers, skills, and perceived skills. Self-efficacy is often a crucial determinant in changing health behavior.

**Table 6.11**    Methods to Change Skills, Capability, and Self-Efficacy and to Overcome Barriers

| Method (Related Theories and References) | Definition | Parameters | Examples |
|---|---|---|---|
| **Guided practice** (Social Cognitive Theory; Theories of Self-Regulation: Kelder et al., 2015) | Prompting individuals to rehearse and repeat the behavior various times, discuss the experience, and provide feedback. | Subskill demonstration, instruction, and enactment with individual feedback; requires supervision by an experienced person; some environmental changes cannot be rehearsed. | The trainer first models the target behavior a number of times and then asks the trainees to do the same a number of times. The trainer gives brief comments on the trainees' performances, emphasizing aspects done well. |
| **Enactive mastery experiences** (Social Cognitive Theory; Theories of Self-Regulation: Kelder et al., 2015) | Providing increasingly challenging tasks with feedback to serve as indicators of capability. | Requires willingness to accept feedback. | After the students are taught the necessary know-how of intervening in bullying situations, they perform the new skills in a simulated setting in order to experience their mastery at handling bullying class mates. |
| **Verbal persuasion** (Social Cognitive Theory; Theories of Self-Regulation: Kelder et al., 2015) | Using messages that suggest that the participant possesses certain capabilities. | Credible source. | Teachers were shown a videotape on which teachers like them discussed their successful experiences in the regular classroom using the intervention with difficult-to-teach children. |
| **Improving physical and emotional states** (Social Cognitive Theory: Kelder et al., 2015) | Prompting interpretation of enhancement or reduction of physiological and affective states, to judge own capabilities. | Must carefully interpret and manage emotional states. | Students in a public speaking class are taught to breathe deeply and relax prior to their presentation. They label the anxiety they feel as excitement. Reduce stress and depression while building positive emotions—as when fear is labeled as excitement. |
| **Reattribution training** (Attribution Theory and Relapse Prevention Theory; Theories of Self-Regulation: Marlatt & Donovan, 2005) | Helping people reinterpret previous failures in terms of unstable attributions and previous successes in terms of stable attributions. | Requires counseling or bibliotherapy to make unstable and external attributions for failure. | The counselor suggests that a smoker's relapse was due to a temporary condition and that she can learn from this experience to stay off cigarettes. |
| **Self-monitoring of behavior** (Theories of Self-Regulation: Creer, 2000) | Prompting the person to keep a record of specified behavior(s). | The monitoring must be of the specific behavior (that is, not of a physiological state or health outcome). The data must be interpreted and used. The reward must be reinforcing to the individual. | Patients keep a diary on their therapy adherence in order to find out when and why medication is missed. |

**Table 6.11**    *(Continued)*

| Method (Related Theories and References) | Definition | Parameters | Examples |
| --- | --- | --- | --- |
| **Provide contingent rewards** (Theories of Learning; Theories of Self-Regulation: Bandura, 1986) | Praising, encouraging, or providing material rewards that are explicitly linked to the achievement of specified behaviors. | Rewards need to be tailored to the individual, group or organization, to follow the behavior in time, and to be seen as a consequence of the behavior. | Smokers who are trying quit smoking receive monetary vouchers for breath samples with carbon monoxide (CO) levels of 8 ppm or less. |
| **Cue altering** (Theories of Automatic, Impulsive, and Habitual Behavior; Theories of Self-Regulation: Achtziger, Gollwitzer, & Sheeran, 2008) | Teaching changing a stimulus, either consciously or unconsciously perceived, that elicits or signals a behavior. | Existing positive intention. | Dieters change the route they take walking to work in order to avoid easy access to snack shops. |
| **Public commitment** (Theories of Automatic, Impulsive, and Habitual Behavior: Ajzen et al., 2009) | Stimulating pledging, promising, or engaging oneself to perform the healthful behavior and announcing that decision to others. | Needs to be a public announcement; may include contracting. | High school students sign individual contracts not to smoke, which are then placed on the classroom wall for all to see. |
| **Goal setting** (Goal-Setting Theory; Theories of Self-Regulation: Latham & Locke, 2007) | Prompting planning what the person will do, including a definition of goal-directed behaviors that result in the target behavior. | Commitment to the goal; goals that are difficult but available within the individual's skill level. | Dietician and patient discuss the goal for the next meeting, deciding on a goal that is acceptable to the patient and to the dietician. |
| **Set graded tasks** (Social Cognitive Theory; Theories of Self Regulation: Kelder et al., 2015) | Setting easy tasks and increase difficulty until target behavior is performed. | The final behavior can be reduced to easier but increasingly difficult subbehaviors. | Physiotherapist and patient discuss increasingly intensive exercises for the patient in order to gradually build up the patient's condition. |
| **Planning coping responses** (Attribution Theory and Relapse Prevention Theory; Theories of Self-Regulation: Marlatt & Donovan, 2005) | Prompting participants to list potential barriers and ways to overcome these. | Identification of high-risk situations and practice of coping response. | The HIV nurse and the patient define the causes of nonadherence (lack of understanding, lack of motivation, insufficient action plan, barriers). Then the HIV nurse and the patient formulate solutions to solve or avoid the causes for nonadherence. |

When people are motivated, the remaining question is whether they are able and feel confident to change their behavior. Self-efficacy is a determinant for the precursors of behavior—intention, preparation to act, and decision to act—but it also can directly influence implementation and maintenance of behavior change. Self-efficacy and related concepts are all personal determinants, but there is a distinction between perceptions (e.g., perceived skills) and reality (e.g., real skills). Even with sufficient real skills, people may not try the new behavior when their perceived skills are low. And people with high perceived skills may fail because they have insufficient real skills. Methods to improve self-efficacy are therefore often methods that also improve real skills.

**Methods to Reduce Public Stigma**    The last table on changing individual behavior, Table 6.12, presents methods to reduce stigma. Stigma is very difficult to change (Paluck & Green, 2009), but there are methods that may be successful under certain circumstances. Therefore, sticking to the parameters is especially crucial.

### *Methods for Changing Environmental Conditions*

This section first lists basic methods for change that can be applied at all environmental levels and then methods related to environmental conditions at each ecological level. These tables refer the reader back to earlier tables of methods for both individual and general determinants, indicating that these methods can be used to change the environmental condition or that the individual level methods are embedded in the environmental change methods. Planners should note that some change methods at the individual level are also useful at most environmental levels. Skills training by guided practice (see Table 6.11), for example, can be applied in almost any method directed at changing an environmental agent's behavior, even though the form and content of the training may be different than when this method is applied at the strictly individual level.

**Basic Methods for Change of Environmental Conditions**    Table 6.13 lists basic methods at the environmental level for the health promoter: systems change, participatory problem solving, coercion, advocacy and lobbying, modeling, and technical assistance. Intervention planners should always consider these methods when identifying promising methods for change at all environmental levels. See Chapter 3 for the theoretical and empirical background for these basic methods.

**Methods to Change Social Norms**    Table 6.14 presents methods for changing social norms. Chapter 3 presented social norms theory as a community-level theory. However, social norms are influential at all levels. In Table 6.10 we summarized the methods to change social influence, of which social norms are a relevant form. There, the focus was on the individual's perception of, and coping with, social norms, whereas here the focus is on changing the norms themselves.

**Table 6.12**    Methods to Reduce Public Stigma

| Method (Related Theories and References) | Definition | Parameters | Examples |
|---|---|---|---|
| **Stereotype-inconsistent information** (Theories of Stigma and Discrimination: Bos, Schaalma, & Pryor, 2008) | Providing positive examples from the stigmatized group. | Only effective when there are many different examples. Examples are not too discrepant from original stereotype. | Positive portrayals of stigmatized individuals in mass media or leaflets. |
| **Interpersonal contact** (Theories of Stigma and Discrimination: Pettigrew & Tropp, 2006) | Bringing people in contact with members of the stigmatized group. | Requires positive experiences. Most effective when: no status differences; externally sanctioned; intensive contact; common or shared goals. | Presentations by stigmatized persons in educational interventions. |
| **Empathy training** (Theories of Stigma and Discrimination: Batson et al., 2002) | Stimulating people to empathize with another person, i.e., imagine how the other person would feel. | Requires being able and willing to identify with the stigmatized person. Imagine how the other person would feel (this leads to empathy). Do not imagine how you would feel (this leads to both empathy and distress). | Personal stories of experiences of stigmatized individuals. |
| **Cooperative learning** (Theories of Stigma and Discrimination: Aronson, 2015) | Engineering lessons in a way that students must learn from one another. | Requires careful organization of lesson information distribution. | Teachers give each student one piece of the lesson plan, so that good comprehension requires students to collaborate. |
| **Conscious regulation of impulsive stereotyping and prejudice** (Theories of Stigma and Discrimination: Bos et al., 2008) | Forcing oneself to control impulsive negative reactions related to stigma. | Mere suppression almost always leads to counterproductive effects and is not advisable. Conscious self-regulation of automatic stereotyping can be used effectively. | Participants practice saying "Stop thinking this way" to themselves as they watch videos of stigmatizing people. |
| **Reducing inequalities of class, race, gender and sexuality** (Theories of Stigma and Discrimination: Link & Phelan, 2001) | *See methods for changes at higher environmental levels (Tables 9-14).* | | Mobilizing social support, community organizing, empowerment of stigmatized persons, agenda setting, creating and enforcing laws and regulations, and threatening with coercion. |

## Methods to Change Social Support and Social Networks    Table 6.15 describes methods at the interpersonal level:

1. to change social networks so that they offer social support more effectively to their members,

2. to help members mobilize support from their networks, and

3. to link members with other networks.

**Table 6.13**    Basic Methods for Change of Environmental Conditions

| Method (Related Theories and References) | Definition | Parameters | Examples |
|---|---|---|---|
| **Systems change** (Systems Theory: Best et al., 2012; National Cancer Institute, 2007) | Interacting with the environment to change the elements and relationship among elements of a system at any level, especially through dialogue with stakeholders, action, and learning through feedback. | Methods and actors depend on the level of the system. | A city's transportation department created bicycle lanes on streets to encourage people to ride bicycles to work as a result of a stakeholder advisory committee's recommendations. The committee monitored the use of the bicycle lanes and held a focus group of bicyclists about their experiences. |
| **Participatory problem solving** (Organizational Development Theories; Social Capital Theory; Models of Community Organization: Butterfoss et al., 2008; Cummings & Worley, 2014; Wallerstein et al., 2015) | Diagnosing the problem, Generating potential solutions, developing priorities, making an action plan, and obtaining feedback after implementing the plan. | Requires willingness by the health promoter or convener to accept the participants as equals and as having a high level of influence; requires target group to possess appropriate motivation and skills. Will often include goal setting, facilitation, feedback and consciousness raising. | A health promotion consultant assists employees of a small company to identify the level of perceived work stress and sources of work stress, to develop a plan with management support to address sources of stress and provide coping strategies, to implement the plan, and to monitor perceived work stress. |
| **Coercion** (Theories of Power: Freudenberg & Tsui, 2014; Turner, 2005) | Attempting to control others against their will. | Requires or creates a power differential. | Health promotion activists organize a consumer boycott of a company that sells formula in developing countries. |
| **Advocacy and lobbying** (Stage Theory of Organizational Change; Models of Community Organization; Agenda-Building Theory; Multiple Streams Theory: Christoffel, 2000; Galer-Unti, Tappe, & Lachenmayr, 2004; Kingdon, 2003; Wallack, Dorfman, Jernigan, & Themba,1993; Weible, Sabatier, & McQueen, 2009) | Arguing and mobilizing resources on behalf of a particular change; giving aid to a cause; active support for a cause or position. | Form of advocacy must match style and tactics of the people, communities or organizations represented, and the nature of the issue; includes policy advocacy; often tailored to a specific environmental agent. Will often include persuasive communication, information about others' approval, and consciousness raising. | Members of the American Public Health Association use the organization's action alert system to contact their legislators to urge them to vote for pending health care reform legislation. |
| **Modeling** (Social Cognitive Theory; Organizational Development Theories; Diffusion of Innovations Theory; Empowerment Theory: Bandura, 1997; Kelder et al., 2015; Rogers, 2003) | Providing an appropriate model being reinforced for the desired action. | Appropriate models will vary by level, including group members and organizational, community, and policy change agents. | An article in the state medical journal highlights the experience of a city hospital emergency department that has instituted routine HIV testing, found new cases of HIV that would have gone undetected, and received recognition from the state's HIV Community Planning Group. |

**Table 6.13**     *(Continued)*

| Method (Related Theories and References) | Definition | Parameters | Examples |
|---|---|---|---|
| **Technical assistance** (Organizational Development Theories, Diffusion of Innovations Theory, Social Capital Theory, Models of Community Organization: Flashpohle, Duffy, Wandersman, Stillman, & Maras, 2008; C. Mitchell & LaGory, 2002) | Providing technical means to achieve desired behavior. | Nature of technical assistance will vary by environmental level, but must fit needs, culture, and resources of the recipient. | A health department liaison helps a community health center design recruitment procedures, training, and supervisory guidelines as they establish a new lay health worker program. |

**Table 6.14**     Methods to Change Social Norms

| Method (Related Theories and References) | Definition | Parameters | Examples |
|---|---|---|---|
| **Mass media role-modeling** (Diffusion of Innovations Theory; Social Cognitive Theory; Social norm theories: Bandura, 1997; Rogers, 2003) | Providing appropriate models being reinforced for the desired action through the mass media. | Conditions for modeling; conditions for persuasive communication (see Table 1). | A feature story about mammography screening on the news includes a woman who caught the cancer early by having routine mammogram. The cancer was removed by lumpectomy. |
| **Entertainment education** (Diffusion of Innovations Theory; Social norm theories: Moyer-Gusé, 2008; Petraglia, 2007; Shen & Han, 2014; Wilkin et al., 2007) | Providing a form of entertainment designed to educate (about health behavior) as well as to entertain. | Consideration of source and channel; balance of media professional's and health promoter's needs. | A soap opera has a storyline about a lead character's being arrested for drinking and driving. |
| **Behavioral journalism** (Diffusion of Innovations Theory; Social Cognitive Theory; Social norm theories: McAlister, 1991; McAlister et al., 2000; Ramirez et al., 1999; Reininger et al., 2010) | Using by the mass and local media of appropriate role-model stories of behavior change based on authentic interviews with the target group. | Adequate role models from the community and elicitation interviews to describe the behavior and the positive outcome. | Baseball card-size cards with a picture and a short story concerning how a woman got her boyfriend to willingly use a condom are part of a sex education program for runaway teens. |
| **Mobilizing social networks** (Theories of Social Networks and Social Support; Social norm theories: Valente, 2015) | Encouraging social networks to provide informational, emotional, appraisal, and instrumental support. | Availability of social network and potential support givers. Will often include information about others' approval, facilitation, and persuasive communication. | Parents are coached on how to make their negative views about smoking clear to their children as part of a tobacco prevention program. |

**Table 6.15**   Methods to Change Social Support and Social Networks

| Method (Related Theories and References) | Definition | Parameters | Examples |
|---|---|---|---|
| **Enhancing network linkages** (Theories of Social Networks and Social Support: Holt-Lundstad & Uchino, 2015; Valente, 2015) | Training network members to provide support and members of the target group to mobilize and maintain their networks. | Available network. | A patient educator helps a patient who has had a stroke and her family members to make plans for the patient to return home. The plans include linking to a patient support group and community day care. |
| **Developing new social network linkages** (Theories of Social Networks and Social Support: Holt-Lundstad & Uchino, 2015; Valente, 2015) | Linking members to new networks by mentor programs, buddy systems, and self-help groups. | Willingness of networks to reach out; availability of networks that can provide appropriate support and linkage agents. | Volunteers who are breast cancer survivors are linked to newly diagnosed patients to provide emotional and informational support. |
| **Use of lay health workers; peer education** (Theories of Social Networks and Social Support; Models of Community Organization: Eng, Rhodes, & Parker, 2009; Tolli, 2012) | Mobilizing members of the target population to serve as boundary spanners, credible sources of information, and role models. | Natural helpers in community with opinion leader status and availability to volunteer for training. | *Promotoras* from a local clinic provide information and outreach to community members at risk for diabetes. |

Networks can engage in participatory problem-solving processes aimed at finding ways to solve specific problems of individuals, families, or communities. We highlight the use of lay health workers specifically (Eng et al., 2009; Tolli, 2012). These are natural helpers (community members to whom other persons turn for advice, emotional support, and tangible aid) who receive special training to support others, including linking them to the formal service delivery system.

**Methods to Change Organizations**   Table 6.16 presents methods from organizational change theories, including organizational development, the Stage Theory of Organizational Change, Diffusion of Innovations Theory (DIT), and Stakeholder Theory. These include organizational processes, such as participatory problem solving and team building, which can create changes in organizational norms and practices (Butterfoss et al., 2008). DIT and the Stage Theory of Organizational Change provide methods that can influence the adoption, implementation, and continuation innovations such as health promotion programs. Methods from Stakeholder Theory focus on using influence from external agents to promote organizational change.

**Table 6.16**  Methods to Change Organizations

| Method (Related Theories and References) | Definition | Parameters | Examples |
|---|---|---|---|
| **Sense-making** (Organizational Development Theory: Weick & Quinn, 1999) | Leaders reinterpret and relabel processes in organization, create meaning through dialogue, and model and redirect change. | Used for continuous change, including culture change. | A supervisor in a hospital talks to his staff about the positive aspects of finding and correcting mistakes in documentation of medication administration. |
| **Organizational diagnosis and feedback** (Organizational Development Theory: Cummings & Worley, 2014) | Assessing of organizational structures and employees' beliefs and attitudes, desired outcomes, and readiness to take action, using surveys and other methods. | Methods appropriate to organizational characteristics, e.g., size and information technology. Will often include feedback and consciousness raising. | An organizational consultant conducts a survey of employees' health behaviors and determinants and holds focus groups of employees to review the results and plan for health promotion programs. |
| **Team building and human relations training** (Organizational Development Theory: Cummings & Worley, 2014) | Grouping development activities based on the values of human potential, participation, and development. | Compatible with the culture. | Participants in a retreat work interdependently to solve a puzzle. |
| **Structural redesign** (Organizational Development Theory: Cummings & Worley, 2014; Jones, 2004) | Change organizational elements such as formal statements of organizational philosophy, communication flow, reward systems, job descriptions, and lines of authority. | Management authority and agreement. | A health promotion consultant works with an organization to renew the organizational vision statement to include the health of employees. |
| **Increasing stakeholder influence** (Stakeholder Theory: Brown, Bammer, Batliwala, & Kunreuther, 2003; Kok, Gurabardhi, Gottlieb, & Zijlstra, 2015; R. K. Mitchell, Agle, & Wood, 1997) | Increase stakeholder power, legitimacy, and urgency, often by forming coalitions and using community development and social action to change an organization's policies. | The focal organization perceives that the external organization or group is one of its stakeholders. | A community group uses media advocacy to highlight the groundwater pollution by gas storage tanks located in the community and to demand that the tanks be moved by the gas company that owns them. |

**Methods to Change Communities**    Table 6.17 summarizes methods to promote community change. These include problem-posing education or conscientization, community assessment, community development, social action, forming coalitions, social planning, and framing to shift perspectives. See Chapter 3. The skillful community organizer selects methods that fit the context of the community and the key issues to be addressed. These often shift over time. The community methods relate to two types of

**Table 6.17**    Methods to Change Communities

| Method (Related Theories and References) | Definition | Parameters | Examples |
|---|---|---|---|
| **Problem-posing education** (Conscientization Theory; Empowerment Theory: Freire, 1973a,1973b; Wallerstein, Sanchez, & Velarde, 2004) | Participatory analysis using critical reflection, self-disclosure, and dialogue regarding the social forces underlying a problem and a commitment to change self and community. | A safe environment for participation and disclosure; a critical stance. | In facilitated small-group discussion, adolescents share the effects of their own and others' alcohol abuse on their lives. They reflect on what this means both personally and to their community. They ask, "What can we do about this?" and take action. |
| **Community assessment** (Models of Community Organization: Rothman, 2004) | Assessing a community's assets and needs, with feedback of results to the community. | Requires expert assistance and possibilities for feedback. | Community members, with technical assistance from the health department, used surveys, door-to-door interviewing, and community asset mapping to conduct a community assessment. The findings were presented and discussed at a community-wide meeting. |
| **Community development** (Models of Community Organization; Theories of Power: Minkler & Wallerstein, 2008; Rothman, 2004; Wallerstein et al., 2015) | A form of community organization, based on consensus, in which power is shared equally and members engage together in participatory problem solving. | Starting where the community is; may be grassroots or professional driven. Will often include consciousness raising, facilitation, goal setting, and information about others' approval. | A community organizer convenes a task force of representatives of the school board, the mayor's office, the disenfranchised community, and the city council member representing the community to discuss the findings of a report documenting inequities in the schools and to make plans to address them. |
| **Social action** (Theories of Power; Stakeholder Theory; Kok et al., 2015; Minkler & Wallerstein, 2012; Rothman, 2004; Wallerstein et al., 2015) | A form of community organization, based in conflict, in which disenfranchised people wrest power from the official power. | Starting where the community is; may be grassroots or professional driven. Will often include consciousness raising, persuasive communication, information about others' approval, and modeling. | A community organizer works with a low-income community that has identified a need to improve educational resources available to their children. They document the inequities in the schools and extracurricular programs across the city, present their findings, and challenge the school board to act on them in a press conference. They organize community members to attend the next school board meeting to demand that this inequality be redressed. |

**Table 6.17**    *(Continued)*

| Method (Related Theories and References) | Definition | Parameters | Examples |
|---|---|---|---|
| **Forming coalitions** (Models of Community Organization; Social Capital Theory: Butterfoss, 2007; Butterfoss & Kegler, 2009; Clavier & De Leeuw, 2013) | Forming an alliance among individuals or organizations, during which they cooperate in joint action to reach a goal in their own self-interests. | Requires collaboration across various agendas; requires attention to stages of partnership development. Will often include persuasive communication, consciousness raising, goal setting, facilitation, and information about others' approval. | A grant application requires that a community develop a tobacco prevention coalition with representatives from public health, education, voluntary health associations, law enforcement, businesses, the health care sector, and other community groups to address the issue of youth smoking. |
| **Social planning** (Models of Community Organization: Rothman, 2004) | Using information based on research to address issues. | Requires credible source of the information. | The health department planner presented epidemiological data on HIV/AIDS prevalence and trends to the Prevention Planning Group as they selected priority populations for programs. |
| **Framing to shift perspectives** (Models of Community Organization: Snow, 2004) | Assigning meaning and interpretation to relevant events and conditions in order to mobilize potential constituents, gain bystander support, and demobilize antagonists. | Match with culture. | Community organizers in tobacco prevention frame youth smoking as the result of heavy targeted advertising by the tobacco industry rather than as an individual decision. |

interventions: (a) those implemented by the health promoter with the community to develop empowerment and community capacity, and (b) those implemented by the community toward the environmental agent. For example, the health promoters carry out a facilitated community intervention designed to assist the community in understanding the issues it must face, setting priorities, and developing and implementing action plans to address the key issues. Then the community implements the action plan, using methods of change appropriate to the environmental agent and desired change. This may involve individuals, organizations, and government. We discuss specific methods for political change in the next section.

**Methods to Change Policy**    Political change takes place using many of the methods for individual, organizational, and community change in the earlier tables. However, these methods should be applied in the context of theories that explain how policy is formulated, implemented, and modified. In Chapter 3 we discussed the Multiple Streams Theory and

**Table 6.18**    Methods to Change Policy

| Method (Related Theories and References) | Definition | Parameters | Examples |
|---|---|---|---|
| **Media advocacy** (Models of Community Organization: Dorfman & Krasnow, 2014; Wallack, 2008; Wallack et al., 1993) | Expose environmental agents' behaviors in the mass media to order to get them to improve health-related conditions. A type of advocacy. | Requires the media to approve the news value of the message and accept the message without changing its essential content. | A public-interest group holds a press conference to focus attention on the serving sizes of and fat and calories in foods served in fast food restaurants; how that contributes to the obesity epidemic; and what the restaurants, as responsible community businesses, should do. |
| **Agenda setting** (Multiple Streams Theory, Advocacy Coalition Theory, Theories of Power: Clavier & De Leeuw, 2013; Sabatier, 2003; Weible, 2008; Weible et al., 2009) | Process of moving an issue to the political agenda for action; may make use of broad policy advocacy coalitions and media advocacy. | Requires appropriate timing (see policy window) and collaboration of (media) gatekeepers. Will often include persuasive communication and consciousness raising. | A state child health advocacy group developed a position paper on the expansion of the child health insurance program. They released the report to the media and held meetings with key state legislators on the recommendations. |
| **Timing to coincide with policy windows** (Multiple Streams Theory: Kingdon, 2003; Zahariadis, 2007) | Advocating policy when politics, problems, and policy solutions are aligned to be receptive to a policy issue. | Requires an astute policy advocate who is well prepared | Health care reform advocates in the United States began to develop coalitions and position papers with the election of a president known to be supportive of that issue. |
| **Creating and enforcing laws and regulations** (Multiple Streams Theory, Theories of Power: Clavier & De Leeuw, 2013; Kingdon, 2003; Longest, 2006) | Forcing compliance or dictating or precluding choices. Sometimes Implementing existing laws to accomplish change. Laws and regulations may also provide incentives. | Requires unequal power and availability of control and sanctions. | Based on a citizen group's request the police department began to enforce the loitering ordinance to reduce drug-related activity in the community. |

the Advocacy Coalition Framework. These theories provide insight into when to use various individual and community influence methods, such as media advocacy, agenda setting, timing to coincide with policy windows, and creating and enforcing laws and regulations (see Table 6.18).

## Moving From Methods to Applications

The third task in Step 3 is to select or design practical applications to operationalize change methods.

One change method may be accomplished by many applications, and the planner must decide which applications best fit the situation's context. The Web-based case studies give examples of the links between objectives, methods, applications, and programs (see Publisher's website www.wiley.com/go/bartholomew4e). The first challenge of this task for most health promoters is how to come up with creative practical applications. Some planning groups may feel less than creative at this point because they have been grappling with the science of intervention—describing the problem and gathering theory and evidence on which to base the intervention. This task, along with the first task in this step, require stepping back from the details of program planning to freely discuss all the ideas that have been bubbling up for intervention applications.

### *How to Think About Applications*

After working on the first two tasks of this step, planners will have a sense of how they will deliver their program and a sense of what theory- and evidence-based methods the program will contain. They can think about the change methods as the program's *active ingredients*, and the active ingredients need to be presented in practical applications. For example, the method of modeling might be presented as a role model story in print, or as a personal testimonial in person or online—or in any number of creative applications. The core of an application is the messages that will be processed by the target group for that application. Spending time with members of the intervention populations and potential program implementers will be a great help for thinking about applications and for writing the messages in the applications in Step 4 (See Chapter 7). Suitable applications will depend greatly on to whom and where the program is being delivered. For example, the Cystic Fibrosis Family Education Program (CF FEP) (Bartholomew et al., 1991) included many SCT constructs, so the planning team might logically have thought of applications that included a lot of interaction, such as group sessions and role playing for modeling. However, the team knew from having met with parents and adolescents during the needs assessment that they could reach only about 25 percent of the parent intervention group and almost none of the adolescents in a group setting. They therefore used applications such as role-model stories in newsletters, and they integrated delivery into families' clinical encounters. These types of application decisions, based on formative work, are very important. For example, Schaalma and colleagues (Schaalma, Kok, Poelman, & Reinders, 1994; Schaalma et al., 2004) describe trying to operationalize modeling with role playing as part of an HIV-prevention program in vocational schools. The teachers, however, had a different idea. They were so uncomfortable with organizing and moderating role playing that the planners knew they had to choose another application.

The following section provides examples of program elements that illustrate the translation of methods to applications with careful attention to theoretical parameters, the conditions under which a program should work.

### Stick to the Theoretical Parameters of Change Methods

The methods tables presented earlier provided considerations for effective use for each method. These considerations included theoretical parameters and, particularly at the environmental levels, characteristics of the context that program planners must take into account. The challenge for health-promotion program planners is to design creative intervention applications that fit the context and characteristics of the program participants while ensuring that the applications also address the parameters for the selected methods.

The following is an example of an intervention that failed to use theory correctly: One practical application frequently proposed for school-based programs aimed at the prevention of drug abuse is to have former drug users warn students about the dangers of drugs. This activity is very popular among students, teachers, parents, school boards, and politicians. However, evaluation studies have shown that this application may lead to a significant increase in drug use among students (de Haes, 1987). The program planners made two mistakes in translating the method of modeling into a practical application. First, the former drug users provide an incorrect model for the students by showing that even people who start using drugs may end up in a very respectable position—in this case, lecturing in schools. This mistake suggests inattention to parameters (i.e., for role modeling). The second mistake is that the focus of the model's message is on the dangers of drug use, whereas the most important determinants of drug use initiation are decision-making skills, skills to resist social pressure, and self-efficacy for those skills. In this case, program planners did not adequately use evidence in the form of theory and empirical data. They should have focused on interventions dealing with social norms and social-cognitive skills (L. W. Peters, Kok, Ten Dam, Buijs, & Paulussen, 2009). This second example suggests that the model focused on the wrong determinants and perhaps also that other change methods may have been more appropriate.

### Examples of Translating Methods to Applications

The following are examples of adequate theory use in translating methods to applications.

**Modeling**   Developers of the Dutch HIV-prevention program chose modeling as a change methods for the following objective: "Adolescents express their confidence in successfully negotiating condom use with a sex partner" (Schaalma & Kok, 2001, p. 366). Modeling from Social Cognitive Theory (see Chapter 2) is a method with the potential to increase self-efficacy (the determinant in the change objective). Bandura (1997) and Kelder et al. (2015) are sources for understanding the method and for discovering that modeling is effective under specific conditions or parameters:

- The learner identifies with the model
- The model demonstrates feasible subskills
- The model receives reinforcement
- The observer perceives a coping model, not a mastery model

Using modeling in the program would be effective only when the parameters for this method are translated to the practical application. As part of their program, Schaalma and colleagues developed video scenes, in which models demonstrated skills for negotiating condom use with partners. These skills, which were taught earlier in the program, included rejection, repeated rejection with arguments, postponement, making excuses, avoiding the issue, and counterposing (Evans, Getz, & Raines, 1991; Schaalma et al., 2004). The models were carefully selected to serve as identifiable models for the priority population. In all scenes the modeled behavior was identifiable, and the models were rewarded for the behavior with a positive ending. The models were coping models; they were clearly struggling a bit with their task of persuading their partners to use a condom. Keep in mind that these scenes were only a part of the program, in which various methods for many objectives were translated into practical applications within an integrated program.

**Active Learning**    Schaalma and colleagues presented their models in a context of active learning. For example, interventionists presented video scenes of high-risk situations and stopped the scenes after the situation had developed so that students could elaborate on what they would do in the situation or give advice to the role model actor. After the participation, the video continued, and the students observed the scene's further development and ending. Again, the group discussed the scene's development. Active learning may be effective in almost any change method, as long as the situation provides sufficient motivation, information, time for elaboration, and skills-related advice. The following example presents one scene from the video, a dating situation in which an adolescent girl stands up to social pressure from her date about not going home on time. Note that the role model uses techniques about how to resist social pressure that were taught earlier in the program: rejection, repeated rejection with arguments, and counterposing.

## SCENE FROM HIV-PREVENTION ACTIVE LEARNING VIDEO

*Video scene: In the discotheque*

*Boy*:  Would you like another drink?

*Girl*:  No, I have to go home.

*Boy*:  Come on, don't be lame.

*Girl*:  No, I've got to be home at twelve.

*Boy*:  This is a great tune, let's dance.

> On screen: Assignment. Sasja really likes Mike. How can she make clear that she still wants to be home at midnight? How will Mike react? (Video stops, students discuss possible effective reactions. Video starts again.)

*Boy*:  Don't you care about me anymore?

*Girl*:  Yes, but that's not the point. They'll get on my case again if I don't get in before midnight.

*Boy*:  Come on, it can't be that bad.

*Girl*:  How do you know? I just want to go home. Besides, you'll ruin the whole evening if you're going to sulk.
(Boy sinks to his knees in feigned apology.)

*Girl*:  (laughs) Come on, if I'm late, you'll be kneeling for my dad on Saturday.

*Boy*:  So, you'll come on Saturday?

*Girl*:  That's the plan.

*Boy*:  Let's go then.

In this example, modeling was combined with active learning. The developers took into consideration the parameters for the methods including identification, skills demonstration, reinforcement (happy ending), coping model, information (on negotiation skills), and time for elaboration. However, the parameter of motivation may have been underrepresented. Skills training often needs to be combined with methods to enhance motivation. In this case, the health promoters might have used several methods for increasing HIV-risk awareness and creating an attitude favoring reduction of sexual risk: risk-scenario information, anticipated regret, and fear arousal, among others.

**Risk Perception Information**    Another change objective in the HIV-prevention school program was: "Adolescents recognize the possibility of ending up in situations in which contracting HIV or a sexually transmitted infection cannot be ruled out" (Schaalma & Kok, 2001, p. 365). Here the determinant is risk perception. The developers turned to theories on risk perception and risk communication for methods to improve personal risk perception. These theories suggest the provision of risk information and risk feedback, message framing, self-reevaluation, and fear arousal. For instance, Hendrickx, Vlek, and Oppewal (1989) state that people may base their risk judgments on information that aids the construction of an image of the ways in which a particular outcome may occur. An essential parameter for this method is that the information includes a plausible and imaginable scenario with a cause and an outcome, instead of only an outcome. Therefore, the peer models in the HIV-prevention program presented a series of scenarios in which they described how they found themselves in risky situations (e.g., a sexual relationship over the summer holidays). These scenarios clearly presented a cause and an effect to make these contingencies more likely. The method might have been even more effective if the students could have generated their own scenario; however, choosing from multiple risk scenarios has also shown to be effective (Mevissen, Meertens, Ruiter, & Schaalma, 2010; Mevissen, et al., 2009).

**Anticipated Regret**   Anticipated regret (Abraham & Sheeran, 2004; Richard et al., 1995) is a method for attitude change. The Reasoned Action Approach suggests insight into relevant beliefs as the basis of attitude change methods (Fishbein & Ajzen, 2010). Schaalma and colleagues (Schaalma et al., 1994; Schaalma & Kok, 2001) used various methods to change beliefs, for example, anticipated regret, active processing of information, linkage of beliefs with enduring values, and association of the attitude object with positive stimuli. The risk-scenario information we discussed earlier may be combined with the method of anticipated regret: asking people to imagine how they would feel after risky behavior such as having had unsafe sex. The parameter for anticipated regret is that the regret question should stimulate imagery.

**Fear Arousal**   Many health promotion interventions use some kind of fear-arousing message to promote safer behavior. Theories of fear-arousing communication and recent meta-analyses suggest that although fear arousal may enhance the motivation to avert the threat, acceptance of health recommendations is mainly dependent on people's outcome expectations regarding the recommendations (What will happen if I follow the recommendations?) and their self-efficacy (How confident am I that I can do the recommendations?). In addition, high levels of fear may easily inhibit persuasion through processes of denial and defensive avoidance especially when response efficacy or self-efficacy is low. Thus, when using fear arousal, program developers should always provide coping methods for reducing the perceived threat and teach the skills for applying these coping methods (G. Y. Peters, Ruiter, & Kok, 2013; Ruiter et al., 2014).

One way that fear appeals may be better able to motivate people into precautionary action is to include recommendations that can be easily performed, such as calling a help line. First, motivate people by presenting threatening information, and second, provide specific instructions about what to do. The current state of the art with respect to fear arousal in health promotion suggests that health promoters should be rather reserved in scaring their participants. Typically, of the four information components composing a fear appeal, severity information has been found to be the weakest predictor of protection motivation as compared to susceptibility information and information about the effectiveness and feasibility of recommended action. The optimal application might be a combination of creating personal risk awareness, without arousing too much fear, and developing skills for the desired behavior change (Ruiter et al., 2014).

Combinations of risk-scenario information, anticipated regret, and fear arousal may promote risk awareness and attitude change. In the following example, these three methods are combined in one video scene, again using modeling. This part of the video shows a series of scenes in which students interview fellow students about safe sex. The example interview is introduced as a story of a girl who had contracted a chlamydia infection. Her boyfriend is with her.

| | |
|---|---|
| *Girl*: | I wasn't with him [current boyfriend] last year. It was a boy I fell in love with on my holiday. So we ended up in bed. I was prepared and had brought some condoms, but he refused to use them. He kept on saying, "Trust me, no AIDS." He was very persistent. "It's okay to do it without, just once." It was so stupid. But he was such a hunk. I couldn't pass him up. I've got a much bigger hunk now (looks at current boyfriend). What's more, the boy looked very clean. But I was so stupid. I slept with him without using a condom. I was on the pill at the time. |
| *Interviewer*: | But why did you do it? It's risky as hell. |
| *Girl*: | I didn't know what to think anymore. I thought, "Maybe it won't come to that." I thought, "As long as I'm careful." And I was afraid if I'd turn him down. I was doing it for him, basically. It was brought home to me later how stupid it was. I was pretty scared afterward. |

| | |
|---|---|
| | And sure enough I got a discharge. I went to a doctor, who said I had chlamydia. I was petrified. It can make you infertile. |
| *Interviewer:* | That would mean that you could never have children! |
| *Girl:* | I acted quickly, so it wasn't that bad. I was so angry with him afterward for saying that he cared but refusing to use a condom. Of course, I was angry at myself as well. I was stupid. |
| *Interviewer:* | So, now you always use a condom? |
| *Girl and Boy:* | Yes! |
| *Interviewer (to boyfriend):* | I guess you don't agree with the holiday guy? |
| *Boyfriend:* | No, I was glad she brought it up. |
| *Interviewer:* | What do you mean? |
| *Boyfriend:* | She mentioned it first. I was worried about asking her about condoms. I was afraid she'd think I jump into bed with any girl. |
| *Girl:* | Nonsense, I think it's great if a boy brings it up. It means that he really cares about you. I like boys who can talk about it. And sex is more fun if you know you are safe. No worries the next day. |
| *Boyfriend:* | You bet. She takes care of the pill, and I take care of the condoms. We've got a nice condom joke (both start laughing). |
| *Interviewer:* | Are you going to let me in on it? |
| *Boyfriend:* | Before we make love ... I say I've got to put on a CD! |
| *Interviewer:* | That's a good one. I've got to remember that. |

In the example the source of the risk-scenario information combined with anticipated regret and fear arousal is a peer, representing another example of modeling. The developers took all the parameters into account: scenario imagery, cause and outcome, regret imagery, personal susceptibility, outcome expectations, and self-efficacy. Moreover, the parameters for modeling, such as reinforcement of the desired behavior were met. A careful analysis of the parameters makes clear that methods for risk awareness and attitude change have to be combined with methods for self-efficacy improvement and skills training. People need to be motivated for active learning and skills training, but they also need to be self-efficacious for opening up to unpleasant information (Bandura, 1997).

## *Methods and Applications at Different Levels*

Translating methods into applications for interventions to change environmental conditions, such as those directed toward social networks, organizations, communities, and policy makers, brings in some special considerations. At each of these levels, the environmental agent is influenced by methods addressing change objectives derived from the person's role. For example, outcome expectations for legislators related to voting to fund mammograms for low-income women might relate to constituent response or to expectations of improved constituent health.

The use of methods and practical applications to change determinants vary with ecological level. Health promoters can use the same methods with environmental agents that they direct toward individuals to increase knowledge, awareness, attitudes, skills, and social influence. However, at the environmental level these methods are often packaged into broader methods or processes that take into account the level and context of the situation. These broader methods include participatory problem solving, advocacy, or organizational development. For example, participatory problem solving as an environmental change method includes basic individual methods and those specific to knowledge change, attitude change, skills building, self-efficacy and collective efficacy, and other individual-level determinants. It includes diagnosing the problem, generating potential solutions, developing priorities, making an action plan, and obtaining feedback after implementing the plan. At the social network level, the application might take the form of calling together the family, friends, and helpers of an older person living alone for a meeting to discuss what the situation is and how they can come together to handle increasing needs for activities of daily living. At the organizational level, an intervention to improve employee morale might include conducting a survey of employee attitudes, giving feedback on the findings to employees and managers, holding small-group discussions of what the findings mean and how to address them, discussing the importance and changeability of the proposed activities, setting priorities, putting the changes into place, and getting feedback concerning their effectiveness through focus groups and surveys. At the community level, the application might be a workshop to develop a strategic plan for a community problem, such as obesity. Persons representing government and other organizations in the community meet with residents with a stake in the issue to discuss data concerning the problem, possible solutions, and available community resources. They brainstorm and evaluate applications for solutions, prioritize them, and develop action plans using committees for different community sectors.

The approach used for adoption and implementation of the Put Prevention Into Practice program by Texas primary care clinics is an example of an organizational intervention using participatory problem solving (Murphy-Smith, Meyer, Hitt, Taylor-Seehafer, & Tyler, 2004; Tyler, Taylor-Seehafer, & Murphy-Smith, 2004). The program comprises discussion and reflection on practice change; advisory committee guidance for change policies, space, continuing education, systems for prescreening charts, clinic flow, referral protocols, and quality measures; and office-based tools, including a guide to preventive services, a health-risk profile, a flow sheet of dates of services and counseling with findings, and patient education materials, all intended to support the provision of clinical preventive services (Gottlieb, Huang, Blozis, Guo, & Murphy Smith, 2001).

Combining change methods may result in greater environmental impact. For example, in 2004, to address growing concerns about childhood obesity in Latvia, key stakeholders used a variety of methods and applications to influence government legislation. School directors and parent groups applied participatory problem-solving methods to circumvent exclusive contracts with international soft drink companies by purchasing only water products. Nongovernmental organizations, civil society groups, and nutrition specialists applied media advocacy to raise the issue of obesity and healthy diet in the public domain. These approaches led to legislative action in 2006 to ban certain foods and drinks in schools (Knai, McKee, & Pudule, 2010).

In the T.L.L. Temple Foundation stroke project (see publisher's website www.wiley.com/go/bartholomew4e), program planners used multiple methods and applications to target behavior change in health care providers (see Table 6.19). These included:

- Organizational change consultation to assess awareness, increase perceptions of need, and diagnose needed support for change in EDs and EMS. (Most hospitals and EMS needed support for getting revised stroke care guidelines in place, including individualized guideline development and staff training.)

- Skill training individualized to the provider and the setting

- Reinforcement for using new treatment protocols through newsletters and newspaper stories of successes

The community advisory committee helped to generate change methods and applications and to provide local role models. Program planners wanted to use locally recognizable role models who had experienced stroke and recovered, for example, the mayor of Lufkin, to enhance the salience of the intervention in the local community.

**Table 6.19**  Methods and Applications for Emergency Department Matrices in the T.L.L. Temple Foundation Stroke Project

| Determinants and Change Objectives | Methods | Applications |
|---|---|---|
| Knowledge of rtPA study results | Persuasive communication Elaboration | Presentations at medical staff meetings, committee meetings<br>Newsletters delivered to emergency departments (EDs) with science articles and news |
| Skills & self-efficacy for stroke workup | Modeling Guided practice | Training in EDs<br>Community mock stroke activity |
| Perceived social norms and standard of care to lower stroke workup times | Cues to action Modeling Social comparison Reinforcement | Newspaper articles of treatment of stroke patients by hospitals in the community<br>Provision of national association guidelines |
| Perceived social norms and standard of care to treat stroke | Information about others' approval Social comparison Facilitation | Newspaper articles of treatment of stroke patients by hospitals in the community<br>Provision of national association guidelines |
| Outcome expectations, attitude | Mass media role-modeling Feedback | Newsletters delivered to EDs with role-model stories of physicians treating patients who had good recovery and reports on treated patients |
| System barriers | Organizational diagnosis and feedback | Meetings with hospital teams – including administration, ED medical and nursing directors, and physicians – to plan rtPA use, discuss barriers, and develop protocols |

## Where Have All the Objectives Gone?

At the end of Intervention Mapping Step 3, the planner has moved from objectives to program ideas, methods, parameters, and applications. During that process, the planner has made many decisions, from theoretical and practical perspectives. The planner has estimated the strength of the evidence of methods and the feasibility of applications. The planner has anticipated issues in implementation by program users. At this point it is necessary to ensure that all the objectives that were selected for the program are still matched in the current list of applications. If that is the case, the planner may continue to the next step; if not, the planner has to decide whether to leave some objectives out or to go back and develop methods and applications to cover the neglected objectives.

In previous tasks in Step 3, we suggested that the planner make a list of change objectives for each determinant in each of the matrices. In this final task for Step 3, the planning group should return to this list to check that the selected methods or designated applications address each objective. This is done to ensure that the planning group has not overlooked any of the change objectives. If any of the objectives have been missed, the planning team should either address the objectives by linking them to methods and applications for other change objectives associated with the determinant, or go back through the preceding tasks to select additional methods or applications for the missing objectives.

## Planning for Process Evaluation

The choice of appropriate change methods and applications for a program will have a lot to do with whether the program is effective or not. However, the direct implications for evaluation of the methods and application choices are in the process evaluation. The process evaluation includes whether the theoretical methods that have been chosen are based on evidence and theory to support that they can produce changes in the determinants and change objectives from the matrices. Another question is whether the methods have been operationalized in ways that adhere to the parameters or the assumptions inherent in the use of the proposed theoretical change methods. For example, parameters for modeling would include whether the participants can identify with a role model and whether the model is reinforced for the behavior that is performed. Finally, a process evaluation question that relates to this step is whether the correct methods and parameters are apparent in the applications that are ultimately delivered to participants.

---

### BOX 6.2.  IT'S YOUR GAME . . . KEEP IT REAL

In Step 3 the planning group for It's Your Game . . . Keep It Real built upon their previous work from Steps 1 and 2 to generate ideas for a multicomponent, multimedia program. They developed program themes, drafted a scope and sequence with adolescent and parent components, and selected theory- and evidence-based change methods and applications to influence their behavioral and environmental objectives.

**The first task in Step 3 is to generate ideas for program themes, components, scope, and sequence.**

The planning group and youth advisory group that we described in Chapter 4's It's Your Game Box helped to generate ideas for program planning. Research staff also conducted focus groups with adolescents from the at-risk group to ensure that program ideas that would be relevant and engaging for youth. Students advised not to use the word "abstinence" in program activities but rather to focus on giving youth the knowledge and skills they needed to make healthy decisions in life. From these conversations, the planning group developed the overall program theme of It's Your Game . . . Keep It Real, with "your game" equating to "your life," and the student being the most important player in his or her game. "Keeping It Real" came directly from the youth vernacular, with meanings of, "telling it like it is, being respectful, being responsible, doing the right thing, being yourself, and being healthy and happy." Just as games have rules about how to win, so youth need personal rules to make healthy decisions. Thus, the planners developed a subtheme founded on a self-regulatory, decision-making paradigm: *select* (students select their personal rules or limits), *detect* (students recognize challenges to these rules), *protect* (students avoid situations which challenge these rules and use refusal skills to protect these rules). These steps—select, detect, and protect—operationalized performance objectives from the Step 2 matrices.

Building on the characteristics of effective sexual health education programs (Kirby, 2001, 2007), the planning team set about developing a program that was interactive, delivered clear messages about sexual behavior, included age-appropriate instructional methods, integrated skill-building activities, used personalization, reinforced key messages, and lasted for a sufficient duration. They also recognized that using a multimedia approach was critical for youth engagement (Lenhart, Arafeh, & Smith, 2008; Rideout, 2001). Technology-based interventions offer the ability to tailor activities by sexual experience, which was particularly important in middle schools where the small proportion of sexually experienced students may require different instruction compared to nonsexually experienced students. Thus, the group proposed to utilize multiple communication channels (interpersonal and mediated) and delivery vehicles including group-based classroom lessons, individual journaling, computer-based lessons with some activities tailored by gender and sexual experience, parent-child take-home activities, and parent newsletters.

The planners divided the content into twenty-four, 50-minute lessons, with 12 lessons in seventh grade and 12 lessons in eighth grade. Each grade level included three take-home activities to facilitate parent-child communication and a parent newsletter, which addressed parent-child communication and monitoring objectives. Group- and computer-based lessons were interspersed. Students accessed the computer lessons one-on-one; these lessons included activities designed to personalize and reinforce activities in the group-based classroom lessons.

The scope and sequence depicted in Table 6.20 illustrates the breadth and amount of content in the It's Your Game curriculum (scope) and the order in which the content was delivered (sequence). Initial seventh grade lessons addressed topics such as healthy friendships and how to apply the select, detect, protect paradigm to set personal rules for general risk behaviors (e.g., not using drugs and not stealing). Later seventh grade lessons helped students apply the paradigm more specifically to sexual situations. The eighth-grade lessons continued to apply the paradigm to sexual situations along with activities on healthy dating relationships and contraception and HIV, STIs, and pregnancy testing messages for all students.

**The second and third tasks in Step 3 involve choosing theory- and evidence-based methods and practical applications to influence change in the behavior and environmental objectives.**

The planning team selected theory-based change methods that had been shown to be effective for adolescent sexual health education (Coyle et al., 1996; Coyle, Kirby, Marin,

**Table 6.20**   Scope and Sequence for It's Your Game . . . Keep It Real

| Youth Component | | | |
|---|---|---|---|
| **7th Grade Lessons** | **Vehicle** | **8th Grade Lessons** | **Vehicle** |
| 1 It's Your Game . . . Pre-Game Show<br>• Set short & long term goals | Group | 1 It's Your Game . . . Pre-Game Show<br>• Set short & long term goals | Group |
| 2 Keeping It Real . . . Among Friends<br>• Define qualities of healthy friendships<br>• Practice evaluating friendships | Group | 2 Keeping It Real . . . Consequences of Pregnancy<br>• Personalize risk of getting pregnant<br>• Identify the social, emotional, & physical consequences of getting pregnant<br>• Describe the impact of pregnancy on a teen's life and future | Group |
| 3 Keeping It Real . . . Among Friends<br>• Practice evaluating friendships<br>• Resist social pressure to have an unhealthy friendships | Computer | 3 Keeping It Real . . . Consequences of HIV/STIs<br>• Examine the impact HIV and other STIs may have on their lives and future<br>• State physical, social, and emotional consequences of being infected with HIV or other STIs | Computer |
| 4 It's Your Game . . . Playing by Your Rules<br>• Describe what a personal rule is<br>• Describe steps necessary to play by your rules ("Select, Detect, Protect") | Group | 4 Keeping It Real . . . About STIs<br>• Describe the types, modes of transmission, and symptoms of STIs<br>• State importance of seeing a health care provider & getting tested for HIV/STI and pregnancy, if sexually active | Group |
| 5 It's Your Game . . . Playing by Your Rules<br>• Detect situations that may challenge personal rules | Computer | 5 Keeping It Real . . . Risk Reduction Strategies<br>• Describe importance of using condoms to reduce risk of HIV/STIs or pregnancy<br>• Identify the correct steps for condom use<br>• Describe different contraceptive methods and failure rates | Computer |

(continued)

**Table 6.20**    *(Continued)*

| Youth Component | | | |
|---|---|---|---|
| **7th Grade Lessons** | **Vehicle** | **8th Grade Lessons** | **Vehicle** |
| 6  Protecting Your Rules . . . A Clear No<br>• Describe characteristics of refusal skills<br>• Use refusal skills to help maintain personal rules | Group | 6  Playing by the Game Rule . . . A Review<br>• Review how to "Select, Detect, Protect"<br>• Practice using refusal skills to protect personal rules for sex in different situations | Group |
| 7  Protecting Your Rules . . . Alternative Actions<br>• Review characteristics of refusal skills<br>• Use refusal skills to help maintain personal rules | Computer | 7  Playing by the Game Rule . . . A Review<br>• Review effective refusal skills<br>• Practice using refusal skills to protect personal limits in different situations | Computer |
| 8  Know Your Body<br>• Describe puberty, reproductive systems, menstruation<br>• Define sexual activity & consequences | Computer | 8  Keeping It Real . . . Healthy Dating Relationships<br>• Evaluate healthy/unhealthy dating relationships<br>• Identify personal values and expectations for dating relationships | Group |
| 9  Keeping It Real . . . For Yourself<br>• State the social, emotional, & physical consequences of having/not having sex<br>• Personalize reasons for waiting to have sex | Group | 9  Keeping It Real . . . Healthy Dating Relationships<br>• Evaluate healthy/unhealthy dating relationships<br>• State importance of respecting other people's rules in dating relationships | Computer |
| 10  Playing by Your Rules . . . Regarding Sex<br>• Practice how to "Select, Detect, Protect"<br>• Identify reasons for choosing to wait to have sex | Computer | 10  Playing by Your Rules . . . Regarding Sex<br>• Review "Select, Detect, Protect"<br>• Practice using refusal skills to protect personal rules about sex | Group |

*(continued)*

**Table 6.20**    (*Continued*)

| Youth Component | | | |
|---|---|---|---|
| **7th Grade Lessons** | **Vehicle** | **8th Grade Lessons** | **Vehicle** |
| 11  Protecting Your Rules . . . Regarding Sex<br>• Review characteristics of refusal skills<br>• Practice using refusal skills to protect personal limit to wait to have sex | Group | 11  It's Your Game . . . Free Time<br>• Review past computer program activities<br>• Describe what they have learned from computer activities | Computer |
| 12  It's Your Game . . . Post Game Show<br>• Describe what they have learned from the program<br>• Describe how they will use what they have learned in the future | Group | 12  It's Your Game . . . Post Game Show<br>• Describe what they have learned from the program<br>• Describe how they will use what they have learned in the future<br>• Personalize commitment to make responsible decisions to reduce risk of HIV/STIs, & pregnancy | Group |
| **Parent-Student Take-Home Activities** | | | |
| • Real friends<br>• Protecting Your Rules . . . Using A Clear NO<br>• Keeping It Real . . . About Sex | Worksheet<br>Group debriefing | • Keeping It Real . . . About Sex<br>• Keeping It Real . . . Dating Relationships<br>• It's Your Game . . . Keep It Real | Worksheet<br>Group debriefing |
| **Parent Component** | | | |
| • Parent-child communication<br>• Overview of It's Your Game<br>• Tips for talking with your teen<br>• Communication is the key | Newsletter | • Parental monitoring<br>• Setting limits for teens<br>• Knowing your child's friends and their parents<br>• Staying involved in your teen's life | Newsletter |

Gomez, & Gregorich, 2004) and matched them to specific determinants and change objectives in the matrices for youth and parents (Tables 6.20 and 6.21). As the tables indicate, the methods were quite similar for the adolescent and parent components; however, the practical applications were often different. Even though the matrices were different, the determinants were similar, which accounts for the similarity of methods.

**Table 6.21**    Sample of Methods and Applications for Students From It's Your Game . . . Keep It Real

| Behavioral Outcome | Determinants and Change Objectives | Method | Application |
|---|---|---|---|
| Choose not to have sex | Knowledge of consequences of oral, anal, and vaginal sex | Information | Quizzes & games about sex, reproduction, and HIV/STI transmission |
| | | Modeling | Role model story of teen parents |
| | | | Peer videos of teen parents, and HIV+ youth |
| | Knowledge of effective refusal skills | Demonstration | Facilitator demonstrates effective and ineffective refusal skills |
| | Skills & self-efficacy to select personal rules about sex | Chunking | Select, Detect, Protect mnemonic device |
| | | Modeling | MTV style "real world" video series – characters select personal rules about sex |
| | | Goal setting | Setting short- and long-term goals |
| | Skills & self-efficacy to avoid risky situations / refuse sex | Guided practice | Role plays on avoiding or getting out of risky situations / saying no to sex |
| | | | Responding to pressure lines |
| | Normative beliefs about choosing not to have sex | Modeling | Peer video on reasons not to have sex |
| | | Discussion | Take-home activity - talk to parent about selecting personal rules about sex |
| | Outcome expectations about refusing sex | Anticipated regret | Journal activity – anticipating consequences of unwanted sex |
| | | Goal setting | Setting short- and long-term goals |
| | | Social support | Take-home activity – talk to parent about handling social pressures to have sex |
| Have healthy relationships with their friends, girlfriends, or boyfriends | Knowledge of characteristics of healthy and unhealthy dating relationships | Information | Quiz on characteristics of healthy and unhealthy dating relationships |
| | Skills & self-efficacy to evaluate dating relationships | Scenario-based risk information | Mock TV dating game show – evaluate healthy/unhealthy characteristics of potential dates |
| | Normative beliefs about avoiding unhealthy dating relationships | Modeling | Peer video on expectations for healthy dating relationships |
| | | Discussion | Take-home activity – talk to parent about how boyfriends/girlfriends should treat each other |
| | Gender role norms about healthy dating relationships | Modeling | Role model stories about how different couples treat each other |
| | | Discussion | Group processing of role model stories |

**Table 6.21**    (*Continued*)

| Behavioral Outcome | Determinants and Change Objectives | Method | Application |
|---|---|---|---|
| Use condoms correctly and consistently if having sex* | Knowledge about correct condom use | Information | Quiz on correct condom use |
| | | | Animated cartoon on steps to correct condom use |
| | Skills & self-efficacy for negotiating condom use | Skills training | Help animated cartoon couple to use effective condom negotiation skills |
| | Skills & self-efficacy for using condom correctly | Guided practice | Place condom use steps in correct order |
| | Normative beliefs about condom use | Modeling | Peer video on importance of using condoms |
| | Outcome expectations about condom use | Modeling | MTV style "real world" video series – characters choose to use condoms to reduce risk of pregnancy and STIs |

*Condom use applications were restricted to computer-based lessons to reduce potential embarrassment for middle school students and teachers

**Table 6.22**    Sample of Methods and Applications for Parents From It's Your Game . . . Keep It Real

| Environmental Outcome | Determinants and Change Objectives | Method | Application |
|---|---|---|---|
| Communicate with child about dating and sexual health topics | Knowledge that parents can influence child's dating and sexual behavior | Information | Credible expert provides data on parental influence on teen behavior |
| | | Modeling | Role model story of parent who talked with child and had positive outcomes |
| | Skills & self-efficacy to listen calmly and nonjudgmentally | Skills training | Ten tips for talking with your teen |
| | Perceived barriers to discussing dating and sexual health topics with child | Modeling | Role model story of parent who talked with child and had positive outcomes |
| | | Skills training | Ten tips for talking with your teen |
| | | Planning coping responses | Credible expert provides advice that some embarrassment is normal |
| | Perceived susceptibility of child's risk of experiencing dating violence, pregnancy, HIV, or STIs | Information | Statistics on teen dating violence, teen births, and HIV/STIs |

**Table 6.22** *(Continued)*

| Environmental Outcome | Determinants and Change Objectives | Method | Application |
|---|---|---|---|
| Monitor child's time, friendships, and dating activities | Knowledge of child's friends and activities | Active learning | Quiz on child's friends (check answers with child) |
| | | Chunking | Mnemonic device - Four Ws (where, what, who, when) |
| | Skills and self-efficacy to monitor child's friends and activities | Guided practice | Step-by-step tips on "Staying Involved in Your Teen's Life" and "Knowing Your Child's Friends and Their Parents" |
| | Perceived barriers to monitoring child's friends and activities | Scenario-based risk information | Credible expert responds to situation in which child does not follow rules |
| | | Planning coping responses | Tips on how to cope when parent has trouble discussing monitoring effectively with child |
| | Outcome expectations for monitoring child's friends and activities | Anticipated regret | Role model story showing potential dangers of not monitoring child's friends and activities |

To assure that they had methods and applications to cover all the change objectives from all the matrices and to assure that all applications contained well-translated methods, the planning group organized design documents (see Chapter 7 for more detail) for each application that covered intended methods and the change objectives that were to be influenced by each method.

The other important issue when designing applications is to ensure that as the methods are translated, the parameters under which a particular method could be expected to be effective are present. For example, in order to be effective, the role-model stories had to be credible so that youth and parents could identify with them; the behaviors that were desired needed to be clearly discernible; and the role model had to be reinforced. The planners had to keep these parameters in mind for every application that included a role model—for example, videos and newsletter stories. The youth advisory group reviewed all scripts and story boards (see Chapter 7) as they were developed to ensure that the role models and situations were credible.

## Summary

This chapter explained creative, theory- and evidence-based program design. We discussed the importance of all program components having theoretical behavior change methods as well as practical applications;

at both the individual level and the environmental level. Planners first generate program ideas with the planning group. They describe program themes, components, scope, and sequence. Then they choose theory-based change methods to address program objectives, applying the core processes provided in Chapter 1. Tables of methods in this chapter provided definitions, parameters for application, and examples at individual and environmental levels. In the last task planners select or design practical applications of change methods. The chapter emphasized the importance of applying the methods correctly using the parameters for use.

## Discussion Questions and Learning Activities

1. Describe and give examples of program structures including: themes, components, scope, sequence, and delivery vehicles.

2. Explain the characteristics that distinguish theoretical methods from practical applications. Give examples of theoretical methods and related practical applications.

3. Discuss why it is important to review program ideas with intended program participants before making decisions on what methods and practical applications will be used to plan the interventions.

4. Describe how core processes can be used to choose theoretical methods. Give an example of a question that can be asked to guide the use of core processes to choose theoretical methods.

5. Discuss examples of basic methods that can be applied at the individual level and examples that can be applied at environmental levels of intervention.

6. For each of the following categories of determinants or environmental change, select one method and describe the parameters for use that are critical for the method to influence a change: knowledge, awareness and risk perception, habits and automatic behavior, attitudes, social influence, skills and self-efficacy, social norms, organizational change, community change, and policy change.

7. Describe your ideas for organizing methods and applications into an intervention program.

8. For each of the theoretical methods selected for the intervention, discuss the parameters that would have to be considered to ensure that the application of the methods would likely be effective in changing the determinants of behavior and environmental outcomes.

# References

Abraham, C., & Graham-Rowe, E. (2009). Are worksite interventions effective in increasing physical activity? A systematic review and meta-analysis. *Health Psychology Review, 3*(1), 108–144.

Abraham, C., & Michie, S. (2008). A taxonomy of behavior change techniques used in interventions. *Health Psychology, 27*(3), 379–387.

Abraham, C., & Sheeran, P. (2004). Deciding to exercise: The role of anticipated regret. *British Journal of Health Psychology, 9*(2), 269–278.

Achtziger, A., Gollwitzer, P. M., & Sheeran, P. (2008). Implementation intentions and shielding goal striving from unwanted thoughts and feelings. *Personality & Social Psychology Bulletin, 34*(3), 381–393.

Ajzen, I., Czasch, C., & Flood, M. G. (2009). From intentions to behavior: Implementation intention, commitment, and conscientiousness. *Journal of Applied Social Psychology, 39*(6), 1356–1372.

Aronson, E. (2015). Jigsaw classroom. Retrieved from http://www.jigsaw.org/

Atkinson, N. L., & Gold, R. S. (2002). The promise and challenge of eHealth interventions. *American Journal of Health Behavior, 26*(6), 494–503.

Bandura, A. (1986). *Social foundations of thought and action: A Social Cognitive Theory*. Englewood Cliffs, NJ: Prentice-Hall.

Bandura, A. (1997). *Self-efficacy: The exercise of control*. New York, NY: W.H. Freeman.

Baranowski, T., Buday, R., Thompson, D. I., & Baranowski, J. (2008). Playing for real: Video games and stories for health-related behavior change. *American Journal of Preventive Medicine, 34*(1), 74–82. e10.

Bartholomew, L. K., Czyzewski, D. I., Swank, P. R., McCormick, L., & Parcel, G. S. (2000a). Maximizing the impact of the cystic fibrosis family education program: Factors related to program diffusion. *Family & Community Health, 22*(4), 27–47.

Bartholomew, L., Gold, R., Parcel, G., Czyzewski, D., Sockrider, M., Fernández, M., ... Swank, P. (2000b). Watch, Discover, Think, and Act: Evaluation of computer assisted instruction to improve asthma self-management in inner-city children. *Patient Education and Counseling, 39*(2), 269–280.

Bartholomew, L. K., Markham, C. M., Ruiter, R. A. C., Fernández, M. E., Kok, G., & Parcel, G. S. (2016). *Planning health promotion programs: An Intervention Mapping approach* (4th ed.). San Francisco: CA: Jossey-Bass.

Bartholomew, L. K., Parcel, G. S., Kok, G., & Gottlieb, N. H. (2001). *Planning health promotion programs: An Intervention Mapping approach* (1st ed.). San Francisco: CA: Jossey-Bass.

Bartholomew, L. K., Parcel, G. S., Kok, G., & Gottlieb, N. H. (2006). *Planning health promotion programs: An Intervention Mapping approach* (2nd ed.). San Francisco: CA: Jossey-Bass.

Bartholomew, L. K., Parcel, G. S., Kok, G., Gottlieb, N. H., & Fernández, M. E. (2011). *Planning health promotion programs: An Intervention Mapping approach* (3rd ed.). San Francisco: CA: Jossey-Bass.

Bartholomew, L. K., Parcel, G. S., Seilheimer, D. K., Czyzewski, D., Spinelli, S. H., & Congdon, B. (1991). Development of a health education program to promote the self-management of cystic fibrosis. *Health Education & Behavior*, *18*(4), 429–443.

Bartholomew, L., Shegog, R., Parcel, G., Gold, R., Fernández, M., Czyzewski, D., ... Berlin, N. (2000c). Watch, discover, think, and act: A model for patient education program development. *Patient Education and Counseling*, *39*(2), 253–268.

Batson, C. D., Chang, J., Orr, R., & Rowland, J. (2002). Empathy, attitudes, and action: Can feeling for a member of a stigmatized group motivate one to help the group? *Personality and Social Psychology Bulletin*, *28*(12), 1656–1666.

Begley, C., Shegog, R., Harding, A., Goldsmith, C., Hope, O., & Newmark, M. (2015). Longitudinal feasibility of MINDSET: A clinic decision aid for epilepsy self-management. *Epilepsy & Behavior*, *44*, 143–150.

Bender, J. L., Yue, R. Y., To, M. J., Deacken, L., & Jadad, A. R. (2013). A lot of action, but not in the right direction: Systematic review and content analysis of smartphone applications for the prevention, detection, and management of cancer. *Journal of Medical Internet Research*, *15*(12), e287.

Best, A., Greenhalgh, T., Lewis, S., Saul, J. E., Carroll, S., & Bitz, J. (2012). Large system transformation in health care: A realist review. *Milbank Quarterly*, *90*(3), 421–456.

Bos, A. E., Schaalma, H. P., & Pryor, J. B. (2008). Reducing AIDS-related stigma in developing countries: The importance of theory-and evidence-based interventions. *Psychology, Health & Medicine*, *13*(4), 450–460.

Brown, L. D., Bammer, G., Batliwala, S., & Kunreuther, F. (2003). Framing practice-research engagement for democratizing knowledge. *Action Research*, *1*(1), 81–102.

Brug, J., Steenhuis, I., van Assema, P., & de Vries, H. (1996). The impact of a computer-tailored nutrition intervention. *Preventive Medicine*, *25*(3), 236–242.

Butterfoss, F. D. (2007). *Coalitions and partnerships in community health*. Hoboken, NJ: John Wiley & Sons.

Butterfoss, F. D., & Kegler, M. C. (2009). The community coalition action theory. In R. J. DiClemente, R. A. Crosby, & M. C. Kegler (Eds.), *Emerging theories in health promotion practice and research* (2nd ed., pp. 237–276). San Francisco, CA: Jossey-Bass.

Butterfoss, F. D., Kegler, M. C., & Francisco, V. T. (2008). Mobilizing organizations for health promotion: Theories of organizational change. In K. Glanz, B. K. Rimer, & K. Viswanath (Eds.), *Health behavior and health education: Theory, research, and practice* (4th ed., pp. 335–362). San Francisco, CA: Jossey-Bass.

Chang, T., Chopra, V., Zhang, C., & Woolford, S. J. (2013). The role of social media in online weight management: Systematic review. *Journal of Medical Internet Research*, *15*(11), e262.

Cheng, H., Kotler, P., & Lee, N. R. (Eds.). (2011). *Social marketing for public health: Global trends and success stories*. Sudbury, MA: Jones and Bartlett Publishers, LLC.

Christoffel, K. K. (2000). Public health advocacy: Process and product. *American Journal of Public Health, 90*(5), 722–726.

Cialdini, R. B. (2008). *Influence: Science and practice.* Needham Heights, MA: Allyn & Bacon.

Clavier, C., & De Leeuw, E. (Eds.). (2013). *Health promotion and the policy process.* Oxford, England: Oxford University Press.

Cohen, G. L., & Sherman, D. K. (2014). The psychology of change: Self-affirmation and social psychological intervention. *Annual Review of Psychology, 65*, 333–371.

Cole-Lewis, H., & Kershaw, T. (2010). Text messaging as a tool for behavior change in disease prevention and management. *Epidemiologic Reviews, 32*, 56–69.

Coyle, K. K., Kirby, D. B., Marin, B. V., Gomez, C. A., & Gregorich, S. E. (2004). Draw the Line/Respect the Line: A randomized trial of a middle school intervention to reduce sexual risk behaviors. *American Journal of Public Health, 94*(5), 843–851.

Coyle, K. K., Kirby, D., Parcel, G., Basen-Engquist, K., Banspach, S., Rugg, D., & Weil, M. (1996). Safer Choices: A multicomponent school-based HIV/STD and pregnancy prevention program for adolescents. *The Journal of School Health, 66*(3), 89–94.

Crano, W. D., & Prislin, R. (Eds.). (2011). *Attitudes and attitude change.* New York, NY: Psychology Press.

Creer, T. L. (2000). Self-management of chronic illness. In M. Boekaerts, P. R. Pintrich, & M. Zeidner (Eds.), *Handbook of self-regulation* (pp. 601–629). San Diego, CA: Academic Press.

Cummings, T. G., & Worley, C. G. (2014). *Organization development and change* (10th ed.). Mason, OH: South-Western Cengage Learning.

de Bono, E. (2015). *Lateral thinking: Creativity step by step.* New York, NY: Harper Colophon.

de Bono, E. (2006). *De Bono's thinking course: Powerful ways to transform your thinking.* Newmarket, Ontario: Pearson Education Canada.

de Bono, E. (2008). *Six frames: For thinking about information.* London, UK: Vermilion.

de Bruin, M., Crutzen, R., & Peters, G. Y. (2015). Everything should be as simple as possible, but this will still be complex: A reply to various commentaries on IPEBA. *Health Psychology Review, 9*(1), 38–41.

de Bruin, M., Viechtbauer, W., Schaalma, H. P., Kok, G., Abraham, C., & Hospers, H. J. (2010). Standard care impact on effects of highly active antiretroviral therapy adherence interventions: A meta-analysis of randomized controlled trials. *Archives of Internal Medicine, 170*(3), 240–250.

De Craemer, M., De Decker, E., De Bourdeaudhuij, I., Verloigne, M., Duvinage, K., Koletzko, B., ... Cardon, G. (2014). Applying the Intervention Mapping protocol to develop a kindergarten-based, family-involved intervention to increase European preschool children's physical activity levels: The ToyBox-Study. *Obesity Reviews, 15*, 14–26.

De Decker, E., De Craemer, M., De Bourdeaudhuij, I., Verbestel, V., Duvinage, K., Iotova, V., ... Cardon, G. (2014). Using the Intervention Mapping protocol to reduce European preschoolers' sedentary behavior, an application to the ToyBox-Study. *International Journal of Behavioral Nutrition & Physical Activity*, *11*(1), 1–35.

De Haes, W. F. (1987). Looking for effective drug education programmes: Fifteen years' exploration of the effects of different drug education programs. *Health Education Research*, *2*(4), 433–438.

de Ridder, D. (2014). Nudging for beginners: A shortlist of issues in urgent needs research. *The European Health Psychologist*, *16*(1), 2–5.

DeSmet, A., Van Ryckeghem, D., Compernolle, S., Baranowski, T., Thompson, D., Crombez, G., ... Van Cleemput, K. (2014). A meta-analysis of serious digital games for healthy lifestyle promotion. *Preventive Medicine*, *69*, 95–107.

de Vries, H., & Brug, J. (1999). Computer-tailored interventions motivating people to adopt health promoting behaviours: Introduction to a new approach. *Patient Education and Counseling*, *36*(2), 99–105.

Diamond, A. (2013). Executive functions. *Annual Review of Psychology*, *64*, 135–168.

DiClemente, R. J., Crosby, R. A., & Kegler, M. (2009). *Emerging theories in health promotion practice and research*. Hoboken, NJ: John Wiley & Sons.

Dijkstra, A., & de Vries, H. (1999). The development of computer-generated tailored interventions. *Patient Education and Counseling*, *36*(2), 193–203.

Dorfman, L., & Krasnow, I. D. (2014). Public health and media advocacy. *Annual Review of Public Health*, *35*, 293–306.

Edberg, M., & APA Publications and Communications Board Working Group on Journal Article Reporting Standards. (2007). *Essentials of health behavior: Social and behavioral theory in public health*. London, UK: Jones & Bartlett.

Eng, E., Rhodes, S. D., & Parker, E. (2009). Natural helper models to enhance a community's health and competence. In R. J. DiClemente, R. A. Crosby, & M. C. Kegler (Eds.), *Emerging theories in health promotion practice and research* (2nd ed., pp. 303–330). San Francisco, CA: Jossey-Bass.

Evans, R., Getz, J., & Raines, B. (1991). Theory-guided models on prevention of AIDS in adolescents. Paper Presented at the Science Weekend of the American Psychological Association, San Francisco, CA.

Evans, R., Getz, J., & Raines, B. (1992). Applying social inoculation concepts to prevention of HIV/AIDS in adolescents: Just say no is obviously not enough. Paper Presented at the Meeting of the Society of Behavioral Medicine, New York, NY.

Fernández, M. E., Gonzales, A., Tortolero-Luna, G., Partida, S., & Bartholomew, L. K. (2005). Using Intervention Mapping to develop a breast and cervical cancer screening program for Hispanic farmworkers: Cultivando La Salud. *Health Promotion Practice*, *6*(4), 394–404.

Fishbein, M., & Ajzen, I. (2010). *Predicting and changing behaviour: The Reasoned Action Approach*. New York, NY: Taylor & Francis.

Fishbein, M., & Cappella, J. N. (2006). The role of theory in developing effective health communications. *Journal of Communication*, *56*(S1), S1–S17.

Fjeldsoe, B. S., Marshall, A. L., & Miller, Y. D. (2009). Behavior change interventions delivered by mobile telephone short-message service. *American Journal of Preventive Medicine, 36*(2), 165–173.

Flaspohler, P., Duffy, J., Wandersman, A., Stillman, L., & Maras, M. A. (2008). Unpacking prevention capacity: An intersection of research-to-practice models and community-centered models. *American Journal of Community Psychology, 41*(3–4), 182–196.

Forsyth, D. R. (2014). *Group dynamics* (6th ed.). Belmont, CA: Wadsworth Cengage Learning.

Freire, P. (1973a). *Education for critical consciousness.* New York, NY: Seabury Press.

Freire, P. (1973b). *Pedagogy of the oppressed.* New York, NY: Seabury Press.

Freudenberg, N., & Tsui, E. (2014). Evidence, power, and policy change in community-based participatory research. *American Journal of Public Health, 104*(1), 11–14.

Friedman, R. H., Stollerman, J. E., Mahoney, D. M., & Rozenblyum, L. (1997). The virtual visit: Using telecommunications technology to take care of patients. *Journal of the American Medical Informatics Association, 4*(6), 413–425.

Galer-Unti, R. A., Tappe, M. K., & Lachenmayr, S. (2004). Advocacy 101: Getting started in health education advocacy. *Health Promotion Practice, 5*(3), 280–288.

Gedney, K., & Fultz, P. (1988). *The complete guide to creating successful brochures.* Asher-Gallant Press.

Glanz, K., & Bishop, D. B. (2010). The role of behavioral science theory in development and implementation of public health interventions. *Annual Review of Public Health, 31*, 399–418.

Glanz, K., Rimer, B. K., & Viswanath, K. (Eds.). (2015). *Health behavior: Theory, research, and practice* (5th ed.). San Francisco, CA: Jossey-Bass.

Gobet, F., Lane, P. C., Croker, S., Cheng, P. C., Jones, G., Oliver, I., & Pine, J. M. (2001). Chunking mechanisms in human learning. *Trends in Cognitive Sciences, 5*(6), 236–243.

Godden, D. R., & Baddeley, A. D. (1975). Context-dependent memory in two natural environments: On land and underwater. *British Journal of Psychology, 66*(3), 325–331.

Gold, J., Pedrana, A. E., Sacks-Davis, R., Hellard, M. E., Chang, S., Howard, S., ... Stoove, M. A. (2011). A systematic examination of the use of online social networking sites for sexual health promotion. *BMC Public Health, 11*, 583.

Gollwitzer, P. M., & Sheeran, P. (2006). Implementation intentions and goal achievement: A meta-analysis of effects and processes. *Advances in Experimental Social Psychology, 38*, 69–119.

Goodson, P. (2009). *Theory in health promotion research and practice: Thinking outside the box.* London, UK: Jones & Bartlett.

Gottlieb, N. H., Huang, P. P., Blozis, S. A., Guo, J., & Murphy Smith, M. (2001). The impact of put prevention into practice on selected clinical preventive services in five Texas sites. *American Journal of Preventive Medicine, 21*(1), 35–40.

Griffiths, F., Lindenmeyer, A., Powell, J., Lowe, P., & Thorogood, M. (2006). Why are health care interventions delivered over the internet? A systematic review of the published literature. *Journal of Medical Internet Research, 8*(2), e10.

Gurol-Urganci, I., de Jongh, T., Vodopivec-Jamsek, V., Atun, R., & Car, J. (2013). Mobile phone messaging reminders for attendance at healthcare appointments. *Cochrane Database of Systematic Reviews, 12*, CD007458.

Gustafson, D., Bosworth, K., Chewning, B., & Hawkins, R. (1987). Computer-based health promotion: Combining technological advances with problem-solving techniques to effect successful health behavior changes. *Annual Review of Public Health, 8*(1), 387–415.

Gustafson, D. H., Hawkins, R. P., Boberg, E. W., McTavish, F., Owens, B., Wise, M., ... Pingree, S. (2002). CHESS: 10 years of research and development in consumer health informatics for broad populations, including the underserved. *International Journal of Medical Informatics, 65*(3), 169–177.

Gustafson, D., Wise, M., McTavish, F., Taylor, J. O., Wolberg, W., Stewart, J., ... Bosworth, K. (1994). Development and pilot evaluation of a computer-based support system for women with breast cancer. *Journal of Psychosocial Oncology, 11*(4), 69–93.

Hawkes, A. L., Atherton, J., Taylor, C. B., Scuffham, P., Eadie, K., Miller, N. H., & Oldenburg, B. (2009). Randomised controlled trial of a secondary prevention program for myocardial infarction patients ('ProActive Heart'): Study protocol. *BMC Cardiovascular Disorders, 9*(1), 16.

Hawkins, R. P., Kreuter, M., Resnicow, K., Fishbein, M., & Dijkstra, A. (2008). Understanding tailoring in communicating about health. *Health Education Research, 23*(3), 454–466.

Head, K. J., Noar, S. M., Iannarino, N. T., & Harrington, N. G. (2013). Efficacy of text messaging-based interventions for health promotion: A meta-analysis. *Social Science & Medicine, 97*, 41–48.

Heinen, M., Bartholomew, L. K., Wensing, M., Van de Kerkhof, P., & Van Achterberg, T. (2005). Lively Legs, the development of a lifestyle program for leg ulcer patients. *16th International Nursing Research Congress.*

Heinen, M. M., Bartholomew, L. K., Wensing, M., van de Kerkhof, P., & van Achterberg, T. (2006). Supporting adherence and healthy lifestyles in leg ulcer patients: Systematic development of the Lively Legs program for dermatology outpatient clinics. *Patient Education and Counseling, 61*(2), 279–291.

Heinen, M., Borm, G., van der Vleuten, C., Evers, A., Oostendorp, R., & van Achterberg, T. (2012). The Lively Legs self-management programme increased physical activity and reduced wound days in leg ulcer patients: Results from a randomized controlled trial. *International Journal of Nursing Studies, 49*(2), 151–161.

Hendrickx, L., Vlek, C., & Oppewal, H. (1989). Relative importance of scenario information and frequency information in the judgment of risk. *Acta Psychologica, 72*(1), 41–63.

Hernandez, B. F., Peskin, M., Shegog, R., Markham, C., Johnson, K., Ratliff, E. A., ... Tortolero, S. R. (2011). Choosing and maintaining programs for sex education in schools: The CHAMPSS model. *Journal of Applied Research on Children: Informing Policy for Children at Risk, 2*(2), 7.

Hieftje, K., Edelman, E. J., Camenga, D. R., & Fiellin, L. E. (2013). Electronic media–based health interventions promoting behavior change in youth: A systematic review. *JAMA Pediatrics, 167*(6), 574–580.

Hofmann, W., Friese, M., & Wiers, R. W. (2008). Impulsive versus reflective influences on health behavior: A theoretical framework and empirical review. *Health Psychology Review, 2*(2), 111–137.

Holt-Lunstad, J., & Uchino, B. (2015). Social support and health behavior. In K. Glanz, B. Rimer, & K. Viswanath (Eds.), *Health behavior: Theory, research and practice* (5th ed.). San Francisco, CA: Jossey-Bass.

Huang, J. S., Gottschalk, M., Pian, M., Dillon, L., Barajas, D., & Bartholomew, L. K. (2011). Transition to adult care: Systematic assessment of adolescents with chronic illnesses and their medical teams. *The Journal of Pediatrics, 159*(6), 994–998. e2.

Huang, J. S., Terrones, L., Tompane, T., Dillon, L., Pian, M., Gottschalk, M., ... Bartholomew, L. K. (2014). Preparing adolescents with chronic disease for transition to adult care: A technology program. *Pediatrics, 133*(6), e1639–e1646.

Jones, G. R. (2004). *Organizational theory, design, and change* (4th ed.). Upper Saddle River, NJ: Pearson/Prentice-Hall.

Kato, P. M. (2010). Video games in health care: Closing the gap. *Review of General Psychology, 14*(2), 113.

Kazdin, A. E. (2012). *Behavior modification in applied settings* (7th ed.). Long Grove, IL: Waveland Press.

Kelder, S., Hoelscher, D., & Perry, C. L. (2015). How individuals, environments, and health behaviour interact: Social Cognitive Theory. In K. Glanz, B. K. Rimer, & K. Viswanath (Eds.), *Health behavior: Theory, research, and practice* (5th ed., pp. 285–325). San Francisco, CA: Jossey-Bass.

Khan, L. K., Sobush, K., Keener, D., Goodman, K., Lowry, A., Kakietek, J., & Zaro, S. (2009). Recommended community strategies and measurements to prevent obesity in the United States. *Morbidity and Mortality Weekly Report, 58*(RR07), 1–26.

Kingdon, J. W. (2003). *Agenda, alternatives, and public policies* (2nd ed.). New York, NY: Longman.

Kirby, D. (2001). Understanding what works and what doesn't in reducing adolescent sexual risk-taking. *Family Planning Perspectives, 33*(6), 276–281.

Kirby, D. (2007). *Emerging answers 2007: Research findings on programs to reduce teen pregnancy and sexually transmitted diseases.* Washington, D.C.: The National Campaign to Prevent Teen and Unplanned Pregnancy.

Knai, C., McKee, M., & Pudule, I. (2011). Soft drinks and obesity in Latvia: A stakeholder analysis. *European Journal of Public Health, 21*(3), 295–299.

Kohl, L. F., Crutzen, R., & de Vries, N. K. (2013). Online prevention aimed at lifestyle behaviors: A systematic review of reviews. *Journal of Medical Internet Research, 15*(7), e146.

Kok, G., Gottlieb, N. H., Commers, M., & Smerecnik, C. (2008). The ecological approach in health promotion programs: A decade later. *American Journal of Health Promotion, 22*(6), 437–442.

Kok, G., Gottlieb, N. H., Panne, R., & Smerecnik, C. (2012). Methods for environmental change; an exploratory study. *BMC Public Health, 12,* 1037.

Kok, G., Gottlieb, N. H., Peters, G.-J. Y., Mullen, P. D., Parcel, G. S., Ruiter, R. A. C., ... Bartholomew, L. K. (2015). A taxonomy of behavior change methods: an Intervention Mapping approach. *Health Psychology Review.* Advance online publication. doi: 10.1080/17437199.2015.1077155.

Kok, G., Gurabardhi, Z., Gottlieb, N. H., & Zijlstra, F. R. H. (2015). Influencing organizations to promote health: Applying stakeholder theory. *Health Education & Behavior, 42*(IS), 123S–132S.

Kok, G., Harterink, P., Vriens, P., de Zwart, O., & Hospers, H. J. (2006). The Gay Cruise: Developing a theory- and evidence-based internet HIV-prevention intervention. *Sexuality Research & Social Policy, 3*(2), 52–67.

Kok, G., Schaalma, H., Ruiter, R. A. C., van Empelen, P., & Brug, J. (2004). Intervention Mapping: Protocol for applying health psychology theory to prevention programmes. *Journal of Health Psychology, 9*(1), 85–98.

Kools, M. (2012). Making written materials easy to use. In C. Abraham & M. Kools (Eds.), *Writing health communication: An evidence-based guide* (pp. 43–62). London, United Kingdom: Sage.

Kools, M., van de Wiel, M. W., Ruiter, R. A. C., Crüts, A., & Kok, G. (2006). The effect of graphic organizers on subjective and objective comprehension of a health education text. *Health Education & Behavior, 33*(6), 760–772.

Krebs, P., Prochaska, J. O., & Rossi, J. S. (2010). A meta-analysis of computer-tailored interventions for health behavior change. *Preventive Medicine, 51*(3), 214–221.

Kreuter, M. W., & McClure, S. M. (2004). The role of culture in health communication. *Annual Review of Public Health, 25,* 439–455.

Kreuter, M. W., Strecher, V. J., & Glassman, B. (1999). One size does not fit all: The case for tailoring print materials. *Annals of Behavioral Medicine, 21*(4), 276–283.

Latham, G. P., & Locke, E. A. (2007). New developments in and directions for goal-setting research. *European Psychologist, 12*(4), 290.

Lenhart, A., Arafeh, S., & Smith, A. (2008). *Writing, technology and teens.* Retrieved from http://www.pewinternet.org/2008/04/24/writing-technology-and-teens/

Link, B. G., & Phelan, J. C. (2001). Conceptualizing stigma. *Annual Review of Sociology, 17,* 363–385.

Long, T., Taubenheim, A. M., Wayman, J., Temple, S., & Ruoff, B. A. (2008). The heart truth: Using the power of branding and social marketing to increase awareness of heart disease in women. *Social Marketing Quarterly, 14*(3), 3–29.

Longest, B. B. (2006). *Health policymaking in the United States* (4th ed.). Chicago, IL: Health Administration Press.

Lu, A. S., Kharrazi, H., Gharghabi, F., & Thompson, D. (2013). A systematic review of health videogames on childhood obesity prevention and intervention. *Games for Health: Research, Development, and Clinical Applications, 2*(3), 131–141.

Lustria, M. L. A., Cortese, J., Noar, S. M., & Glueckauf, R. L. (2009). Computer-tailored health interventions delivered over the web: Review and analysis of key components. *Patient Education and Counseling, 74*(2), 156–173.

Maher, C. A., Lewis, L. K., Ferrar, K., Marshall, S., De Bourdeaudhuij, I., & Vandelanotte, C. (2014). Are health behavior change interventions that use online social networks effective? A systematic review. *Journal of Medical Internet Research, 16*(2), e40.

Maibach, E. W., & Cotton, D. (1995). Moving people to behavior change: A staged social cognitive approach to message design. In E. W. Maibach & R. L. Parrott (Eds.), *Designing health messages: Approaches from communication theory and public health practice* (pp. 41–64). Thousand Oaks, CA: Sage.

Maon, F., Lindgreen, A., & Swaen, V. (2009). Designing and implementing corporate social responsibility: An integrative framework grounded in theory and practice. *Journal of Business Ethics, 87*(1), 71–89.

Marlatt, G. A., & Donovan, D. M. (Eds.). (2005). *Relapse prevention: Maintenance strategies in the treatment of addictive behaviors* (2nd ed.). New York, NY: Guilford.

McAlister, A. L. (1991). Population behavior change: A theory-based approach. *Journal of Public Health Policy, 12*(3), 345–361.

McAlister, A., Johnson, W., Guenther-Grey, C., Fishbein, M., Higgins, D., & O'Reilly, K. (2000). Behavioral journalism for HIV prevention: Community newsletters influence risk-related attitudes and behavior. *Journalism & Mass Communication Quarterly, 77*(1), 143–159.

McCullum, C., Pelletier, D., Barr, D., Wilkins, J., & Habicht, J. P. (2004). Mechanisms of power within a community-based food security planning process. *Health Education & Behavior, 31*(2), 206–222.

McGuire, W. J. (2001). Input and output variables currently promising for constructing persuasive communications. In R. E. Rice & C. K. Atkin (Eds.), *Public communication campaigns* (3rd ed., pp. 22–48). Thousand Oaks, CA: Sage.

McLean, G. N. (2005). *Organiztional development: Principles, processes, performance.* San Francisco, CA: Berrett-Koehler.

McSweeney, F. K., & Murphy, E. S. (2014). *The Wiley Blackwell handbook of operant and classical conditioning.* Chichester, United Kingdom: John Wiley & Sons.

Mevissen, F. E., Meertens, R. M., Ruiter, R. A. C., Feenstra, H., & Schaalma, H. P. (2009). HIV/STI risk communication: The effects of scenario-based risk information and frequency-based risk information on perceived susceptibility to chlamydia and HIV. *Journal of Health Psychology, 14*(1), 78–87.

Mevissen, F. E., Meertens, R. M., Ruiter, R. A. C., & Schaalma, H. P. (2010). Testing implicit assumptions and explicit recommendations: The effects of probability information on risk perception. *Journal of Health Communication, 15*(6), 578–589.

Michie, S., Ashford, S., Sniehotta, F. F., Dombrowski, S. U., Bishop, A., & French, D. P. (2011). A refined taxonomy of behaviour change techniques to help people change their physical activity and healthy eating behaviours: The CALO-RE taxonomy. *Psychology & Health, 26*(11), 1479–1498.

Michie, S., Richardson, M., Johnston, M., Abraham, C., Francis, J., Hardeman, W., ... Wood, C. E. (2013). The behavior change technique taxonomy (v1) of 93 hierarchically clustered techniques: Building an international consensus for the reporting of behavior change interventions. *Annals of Behavioral Medicine, 46*(1), 81–95.

Migneault, J. P., Farzanfar, R., Wright, J. A., & Friedman, R. H. (2006). How to write health dialog for a talking computer. *Journal of Biomedical Informatics, 39*(5), 468–481.

Mikolajczak, J., Kok, G., & Hospers, H. J. (2008). Queermasters: Developing a theory- and evidence-based internet HIV-prevention intervention to promote HIV-testing among men who have sex with men (MSM). *Applied Psychology: An International Review, 57*(4), 681–697.

Miller, W. R., & Rollnick, S. (2012). *Motivational interviewing: Helping people change* (3rd ed.). New York, NY: Guilford press.

Minkler, M. (Ed.). (2012). *Community organizing and community building for health and welfare* (3rd ed.). New Brunswick, NJ: Rutgers University Press.

Minkler, M., & Wallerstein, N. (Eds.). (2008). *Community-based participatory research for health: From process to outcomes* (2nd ed.). San Francisco, CA: Jossey-Bass.

Mitchell, C. U., & LaGory, M. (2002). Social capital and mental distress in an impoverished community. *City & Community, 1*(2), 199–222.

Mitchell, R. K., Agle, B. R., & Wood, D. J. (1997). Toward a theory of stakeholder identification and salience: Defining the principle of who and what really counts. *Academy of Management Review, 22*(4), 853–886.

Mollen, S., Ruiter, R. A. C., & Kok, G. (2010). Current issues and new directions in psychology and health: What are the oughts? The adverse effects of using social norms in health communication. *Psychology & Health, 25*(3), 265–270.

Montaño, D. E., & Kasprzyk, D. (2015). Theory of Reasoned Action, Theory of Planned Behavior, and the Integrated Behavioral Model. In K. Glanz, B. K. Rimer, & K. Viswanath (Eds.), *Health behavior: Theory, research, and practice* (5th ed., pp. 168–222). San Francisco, CA: Jossey-Bass.

Mosca, L., Mochari-Greenberger, H., Dolor, R. J., Newby, L. K., & Robb, K. J. (2010). Twelve-year follow-up of American women's awareness of cardiovascular disease risk and barriers to heart health. *Circulation. Cardiovascular Quality and Outcomes, 3*(2), 120–127.

Moyer-Gusé, E. (2008). Toward a theory of entertainment persuasion: Explaining the persuasive effects of Entertainment-Education messages. *Communication Theory, 18*(3), 407–425.

Murphy-Smith, M., Meyer, B., Hitt, J., Taylor-Seehafer, M. A., & Tyler, D. O. (2004). Put prevention into practice implementation model: Translating practice into theory. *Journal of Public Health Management and Practice, 10*(2), 109–115.

Napolitano, M. A., & Marcus, B. H. (2002). Targeting and tailoring physical activity information using print and information technologies. *Exercise and Sport Sciences Reviews, 30*(3), 122–128.

National Cancer Institute. (2007). *Greater than the sum: Systems thinking in tobacco control (Publication no. 06-6085, Tobacco Control Monograph no. 18).* Bethesda, MD: US Department of Health and Human Services, National Institutes of Health, National Cancer Institute.

Ng, J. Y., Ntoumanis, N., Thøgersen-Ntoumani, C., Deci, E. L., Ryan, R. M., Duda, J. L., & Williams, G. C. (2012). Self-Determination Theory applied to health contexts: A meta-analysis. *Perspectives on Psychological Science, 7*(4), 325–340.

Noar, S. M., Benac, C. N., & Harris, M. S. (2007). Does tailoring matter? Meta-analytic review of tailored print health behavior change interventions. *Psychological Bulletin, 133*(4), 673.

Paluck, E. L., & Green, D. P. (2009). Prejudice reduction: What works? A review and assessment of research and practice. *Annual Review of Psychology, 60*, 339–367.

Payne, H. E., Lister, C., West, J. H., & Bernhardt, J. M. (2015). Behavioral functionality of mobile apps in health interventions: A systematic review of the literature. *JMIR mHealth and uHealth, 3*(1), e20.

Perry, C. L., Sellers, D. E., Johnson, C., Perdersen, S., Bachman, K. J., Parcel, G. S., … Cook, K. (1997). The Child and Adolescent Trial for Cardiovascular Health (CATCH): Intervention, implementation, and feasibility for elementary schools in the United States. *Health Education and Behavior, 24*, 716–735.

Peters, G. Y., de Bruin, M., & Crutzen, R. (2015). Everything should be as simple as possible, but no simpler: Towards a protocol for accumulating evidence regarding the active content of health behaviour change interventions. *Health Psychology Review, 9*(1), 1–14.

Peters, G. Y., Ruiter, R. A. C., & Kok, G. (2013). Threatening communication: A critical re-analysis and a revised meta-analytic test of fear appeal theory. *Health Psychology Review, 7*(sup1), S8–S31.

Peters, G. Y., Ruiter, R. A. C., & Kok, G. (2014). Threatening communication: A qualitative study of fear appeal effectiveness beliefs among intervention developers, policymakers, politicians, scientists, and advertising professionals. *International Journal of Psychology, 49*(2), 71–79.

Peters, L. W., Kok, G., Ten Dam, G. T., Buijs, G. J., & Paulussen, T. G. (2009). Effective elements of school health promotion across behavioral domains: A systematic review of reviews. *BMC Public Health, 9*, 182.

Petraglia, J. (2007). Narrative intervention in behavior and public health. *Journal of Health Communication, 12*(5), 493–505.

Pettigrew, T. F., & Tropp, L. R. (2006). A meta-analytic test of intergroup contact theory. *Journal of Personality and Social Psychology, 90*(5), 751.

Petty, R. E., Barden, J., & Wheeler, S. C. (2009). The Elaboration Likelihood Model of persuasion: Developing health promotions for sustained behavioral change. In R. J. DiClemente, R. A. Crosby, & M. Kegler (Eds.), *Emerging theories in health promotion practice and research* (2nd ed., pp. 185–214). San Francisco, CA: Jossey-Bass.

Petty, R., & Cacioppo, J. T. (2012). *Communication and persuasion: Central and peripheral routes to attitude change.* New York, NY: Springer Science & Business Media.

Petty, R. E., & Wegener, D. T. (1998). Attitude change: Multiple roles for persuasive variables. In D. T. Gilbert, S. T. Fiske, & G. Lindzey (Eds.), *The handbook of social psychology* (4th ed., pp. 323–390). Boston, MA: McGraw-Hill.

Pietrzak, E., Pullman, S., & McGuire, A. (2014). Using virtual reality and videogames for traumatic brain injury rehabilitation: A structured literature review. *Games for Health: Research, Development, and Clinical Applications, 3*(4), 202–214.

Piette, J. D., Mendoza-Avelares, M. O., Ganser, M., Mohamed, M., Marinec, N., & Krishnan, S. (2011). A preliminary study of a cloud-computing model for chronic illness self-care support in an underdeveloped country. *American Journal of Preventive Medicine, 40*(6), 629–632.

Porras, J. I., & Robertson, P. J. (1987). Organizational development theory: A typology and evaluation. In R. W. Woodman & W. A. Pasmore (Eds.), *Research in organizational change and development* (vol. 1; pp. 1–57). Greenwich, CT: JAI Press.

Portnoy, D. B., Scott-Sheldon, L. A., Johnson, B. T., & Carey, M. P. (2008). Computer-delivered interventions for health promotion and behavioral risk reduction: A meta-analysis of 75 randomized controlled trials, 1988–2007. *Preventive Medicine, 47*(1), 3–16.

Prochaska, J. O., Redding, C. A., & Evers, K. E. (2015). The transtheoretical model of stages of change. In K. Glanz, B. K. Rimer, & K. Viswanath (Eds.), *Health behavior: Theory, research, and practice* (5th ed., pp. 168–222). San Francisco, CA: Jossey-Bass.

Prokhorov, A. V., Kelder, S. H., Shegog, R., Murray, N., Peters, R., Jr., Agurcia-Parker, C., ... Marani, S. (2008). Impact of a smoking prevention interactive experience (ASPIRE), an interactive, multimedia smoking prevention and cessation curriculum for culturally diverse high-school students. *Nicotine & Tobacco Research, 10*(9), 1477–1485.

Ramelson, H. Z., Friedman, R. H., & Ockene, J. K. (1999). An automated telephone-based smoking cessation education and counseling system. *Patient Education and Counseling, 36*(2), 131–144.

Ramirez, A. G., Villarreal, R., Mcalister, A., Gallion, K. J., Suarez, L., & Gomez, P. (1999). Advancing the role of participatory communication in the diffusion of cancer screening among Hispanics. *Journal of Health Communication, 4*(1), 31–36.

Randolph, W., & Viswanath, K. (2004). Lessons learned from public health mass media campaigns: Marketing health in a crowded media world. *Annual Review of Public Health, 25*, 419–437.

Reininger, B. M., Barroso, C. S., Mitchell-Bennett, L., Cantu, E., Fernandez, M. E., Gonzalez, D. A., ... McAlister, A. (2010). Process evaluation and participatory methods in an obesity-prevention media campaign for Mexican Americans. *Health Promotion Practice, 11*(3), 347–357.

Richard, R., Pligt, J., & de Vries, N. (1995). Anticipated affective reactions and prevention of AIDS. *British Journal of Social Psychology, 34*(1), 9–21.

Rideout, V. (2001). *Generation rx.com: How young people use the internet for health information. Kaiser Family Foundation survey.* Menlo Park, CA: Henry J. Kaiser Family Foundation.

Robbins, S. J., Schwartz, B., & Wasserman, E. A. (2001). *Psychology of learning and behavior* (5th ed.). New York, NY: Norton.

Rogers, E. M. (2003). *Diffusion of innovations* (5th ed.). New York, NY: Free Press.

Rothman, J. (2004). Three models of community organization practice, their mixing and phasing. In F. M. Cox, J. L. Erlich, J. Rotherman, & J. E. Tropman (Eds.), *Strategies of community organization: A book of readings* (3rd ed.). Itasca, IL: F.E. Peacock.

Ruiter, R. A. C., Kessels, L. T., Peters, G. Y., & Kok, G. (2014). Sixty years of fear appeal research: Current state of the evidence. *International Journal of Psychology, 49*(2), 63–70.

Ryan, R. M., & Deci, E. L. (2000). Self-Determination Theory and the facilitation of intrinsic motivation, social development, and well-being. *American Psychologist, 55*(1), 68.

Sabatier, P. A. (2003). Policy change over a decade or more. In P. R. Lee, C. L. Estes, & F. M. Rodriguez (Eds.), *The nation's health* (pp. 143–174). Sudbury, MA: Jones and Bartlett.

Schaalma, H. P., Abraham, C., Gillmore, M. R., & Kok, G. (2004). Sex education as health promotion: What does it take? *Archives of Sexual Behavior, 33*(3), 259–269.

Schaalma, H., & Kok, G. (2001). A school AIDS prevention program in the Netherlands. *Intervention Mapping: Designing theory- and evidence-based health promotion programs* (pp. 353–386). Mountain View, CA, Mayfield.

Schaalma, H., & Kok, G. (2009). Decoding health education interventions: The times are a-changin'. *Psychology and Health, 24*(1), 5–9.

Schaalma, H., Kok, G., Poelman, J., & Reinders, J. (1994). The development of AIDS education for Dutch secondary schools: A systematic approach. In D. R. Rutter (Ed.), *The social psychology of health and safety: European perspectives* (pp. 175–194). Aldershot, United Kingdom: Avebury.

Shaw, B., Gustafson, D. H., Hawkins, R., McTavish, F., McDowell, H., Pingree, S., & Ballard, D. (2006). How underserved breast cancer patients use and benefit from eHealth programs implications for closing the digital divide. *American Behavioral Scientist, 49*(6), 823–834.

Shegog, R., Bartholomew, L. K., Gold, R. S., Pierrel, E., Parcel, G. S., Sockrider, M. M. et al. (1999). *Self-management education for pediatric chronic disease: A description of the Watch, Discover, Think, and Act asthma computer program.* Unpublished manuscript.

Shegog, R., Bartholomew, L. K., Sockrider, M. M., Czyzewski, D. I., Pilney, S., Mullen, P. D., & Abramson, S. L. (2006). Computer-based decision support for pediatric asthma management: Description and feasibility of the Stop Asthma clinical system. *Health Informatics Journal, 12*(4), 259–273.

Shegog, R., Begley, C. E., Harding, A., Dubinsky, S., Goldsmith, C., Hope, O., & Newmark, M. (2013b). Description and feasibility of MINDSET: A clinic decision aid for epilepsy self-management. *Epilepsy & Behavior, 29*(3), 527–536.

Shen, F., & Han, J. (2014). Effectiveness of entertainment education in communicating health information: A systematic review. *Asian Journal of Communication, 24*(6), 605–616.

Skinner, C. S., Tiro, J., & Champion, V. L. (2015). The Health Belief Model. In K. Glanz, B. K. Rimer, & K. Viswanath (Eds.), *Health behavior and health education: Theory, research, and practice* (5th ed., pp. 131–167). San Francisco, CA: Jossey-Bass.

Smith, R. M. (2008). *Conquering the content: A step-by-step guide to web-based course development.* San Francisco, CA: Jossey-Bass.

Snow, D. A. (2004). Framing processes, ideology, and discursive fields. In D. A. Snow, S. A. Soule, & H. Kriesi (Eds.), *Blackwell companion to social movements* (pp. 380–412). Oxford, United Kingdom: Blackwell.

Soet, J. E., & Basch, C. E. (1997). The telephone as a communication medium for health education. *Health Education & Behavior, 24*(6), 759–772.

Steen, R. G. (2007). *The evolving brain: The known and the unknown* (illustrated ed.). Amherst, NY: Prometheus Books.

Storey, J. D., Hess, R., & Saffitz, G. (2015). Social marketing. In K. Glanz, B. K. Rimer, & K. Viswanath (Eds.), *Health behavior: Theory, research, and practice* (5th ed., pp. 745). San Francisco, CA: Jossey-Bass.

Suls, J., Martin, R., & Wheeler, L. (2002). Social comparison: Why, with whom, and with what effect? *Current Directions in Psychological Science, 11*(5), 159–163.

Ten Hoor, G. A., Peters, G. J., Kalagi, J., de Groot, L., Grootjans, K., Huschens, A., ... Kok, G. (2012). Reactions to threatening health messages. *BMC Public Health, 12*, 1011.

Thaler, R. H., & Sunstein, C. R. (2008). *Nudge.* New Haven, CT: Yale University Press.

Tolli, M. V. (2012). Effectiveness of peer education interventions for HIV prevention, adolescent pregnancy prevention and sexual health promotion for young people: A systematic review of European studies. *Health Education Research, 27*(5), 904–913.

Turner, J. C. (2005). Explaining the nature of power: A three-process theory. *European Journal of Social Psychology, 35*(1), 1–22.

Tyler, D. O., Taylor-Seehafer, M. A., & Murphy-Smith, M. (2004). Utilizing "PPIP Texas style!" in a medically underserved population. *Journal of Public Health Management and Practice, 10*(2), 100–108.

Valente, T. (2015). Social networks and health behavior. In K. Glanz., B. Rimer, & K. Viswanath (Eds.), *Health behavior: Theory, research and practice* (5th ed.). San Francisco, CA: Jossey-Bass.

van Achterberg, T., Huisman-de Waal, G. G., Ketelaar, N. A., Oostendorp, R. A., Jacobs, J. E., & Wollersheim, H. C. (2011). How to promote healthy behaviours in patients? An overview of evidence for behaviour change techniques. *Health Promotion International, 26*(2), 148.

van de Glind, I. M., Heinen, M. M., Evers, A. W., Wensing, M., & van Achterberg, T. (2012). Factors influencing the implementation of a lifestyle counseling program in patients with venous leg ulcers: A multiple case study. *Implement Science, 7*, 104.

Van't Riet, J., Cox, A. D., Cox, D., Zimet, G. D., De Bruijn, G., Van den Putte, B., ... Ruiter, R. A. C. (2014). Does perceived risk influence the effects of message framing? A new investigation of a widely held notion. *Psychology & Health, 29*(8), 933–949.

Verplanken, B., & Aarts, H. (1999). Habit, attitude, and planned behaviour: Is habit an empty construct or an interesting case of goal-directed automaticity? *European Review of Social Psychology, 10*(1), 101–134.

Vollmer Dahlke, D., Fair, K., Hong, Y. A., Beaudoin, C. E., Pulczinski, J., & Ory, M. G. (2015). Apps seeking theories: Results of a study on the use of health behavior change theories in cancer survivorship mobile apps. *JMIR mHealth and uHealth, 3*(1), e31.

Wallack, L. (2008). Media advocacy: A strategy for empowering people and communities. In M. Minkler (Ed.), *Community organizing and community building for health* (2nd ed., pp. 419–432). New Brunswick, NJ: Rutgers University Press.

Wallack, L., Dorfman, L., Jernigan, D., & Themba, M. (1993). *Media advocacy and public health: Power for prevention*. Thousand Oaks, CA: Sage.

Wallerstein, N., Minkler, M., Carter-Edwards, L., Avila, M., & Sanchez, V. (2015). Improving health through community engagement and community building. In K. Glanz, B. Rimer, & K. Viswanath (Eds.), *Health behavior: Theory, research, and practice* (5th ed.). San Francisco, CA: Jossey-Bass.

Wallerstein, N., Sanchez, V., & Velarde, L. (2004). Freirian praxis in health education and community organizing: A case study of an adolescent prevention program. In M. Minkler (Ed.), *Community organizing and community building for health* (2nd ed., pp. 218–236). Piscataway, NJ: Rutgers University Press.

Walthouwer, M. J. L., Oenema, A., Soetens, K., Lechner, L., & de Vries, H. (2013). Systematic development of a text-driven and a video-driven web-based computer-tailored obesity prevention intervention. *BMC Public Health, 13*, 978.

Weible, C. M. (2008). Expert-based information and policy subsystems: A review and synthesis. *Policy Studies Journal, 36*(4), 615–635.

Weible, C. M., Sabatier, P. A., & McQueen, K. (2009). Themes and variations: Taking stock of the Advocacy Coalition Framework. *Policy Studies Journal, 37*(1), 121–140.

Weick, K. E., & Quinn, R. E. (1999). Organizational change and development. *Annual Review of Psychology, 50*(1), 361–386.

Weinstein, N. D., Sandman, P. M., & Blalock, S. J. (2008). The precaution adoption process model. In K. Glanz, F. M. Lewis, & B. K. Rimer (Eds.), *Health behavior and health education: Theory, research, and practice* (4th ed., pp. 123–165). San Francisco, CA: Jossey-Bass.

Werrij, M. Q., Ruiter, R. A. C., Riet, J. V. T., & de Vries, H. (2012). Message framing. In C. Abraham & M. Kools (Eds.), *Writing health communication: An evidence-based guide* (pp. 134–143). London, United Kingdom: Sage.

Whittaker, R., Borland, R., Bullen, C., Lin, R. B., McRobbie, H., & Rodgers, A. (2009). Mobile phone-based interventions for smoking cessation. *Cochrane Database of Systematic Reviews, 4.*

Wilkin, H. A., Valente, T. W., Murphy, S., Cody, M. J., Huang, G., & Beck, V. (2007). Does entertainment-education work with Latinos in the United States? Identification and the effects of a telenovela breast cancer storyline. *Journal of Health Communication, 12*(5), 455–469.

Wood, W., & Neal, D. T. (2007). A new look at habits and the habit-goal interface. *Psychological Review, 114*(4), 843.

World Health Organization Regional Office for Europe. (2002). Community participation in local health and sustainable development approaches and techniques. Retrieved from http://www.euro.who.int/__data/assets/pdf_file/0013/101065/E78652.pdf

Wright, P. (2012). Using graphics effectively in text. In C. Abraham & M. Kools (Eds.), *Writing health communication: An evidence-based guide* (pp. 62–82). London, United Kingdom: Sage.

Zahariadis, N. (2007). The multiple streams framework: Structure, limitations, prospects. In P. A. Sabatier (Ed.), *Theories of the policy process* (2nd ed., pp. 65–92). Boulder, CO: Westview Press.

Zajonc, R. B. (2001). Mere exposure: A gateway to the subliminal. *Current Directions in Psychological Science, 10*(6), 224–228.

# INTERVENTION MAPPING STEP 4

*Program Production*

## Competency

- Use information from Steps 1–3 to produce program materials.

The purpose of this chapter is to enable program planners to produce creative program messages, materials, and protocols in support of health promotion programs. The materials are based on the program plan from Step 3. The program will often be multicomponent, with complex activities to address the needs of both at-risk groups and environmental agents, with each part of the program typically supported by materials such as computer programs, flip charts, text messages, and other resources. The goal is that these materials are creative, effective pieces that promote and support key messages of the planned behavioral- and environmental-change program. A challenge in this step is one of translation: designing the support materials so that the methods and practical applications are effectively operationalized and the change objectives accomplished.

The planning steps completed to this point have created the foundation for production of creative materials. Materials will emerge from the thinking captured in the matrix development and the selection of change methods and practical applications. In particular, the program materials should represent the parameters that pertain to the selected change methods (see Chapter 6). For example, if a planning team decides to use modeling (method), they must ensure that their program's role-model stories (practical application) include models with which participants can identify (parameter). The end product of this step should be materials that remain true to the planning in Steps 1, 2, and 3.

Another challenge of this step is to ensure that the final program "fits" with both the populations for whom it is intended and within the context(s) or setting(s) in which it will be delivered. Health educators can use this step in the planning process to obtain further input from potential participants, program adopters, and implementers. This step focuses on the health promotion program that is directed to the priority population and related environmental agents; the next step (Step 5) focuses on program materials for program adopters and implementers (see Chapter 8).

## Perspectives

Our perspective in this chapter is to encourage adherence to the plans from the previous steps to create engaging and culturally relevant materials. The program materials should be feasible to implement and should fit with the intervention context and setting.

### Using Steps 1, 2, and 3

Steps 1, 2, and 3 will inform the work to be completed in Step 4. In Step 2, the planners developed matrices of change objectives for the at-risk group and environmental agents. In Step 3, they identified methods and practical applications for each matrix, and generated an initial program scope, sequence, and themes. Now, they will produce messages and materials that will bring these ideas to life. There are multiple strategies for moving forward depending on budget and time frame. Sometimes, the planning team will be able to locate existing materials that match the objectives, change methods, and applications identified in previous steps; other times, the team will produce original material. Such production always requires plans (design documents) to ensure that program messages and materials meet the intervention specifications. Production sometimes requires creative consultants such as writers, graphic designers, and videographers. Working with these new team members will also require guidance from detailed planning documents.

### Designing for Implementation

As planners design program components and materials, they should continue to consider the intervention context and setting. They will want to involve potential participants in the program design. Also, if potential program adopters and implementers have not been involved on the planning team to this point, planners will need to recruit them to understand aspects of the implementation setting important to program design. These individuals can help planners understand what materials can be delivered feasibly and to further explore preferences of potential participants. They can also help planners consider aspects of program materials that are attractive to implementers such as low complexity, good fit with organizational routines, resource conserving, and easy to try (see Chapter 8). Seeing characteristics of materials and activities from the viewpoint of potential gatekeepers is important for both the initial implementation of the intervention and the later wide scale dissemination of a program that has been shown to be effective.

## Tasks for Step 4

## Refining Program Structure and Organization

The first task completed in Step 3 (i.e., generating program themes, components, scope, and sequence) lays the foundation for the task at hand. At this point, planners should have preliminary plans for program components, the order of presentation, and the change methods and practical applications to be included. Issues that have to be dealt with now are best summarized as a "reality check."

*The first task in Step 4 is to refine the program structure and organization that were generated in Step 3.*

### *Reaching the Intended Program Participants*

Program materials and activities are not the "program"; they support the program. They represent the interaction of the program participants with the change methods. They are what the participants see, do, read, hear, and feel as a part of the intervention. The first part of the "reality check" is to answer the question of feasibility. Where are potential program participants going to interact with the program? Is the planning group sure that participants will come into contact with what is planned? For example, planners may want to use a method that encourages social support enhancement by expanding the networks of families of chronically ill children. They might initially think of holding support groups, but they must ensure that they can reach their intended participants with this method.

### *Checking Budget and Time Constraints*

In Step 3, planners developed initial ideas for program components and what materials are needed to support them. For example, if part of a program will be incorporated into a school curriculum, what materials are needed for a teacher to effectively and efficiently deliver the curriculum? At this point, the planning team will need to develop final ideas that include reliable estimates of budget and time for development as well as budget and time for implementation. Are the program components and materials feasible given budget and time constraints? If not, the program structure and organization might need to be refined and priority messages, materials, and activities reconsidered. However, at this (and all) phases of program planning and production, health promoters must be sure that they do not lose change methods that cover all of the change objectives specified in Step 2.

Continuing the illustration of the school curriculum: The planning team will determine dose—how much material can be delivered and cognitively processed in one class hour and how many class hours can realistically be devoted to a health promotion program within a school semester or year? Sometimes considering these issues will bring up needed changes at the environmental level to facilitate implementation of the health promotion program. Making new plans to change the environment will require negotiations with stakeholders and refinement of the time line.

In general, if the planning group considers feasibility in terms of producing and delivering materials during Step 3, then no dramatic changes in program structure and organization are expected. Nevertheless, this task is crucial prior to preparing plans for program materials, as it helps to prevent issues from arising during the materials production process.

## Preparing Plans for Program Materials

The second task in Step 4 is preparing production plans (design documents).

In Step 4, program planners prepare production plans, or design documents, for all program materials. These documents will guide production to ensure that program materials and activities are culturally relevant, meet the program objectives, and follow the parameters for use of their selected change methods and practical applications.

### *Aiming at Cultural Relevance*

If program plans are not culturally grounded at this point in the planning process, the project is in trouble. If following Intervention Mapping, from the program's inception and through each step, the planning team will have involved community members. The team will have taken into account culture by fully describing the causes of health problems in specific groups (Step 1), suggesting what should change among members of the groups and in their environments (Step 2), and thinking about change method and practical applications with the potential program participants in mind (Step 3). However, the issues of cultural relevance resurface when the planning team begins to design materials. Resnicow, Baranowski, Ahluwalia, and Braithwaite (1999) define cultural sensitivity (referred to here as cultural relevance) as "the extent to which ethnic/cultural, characteristics, experience, norms, values, behavioral patterns and beliefs of a priority population as well as relevant historical, environmental, and social forces are incorporated in the design, delivery, and evaluation of targeted health promotion materials and programs" (p. 13). Even though there is sparse evidence about the impact of cultural relevance on the effectiveness of health promotion interventions or materials, there is expert agreement that cultural relevance is closely related to the principle of participation in program development and is a good thing (Davis, Peterson, Rothschild, & Resnicow, 2011; Kreuter et al., 2004; Kreuter et al., 2005; Resnicow et al., 1999; Resnicow et al., 2009).

Resnicow and colleagues (1999) define two primary dimensions of culture that are relevant to program development: deep structure and surface structure. Deep structure refers to the factors that influence the health behavior in the intervention's proposed recipients. According to Deshpande and colleagues (2009) aspects of culture that are relevant to the study of and intervention in health behavior include, "family relationships, rules for emotional expression, communication and affective styles, collectivism, individualism, spirituality and religiosity, myths, time orientation, ethnic identity, level of acculturation, resilience, medical mistrust and . . . coping behavior" (Deshpande, Sanders, Thompson, Vaughn, & Kreuter, 2009, p. 257). In the process of planning programs with Intervention Mapping, these aspects can influence what behaviors, environmental conditions, performance objectives, and determinants become the program focus. We hope that it is clear that if planners have not characterized these factors correctly to this point, attention to cultural relevance of materials is unlikely to be effective because the program will not have salience to the intended cultural group.

Assuming that the planning team has brought to bear the insights of the cultural group to the behaviors and determinants and the methods that can change them, they can turn their attention to surface structure and the creation of materials. Surface structure comprises the superficial but still important characteristics of a cultural group such as familiar people, language, music, clothing, and so on.

Kreuter, Lukwago, Bucholtz, Clark, and Sanders-Thompson (2003) propose five categories of mechanisms by which health promoters can work to achieve attention to both surface and deeper aspects of culture in their program planning:

- Peripheral processes match materials' characteristics to the culture's surface characteristics. This attempt to make materials familiar and comfortable to the intended audience relies heavily on visual aspects of production (Kostelnick, 1996; Moriarty, 1994; Shiffman, 1994).

- Evidential strategies remind the cultural group of the health problem's significance to them: for example, "African American children suffer twice the hospitalizations for asthma as white children."

- Linguistic strategies provide programs and materials in the language of the cultural group.

- Constituent-involving approaches cover several strategies for involving the intended program group, including hiring staff from the cultural group, using lay health workers from the group, and continuing to work with the group as members of the planning team.

- Sociocultural strategies embed health education in the context of broader cultural values and issues.

## Conducting Formative Research

Formative (preproduction) research elucidates characteristics of the intended participants' needs, cultural preferences, knowledge, attitudes, beliefs, and health literacy that relate to message, medium, and situation; production testing (pretesting—see Task 4 below), on the other hand, is a process in which prototypes of program materials are tested for audience reaction and to determine whether tailoring or targeting is needed (Atkin & Freimouth, 1989; Baranowski, Cerin, & Baranowski, 2009; Bellows, Anderson, Gould, & Auld, 2008; Cullen & Thompson, 2008; Sorensen et al., 2004; Vu, Murrie, Gonzalez, & Jobe, 2006; Young et al., 2006; Zapka, Lemon, Estabrook, & Jolicoeur, 2007). Regardless of the population's demographic, cultural, or clinical background, the conduct of formative research is an important step in the design of effective health materials.

In the preproduction research phase, the team may explore interpersonal as well as media channels to identify the best methods for intervention delivery to the participant population. Preproduction testing can include both informal feedback and ratings of sources, messages, themes, persuasive arguments, and stylistic devices. Focus groups are a widely used mechanism for preproduction testing (Della, DeJoy, Goetzel, Ozminkowski, & Wilson, 2008; Gilmore & Campbell, 2005; Krueger & Casey, 2009; M. G. Wilson et al., 2007; Wyatt, Krauskopf & Davidson, 2008; Young et al., 2006). For example, Rhee and colleagues used focus groups with adolescents to assess needs and learning preferences in planning a comprehensive asthma Internet site (Rhee, Wyatt, & Wenzel, 2006). Focus groups, typically held with 8 to 12 participants, allow for the review of concepts, messages, and materials with the participant population. A second method for identification of message needs and vehicle appropriateness are cognitive interviews, which allow you to better understand individual use and processing of information presented within your methods (Wilson, 1999).

**Culture-Oriented Formative Research** Formative research should include specific exploration of cultural issues (Bentley, et al., 2014; Horner et al., 2008). Resnicow and colleagues (1999) describe preproduction design of culturally oriented materials. They use focus groups, for example, "to explore the thoughts, feelings, experience, associations, language, assumptions, etc. regarding the target health behavior" (p. 15), allowing for identification and integration of the specific language of communities in messages. They suggest exploratory research with both the population group of interest and with a comparison group to clarify and determine the importance of ethnic differences. For example, Resnicow and colleagues (2009) developed a tailoring algorithm that included ethnic identity for newsletters to promote fruit and vegetable intake among African American adults. From formative research, they identified five ethnic identities that loosely corresponded to Black American, Afrocentric, Bicultural, Multicultural, and Assimilated. Results from a randomized controlled trial demonstrated that although the overall between-group effects were not significant, tailoring on ethnic identity may have improved the intervention's impact for some African American subgroups (Resincow et al., 2009). Programs should be culturally grounded to expand reach and acceptability and better promote targeted behavioral changes.

## *Developing Design Documents*

Whether the planning team hires creative consultants or produces materials themselves, they will need documents to convey the team's intent in detail to those who write or select content from available resources and design graphics and other communications. There are two basic types of design documents:

- A set of design documents from the planning team to the production team (whether the production team is member of planning team or creative consultants who are new to the project at this stage).

- A series of production design documents from the production team to the planning team showing detail about the creative translation of plans into materials and activities.

The first design documents the planning team will share with the production team is a project prospectus that gives the length of the product, a brief description of the audience, the way that the user will interact with the product, the purpose of the piece (the intended impact), the central messages, and the expected budget.

A second document from the planning team is the set of matrices from Step 2. Some teams highlight each set of change objectives as they pertain to each material or activity. A variety of highlighter colors are good for this purpose.

The design documents then become more specific with one document for each material. For example, Table 7.1 provides an overview of the materials developed for the community component of the T.L.L. Temple Foundation Stroke Project with highlights from each of their design documents (Morgenstern et al., 2003; 2002). (See publisher's website for the stroke case study; www.wiley.com/go/bartholomew4e). This project delivered methods through a series of billboards, public service announcements, brochures, one-to-one trainings, newspaper stories, and newsletters directed at community members. Each material had its own specific format and messages. Table 7.2 provides additional design document details for two of these community component materials, and for two materials

**Table 7.1**    Design Document Highlights From the T.L.L. Temple Foundation Stroke Project—Community Component Materials

| Material | Design Document Highlights |
|---|---|
| Billboard | Recognize community role models participating fully in life after stroke |
| | Is there life after stroke? (outcome expectations) |
| | Every minute counts – Call 911 (behavioral capability) |
| Public Service Announcement (PSA)<br>Time One – Bystander<br>Response – Television | Use actors to depict response to stroke |
| | Show rapid treatment |
| | Show recovery |
| | Reinforce bystander for acting |
| PSA Time One – Physician<br>Response – Television | Show physician saying that his patients should call 911 |
| | Stroke is an emergency |
| | Reviewing symptoms |
| PSA Time One – Radio | Same as above for TV |
| Brochure | Symptoms |
| | Call 911 |
| | Treatment results in better outcomes |
| One-to-One Training | Script with symptoms |
| | Call 911 |
| | Treatment results in better outcomes |
| PSAs Time Two - Television | Same as above with actual local cases |
| Newspaper Story – Intro Type | What is the T.L.L. Temple Stroke Project? |
| | What the community can expect |
| | Stroke is an emergency |
| | Call 911 |
| Newsletter Story – Stroke Code | Coverage of local hospitals and EMS practicing stroke response |
| Newsletter Story – Symptom<br>Recognition and Response | Stoke symptoms |
| | Call 911 |
| | New medication leads to better outcomes |
| Newsletter Story – Success Story | Local individual experienced stroke |
| | Reiteration of symptoms |
| | Bystander / significant other called 911 |
| | Good outcome |

**Table 7.2**    Additional Design Document Details for the Stroke Project

| Proposed Vehicle | Change Objectives Grouped by Determinant | Methods and Practical Applications | Message Content |
|---|---|---|---|
| **Community Member; Bystander** | | | |
| Billboard | **Knowledge:** Describe importance of calling 911 for stroke symptoms | Information transfer | Call 911; Every minute counts |
| | **Outcome expectations:** Expect that getting to the emergency department fast will allow treatment to minimize effects of stroke | Modeling through recognizable community member | Is there treatment for stroke? (Ask Annon Card, stroke victim, who is playing golf) |
| Newspaper Story | **Knowledge:** Lists symptoms; describes to call 911 | Information transfer | Every minute counts; Symptom list |
| | **Skills:** Recognize symptoms | Modeling; Information transfer | Symptom list and someone responding to symptoms |
| | **Outcome Expectations:** Describes that treatment can prevent disability | Modeling through role model story with vicarious reinforcement | Some bystander or significant other does the right thing; the patient is treated; the outcome is good |
| **Emergency Department Staff and Physicians; Community Physicians** | | | |
| Newspaper Article | **Social norms:** Recognize that other physicians in the community respond rapidly to symptoms of stroke; believe that other emergency departments are lowering their workup times for stroke | Modeling through role-model stories and testimonials | I had a stroke patient who got to the hospital on time; the hospital emergency department treated my patient |
| | **Outcome expectations:** Expect that stroke patients (especially those presenting with moderate disability) can recover function with acute treatment of stroke | Modeling through role-model stories and testimonials | I wasn't sure about this new treatment before, but I am really pleased with the improvement I saw in my patient |
| | **Reinforcement:** Prepare and share patient success stories because there may be a lack of feedback to emergency department staff | Modeling through role-model stories and testimonials | From the patient or family's point of view: I am back (or my family member is back) to full functioning. The doctor saved our quality of life by acting quickly |
| Newsletter | **Knowledge:** Describe the results of the rt-PA clinical trial | Information transfer – science article | Stroke clinical trial article and references |
| | **Social Norms:** Recognize that other EDs are lowering work up times and treating patients | Modeling through physician testimonials | Article from physician's view point of actual treated case |
| | **Reinforcement:** Recognize that patient did well after treatment | Reinforcement through patient stories | Article about patient treated in ED |
| | **Outcome Expectation:** Recognize that when work-up times are lowered patients can get function-saving treatment | Modeling through actual hospital role model stories | Article about patient treated in the ED |

developed for emergency department staff and community physicians. It denotes the change objectives, change methods and practical applications, and first drafts of the messages to be contained in the materials they were planning.

Preparing design documents for materials, activities, and messages that are mediated by interactive technology such as computers, telephones, or social media may be more complex than for other types of materials. For example, a computer program requires a description of purpose, functions, features, and context or use. It also requires flowcharts depicting the sequence of content and branching logic depending on the learner's input (what the learner will experience and its order), screen maps depicting how the screen contents are arrayed with functional definitions of screen components (what the learner will see and do), and scripts and storyboards (a written list of audio and visuals of each embedded animation, video, quiz, or other interactive activity). Figure 7.1 presents the top level flowchart for the Management Information Decision-Support Epilepsy Tool (MINDSET), a tablet-based program to provide real-time self-management decision support to patients living with epilepsy and their health care providers (Shegog et al., 2013) (see publisher's website, epilepsy case study; www .wiley.com/go/bartholomew4e). The theoretical framework for MINDSET

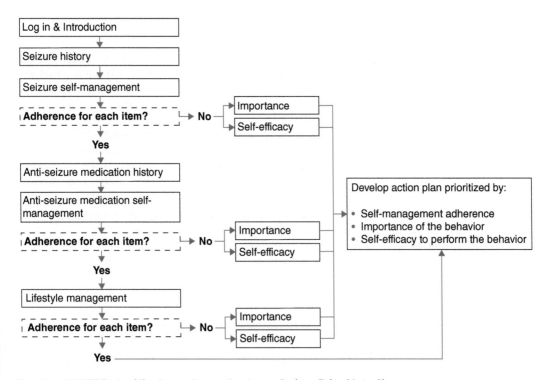

**Figure 7.1**  MINDSET Top Level Flow Diagram Depicting Data Input to Produce a Tailored Action Plan

is based in Social Cognitive Theory (Bandura, 1986), self-regulation models (Bandura, 1986; Clark, 2003), the 5-A's model of behavioral change (Glasgow, Bull, Piette, & Steiner, 2004), motivational enhancement therapy (Velasquez, Gaddy-Maurer, Crouch, & DiClemente, 2001), quality-of-care criteria (Fountain et al., 2011), and clinical guidelines for epilepsy (American Epilepsy Society, 2004). The team developed the flowchart to establish the function of MINDSET for the programmer, depicting the steps in the development of a tailored self-management action plan focused on seizure management, antiseizure medication adherence, and lifestyle management. The action plan prioritized recommendations based on data input by the patient based on validated measures of self-management adherence, importance of specific behaviors, and self-efficacy to perform the behaviors (Figure 7.2). The planning team then worked from the matrices to develop more detailed flowcharts and screen maps that outlined the data input process for each measure and the generation of tailored decision support recommendations (Figures 7.3 and 7.4).

The production design documents that flow from the production team to the planning team are usually more than written words. They might be written, as in a concept for a videotape, or they might be a combination of words and pictures, as in a storyboard or a rough sketch of a layout. They also might be illustrations or photographs in a layout or rough-cut videotape. These documents are all elements of conveying the creative person's image of the final product as it is developed first in the mind of that person and then in some medium. The number of these intermediate

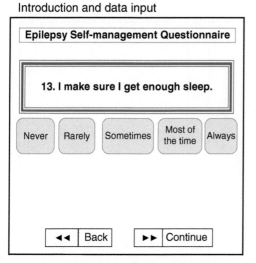

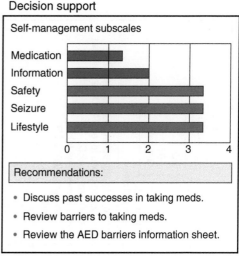

**Figure 7.2**  Example Draft Screen Map Mock-Ups for MINDSET

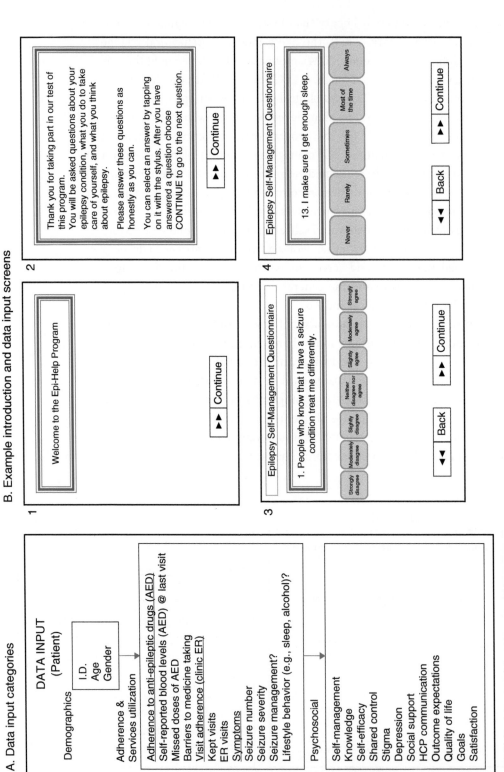

**Figure 7.3** Flowchart and Screen Maps Outlining the Data Input Process for MINDSET

Decision support for the patient and clinician comprises:

- Patient profile confirming data
- Graphic summary with alerts
- Recommendations for action
- Cues to promote patient-clinician communication

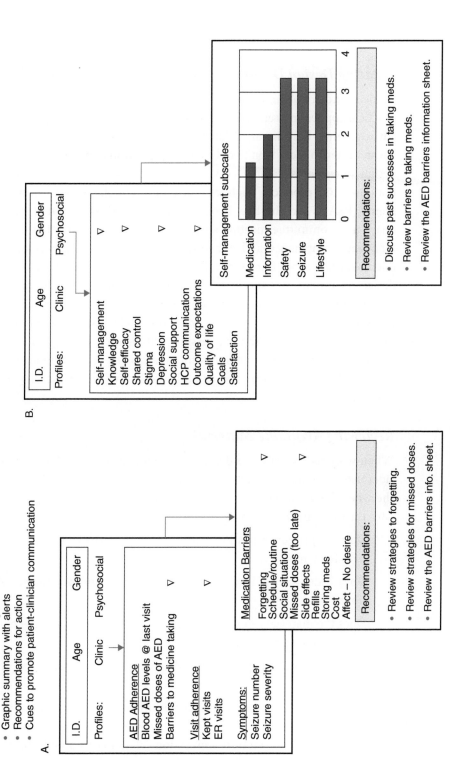

**Figure 7.4** Screen Maps Outlining the Generation of Tailored Decision Support Recommendations for MINDSET

production design documents that the health educator requires will affect the budget.

## Creating Design Documents for Community Processes

Readers who are planning an intervention that includes such methods and practical applications as policy development, coalition building, and media advocacy may be thinking: "All this discussion about design documents doesn't refer to me! I won't be developing traditional materials." However, design documents can be very helpful to guide program components that are not products such as videotapes, public service announcements (PSAs), and the like. Products can be processes such as advisory board and committee meeting structure and function, coalition development and maintenance, and lobbying. Each of these products needs a design document and sometimes more than one. Coalitions, for example, need a design document that specifies how coalition members will be recruited, how meetings will be run, and how minutes or meeting summaries will be constructed and delivered. A coalition might also need training for membership, and the training session will require a design document. Not only can such documents prevent breakdowns in communication but they can also make the processes smooth, productive, and reinforcing for the participants.

## Reviewing Available Material

When working on materials design documents planners will want to consider using existing materials or parts of materials rather than "reinventing the wheel." The team may want to start the review of existing materials with the following questions:

- Does the proposed existing material enable the relevant change objectives to be met?

- Does it deliver the intended change methods and practical applications?

- Does the material represent the correct surface aspects of the culture of the intended audience?

- Does the material fit into the planned scope and sequence of the program?

To determine whether the available materials are appropriate, the planning team reviews existing materials against the program matrices and lists of methods and practical applications. The match should be almost perfect and any gaps in addressing change objectives should be clearly identified. If gaps exist, the team will have to determine whether the gaps can be filled. Questions to ask during this level of review include the following:

• Are all the messages that are needed to influence change objectives included? If not, is there a sufficient presentation of key messages or can the team develop additional materials to address change objectives?

• Are the required change methods executed with the appropriate parameters? For example, do role-model stories use coping models, and are they derived from a group that matches the community on important characteristics?

It is difficult to make all these matches, but sometimes parts of existing programs work well and will provide a base for development of any materials to address gaps.

**Determining Suitability**    Existing materials that match change objectives, methods, and practical applications can be reviewed for production quality and suitability (Allies Against Asthma & Center for Managing Chronic Disease, n.d.; Doak, Doak, & Root, 1996; U.S. National Library of Medicine, 2013). The Suitability Assessment of Materials (SAM) is one framework for reviewing and improving the appropriateness of health education materials (Daley, Cowan, Nollen, Greiner, & Choi, 2009; Doak et al., 1996; Kaphingst, Zanfini, & Emmons, 2006; Neuhauser, Rothschild, Graham, Ivey, & Konishi, 2009; Shieh & Hosei, 2008) (Table 7.3). For example, Kaphingst and colleagues reviewed 19 colorectal cancer screening websites and found problems with lack of summary presentation, visual crowding, inappropriate type size, and lack of interactive features (Kaphingst et al., 2006). SAM guides the scoring of materials in six categories: content, literacy demand, graphics, layout and typography, learning stimulation, and cultural appropriateness. This yields a final score and indicates whether the materials are superior, adequate, or not suitable.

One factor that is often missed in assessment of materials is their appropriateness in terms of showing nonstereotypical power and social relations. Program developers should note whether there is anything stereotypical about the materials. For example, are only mothers portrayed giving certain kinds of care to children? Does the text make inappropriate assumptions as to the reader's socioeconomic status or environmental resources? Are certain social roles inequitably portrayed based on characteristics such as gender?

**Determining Availability**    Prior to the full review and evaluation of identified program materials, the planner should determine whether the materials are available in the quantity needed, in the appropriate

**Table 7.3**    Suitability Assessment of Materials Rationale

| Factor to Be Rated | Considerations for Rating |
|---|---|
| **Content** | |
| Purpose is evident. | Readers should be able to readily discern the purpose. |
| Content is about behaviors. | The content is about what the reader is expected to do without superfluous information. |
| Scope is limited. | The scope is limited to the objectives. |
| Summary or review is included. | Reviews help the reader process the main points. |
| **Literacy Demand** | |
| Reading grade level. | Ninth grade or more is usually not suitable; grade should match the intended readers' competence. |
| Writing style, active voice. | Text should be active voice and conversational with simple sentences. |
| Vocabulary uses common words. | Common explicit words should be used. Imagery words are good. Concept and category words are avoided or examples are used. |
| Context is given first. | Tell the purpose first. |
| Learning aids via advance organizers. | Headers, topic captions, and statements of what will be presented help orient the reader and aid encoding to memory. |
| **Graphics** | |
| Cover graphic shows purpose. | The first thing the reader sees may determine attitude. It should portray the purpose, be friendly, and get attention. |
| Type of graphics. | Illustrations should be familiar, age appropriate, without symbols and distracting details. |
| Relevance of illustrations. | Illustrations should tell the key messages visually with no distractions. |
| Lists, tables, figures explained. | Graphics must include step-by-step directions for interpretation. |
| Captions used for graphics. | Graphics should tell the reader what the graphic is and where to focus. |
| **Layout and Typography** | |
| Layout factors. | Most of the following should be present: low gloss paper, high contrast of paper and ink, consistent information flow, visual cues such as shading or arrows to guide the reader, illustrations next to text, adequate white space, appropriate/nondistracting use of color. |
| Typography. | Text is uppercase and lowercase, type is serif, type is at least 12 point, typographic cues such as size, color emphasize key points, no all caps. |
| Subheads and "chunking" of information. | Lists should be grouped so that people do not have to remember more than a few points. |
| **Learning Stimulation, Motivation** | |
| Interaction used | Enhances central processing to solve problems, respond to open ended questions, make choices. |
| Behaviors are modeled, specific, and reinforced. | Learner must be able to distinguish and practice the exact behaviors to be learned. |
| Self-efficacy is enhanced | People are more able to engage in the task and persist when they are confident about their task-related ability. |
| **Cultural Appropriateness** | |
| Match in logic, language, experience | Matching will facilitate engagement, reading, and learning. |
| Culturally relevant images and examples | All learning materials should present recognizable images and present the culture in positive ways. |

time frame, and at an acceptable cost. Some governmental, foundation, and community-based organizations allow reproduction for educational or community-based distribution while others may require a fee for use. Some materials may be available in electronic form—for instance, as a PDF file—over the Internet, and can be downloaded for reproduction. If a material is adapted or reproduced, planners should assure that all copyrights, adaptations, and permissions are acknowledged on every piece; and it is appropriate to provide courtesy copies to the people who created the original materials.

**Determining Reading Level**    Another factor to assess for both newly designed and adapted materials is the general readability and reading level of the materials. Reading levels indicate a grade level beyond which the message is likely to be difficult to decipher. Two issues should be addressed: What should the reading level be for a program's intended audience? What is the actual reading level of the material?

Many adults with low reading skills do not recognize their limitation and may not seek help with reading tasks (Chew et al., 2008; Harvard T.H. Chan School of Public Health, 2015; Haun, Valerio, McCormack, Sørensen, & Paasche-Orlow, 2014; Kirsch, Jungeblut, Jenkins, & Kolstad, 1993). Poor readers share certain characteristics that should be considered when identifying the reading level needs of program participants. Poor readers often decode one word at a time, skip over words, and fail to categorize information. They also often miss the context of the information and they fail to make inferences from data (Doak et al., 1996).

Limited literacy and limited health literacy, including the ability to use formal oral language, has implications for health status including disease outcomes (Baker et al., 2007; Berkman, Sheridan, Donahue, Halpern, & Crotty, 2011; Harrington & Valerio, 2014; Institute of Medicine, Committee on Health Literacy, 2004; National Institutes of Health, 2003; Osborne, 2005; Schwartzberg, VanGeest, & Wang, 2005; Zarcadoolas, Pleasant, & Greer, 2006). The overestimation of a patient's ability to understand medical instructions may contribute to health disparities (Harrington & Valerio, 2014; Kelly & Haidet, 2007). The mechanisms of the link between literacy, health literacy, and health status include access and utilization of health care, patient-provider relationship, and self-care (Harrington & Valerio, 2014; Haun et al., 2014; McCormick, Haun, Sørensen, & Valerio, 2013; Paasche-Orlow & Wolf, 2007).

Studies have addressed whether materials are written at levels that patients can be expected to read and have found that many health and health care topics are designed, implemented, and disseminated at levels beyond patient skills: for example, medication instructions (Estrada,

Hryniewicz, Higgs, Collins, & Byrd, 2000; Estrada, Martin-Hryniewicz, Peek, Collins, & Byrd, 2004), cancer information (Helitzer, Hollis, Cotner, & Oestreicher, 2009; Kaphingst, et al., 2006), domestic violence information (Yick, 2008), Medicaid application enrollment forms (J. M. Wilson, Wallace, & DeVoe, 2009), and patient education for such chronic diseases as diabetes, arthritis, and epilepsy (Foster & Rhoney, 2002; Hill-Briggs & Smith, 2008; Ratanawongsa et al., 2012).

The most reliable way to determine what the reading level of any print materials should be is to assess the health literacy of the intended program participants (Institute of Medicine, Committee on Health Literacy, 2004). This is commonly done in patient education settings and less commonly practiced in community settings, although short assessments based on instruments such as the Rapid Estimate of Adult Literacy in Medicine (REALM) or the Test of Functional Health Literacy in Adults (TOFHLA) or Short-TOFHLA (Baker, Williams, & Nurss, 1995; Parker, Baker, Williams, & Nurss, 1995) may be feasible.

The second issue is how to assess the reading level of a document. Many techniques are available; most are based on formulas that assess the average number of words in a sentence and the average number of syllables in a word. The former is used as a measure of complexity and the latter as a measure of vocabulary level. Many word processing and grammar-checking programs will now calculate and report a reading level; however, the programs are still using algorithms. Common assessments include the SMOG formula, the Fry Readability Graph, the Flesch Reading Ease score, and the Flesch-Kincaid grade level (Flesch, 1974; Fry, 1977; Indian Health Service, n.d.; McLaughlin, 1969). Many health educators find it simplest to use the protocols included with Microsoft Word. A different approach to assessing document complexity is the PMOST/KIRSCH document readability formula, which looks at both the organizational pattern (simple list, combined list, intersected list, nested list) and density (number of labels and number of items) (Mosenthal & Kirsch, 1998). This formula is an attempt to evaluate the readability of charts, graphs, tables, forms, and other nonlinear presentations of written words. In conjunction with Tufte's work on visual display (1997), it may prove a useful adjunct to standard reading-level formulas. These various protocols will not necessarily give comparable results; planners may want to pick one protocol and use it consistently. By using one protocol across all program materials, the health educator learns over time to write very close to a target grade level and to edit passages to achieve the target. This understanding may also impact the style of delivery of the program materials in person and guide the emphasis and explanation of specific content and use of information.

Reading level assessments are focused on literacy, but not health literacy. Readability should be addressed and recognized as "necessary" to consider, but planners and program designers should focus as heavily on the interpretation and use of information within the context of proposed change objectives (Centers for Disease Control and Prevention, 2015; U.S. Department of Health and Human Services, Office of Disease Prevention and Health Promotion, 2015).

## *Hiring and Working With Creative Consultants*

In an ideal budgetary world, health educators should take the advice of Balderman (1996), who says that if you weren't trained to do something, don't do it. A creative consultant should be hired when the health educator does not have the specific skill needed to create a component of the program. Commonly used creative resources include graphic and Web designers, graphic studios, copywriters, instructional designers, computer programmers, video and film writers, and video and film directors. In addition, production resources can include photographers, illustrators, talent (models and actors), location search companies, printers, postproduction video editors, and computer programmers.

Experienced health educators talk to people to find the creative or production resources they need. Good sources of referrals are printers or other people who have produced work and can introduce a designer, photographer, or illustrator. Branching out from the health field can often help. Balderman (1996) suggests the following ways to recruit talent to a project:

- Put together a synopsis of the job including approximate budget, length, purpose, concept, and producing agency.

- Send the synopsis with a request for statements of interest. Schedule meetings with the individuals who respond. Interviewing talent is a good way not only to look for help on the current job but also to build a file of possible resources for future work.

- Look at the portfolio of work. Is there any evidence that this person has conveyed the type of message needed and gotten the desired response? Does the planning team like the work? Does the range of previous work of the creative person include the type of work needed for the project?

- Ask about several of the projects in the portfolio. Is a range of budgets represented? Ask the person to talk about each project. If the type of product the team wants is not represented in the portfolio (which is the best of the best), then it is probably not available from this vendor.

Remember that in the circumstance that the team hires a creative consultant, that individual will be designing and creating the material. Health promoters should not have to take over the creative process assuming that they have communicated the intent of the program and or the materials well enough that the creative consultant can bring skills to the team and at the same time create materials that are congruent with the team's previous planning. This scenario implies that the creative consultant should not only be creative but also willing to thoroughly understand the team's intent. When the planning team interviews creative consultants they should pay close attention. How do the consultants present themselves? As salespeople or as people who want to understand the project? Are they too quick to assume that the project is "just like other projects" they have done? Do they seem sensitive to the team's needs and find the planning documents helpful?

A word about second guessing the creative resources: don't. Health educators should give their creative contractors the most understandable background possible and then try not to interfere with their creativity. The opportunity to allow a creative resource to create something independently is one of the reasons for all the planning up to this point. The creative people hired for the project will produce their best effort, and fiddling with it will decrease the quality in some way. It is possible that the person you hire for a project just cannot deliver acceptable work. Some creative people are unable to stay within the project parameters. Planners may encounter the video producer who, no matter what, will try to turn the team's role-model story into her documentary or the graphic designer who wants the team's newsletter to be his award winner. Health educators must know when to end the relationship with the vendor. If the initial ideas, preliminary sketches, or other proposed work are not acceptable, the health educator may want to look for other talent. The health educator might ask for one more attempt from the consultant after clarifying the project intent. But after a couple of unsuccessful tries, the health educator should go back to the hiring process.

The planning team members who are working with creative resources want them to understand the project as well as possible and to wholeheartedly adopt the planning group's intent. The person's creative additions should bring to life rather than override or misinterpret the team's understanding of the problem and its solution. The key to working with the creative production team is to create design documents so that the producers come to fully understand what the planning team intends.

To get started with a creative resource, health educators usually invite him or her to a team meeting to talk about the project once the team can give a fairly consistent message. If possible, the health educator takes the creative person to visit with members of the community. Sometimes the creative person can go to focus groups or interviews. The people that he or she encounters at these meetings may end up in the final materials. In an ideal situation, the designer (or writer or producer) can work with the team almost from the beginning of planning, offering ideas as to format, and serving as an expert witness on what is (and is not) doable. The next best approach is to bring the designer in when the matrices, change methods, and practical applications have been hammered out but before the team has decided on the formats of the support materials. The earlier the designer can enter the process, the more his or her skills will enrich it.

---

**BOX 7.1. MAYOR'S PROJECT**

The mayor's task force was well on its way to the production of support materials for the multicomponent program. The health promoter, while busily looking at portfolios, choosing designers, and trying to understand what the video writer-producer would require in terms of design documents, received a panicky call from the chair of the group working on the community coalition strategy. She and her cochair were in the neighborhood, so the health promoter decided on a spur-of-the-moment, face-to-face discussion of whatever was engendering the panic.

*Group chair:*  Oh my gosh! We had our first coalition organizational meeting, and it was a free-for-all. I couldn't get control of the agenda. I know it is supposed to be a participatory agenda. I've read the books. This was participatory, all right—participatory by one small group! They took over at the beginning, and none of the rest of us could say a thing!

*Cochair:*  Yeah, and one woman felt her ideas were so criticized that she walked out right in the middle of the meeting.

*Group chair:*  Several of our most dedicated supporters stopped me afterward and said they didn't know if they could stand to come back. And on top of all that, we are not sure whether we can develop cohesion with this new group after all the groundwork the planning group has already laid.

The health promoter and the cochairs talked some more about the dynamics of the meeting and then planned a strategy. Before their next meeting, the cochairs put together a couple of coalition meeting design documents. One was on how a participatory agenda would be created by the entire group prior to the meeting; the other was a format for meeting summaries that used the meeting that had just occurred. Finally, they put together the coalition overview and task document that would serve as a beginning for group development and task orientation in the coalition.

The third task in Step 4 is to draft messages and produce preliminary or prototype materials and protocols for the health promotion program.

# Drafting Messages, Materials, and Protocols

## *Writing Program Messages*

In Step 3, the planning team decide on methods that would be included in each program component to address specific change objectives. Each method will be operationalized with multiple health messages and activities and delivered through a variety of channels and vehicles (e.g., an interpersonal counseling session, interactive media, or television). In all cases, messages need to be written. Abraham and Kools (2012) provide detailed guidance on writing health messages.

The messages developed to address and promote the change objectives are informed specifically by data and information from Steps 1–3. The community assessment information identified in Step 1 will allow for an understanding of demographic and clinical characteristics as well as specific clinical information including incidence and prevalence of illness and risk that will allow for writing specific messages to influence determinants of behavior. For example, messages may promote an individual's understanding and knowledge of a specific issue; deliver information to determine an individual's level of susceptibility to the illness; identify the severity of the illness or exposure; or promote intentions to engage in a specific behavior—for example, exercise or the use of condoms.

Many health promotion program materials contain two types of messages. One is a focused message to enable an objective. For example, in the Stroke Project, the team provided some information to influence the change objective regarding behavioral capability for symptom recognition and prompt action by community bystanders/significant others. They recurrently provided messages to promote the community members to recognize stroke symptoms and to take appropriate action, that is, call 911. The second type of message is contextual—not specifically addressing a change objective. For example, contextual messages might set up a scenario, provide information about the program, or provide an engaging narrative. A contextual message might also be related to the health and well-being of the intended audience, though not specifically designed to address the targeted health behavior. For example, in the ToyBox-Study, described in Chapters 5 and 6, which was developed to increase physical activity and reduce sedentary activity among preschool children in Europe, program planners framed the messages for parents and kindergarten teachers from the perspective of being a positive role model for the preschoolers, to facilitate change in the children's behavior.

Messages, a part of all health promotion materials, are focused attempts to effectively promote and accomplish a change objective. The following steps can assist in focusing the planners and health educators through message development:

- Consider the change methods and practical applications that the team has decided on for a particular set of objectives. Identify those that will "fit" together for presentation in a particular vehicle, such as a newspaper story

- Organize all change objectives by determinants, methods, and practical applications to identify the needs for health messages by module

- Draft messages matched to each change objective or combinations of change objectives

- Draft contextual messages that will be incorporated into the vehicle

**Writing to Enhance Cognitive Processing**    The capacity of individual's working memory is limited. Therefore, message writers should promote more cognitive processing and use of information by doing the following:

- Carefully plan (and limit) the number of concepts introduced within a specific module or session and across the program sessions

- Match graphics to messages

- Recognize the prior knowledge of the recipient: use the prior knowledge and fill gaps

- Present old information before new

- Help the recipient make inferences with stimulation of active processes

- Follow an explicit logic in the order of topics, sessions, and sentences within materials

- Make links between sections explicit to the reader, viewer, or listener

- Match the reading level of the intended audience

- Write in the active voice

- Make lists understandable without introductory sentences (e.g., in a list of things people should not do, every item should begin with "Do not")

- Write as clearly as possible (e.g., if the meaning is "do not," copywriters should not use the term *avoid*. Readers often interpret the word to mean "try not to do this, but do it when you have to")

- Present the material in the order in which the reader will need it

- Include only messages in support of the change objectives; remove superfluous material unless it provides an appropriate context

- Use subheads to break up or chunk the text

- Use a careful hierarchy to support comprehension

- Tell the recipient how the material is structured (use advance organizers, see Chapters 2 and 6)

- Use sentences and designs that encourage interaction, such as checklists with boxes that readers can check

- Use one- and two-syllable words and short, simple sentences with definitions of more difficult words in appositional phrases and parenthetical statements

- Provide visual cues

- Use strong topic sentences for paragraphs

**A Cultural Perspective on Writing Messages**    Many cultural characteristics directly influence both how people communicate and how they understand and respond to the health messages they receive. As with the design of other materials, the message writers will want to understand the preferred communication styles of the intended program recipients and will want to pretest the messages with representatives from the community to increase appropriateness. Many aspects of cultural preferences can affect message writing; for example, the structure of arguments (with the main point first or with a buildup to the climax), the use of words, and the standards used to judge credibility.

Health promoters must be particularly careful to clearly understand a cultural communication method before using it. Airhihenbuwa (1994) gives the example of the pitfalls of superficial use of oral culture (ear-to-mouth) versus visual culture (eye-to-object) storytelling methods. He points out that stories are a reciprocal vehicle that depend on the listeners' interaction with the teller to create the learning. Any adaptation that makes this vehicle a one-way street loses the method's power.

On the other hand, he points out that use of a delivery vehicle from outside the culture has different pitfalls. For example, if short messaging service (text messages) is used to convey information in an oral culture, learners will face problems with attention, comprehension, and memory because the learner will first have to learn to use this novel source of information. However, some vehicles may be used in conjunction with others to build a stronger program and reinforce specific messages.

**Translation**    Translation of health education materials into another language is not a trivial matter. Good translation is usually aimed at symmetry: a translation that is loyal to the meaning of the source language while ensuring equal familiarity and colloquiality in both languages. Another term for this symmetry is decentering (from the source language). Decentering implies a de-emphasis of the developer's language in such a way that the system of symbols supersedes a single culture. At best, decentering eliminates the distinction between source and target language. Decentering requires a multistage translation that allows for paraphrasing the meaning of the source materials and of the translation before deciding on a translated version. The translation is then translated back to the original language, and the versions are compared. The process of translation and back translation are continued until the two versions are acceptable. The goal is a dynamic equivalence in which a cultural symbol in the source language is translated into a cultural symbol in the target language that evokes the same functional response from the reader or listener. For example, Werner and Campbell (1973) relate the problem of finding a Navajo word for measles; presenting a list of symptoms might have evoked a more meaningful response than trying to find one word that did not originally exist in a language. They relate an even more significant problem of meaning when they explain that the literal translation of the word meningitis into Navajo would be "the covering of the brain is getting red." The translation period is another good time to work with focus groups to understand the words used to describe certain phenomena. In creating the Spanish version of the Watch, Discover, Think, and Act program, Bartholomew et al. (2000) used focus groups to discover the ways people described asthma and related concepts such as wheezing and inhaler. Some of these words related to asthma had no equivalents in common Spanish.

**Presentation of Medical Terminology**    Sometimes technical material is difficult to write below a fifth-grade level without losing meaning. The inclusion of medical terminology such as cardiovascular disease may be presented and followed by the introduction of the term heart disease. The language and terminology used should not limit the understanding by participants, but promote processing and allow for a greater understanding of diagnosis, care needs, and recommendations. Additionally, copywriters should avoid the trap of replacing commonly heard words with less commonly heard (but shorter or slang) words (e.g., replacing *medicine* with *meds*); doing so may lower the computed reading level but will interfere with comprehension.

## Creating and Choosing Program Visuals—Nontext Messages

Kreuter and colleagues (2003) suggest that visuals, unlike text, can be perceived and understood almost immediately. Visuals should help the materials developer to gain attention, interest, and credibility for the message (Moriarty, Mitchell, & Wells, 2008; Shiffman, 1994; Wells, Burnett, & Moriarty, 2006). Furthermore, the visuals can and should capture elements that are familiar and pleasing to the cultural groups that will use the materials. For example, in the ToyBox-Study, the program planners chose animal characters that were appealing to preschool children as role models in stories and other activities. For example, Little Kangaroo was gender-neutral to encourage both boys and girls to improve their physical activity behavior. The role model character was featured in stories, activities, and take-home posters to model fun ways to be physically active (Duvinage et al., 2014).

In addition to visuals being pleasing to the audience and stimulating interest, Doak and colleagues (1996) argue strongly that visuals should assist the reader with deciphering and remembering a message. According to these authors, the visuals should have the following characteristics:

- Be realistic rather than symbolic
- Be simple with little distracting background
- Be used to reduce text by showing, for example, steps in a procedure
- Show all important elements of a gestalt—for example, the entire body rather than just the chest—so that the reader does not have to struggle with orientation
- Be used to stimulate interaction

### Producing Narrative "Print" Material

Figure 7.5 gives an example of the process involved in producing print materials. Current word processing and publishing software has opened a world of opportunities for text materials and electronic distribution has enabled health promoters to often avoid hard copy distribution. Nevertheless there are several steps in the production. Whoever has the task of production must have read several design documents and must understand the team's intent for the program component by this phase of the process. Designers may benefit from contact with the intended audience for the piece as well. In the production phase, the designer will work with the team to consider the following:

- What design elements or types of copy will the piece have? Examples to consider are levels of subheads, lists, tables, graphs, charts, illustrations, captions, pulled quotes from data or case studies, footnotes or references, interviews, and step-by-step instructions. The more elements there are, the more complicated the design process, though the best result is usually something with a simple design
- When and how will the project need updating? And who will lead?
- What are the costs and constraints?

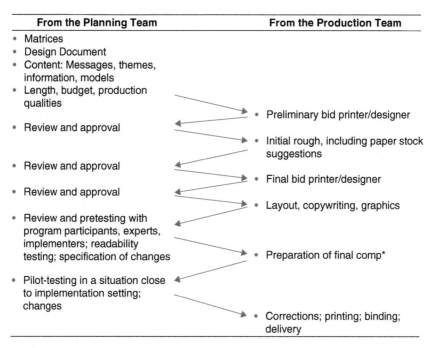

| From the Planning Team | From the Production Team |
| --- | --- |
| • Matrices<br>• Design Document<br>• Content: Messages, themes, information, models<br>• Length, budget, production qualities | • Preliminary bid printer/designer |
| • Review and approval | • Initial rough, including paper stock suggestions |
| • Review and approval | • Final bid printer/designer |
| • Review and approval | • Layout, copywriting, graphics |
| • Review and pretesting with program participants, experts, implementers; readability testing; specification of changes | • Preparation of final comp* |
| • Pilot-testing in a situation close to implementation setting; changes | • Corrections; printing; binding; delivery |

*A comprehensive or "comp" represents the finished product in a more accurate form and detail than a rough. It shows as closely as possible how the final product will look. These are for pretesting and pilot-testing. They may be required but will add to the budget.

**Figure 7.5**  Tasks for Producing a Print Piece

- What are the graphics standards of the organization producing the piece? Color, use of logos, and other materials should be considered

- What process will be used to review the piece by the team?

- For what aspects of the production process is the team responsible?

- Who will produce the camera-ready copy?

- Will the piece be distributed online, photocopied, or printed?

Next, the designer lists all the elements of the design that will be needed to present the important messages within the materials and presents these for review by the planning group. Once a designer provides an acceptable design, the content will have to be edited to conform to it. Remember, asking for changes to a completed design is counterproductive; changing the design will cost more money and decrease the resulting quality.

## Producing Video

Video can be a good way to address some of the readability and presentation problems introduced earlier; in addition most multimedia programs use some video. Most of the production costs for videos are in producing the master. Computer Internet access, smartphones, DVD players, and televisions are ubiquitous in most countries, and the equipment to make a video is also commonplace. Figure 7.6 presents processes in the production of video.

**Contracts and Budgets**    Early in the process, the producer must develop an understanding of what the development team has planned, and optimally the producer has participated in some contacts with the intended audience. An early step in working with a video producer is agreeing on the contract.

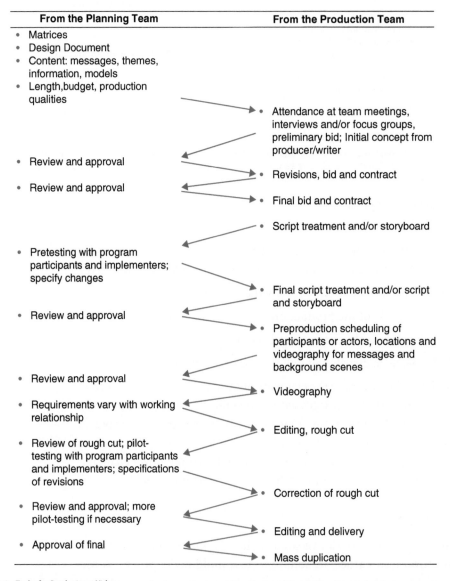

| From the Planning Team | From the Production Team |
|---|---|
| • Matrices | |
| • Design Document | |
| • Content: messages, themes, information, models | |
| • Length, budget, production qualities | |
| | • Attendance at team meetings, interviews and/or focus groups, preliminary bid; Initial concept from producer/writer |
| • Review and approval | |
| | • Revisions, bid and contract |
| • Review and approval | |
| | • Final bid and contract |
| | • Script treatment and/or storyboard |
| • Pretesting with program participants and implementers; specify changes | |
| | • Final script treatment and/or script and storyboard |
| • Review and approval | |
| | • Preproduction scheduling of participants or actors, locations and videography for messages and background scenes |
| • Review and approval | |
| | • Videography |
| • Requirements vary with working relationship | |
| | • Editing, rough cut |
| • Review of rough cut; pilot-testing with program participants and implementers; specifications of revisions | |
| | • Correction of rough cut |
| • Review and approval; more pilot-testing if necessary | |
| | • Editing and delivery |
| • Approval of final | |
| | • Mass duplication |

**Figure 7.6**  Tasks for Producing a Video

The contract and the budget should include a "rough cut" of the video for the team's pretesting, review, and approval. A rough cut is an initial edit of the production prior to final online editing, which is when additional production qualities, such as music, are added to a tape. The planning team can pretest a rough cut with the intended participants and program implementers. The budget must allow for viewing and pretesting at this intermediate stage and for revisions. Members of the planning team should observe the video shoots so that the material included in the rough cut does not come as a surprise. Other examples of contract considerations are casting approval, credits, and copyright. The program development team (not the video producers) should have the assigned copyright so that the organization can recycle the video images from one medium to another. Any artwork bought for the videotape will also have a contract with it that specifies who owns the material. Owning the legal title and custody of the master tape is important. The planning team should obtain from the production company copies of all releases and should make sure that everyone signs a release before filming begins.

**Scripts, Script Treatments, and Storyboards**   A vital component of video production and a centerpiece of work between a planning team and a video producer is the script or script treatment. A script details the audio and visuals for every scene, whereas a script treatment is a "look-and-feel" description of the video and a scene-by-scene sequence of messages. Both scripts and script treatments can include storyboards with the same information plus visuals.

A script is very different from material that is meant to be read; it is meant to be seen and heard. In addition, a video has about 15 seconds to grab the audience's attention, and it has to recapture that attention every few seconds after that. In a video, the picture tells the story and the words complete the messages.

The planning group will want to review the preliminary script carefully to ensure that all elements of the design documents are met (the change objectives, the methods, and parameters for effective delivery of the methods). Reviewing to make sure that the video contains all the planned change methods according to their parameters is a continuing process through production. Many times the planning team will need to educate video producers on important characteristics to make something depicted on video match what is needed to elicit change in the viewer.

After receiving initial approval, the producer can create the final script treatment or script. Script approval prior to shooting is a formal process and a key point in the creative cycle. The planning team will want to list the number of people who should approve the video, because it is easy to underestimate the number of stakeholders (e.g., users, trainers, setting gatekeepers, and program participants). Reshooting can break the budget and in some situations may not even be possible; incorporating changes at the script stage makes more sense. If the same video is needed in more than one language, the script should be translated as soon as the stakeholders have approved the original. For live-action shots, shooting all language versions at the same time can be cost-efficient. For voiceover footage, producers need to allow for the difference in length of the narration and shoot the footage to allow for the longer narration time.

The final script should be compared against the intended change objectives, taking into consideration the available budget, because the more complex the script is or the more difficult it is to shoot, the greater the shooting and editing costs will be. Script approval is also the time for everyone to approve the credits. Although the credits can seem a simple task, if left to the last minute, they will invariably contain errors, and revising credits can be quite time-consuming for the production house.

### Creating a Multimedia Program

Producing a computer-delivered multimedia program contains many of the same production steps as producing a videotape except that it is more complex and involves a computer programmer as a part of the production team. With computer-assisted instruction, the program is able to deliver tailored messages in real time. Depending on the amount of user control, the program can also deliver an individualized learning experience. Because the vehicle has branching pathways for the learner and may contain many different methods and practical applications, the design documents are more complex, as illustrated by the flowcharts (see Figures 7.3 and 7.4 for examples from MINDSET and Figure 7.8 for an example from It's Your Game ... Keep It Real).

## Pretesting, Pilot-Testing, Refining, and Producing Materials

The fourth task in Step 4 is to pretest and pilot-test program materials, and to make revisions prior to overseeing materials' production.

Pretesting is trying out the specific messages and other characteristics of the program materials with the intended participants before final production. Pilot-testing is trying out the program as it will be implemented, with both the implementers and intended participants, prior to the actual implementation. Both pretesting and pilot-testing are crucial to determine whether planning has resulted in appealing, understandable materials, and whether the program can be implemented.

Sometimes program planners do not conduct pretesting and pilot-testing because they are behind schedule. No matter how big the hurry, planners must make time for trying out materials. Sometimes planning teams object to taking time to pretest and pilot-test by pointing out that the planning group already comprises representatives of the potential program participants and implementers. However, representatives, who have been involved in the planning have probably come to value the program that they have developed in a way that biases their objectivity. This step requires going back out into the communities to receive and integrate new feedback. Pilot-testing also provides the opportunity to review the measures that will be used for evaluation.

## *Methods for Pretesting and Pilot Testing*

Table 7.4 presents various pretesting and pilot-testing methods. This is a brief overview, and other sources of information on pretesting will be helpful (Freimuth, Cole, & Kirby, 2011; National Cancer Institute, Center for the Advancement of Health & Robert Wood Johnson Foundation, 2002; National Institutes of Health, 2014; Whittingham, Ruiter, Castermans, Huiberts, & Kok, 2008; Wittingham, Ruiter, Zimbile, & Kok, 2008). The first pretesting that health educators conduct is to test initial program concepts, including key phrases and visuals proposed to portray the main ideas. Focus groups and interviews are good for this purpose. A very important reason for this process is to discover the words, phrases, and vernacular that members of the at-risk group use when discussing the topic. Table 7.4 lists a variety of questions to be answered by pretesting including program participants' responses to messages and materials and perceptions of material characteristics by adopters and implementers (see Chapter 8).

To conduct pretests, the team will execute program components in preliminary formats to test concepts, attention, comprehension, strong and weak points, and personal relevance. The pretest can also assess impact on determinants and can elicit the opinions of potential program adopters and implementers. Before final production, planners can gauge potential objection to sensitive or controversial issues, language, and specific needs of the population. A major question at this stage is how to get materials in final-enough form to be good stimulus material without spending too much extra money. For example, videotapes can be presented in storyboard format, as can PSAs. Radio PSAs can be read aloud, and newsletters can be produced with a word processing program. However, as much of the final product as possible should be included: illustrations, photographs, and graphics for newsletters rather than just the words, for example. It is also important to evaluate individual aspects of materials rather than just the whole.

**Table 7.4** Pretesting and Pilot-Testing Purposes and Methods

| | Concept Testing | Readability Testing | Message Execution | Impact | Adoption/Implementation Characteristics |
|---|---|---|---|---|---|
| **Purpose** | To test the key phrases and visuals that portray the main ideas; to discover vernacular | To estimate school-grade level required to read text | To determine whether program materials and messages are attended to, comprehended, appealing, and culturally relevant | To get a sense of possible impact or to measure impact of change methods and messages on determinants (change objectives). | To determine perceptions of implementers about complexity, trialability, observability, and relative advantage of materials; to predict problems with implementation |
| **Participants** | Program participants and implementers | Program participants | Program participants and implementers | Program participants and implementers | Program adopters and implementers |
| **Research Methods** | Interviews, focus groups, cognitive interviewing | Text and readability formula, word processing program | Interviews, focus groups, questionnaires, cognitive interviewing | Interviews, focus groups, questionnaires, cognitive interviewing (prepost measurement from the determinants columns of the matrices) | Interviews, focus groups, observation of trial implementation |
| **Instructions** | Use concept ideas as stimulus materials; ask people how they would convey an idea | Apply the program or formula to each component | Ask what participants "got" from the material or message (assess identification with "How similar were the thoughts and feelings of these people to yours?") | See Chapter 9 | Ask for review by naïve potential implementers, not those who have worked on development; make the pilot as realistic as possible |
| **Can't Be Used For** | Knowing what will happen with final materials | Knowing whether intended readers will understand text | Estimating impact | Without a comparison group, change is not attributable to the program | Determining perceptions in actual implementation |

## Reviewing Parameters for Change Methods

Regardless of whether program planners elect to develop new materials, use existing materials, or employ some combination of the two, they will want to make sure that the theoretical parameters for operationalizing the change methods and practical applications are met. Chapter 6 presented theoretical parameters under which each change method will be most effective. In Intervention Mapping Step 3, program planners made decisions about theoretical methods and practical applications. For instance, in the development of It's Your Game . . . Keep It Real the developers selected scenario-based risk information as one method for improving skills and self-efficacy for evaluating dating relationships. For the practical application, the developers created a computer-based, mock TV dating game show in which students had to evaluate the healthy and unhealthy characteristics of potential dating situations. In this example, the parameters for the use of scenario-based risk information were that students would find these scenarios plausible and that multiple scenarios would be provided (Mevissen, Meertens, Ruiter, Feenstra, & Schaalma, 2009). Pretesting of the program should provide assurance that these assumptions were met. The developers tested the mock TV show with members of the potential participants and found that all of the scenarios were plausible and believable to the youth. Another assumption for the educational program was that students would pay attention because they think that the program is personally relevant (McGuire, 1986). Again, pretesting addressed this assumption.

## Making Sense of Pretest Data

At every step of pretesting, there is the likelihood of obtaining a lot of information and possibly conflicting opinions. Planers will want to have a plan about how to display data and keep track of recommended changes. For example, a table of pretesting data might include the unit of material and messages being tested, the questions being asked, and an enumeration of the answers. The team will want to know what program participants and implementers think about the program materials, how they respond to materials, and how strongly they hold their opinions. Different types of feedback may lead to different team responses. For example, the team might ask potential implementers of a patient education program to review the materials and find that while the program was being developed, treatment guidelines changed – an obvious need to modify the materials for accuracy. But, what happens when reviewers disagree on design characteristics, cultural relevance, or suitability? The team will have to have a plan for adjudicating recommendations for changes. Furthermore, when decisions are made to change something, the team will need to make sure that the change has not disrupted or eliminated an important element of the program such as a change method. If developers delete activities and change methods, they should attempt to replace them with equally powerful methods and messages, and to address the change objectives with specific practical applications. Making appropriate use of pretest data requires working back through messages, practical applications, and methods to matrices to ensure that changes in the program materials do not leave gaps in the intervention chain of causation.

## Planning for Program Evaluation

Step 4 contributes toward evaluation planning in two ways. The first is related to formative evaluation. We have given an overview of pretesting and pilot testing, evaluation that is conducted while program materials are being developed and that seeks to incorporate into the final materials the opinions of both intended recipients and intended adopters and implementers. The second contribution relates to summative evaluation, and it includes a later assessment of how the audience received the materials during implementation and whether the methods and practical applications were well enough operationalized to have an impact on the change objectives (see Chapter 9).

---

**BOX 7.2. IT'S YOUR GAME . . . KEEP IT REAL PROJECT**

**The first task in Step 4 is to refine the program structure and organization.**

The planning group first reviewed the draft program scope and sequence and proposed delivery vehicles (classroom and computer-based lessons) from Step 3 to ensure the feasibility of implementation in urban middle schools. They solicited feedback from school district and school-level administrators, and middle school health education teachers regarding the feasibility of integrating 12 It's Your Game lessons into the seventh- and eighth-grade health education curriculum, and their ability to provide students with individual access to computers for the computer-based lessons. Stakeholder feedback indicated that implementation would be feasible but would require advanced planning (e.g., teachers would need to modify lesson plans in advance and coordinate with information technology specialists or the librarian to ensure that the necessary time and resources were available).

**The second task in Step 4 is to prepare plans for program materials.**

The planners prepared production plans, or design documents, appropriate for twenty-four 50-minute lessons, with 12 lessons in seventh grade and 12 lessons in eighth grade. The computer-based lessons included interactive skills-training exercises, peer role model videos, and "real world"-style teen serials (*Reel World*) with online student feedback to reinforce and supplement activities in the group-based classroom lessons. Activities within the computer lessons were sequenced to maximize learning: overview of lesson objectives; recap of material from the previous classroom lesson; introduction to a *Reel World* serial (peer modeling), in which a character has to make a decision about a potentially risky situation; interactive activites (e.g., peer video, information, and skill training); questions about the serial (What should the character do?); serial conclusion (character receives reinforcement for making the healthiest decision); and lesson recap (Figure 7.7). Some computer lessons included activities tailored by sexual experience; thus, the design document included instruction on the relevant tailoring points (Figure 7.8).

The planners drafted content for the classroom lessons, student journals, take-home activities, and parent newsletters, all of which included activities to operationalize the specific methods and applications identified in Step 3. Design documents for video- and computer-based activities included the targeted change objectives, methods, and applications; estimated duration; a detailed description of characters and setting; discussion prompts for peer role model videos; and itemized scripts for the *Reel World* serials (Figure 7.9).

**The next task in Step 4 is to draft messages, materials, and protocols.**

The planners wrote content (messages) for all activites and ensured that the parameters of the specified methods were met. For example, the *Reel World* serials used the method of modeling; thus, the planners made sure that each series ended with the main character receiving reinforcement for making a healthy decision (Figure 7.9). They also checked the reading level for the parent newsletters to make sure the language was appropriate for the intended audience. A sample classroom role play activity and parent newsletter pages are presented in Figures 7.10 and 7.11.

The planners hired creative consultants (videographers, postproduction video editors, and computer program developers) to produce the video- and computer-based activities. Preproduction tasks for video development included casting talent, securing locations, collecting props, and scheduling video shoots. Postproduction tasks included working with video editors to include special effects and to ensure that the messages and methods were presented as intended. The planners worked iteratively with the computer program developers and conducted alpha-testing of prototype lessons to ensure that all parameters, tailoring, and other specifications outlined in the design documents were met. Sample screen shots from the computer lesson activities are presented in Figure 7.12.

Finally, the planners drafted curriculum manuals for seventh- and eighth-grade teachers that itemized the timing, materials required, and activities for each lesson.

**The final task in this step is to pretest, refine, and produce program materials.**

The Youth Advisory Group, described in Step 1, pretested drafts of selected student activities (e.g., student role plays and *Reel World* video scripts) to ensure that the language, characters, scenarios, and settings were relevant, realistic, and engaging for urban minority middle school students. As needed, they edited scripts and suggested alternative scenarios.

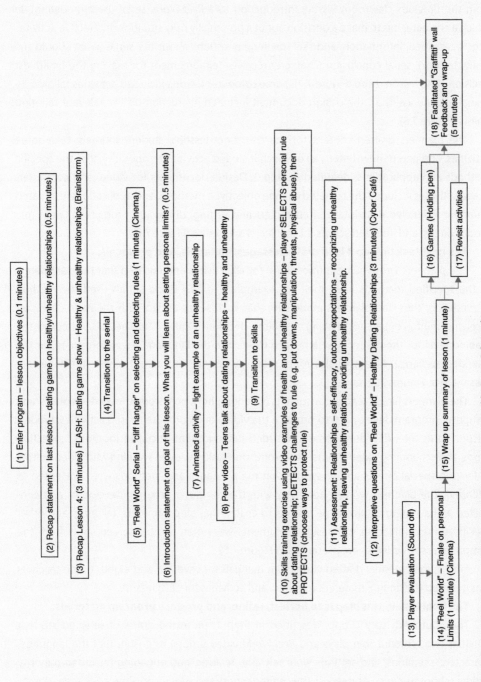

**Figure 7.7** Activity Sequence for an It's Your Game Computer Lesson: Healthy Dating Relationships

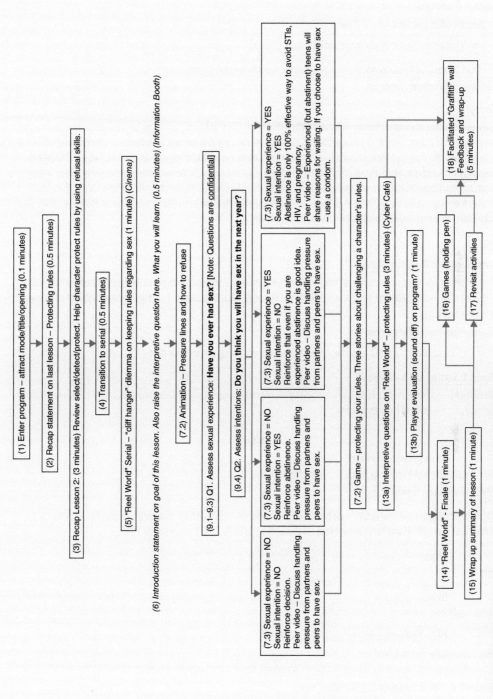

**Figure 7.8** Example of an It's Your Game Computer Lesson Tailored by Sexual Experience

**The Reel World: Eddie's World**

**Change Objectives**

- Describe what a personal rule is. (Select)
- Identify situations that may challenge personal rules. (Detect)

**Method & Practical Application:** Modeling—Real-life teens facing real-life situations
**Estimated Duration:** 10 minutes

**Synopsis:**

Even though Eddie has told his friends, Brian and Nick, earlier in the day that he can't have any friends over because his mom is working and he's taking care of his younger brother, the opposite happens that evening. Nick shows up unannounced with several friends for a party at Eddie's house. Eddie's mom counts on him to look after his younger brother, Gabe, and Eddie has selected this as a personal rule: to protect his brother and be a good role model. Eddie must confront the group of kids at the door, and even though he is somewhat tempted to let his friends in, he protects his personal rule. He tells his friends to leave. Eddie's friends aren't too happy. In the end, Eddie feels good about his decision to take care of his brother. His friend, Brian, sees why Eddie made that decision and has a renewed respect for him.

**PART 1**

**Intro Sequence** (Production Notes)

Before Scene 1, identify characters in a montage: first names, fast-edited sequence with music. End up on character that will be the focus of the serial. [Montage of cut scenes from future episodes, focus on group walking together and highlight names with each character]

Then bring in title: **Eddie's World**

May want to use fast cuts and SFX for some scene transitions to add drama and increase pace

**Scene 1: Setting and Background**

Outside (driveway or sidewalk). Eddie is teaching his younger brother (approx. age 7) Gabe how to ride a bike. Brian and Nick drop by to invite Eddie to party that night.

Fade In

**Eddie** [giving tips to Gabe]:
Hey, Gabe! Don't lean back, whoa, whoa . . . yeah, that's the way. Nice!
[Eddie gives Gabe a thumbs-up.]

[As Gabe is trying out different moves, a car honks and pulls up to the curb. (Can hear thumping bass coming out of the car.) Eddie looks over as Brian and Nick get out of the car and walk up to Eddie. They fist-bump with Eddie.]

**Brian:**
Hey . . .

**Nick:**
What's goin' on . . . ?

**Eddie** [still smiling at Gabe and encouraging him]:
Hey, look at Gabe. Not bad, huh?

**Figure 7.9**  Design Document for a *Reel World* Series

**Two Hours Alone**

**Directions:** Fill in the "You" lines, using clear NO statements, alternative actions, or a combination of both.

**Setting the Stage:**
You are at your partner's house after school. You aren't ready to have sex, and you've said so. You know no one will be home for two hours. You are kissing and touching and your partner lets you know he/she wants to have sex. You don't want to have sex.

**Your Partner:**    I think we should do something more than just kissing and touching.
**You:**    _____
           _____

**Your Partner:**    We don't get many chances to be alone.
**You:**    _____
           _____

**Your Partner:**    I just feel so close to you. That's why I want to have sex with you.
**You:**    _____
           _____

**Your Partner:**    If you loved me as much as I love you, you'd do it.
**You:**    _____
           _____

**Figure 7.10**  Example Role Play Activity From It's Your Game
Reprinted with permission of The University of Texas Health Science Center at Houston, copyright 2000–2014.

All classroom lessons were pilot tested with the priority population. Research staff delivered each classroom lesson to seventh and eight grade students during regular class periods to assess lesson length, to identify difficulty in delivering any activities, and to obtain student feedback. Students completed a brief survey after each lesson with open-ended questions including: Which activities did you like the most/least? Which activities were hard for you to understand? What did you like/not like about the characters in the stories? Were the situations believable for students your age? How can the lessons be improved?

Overall, students reacted favorably to the activities and provided feedback to improve classroom directions and specific activity content. Some lessons ran longer than intended (i.e., beyond a 50-minute class period) indicating the need to abbreviate or delete some activities.

Fourteen seventh- and eighth-grade students from the target population also beta-tested the computer lessons in a simulated classroom setting. They provided feedback on specific activities (Which activities did they like the most/least? How could these lessons be improved?) and usability parameters, including ease of use, credibility, understandability, acceptability, and motivation, using previously validated usability assessment instruments. They also completed pre- and postlesson ratings on the importance of content domains (e.g., the importance of keeping healthy friendships) and self-efficacy to perform targeted behaviors (e.g., self-efficacy to refuse sex and self-efficacy to use a condom).

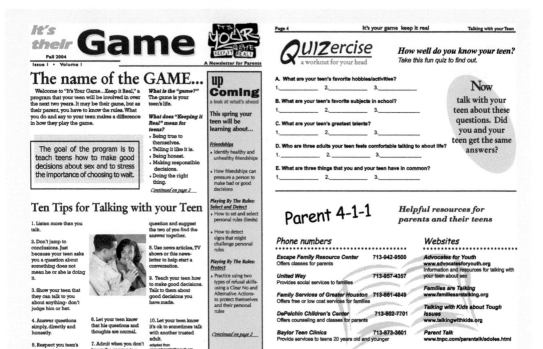

**Figure 7.11**    It's Your Game Parent Newsletter (Sample Pages)

Reprinted with permission of The University of Texas Health Science Center at Houston, copyright 2000–2014.

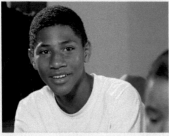

(a) Modeling using peer role models

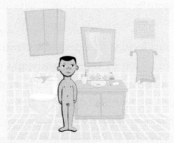

(b) Information transfer using cartoons

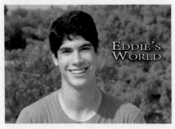

(c) Modeling using real-life serials

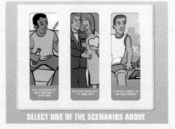

(d) Skills training using scenarios

**Figure 7.12**    Screen Captures Depicting Change Methods and Practical Applications From It's Your Game . . . Keep It Real Computer Activities

Reprinted with permission of The University of Texas Health Science Center at Houston, copyright 2000–2014.

Overall, student feedback was positive. Posttest ratings of importance of program content increased significantly across all content domains (all $p < .05$); self-efficacy ratings for enacting behaviors in these domains also significantly improved (all $p < .05$). Usability parameters were highly rated: 78–100 percent of students rated the It's Your Game computer activities as easy to use; 93 percent perceived the content to be correct and trustworthy; 100 percent agreed that most words in the program were understandable; 71–100 percent rated interface strategies and specific lesson activities as fun, and 93–100 percent rated It's Your Game as helping them make healthy decisions about sexuality (Shegog et al., 2007).

The planning team reviewed these pilot-test data and prioritized revisions based on budget and time constraints prior to the final production of program materials.

## Summary

Chapter 7 presents the process of producing program materials. The purpose of this chapter is to enable the planner to produce creative program components and materials in support of health promotion programs. The program will often be a complex entity with components for both at-risk groups and environmental agents. Each part of the program may be supported by products or materials designed to address the change objectives necessary to influence determinants of the behavior of the at-risk population or environmental agents.

The goal is that these materials are creative, effective pieces of the planned behavior- and environmental-change program (Steps 1, 2, and 3). The planning steps completed to this point should enable production of creative materials that emerge from the thinking captured in the matrix development and the selection of methods and practical applications. As in the other Intervention Mapping steps, in this step it is important to consult with the intended program participants, as well as potential program adopters and implementers, to determine preference for program design. Chapter 7 describes in detail how to organize ideas for program components into design documents that can serve as the guides for production of any materials needed to support the program. Finally, suggestions are made for pretesting program materials and overseeing the final production.

## Discussion Questions and Learning Activities

1. Explain what a design document is and why it is an important part of producing the intervention program.

2. Create an example of a design document that you would use to convey to someone the information needed to produce program materials.

Include communication channels and vehicles, messages, and themes. Match the program component to change objectives, methods, and applications so that the producer of the program materials is clear about what you intend to change.

3. If you propose that the materials are to be tailored, explain how tailoring will be done and on what variables.

4. Explain how you will pretest your program.

5. Explain how cultural issues have played a role in your Intervention Mapping project thus far (e.g., needs assessment, decisions about what should change, performance objectives, and determinants). Describe how cultural considerations will influence your program components and materials.

## References

Abraham, C., & Kools, M. (2012). *Writing health communication: An evidence-based guide*. London, United Kingdom: Sage.

Airhihenbuwa, C. O. (1994). Health promotion and the discourse on culture: Implications for empowerment. *Health Education Quarterly, 21*(3), 345–353.

Allies Against Asthma, & Center for Managing Chronic Disease. (n.d.). Tools for assessing asthma educational materials. Retrieved from http://www.centerformanagingchronicdisease.org/assets/files/Repository/Allies%20Against%20Asthma/Took%20Kit%20for%20Assessing%20Asthma%20Education%20Materials.pdf

American Epilepsy Society, Centers for Disease Control and Prevention (U.S.), Epilepsy Foundation. (2004). Living well with epilepsy II. Report of the 2003 National Conference on Public Health and Epilepsy: Priorities for a public health agenda on epilepsy. Retrieved from http://www.cdc.gov/epilepsy/pdfs/living_well_2003.pdf

Atkin, C. K., & Freimoth, C. (1989). Formative evaluation research in campaign design. In R. E. Rice & C. K. Atkin (Eds.), *Public communication campaigns* (pp. 131–150). Newbury Park, CA: Sage.

Baker, D., Williams, M., & Nurss, J. (1995). The test of functional health literacy in adults: A new instrument for measuring patients' literacy skills. *Journal of General Internal Medicine, 10*, 537–541.

Baker, D. W., Wolf, M. S., Feinglass, J., Thompson, J. A., Gazmararian, J. A., & Huang, J. (2007). Health literacy and mortality among elderly persons. *Archives of Internal Medicine, 167*(14), 1503–1509.

Balderman, B. (1996). *Buying creative services*. Lincolnwood, IL: NTC Publishing Group.

Bandura, A. (1986). *Social foundations of thought and action: A Social Cognitive Theory*. Englewood Cliffs, NJ: Prentice-Hall.

Baranowski, T., Cerin, E., & Baranowski, J. (2009). Steps in the design, development and formative evaluation of obesity prevention-related behavior change trials. *International Journal of Behavioral Nutrition & Physical Activity, 6*, 6.

Bartholomew, L., Shegog, R., Parcel, G., Gold, R., Fernández, M., Czyzewski, D., ... Berlin, N. (2000). Watch, Discover, Think, and Act: A model for patient education program development. *Patient Education and Counseling, 39*(2), 253–268.

Bellows, L., Anderson, J., Gould, S. M., & Auld, G. (2008). Formative research and strategic development of a physical activity component to a social marketing campaign for obesity prevention in preschoolers. *Journal of Community Health, 33*(3), 169–178.

Bentley, M. E., Johnson, S. L., Wasser, H., Creed-Kanashiro, H., Shroff, M., Fernandez Rao, S., & Cunningham, M. (2014). Formative research methods for designing culturally appropriate, integrated child nutrition and development interventions: An overview. *Annals of the New York Academy of Sciences, 1308*(1), 54–67.

Berkman, N. D., Sheridan, S. L., Donahue, K. E., Halpern, D. J., & Crotty, K. (2011). Low health literacy and health outcomes: An updated systematic review. *Annals of Internal Medicine, 155*(2), 97–107.

Centers for Disease Control and Prevention. (2015). Health literacy. Retrieved from http://www.cdc.gov/healthliteracy/

Chew, L. D., Griffin, J. M., Partin, M. R., Noorbaloochi, S., Grill, J. P., Snyder, A., ... VanRyn, M. (2008). Validation of screening questions for limited health literacy in a large VA outpatient population. *Journal of General Internal Medicine, 23*(5), 561–566.

Clark, N. M. (2003). Management of chronic disease by patients. *Annual Review of Public Health, 24*(1), 289–313.

Cullen, K. W., & Thompson, D. (2008). Feasibility of an 8-week African American web-based pilot program promoting healthy eating behaviors: Family Eats. *American Journal of Health Behavior, 32*(1), 40–51.

Daley, C. M., Cowan, P., Nollen, N. L., Greiner, K. A., & Choi, W. S. (2009). Assessing the scientific accuracy, readability, and cultural appropriateness of a culturally targeted smoking cessation program for American Indians. *Health Promotion Practice, 10*(3), 386–393.

Davis, R. E., Peterson, K. E., Rothschild, S. K., & Resnicow, K. (2011). Pushing the envelope for cultural appropriateness: Does evidence support cultural tailoring in type 2 diabetes interventions for Mexican American adults? *The Diabetes Educator, 37*(2), 227–238.

Della, L. J., DeJoy, D. M., Goetzel, R. Z., Ozminkowski, R. J., & Wilson, M. G. (2008). Assessing management support for worksite health promotion: Psychometric analysis of the leading by example (LBE) instrument. *American Journal of Health Promotion, 22*(5), 359–367.

Deshpande, A. D., Sanders Thompson, V. L., Vaughn, K. P., & Kreuter, M. W. (2009). The use of sociocultural constructs in cancer screening research among African Americans. *Cancer Control, 16*(3), 256–265.

Doak, C. C., Doak, L. G., & Root, J. H. (1996). *Teaching patients with low literacy skills* (2nd ed.). Philadelphia, PA: J.B. Lippincott.

Duvinage, K., Ibrügger, S., Kreichauf, S., Wildgruber, A., De Craemer, M., De Decker, E.,... Socha, P. (2014). Developing the intervention material to increase physical activity levels of European preschool children: The ToyBox-Study. *Obesity Reviews, 15*(S3), 27–39.

Estrada, C. A., Hryniewicz, M. M., Higgs, V. B., Collins, C., & Byrd, J. C. (2000). Anticoagulant patient information material is written at high readability levels. *Stroke, 31*(12), 2966–2970.

Estrada, C. A., Martin-Hryniewicz, M., Peek, B. T., Collins, C., & Byrd, J. C. (2004). Literacy and numeracy skills and anticoagulation control. *American Journal of the Medical Sciences, 328*(2), 88–93.

Flesch, R. (1974). *The art of readable writing.* New York, NY: Harper & Row.

Foster, D. R., & Rhoney, D. H. (2002). Readability of printed patient information for epileptic patients. *The Annals of Pharmacotherapy, 36*(12), 1856–1861.

Fountain, N. B., Van Ness, P. C., Swain-Eng, R., Tonn, S., Bever, C. T., Jr., & American Academy of Neurology Epilepsy Measure Development Panel and the American Medical Association-Convened Physician Consortium for Performance Improvement Independent Measure Development Process. (2011). Quality improvement in neurology: AAN epilepsy quality measures: Report of the Quality Measurement and Reporting Subcommittee of the American Academy of Neurology. *Neurology, 76*(1), 94–99.

Freimuth, V., Cole, G., & Kirby, S. (2011). Issues in evaluating mass media-based health communication campaigns. In J. S. Detrani (Ed.), *Mass communication: Issues, perspectives and techniques* (pp. 77–98). Boca Raton, FL: CRC Press.

Fry, E. (1977). Fry's readability graph: Clarifications, validity, and extension to level 17. *Journal of Reading, 21*, 242–252.

Gilmore, G. D., & Campbell, M. D. (2005). *Needs and capacity assessment strategies for health education and health promotion* (3rd ed.). Sudbury, MA: Jones and Bartlett.

Glasgow, R. E., Bull, S. S., Piette, J. D., & Steiner, J. F. (2004). Interactive behavior change technology: A partial solution to the competing demands of primary care. *American Journal of Preventive Medicine, 27*(2), 80–87.

Harrington, K. F., & Valerio, M. A. (2014). A conceptual model of verbal exchange health literacy. *Patient Education and Counseling, 94*(3), 403–410.

Harvard T.H. Chan School of Public Health. (2015). Assessing and developing health materials. Retrieved from http://www.hsph.harvard.edu/healthliteracy/practice/innovative-actions

Haun, J. N., Valerio, M. A., McCormack, L. A., Sørensen, K., & Paasche-Orlow, M. K. (2014). Health literacy measurement: An inventory and descriptive summary of 51 instruments. *Journal of Health Communication, 19*(sup2), 302–333.

Helitzer, D., Hollis, C., Cotner, J., & Oestreicher, N. (2009). Health literacy demands of written health information materials: An assessment of cervical cancer prevention materials. *Cancer Control, 16*(1), 70–78.

Hill-Briggs, F., & Smith, A. S. (2008). Evaluation of diabetes and cardiovascular disease print patient education materials for use with low-health literate populations. *Diabetes Care, 31*(4), 667–671.

Horner, J. R., Romer, D., Vanable, P. A., Salazar, L. F., Carey, M. P., Juzang, I., . . . Stanton, B. (2008). Using culture-centered qualitative formative research to design broadcast messages for HIV prevention for African American adolescents. *Journal of Health Communication, 13*(4), 309–325.

Indian Health Service. (n.d.). Tool 13. Assessing readability level reading formulas. Retrieved from https://www.ihs.gov/healthcommunications/documents/toolkit/Tool13.pdf

Institute of Medicine, Committee on Health Literacy. (2004). *Health literacy: A prescription to end confusion* (Washington, DC ed.) National Academies Press.

Kaphingst, K. A., Zanfini, C. J., & Emmons, K. M. (2006). Accessibility of web sites containing colorectal cancer information to adults with limited literacy (United States). *Cancer Causes & Control, 17*(2), 147–151.

Kelly, P. A., & Haidet, P. (2007). Physician overestimation of patient literacy: A potential source of health care disparities. *Patient Education and Counseling, 66*(1), 119–122.

Kirsch, I., Jungeblut, A., Jenkins, L., & Kolstad, A. (1993). *Adult literacy in America: A first look at the findings of the national adult literacy survey.* Washington, DC: National Center for Education Statistics, US Department of Education.

Kostelnick, C. (1996). Supra-textual design: The visual rhetoric of whole documents. *Technical Communication Quarterly, 5*(1), 9–33.

Kreuter, M. W., Lukwago, S. N., Bucholtz, R. D., Clark, E. M., & Sanders-Thompson, V. (2003). Achieving cultural appropriateness in health promotion programs: Targeted and tailored approaches. *Health Education & Behavior, 30*(2), 133–146.

Kreuter, M. W., Skinner, C. S., Steger-May, K., Holt, C. L., Bucholtz, D. C., Clark, E. M., & Haire-Joshu, D. (2004). Responses to behaviorally vs. culturally tailored cancer communication among African American women. *American Journal of Health Behavior, 28*(3), 195–207.

Kreuter, M. W., Sugg-Skinner, C., Holt, C. L., Clark, E. M., Haire-Joshu, D., Fu, Q., . . . Bucholtz, D. (2005). Cultural tailoring for mammography and fruit and vegetable intake among low-income African-American women in urban public health centers. *Preventive Medicine, 41*(1), 53–62.

Krueger, R. A., & Casey, M. A. (2009). *Focus groups: A practical guide for applied research* (4th ed.). Thousand Oaks, CA: Sage.

McCormack, L., Haun, J., Sørensen, K., & Valerio, M. (2013). Recommendations for advancing health literacy measurement. *Journal of Health Communication, 18*(sup1), 9–14.

McGuire, W. J. (1986). The myth of massive media impact: Savagings and salvagings. In. G. Comstock (Ed.), *Public communication and behavior. Volume 1.* (pp. 173–257). Orlando, FL: Academic Press.

McLaughlin, G. H. (1969). SMOG grading: A new readability formula. *Journal of Reading, 12*(8), 639–646.

Mevissen, F. E., Meertens, R. M., Ruiter, R. A. C., Feenstra, H., & Schaalma, H. P. (2009). HIV/STI risk communication: The effects of scenario-based risk information and frequency-based risk information on perceived susceptibility to chlamydia and HIV. *Journal of Health Psychology, 14*(1), 78–87.

Morgenstern, L. B., Bartholomew, L. K., Grotta, J. C., Staub, L., King, M., & Chan, W. (2003). Sustained benefit of a community and professional intervention to increase acute stroke therapy. *Archives of Internal Medicine, 163*(18), 2198–2202.

Morgenstern, L. B., Staub, L., Chan, W., Wein, T. H., Bartholomew, L. K., King, M., . . . Grotta, J. C. (2002). Improving delivery of acute stroke therapy: The TLL Temple Foundation Stroke Project. *Stroke, 33*(1), 160–166.

Moriarty, S. (1994). Visual communication as a primary system. *Journal of Visual Literacy, 14*(2), 11–21.

Moriarty, S. E., Mitchell, N., & Wells, W. (2008). *Advertising: Principles and practice* (8th ed.). Upper Saddle, NJ: Pearson Prentice-Hall.

Mosenthal, P. B., & Kirsch, I. S. (1998). A new measure for assessing document complexity: The PMOSE/IKIRSCH document readability formula. *Journal of Adolescent & Adult Literacy, 41*(8), 638–657.

National Cancer Institute, Center for the Advancement of Health, & Robert Wood Johnson Foundation. (2002). *Designing for dissemination.* (Conference Summary Report).

National Institutes of Health. (2003). Clear and to the point: Guidelines for using plain language at NIH. Retrieved from http://execsec.od.nih.gov/plainlang/guidelines/index.html

National Institutes of Health. (2014). Clear communication. Retrieved from http://www.nih.gov/clearcommunication/

Neuhauser, L., Rothschild, B., Graham, C., Ivey, S. L., & Konishi, S. (2009). Participatory design of mass health communication in three languages for seniors and people with disabilities on Medicaid. *American Journal of Public Health, 99*(12), 2188–2195.

Osborne, H. (2005). *Health literacy from A to Z: Practical ways to communicate your health.* Sudbury, MA: Jones and Bartlett Publishers.

Paasche-Orlow, M. K., & Wolf, M. S. (2007). The causal pathways linking health literacy to health outcomes. *American Journal of Health Behavior, 31*(Suppl 1), S19–S26.

Parker, R. M., Baker, D. W., Williams, M. V., & Nurss, J. R. (1995). The test of functional health literacy in adults. *Journal of General Internal Medicine, 10*(10), 537–541.

Ratanawongsa, N., Handley, M. A., Quan, J., Sarkar, U., Pfeifer, K., Soria, C., & Schillinger, D. (2012). Quasi-experimental trial of diabetes self-management automated and real-time telephonic support (SMARTSteps) in a Medicaid managed care plan: Study protocol. *BMC Health Services Research, 12*, 22.

Resnicow, K., Baranowski, T., Ahluwalia, J. S., & Braithwaite, R. L. (1999). Cultural sensitivity in public health: Defined and demystified. *Ethnicity & Disease, 9*(1), 10–21.

Resnicow, K., Davis, R., Zhang, N., Strecher, V., Tolsma, D., Calvi, J., . . . Cross, W. E., Jr. (2009). Tailoring a fruit and vegetable intervention on ethnic identity: Results of a randomized study. *Health Psychology, 28*(4), 394.

Rhee, H., Wyatt, T. H., & Wenzel, J. A. (2006). Adolescents with asthma: Learning needs and internet use assessment. *Respiratory Care, 51*(12), 1441–1449.

Schwartzberg, J. G., VanGest, J., & Wang, C. C. (2005). *Understanding health literacy.* Chicago, IL: American Medical Association.

Shegog, R., Begley, C. E., Harding, A., Dubinsky, S., Goldsmith, C., Hope, O., & Newmark, M. (2013). Description and feasibility of MINDSET: A clinic decision aid for epilepsy self-management. *Epilepsy & Behavior, 29*(3), 527–536.

Shegog, R., Markham, C., Peskin, M., Dancel, M., Coton, C., & Tortolero, S. (2007). "It's Your Game": An innovative multimedia virtual world to prevent HIV/STI and pregnancy in middle school youth.

Shieh, C., & Hosei, B. (2008). Printed health information materials: Evaluation of readability and suitability. *Journal of Community Health Nursing, 25*(2), 73–90.

Shiffman, C. B. (1994). Ethnovisual and sociovisual elements of design: Visual dialect as a basis for creativity in public service graphic design. *Journal of Visual Literacy, 14*(2), 23–39.

Sorensen, G., Fagan, P., Hunt, M. K., Stoddard, A. M., Girod, K., Eisenberg, M., & Frazier, L. (2004). Changing channels for tobacco control with youth: Developing an intervention for working teens. *Health Education Research, 19*(3), 250–260.

Tufte, E. R. (1997). *Visual explanations: Images and quantities, evidence and narrative.* Cheshire, CT: Graphics Press.

U.S. Department of Health and Human Services, Office of Disease Prevention and Health Promotion. (2015). Health literacy. Retrieved from http://www.health.gov/communication/literacy/

U.S. National Library of Medicine. (2013). How to write easy-to-read health materials. Retrieved from http://www.nlm.nih.gov/medlineplus/etr.html

Velasquez, M. M., Gaddy-Maurer, G., Crouch, C., & DiClemente, C. C. (2001). *Group treatment for substance abuse: A stages-of-change therapy manual.* New York, NY: Guilford Press.

Vu, M. B., Murrie, D., Gonzalez, V., & Jobe, J. B. (2006). Listening to girls and boys talk about girls' physical activity behaviors. *Health Education & Behavior, 33*(1), 81–96.

Wells, W., Burnett, J., & Moriarty, S. E. (2006). *Advertising: Principles and practice* (7th ed.). Upper Saddle River, NJ: Pearson Prentice-Hall.

Werner, O., & Campbell, D. T. (1973). Translating, working through interpreters, and the problem of decentering. In R. Naroll & R. Cohen (Eds.), *A handbook of methods in cultural anthropology* (pp. 398–422). New York, NY: Columbia University Press.

Whittingham, J. R., Ruiter, R. A. C., Castermans, D., Huiberts, A., & Kok, G. (2008). Designing effective health education materials: Experimental pre-testing of a theory-based brochure to increase knowledge. *Health Education Research, 23*(3), 414–426.

Whittingham, J., Ruiter, R. A. C., Zimbile, F., & Kok, G. (2008). Experimental pretesting of public health campaigns: A case study. *Journal of Health Communication, 13*(3), 216–229.

Wilson, G. (1999). Cognitive interviewing: A "how to" guide. Retrieved from http://appliedresearch.cancer.gov/archive/cognitive/interview.pdf

Wilson, J. M., Wallace, L. S., & DeVoe, J. E. (2009). Are state Medicaid application enrollment forms readable? *Journal of Health Care for the Poor and Underserved, 20*(2), 423–431.

Wilson, M. G., Goetzel, R. Z., Ozminkowski, R. J., DeJoy, D. M., Della, L., Roemer, E. C., ... Baase, C. M. (2007). Using formative research to develop environmental and ecological interventions to address overweight and obesity. *Obesity, 15*(S1), 37S–47S.

Wyatt, T. H., Krauskopf, P. B., & Davidson, R. (2008). Using focus groups for program planning and evaluation. *The Journal of School Nursing, 24*(2), 71–82.

Yick, A. G. (2008). Evaluating readability of domestic violence information found on domestic violence state coalitions' websites. *Journal of Technology in Human Services, 26*(1), 67–75.

Young, D. R., Johnson, C. C., Steckler, A., Gittelsohn, J., Saunders, R. P., Saksvig, B. I., ... McKenzie, T. L. (2006). Data to action: Using formative research to develop intervention programs to increase physical activity in adolescent girls. *Health Education & Behavior, 33*(1), 97–111.

Zapka, J., Lemon, S. C., Estabrook, B. B., & Jolicoeur, D. G. (2007). Keeping a step ahead: Formative phase of a workplace intervention trial to prevent obesity. *Obesity, 15*(S1), 27S–36S.

Zarcadoolas, C., Pleasant, A., & Greer, D. S. (2009). *Advancing health literacy: A framework for understanding and action.* Hoboken, NJ: John Wiley & Sons.

# CHAPTER 8

# INTERVENTION MAPPING STEP 5

*Program Implementation Plan*

## Competency

- Develop an implementation plan to enable adoption, implementation, and maintenance of the health promotion program.

The ultimate impact of a health promotion program depends on both the effectiveness of the program and on its reach in the population. Effective health education and promotion programs will have little impact if they are never used, have limited use, or if they are discontinued while still needed to create the planned health impact (Glasgow, Klesges, Dzewaltowski, Bull, & Estabrooks, 2004a; Klabunde, Riley, Mandelson, Frame, & Brown, 2004; Oldenburg & Glanz, 2008). Without a planned intervention to promote use of the program, the health promotion program may stay on the developers' shelf if the program is not adopted—or on the organization's shelf if the program is adopted but not implemented. Furthermore, if the program is not maintained after initial implementation, it may not produce or sustain the desired outcomes (Damschroder et al., 2009; Klesges, Estabrooks, Dzewaltowski, Bull, & Glasgow, 2005). Throughout this chapter, we refer to interventions to increase program use (adoption, implementation, and/or maintenance) as implementation interventions.

The purpose of this chapter is twofold: (a) to encourage planners to develop programs that include details about how they should be adopted, implemented, and maintained, and (b) to provide a framework for systematic planning of implementation interventions to increase use of existing evidence-based interventions (EBIs; including policies, guidelines, and practices). For new programs,

### LEARNING OBJECTIVES AND TASKS

- Identify potential program implementers
- State outcomes and performance objectives for program use
- Construct matrices of change objectives for program use
- Design implementation interventions

demonstration projects, and research projects, the focus of Step 5 is to plan for initial implementation to ensure that the program is used as intended during evaluation of efficacy or effectiveness. For programs that have already been implemented and evaluated, Step 5 can be used independently of intervention mapping (IM) Steps 1–4 to develop an implementation intervention to enhance dissemination to new sites or to "scale-up" for wide-spread use.

## Perspectives

In the field of health promotion, as in other fields, effective programs, policies, and practices are often available but not used to improve public health (Bero et al., 1998; Brownson et al., 2007a; Jacobs, Dodson, Baker, Deshpande, & Brownson, 2010; Ringwalt et al., 2011; Spoth et al., 2013). Closing the gap between what we know works in health promotion and what is implemented in communities and clinical settings is critical to improving population health (National Cancer Institute, Center for Advancement of Health, Robert Wood Johnson Foundation, 2002). Barriers to broad-scale use of effective health promotion programs include problems during the development and evaluation of a program that limit its acceptability, usability, and real-world relevance, and lack of or inadequate interventions designed to increase program adoption, implementation, and mainte-nance. Intervention Mapping can help planners "design for dissemination" (Brownson, Jacobs, Tabak, Hoehner, & Stamatakis, 2013; Harris et al., 2012; Neta et al., 2015) to ensure that programs are acceptable, relevant, and usable. It can also help planners develop theory- and evidence-based implementation interventions to increase program use. If an existing EBI requires adaptation in addition to an implementation plan, we recommend that the planner follow the steps of a simplified version of IM (IM Adapt) as described in Chapter 10.

### Designing Health Promotion Programs for Dissemination

Several aspects of IM may contribute to creation of an intervention that is both effective and amenable to implementation. One aspect is partici-patory planning to increase the probability that the characteristics of the intervention will be compatible with the needs of the priority population and consistent with the context in which the program will be implemented. Also, the evidence- and theory-based approach of IM helps planners make decisions about program focus, including the behaviors, environmental conditions, and determinants that are most relevant for the priority popu-lation and environmental agents. It also guides planners to select and pretest change methods, practical applications, delivery channels, and materials that fit the priority population, which implementers will find appealing, feasible, and effective. Although planning for program use is positioned as Step 5 in IM, program planners should consider potential factors that will influence the adoption and implementation of the program at each of the preceding steps to ensure that the intervention will be a good fit for potential program participants and implementers.

The design and methods used for program evaluation can also influence practitioners' perspectives about the credibility of the evidence of the program's effectiveness and whether or not it would be appropriate in a "real-world" setting. Recent research guidelines have sought to increase the probability that planners will use evidence. For example, the CONSORT Work Group on Pragmatic Trials (Thorpe et al., 2009; Zwarenstein & Treweek, 2009) developed the Pragmatic Explanatory Continuum Indicator Summary (PRECIS) criteria to provide information about the extent to which a trial is "pragmatic" (broadly applicable) or is "explanatory" (fundamental and focused). The PRECIS consists of dimensions, such as flexibility of the comparison condition and the experimental intervention, practitioner expertise, participant eligibility criteria, and follow-up intensity (Thorpe et al., 2009). Health promotion planners can assess the value of published studies that use the PRECIS criteria in terms of how relevant it may or may not be given their setting. Another example of a framework that strives to increase the value of research for practitioners and decision-makers is based on work by an NIH and Veterans Administration (VA) dissemination and implementation (D&I) workgroup that focused on measurement and reporting. For example, Neta et al. (2015) published a framework, which suggests that trials be pragmatic and adequately report the context, policy climate, organizational settings, delivery details, and incentives. This type of reporting is essential for potential planners to understand the relevance of research evidence for an intervention given their population and setting (Green & Glasgow, 2006). The authors also suggest that published studies should provide more information about the planning of interventions in which planners can understand the program logic, change methods, and practical applications used in evidence-based programs. We further describe some practice-based evaluation approaches, such as pragmatic trials (Glasgow & Riley, 2013), in Chapter 9: Step 6, Evaluation.

## Implementation Interventions to Increase Program Use

Program failure can often be traced to problems with inadequate program adoption and implementation. A review of more than 500 studies of prevention and health promotion programs demonstrated that the level of implementation affected program outcomes (Durlak & DuPre, 2008). Numerous reviews have shown that passive dissemination of evidence-based programs (e.g., publications, mass mailings) has been ineffective to promote program use (Bero et al., 1998; Grimshaw et al., 2001). Although there are efforts to make EBIs available through websites and other resources, these have traditionally been underutilized. In health promotion, we often use systematic planning, theory, evidence, and an ecological approach to develop programs; yet, we rarely use what we know about developing robust programs to plan implementation interventions to ensure that these programs are adopted and used (Bero et al., 1998; Colditz, 2012; Damschroder et al., 2009; Davies, Walker, & Grimshaw, 2010; Proctor et al., 2009). For example, a review of the use of theory in 235 studies that evaluated guideline dissemination and implementation strategies found that only 22 percent had employed theory. Often, researchers describe implementation approaches as single strategies to increase use of an EBI but do not specify the rationale behind the decision to use such an approach (Proctor, Powell, & McMillen, 2013).

Well-conceptualized implementation interventions use theory and evidence to design change methods and practical applications to promote program use. These can help ensure that a program fits the contextual realities of the implementation setting and can be implemented as planned and sustained over time. For example, Glanz, Steffen, Elliott, and O'Riordan (2005) carefully planned a theory- and evidence-informed intervention to disseminate an effective skin-cancer prevention program. This dissemination intervention incorporated methods based on an integration of Social Cognitive Theory (SCT; Bandura, 1986, 2001), Diffusion of Innovations Theory (DIT; Rogers, 1983, 1995), and theories of organizational change (Glanz et al., 2005; Steckler, Goodman, & Kegler, 2002) to create a multicomponent program that targeted organizational as well as individual change. In another example, Donaldson and Poulos (2014) used IM Step 5 to plan an intervention aimed at increasing adoption and implementation among coaches of a neck-injury prevention program for athletes. They applied DIT (Rogers, 2003) to understanding perceived program characteristics and delivery channels. The intervention addressed factors related to adoption and implementation at multiple levels, and the authors noted that using IM Step 5 led them to develop a theory-informed, practical program that was context specific and responsive to stakeholder needs (Donaldson & Poulos, 2014).

In the field of dissemination and implementation research, there sometimes is confusion between the EBI being disseminated and the intervention designed to accelerate its use. Figure 8.1 clarifies the difference between the EBI and the implementation intervention (the oval depicted to the right

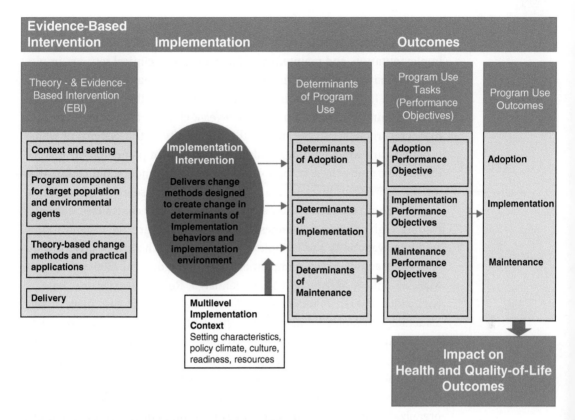

**Figure 8.1**  The EBI and Implementation Intervention Targets and Outcomes

of the EBI). Read from the left, the planning team chooses or develops the EBI, then develops an implementation intervention to influence the determinants of program use—and ultimately adoption, implementation, and maintenance outcomes (far right side of the model). The causal chain of factors for program use interventions is similar to the logic model for health promotion interventions (see Chapter 5, Figure 5.1).

## Using Dissemination and Implementation Frameworks to Inform Step 5

Planners can make use of the implementation science research literature to understand and influence the movement of EBIs into real-world settings (Clavier, Sénéchal, Vibert, & Potvin, 2012; Damschroder et al., 2009; Michie et al., 2005; Michie, Johnston, Francis, Hardeman, & Eccles, 2008; Proctor et al., 2011, 2013). Implementation researchers study factors that influence movement of EBIs from controlled, experimental contexts into delivery contexts where they will be used in existing organizational operations (Rubenstein & Pugh, 2006). Real-world community or health care settings for delivery of new programs typically comprise multiple levels of individuals or groups who need to be involved in program adoption, implementation, and maintenance. For example, in clinical settings, implementers may include individuals in the interpersonal environment (e.g., providers), in the organizational environment (e.g., clinic director), and in the community or social environment (e.g., clinic network/health system managers, regulators). Because of the complexity of the systems in which programs are implemented, health services and implementation science researchers study these complex systems to better understand factors that influence program implementation. For example, researchers have found organizational characteristics, such as larger size, decentralized administration, high interconnectedness and informality, greater organizational resource availability and complexity, and leaders who are positive toward change are associated with implementation (Glasgow et al., 2004a; Glasgow, Marcus, Bull, & Wilson, 2004b; Greenhalgh, Robert, Macfarlane, Bate, & Kyriakidou, 2004). A recent study found that financial resources, strong leadership, organizational climate, and attitudes toward the EBIs were associated with the agency capacity to train providers and implement EBIs (Bonham, Sommerfeld, Willging, & Aarons, 2014). In contrast, characteristics of settings that may act as barriers to adoption include competing demands; imposition of programs from the outside; unstable finances and organizational structure; limited staff time; limited organizational support; low levels of organizational capacity to deliver a program; lack of innovation fit with prevailing practices; and incentives or regulations that work against change (Glasgow et al., 2004a). Over several decades, the work of Rogers (1983, 1995, 2003) and others (Dearing, 2009) has laid the groundwork for how to get programs adopted, implemented, and continued over time. Often this entire process is referred to as diffusion and focuses on initial use of an innovation (see Chapters 2 and 3 for a discussion of DIT). Since the 1980s, researchers have given increasing attention to the processes involved with both program implementation and program continuation (Johnson, Hays, Center, & Daley, 2004; Saunders, Evans, & Joshi, 2005; Scheirer, Shediac, & Cassady, 1995; Shediac-Rizkallah & Bone, 1998). Diffusion has often been described as a staged process of moving from an individual's or organization's becoming aware of an innovation, deciding to adopt it, initially using it, and then maintaining use (Oldenburg & Glanz, 2008), whereas dissemination includes planned systematic efforts to increase program use in a particular population, health care setting, or social system.

More recently, authors have offered new descriptions of the phases of implementation (Proctor et al., 2013). For example, Aarons, Hurlburt, and Horwitz (2011) described four stages: exploration, adoption decision, active implementation, and sustainment. The National Implementation Research Network (NIRN) reviewed more than 2,000 articles on the implementation of programs and identified five interrelated stages of successful implementation: exploration, installation, initial implementation, full implementation, and program sustainability (Fixsen, Naoom, Blase, Friedman, & Wallace, 2005). The exploration stage includes some steps that may precede the decision to adopt a program. It includes the identification of community needs to determine the fit of the program, the assessment of organizational capacity to implement it, the selection of a program to match community needs and available resources, and the understanding of program fidelity and needed adaptation. The addition of the "exploration" stage is important in efforts to search for an existing EBI (see Chapter 10: Adaptation).

Recently, many authors have presented dissemination and implementation frameworks proposing how programs are adopted and implemented, and which types of resources, capacity, and systems influence their use (Damschroeder et al., 2009; Klesges et al., 2005; Mendel, Meredith, Schoenbaum, Sherbourne, & Wells, 2008; Wandersman et al., 2008). These frameworks can support Step 5 by helping the planner to think carefully about implementation outcomes, consider who the adopters and implementers may be, what may influence their actions (personal and contextual factors), and what types of capacity building may be required. There are many frameworks available. Tabak, Khoong, Chambers, and Brownson (2012) reviewed 61 models for dissemination and implementation research, and Moullin, Sabater-Hernández, Fernandez-Llimos, and Benrimoj (2015) identified and categorized 49 implementation frameworks used for innovations in health care. We present the following three examples of frameworks of influences on and outcomes of dissemination and implementation that can be particularly useful in identifying implementation outcomes: Reach, Effectiveness, Adoption, Implementation, and Maintenance (RE-AIM: Glasgow, Vogt, & Boles, 1999); actors and behaviors related to implementation: Interactive Systems Framework (ISF; Wandersman et al., 2008); and contextual and other factors influencing implementation: Consolidated Framework for Implementation Research (Damschroeder et al., 2009). Although these frameworks can help inform decisions about what may influence implementation, none of these provide guidance for how to design interventions that specifically address the factors included in the models. There are only a few examples in the literature of the systematic planning of dissemination interventions (Michie et al., 2005, 2008; Proctor et al., 2011, 2013). IM can serve as an overarching implementation intervention planning framework that can incorporate constructs from other frameworks to inform development decisions at each task. This is analogous to how IM is used to organize theoretical constructs from health behavior models when planning a health promotion program (Steps 1–4).

## Framework Example: RE-AIM

RE-AIM is a framework designed to improve the quality, speed, and public health impact of prevention programs (Glasgow et al., 1999). It was originally developed to promote consistent reporting of research results and for evaluating the overall impact of health promotion programs (Glasgow, Klesges, Dzewaltowski, Estabrooks, & Vogt, 2006). RE-AIM has also been used in program planning to guide decisions during development by helping planners define explicit targets for intervention impact and reach, thus creating a better balance between internal and external validity (Glasgow, McKay, Piette, Reynolds, 2001; Glassgow et al., 1999). RE-AIM has been used to assess program impact across many different behaviors and settings, and to understand the impact of implementation interventions (Akers, Estabrooks, & Davy, 2010; Dunton, Lagloire, & Robertson, 2009; Finch et al., 2011; Gaglio, Shoup, & Glasgow, 2013; Kahwati, Lance, Jones, & Kinsinger, 2011; Kessler et al., 2013; Vick, Duffy, Ewing, Rugen, & Zak, 2013). For example, Sweet and colleagues (2014) used RE-AIM to evaluate multisector partnerships for promoting physical activity. They evaluated implementation strategies applied by the individuals and organizations in national partnerships (Sweet, Ginis, Estabrooks, & Latimer-Cheung, 2014). In another example, a systematic review used RE-AIM to focus the evaluation of evidence-based multilevel interventions to improve obesity-related behaviors in adults (Compernolle et al., 2014). For planners developing implementation interventions using IM Step 5, RE-AIM can help define the various implementation outcomes.

## Framework Example: Interactive Systems Framework

The ISF for dissemination and implementation was developed to help address the gap between research and practice (Noonan, Wilson, & Mercer, 2012). It was designed to help researchers and practitioners have a better understanding of the process of implementation, and the varying levels and actors involved (Wandersman et al., 2008). The ISF describes three systems that work together to advance the implementation of prevention programs. The Prevention Synthesis and Translation System supports summarization of evidence and packaging evidence-based programs so that they can be understood, accessible and easy to use. The Prevention Support System provides general and program-specific training, tools, and technical assistance to increase practitioner and organizational capacity to implement EBIs. The Prevention Delivery System emphasizes the activities to deliver

EBIs and capacity building to make those activities possible (Wandersman et al., 2008). Fernández et al. (2014) describe collaborative activities of the Cancer Prevention and Control Research Network to increase adoption and implementation of evidence-based cancer control interventions framed within the ISF framework. For example, the network developed tools to enhance general and innovation-specific capacity of 211 call centers (delivery system) to implement a referral and navigation program for increasing cancer-control practices among medically underserved individuals. The ISF can help planners as they identify actors in each of the three systems the ISF describes. It can also help planners identify performance objectives for implementation by thinking about what actions may be necessary to enhance general or innovation specific capacity to improve implementation.

## Framework Example: Consolidated Framework for Implementation Research

Developers describe the Consolidated Framework for Implementation Research (CFIR) as an "overarching framework" to support development of implementation theory and assessment of what promotes dissemination in different situations and why (Damschroder et al., 2009; Zulman et al., 2013). To develop the consolidated framework, Damschroder et al. (2009) conducted a systematic review of 19 published theories, models, and frameworks to identify constructs that may influence implementation, have consistent meanings, and be measurable (Greenhalgh et al., 2004). The CFIR constructs are categorized in the following five domains without specifying relationships between them: intervention characteristics (e.g., cost, complexity), outer setting (e.g., external policy and incentives, patient needs, and resources), inner setting (e.g., implementation climate, available resources), characteristics of individuals (e.g., self-efficacy, knowledge and beliefs about the intervention), and implementation process (e.g., planning, reflecting, and evaluating). Program planners can use the CFIR domains to think about their own situations and identify contextual factors that may influence implementation. Thinking about these factors can stimulate identification of implementers and creation of performance objectives to influence the context for implementation. The CFIR also contains constructs found in other theories, such as DIT "characteristics of the innovation," which planners can think about when identifying determinants of implementation behaviors. For example, if an adopter or implementer perceives that the health promotion program has evidence of effectiveness, fits with existing values of the organization, and is better than what is currently being used, they will be more likely to use it.

Many studies have used CFIR constructs for identifying and intervening on factors that may influence implementation (Abbott, Foster, Marin, & Dykes, 2014; Damschroder & Hagedorn, 2011; Damschroder & Lowery, 2013; Ilott, Gerrish, Booth, & Field, 2013; Zulman et al., 2013). For example, Ditty, Landes, Doyle, and Beidas (2014) conducted a mixed method study guided by CFIR to explore the relationship between inner-setting constructs and implementation of an evidence-based behavioral therapy. They found that team cohesion, communication, climate, and supervision were correlated with level of implementation of the evidence-based therapy. Sanchez, Sethi, Santos, and Boockvar (2014) used grounded theory to identify factors influencing implementation of medication reconciliation within a large urban medical center and an affiliated VA hospital resulting in themes organized using CFIR. Chin, Goddu, Ferguson, and Peek (2014) used CFIR to describe a health care community initiative to improve diabetes outcomes by mapping its components to the domains of CFIR. Findings from these types of studies can help implementation planners identify contextual factors that may influence implementation and either include them as intervention targets or measure them as possible moderating variables.

## A Participatory Approach to Implementation Planning

Too often, program developers and evaluators see dissemination as just another step along the "discovery to delivery" continuum in which developers must "push" their products out into the community or clinical setting (Rimer, Glanz, & Rasband, 2001; Wandersman et al., 2008). This perspective may blind them to the need to involve community stakeholders in either the development or implementation of programs. In the case of implementation of tested programs, communities may perceive that the evidence-based interventions that were tested elsewhere are not necessarily appropriate for their context. The "push" perspective also fails to take into account the importance of market "pull" or demand and may not address questions of delivery capacity (National Cancer Institute et al., 2002). In comparison, community-centered approaches begin with a focus on community needs and capacity, and use principles from community-based participatory research (CBPR) to improve program delivery and the translation of research into practice (Tapp & Dulin, 2010; Viswanathan et al., 2004).

Including potential program implementers in planning development and implementation of EBIs can help make programs easier to implement, and can improve the external validity of evaluation research findings (Miller & Shinn, 2005; Trickett, 2011; Wandersman et al., 2008). In Chapter 1, we suggested that potential adopters, implementers, and maintainers of the program should participate in the planning group, and provide input into each aspect of the design and development of the intervention. Planners should not wait until Step 5 of IM to involve potential program adopters and implementers, but they should take time at this point to make sure that potential program users are well represented in the planning group (Peterson, Rogers, Cunningham-Sabo, & Davis, 2007). At this step, when the planning group has designed the program and better understands the requirements for adoption and implementation, it may need to add new members who can represent fresh views from potential program implementers. These new members of the planning group can be seen as a linkage system.

A linkage system, originally described by Havelock (1971) and Orlandi (1986), assure collaborative communications between the program developers and the user group to promote program use. A primary characteristic of a linkage system is the presence of change agents or program champions who bridge the gap between developers and users (Orlandi, 1986; Orlandi, Landers, Weston, & Haley, 1990; Robinson et al., 2005). An examination of seven case studies of how prevention programs or policies were used by communities concluded that program champions or agents linking research resources to the community users moved adoption and implementation forward, and that greater community participation resulted in more advanced utilization (Peterson et al., 2007). The linkage system should provide a means to exchange information and ideas between planners and implementers, to ensure access to the planning process for program implementers, and to facilitate the development of user-friendly programs (Ammerman, Lindquist, Lohr, & Hersey, 2002; Durlak & DuPre, 2008; Havelock, 1971; Johnson et al., 2004; Kocken, Voorham, Brandsma, & Swart, 2001; Kolbe & Iverson, 1981; Orlandi, 1986; Orlandi et al., 1990; Robinson et al., 2005).

Several examples of linkage systems suggest their usefulness in promoting program use. Robinson et al. (2005) examined the utility of linkage systems for the dissemination of the Canadian Heart Health Initiative and found that they resulted in increased health promotion program capacity, delivery, and sustainability in public health organizations. In another example, a linkage system for a trial of activity for adolescent girls (TAAG) facilitated communication between the development team and school and community agency personnel to increase feelings of local ownership of the program. In addition to enabling adoption, implementation, and institutionalization of the TAAG program, program champions facilitated continuation of TAAG after research support ended. In another example, the American Cancer Society (ACS), Midwest Division, served as the linkage system to promote the use of the program, Friend to Friend, to increase mammography (Slater, Finnegan, & Madigan, 2005). The ACS mission, goals, structure, resources, and compatibility with the innovative program made it an excellent linking agent, as did its early involvement in intervention development (Slater et al., 2005).

## Tasks for Step 5

In Step 5, planners do the following: (a) identify program adopters, implementers, and maintainers; (b) state outcomes and performance objective for all three stages of program use; (c) construct matrices of change objectives for implementation interventions; and (d) design implementation interventions. In a sense, the tasks of IM Step 5 are similar to Steps 2, 3, and 4 of IM. The difference in Step 5 is that rather than focusing on the at-risk population and environmental agents, we are concerned with the behaviors and environmental conditions of individuals or groups who adopt the program, those who will use it in every day practice, and those who will maintain it by rolling it into the routine operations of the organization.

### Identifying Program Implementers

The first task in Step 5 is to identify who will do what at each stage of program use.

Although some health education programs may be self-selected and directed by the participants, most require someone to make them available to participants. Programs also require individuals to ensure their continued use and outcomes over time. Often the person or persons who will decide to adopt, and those who will deliver and maintain the program over time will be different. For example, school principals may support adoption of a program but usually will not be the implementer. For example, once a principal adopts a health-promotion curriculum, program implementers might be teachers who present health education programs to students. In a clinical setting, managers might organize review and adoption of new patient education procedures, whereas nurses, dietitians, physicians, or other hands-on providers present the programs to patients. In contrast, some programs, such as those delivered online or via mass media, do not need anyone to implement intervention activities. However, these media-based or online programs still need to reach intended participants, and adopters may be the gatekeepers for mass-media or online distribution systems. For example, program managers at radio stations may not be directly involved in conducting mass-media campaigns, but their support is essential in making sure the program is broadcast.

As they begin Step 5, usually, program planners know the organization or setting in which a program will be adopted and implemented, and can immediately answer the questions below. In some cases, however, Step 5 must start with selecting implementation partners from among several possible venues and organizations. Planners will want to recruit organizations that have a good potential reach to intended program participants (Glasgow et al., 2004b; Klesges et al., 2005; Kreuter et al., 2012; Purnell et al., 2012). Organizations, such as schools, churches, social service organizations, and clinical practice settings typically serve large numbers of individuals who may represent the priority populations intended for the health-promotion program.

Planners will need to understand the organizational structure of adopting agencies to correctly identify individuals who will be making decisions about program use. For example, programs developed for clinic settings to increase mammography screening that include both patient level and provider level components could be adopted by individual primary care clinics or by groups of affiliated clinics, such as Federally Qualified Health Centers, health service collaboratives, or HMOs, that include multiple clinic locations. Before making a decision on the implementing organization, planners will ask how certain characteristics of the organizations, such as size, leadership, readiness for change, and general capacity, may influence implementation. Other elements, such as feasibility, fit with organizational goals and values, and quantity of information or change that an organization can absorb (absorptive capacity) can also be important (Bonham et al., 2014; Cohen & Levinthal, 1990; Flaspohler, Duffy, Wandersman, Stillman, & Maras, 2008; Greenhalgh et al., 2004; Weiner, Amick, & Lee, 2008; Zahra & George, 2002).

Planners will need to understand who the leaders are in organizations and communities because these individuals are often responsible for adoption decisions and can be essential in ensuring proper implementation. Senior management buy-in and support are almost always required for adoption and implementation (Dearing, 2009) in addition to the more focused roles of program champions and opinion leaders as described in classical diffusion theory (Rogers, 1983, 1995). Clear communication about the importance of an innovation and resources for implementation can influence leader support to prepare the organization or community for implementation (Greenhalgh et al., 2004). Once the planning team has made at least a preliminary decision about the setting for program implementation, they will answer the following questions:

- Who will decide to adopt and use the program?
- Which stakeholders will decision makers need to consult?
- Who will make resources available to implement the program?
- Who will implement the program?

- Will the program require different people to implement different components?
- Who will ensure that the program continues as long as it is needed?

## BOX 8.1. MAYOR'S PROJECT

The Mayor's taskforce continues to work on program development. Group members are planning support materials and considering implementation networks. The team has grown into a cohesive working group. Team members have a commitment to inclusivity, and along the way, have added members. Anyone who wanted to work hard on preventing childhood obesity was welcome. For a while, it seemed that every new meeting generated a new member, and every planning success attracted another contingent of community members. The health educator handled this by creating an orientation packet for new members, with information designed to quickly bring a new member up-to-date on the planning milestones the group had accomplished and the alternate paths it had considered. The inclusion fostered by the group was a great characteristic. However, the group members had begun to see themselves as potential program implementers. When the health educator began to hear the words "we" and "us" in relation to implementation, she planned several meetings to cover issues such as program reach and sustainability. The members then began to brainstorm about agencies that might be involved with implementing the program as well as the tasks associated with getting the program used.

The planning committee members were pleased with their efforts to keep an intact linkage with the community. Members who joined the taskforce along the way included representatives of churches, community centers, and advocacy groups. However, as the subgroup on implementation began to list the types of people and agencies that might be involved with the program, they were astounded by who was *not* at the table. Neighborhood social groups, parent organizations, and (interestingly enough) other arms of the mayor's city government that controlled environmental services relevant to physical activity were absent.

The taskforce went back to the community. The members were assigned to recruitment efforts, and the Mayor personally invited her colleagues from other city departments to meet and discuss the history of the child obesity prevention taskforce with her and the health educator. She encouraged department heads to assign both management and neighborhood specialists to the taskforce. Fortunately, the group members prided themselves on inclusivity, and the health educator had been facilitating integration of new individuals all along. The group understood the need to encourage a certain amount of covering old ground and even reinventing programs to integrate these new members, who were so crucial to the linkage system. Soon the group returned to making progress toward planning the adoption, implementation, and sustainability of program objectives.

# Stating Outcomes and Performance Objectives for Program Use

The point of this task is to determine who has to do what to achieve the outcomes of the program being adopted, implemented, and maintained (program use) with acceptable completeness and fidelity. Here, we focus on the development of outcomes and performance objectives for adoption, implementation, and maintenance for two scenarios: (a) a planning team is preparing for the first use of a newly developed program (i.e., have completed the first four steps of IM), or (b) a planning team has selected an EBI and is developing an implementation intervention to support EBI use in a new site or in multiple sites (scale up).

> The second task in Step 5 is to state outcomes and performance objectives for program adoption, implementation, and maintenance.

Program use outcomes are grouped into three stages:

1. *Adoption* is a decision to use a new program (an innovation to the adopting organization), depending on knowledge of the program, awareness of an unmet need, and the decisions to choose and try a certain innovation to meet the perceived need and will be given a trial (adoption can depend on active dissemination of a program).

2. *Implementation* is the use of the program to a "fair trial point," use that is long enough to allow evaluation about whether the innovation meets the perceived need.

3. *Maintenance* is the extent to which the program is continued, and then becomes a part of the normal practices and policies of the adopting organization.

In this task, the program planner states program use outcomes and writes performance objectives for each of these phases. Program use outcomes are similar in concept to the program outcomes stated in Step 2. Instead of stating behavioral outcomes and environmental outcomes, the planners state the expected outcomes for interventions to achieve program adoption, implementation, and maintenance. Examples for each are given in the following section.

## *Stating Outcomes and Performance Objectives for Adoption*

An *innovation* is an idea, practice, or product that is new to the adopter. The adopter may be an individual or an organization. The program that health promoters plan with IM Steps 1–4, developed to promote behavior and environmental change, can be thought of as an innovation because it will be new and will require changes in what individuals and environmental agents do and how they do it.

The adoption of a health education program is the decision to use it. Adoption decision makers or "adopters" can be individuals making an independent decision, such as a clinic director, a school principal, the head of an agency, or the leader of a community-based organization. Adopters can also be groups or organizations that make collective decisions, such as an executive board at a community clinic, a school board, or a patient advocacy group. Adoption in organizational settings may involve multiple levels and usually is a more complex event than is an adoption by individuals. Mendel (2008) presents a framework that depicts multiple levels of health care and community settings including regulatory agencies, insurers, purchasers, and providers (Mendel et al., 2008). Michaels and Green (2013) present a framework describing key concepts and tips for implementing workplace-based wellness programs. They highlight organizational change theories and provide guidance about the types of individuals that may be involved in adoption decisions. Planning teams can benefit from this type of information from the empirical literature when it begins to ask, "What do representatives of these agencies have to do in order to adopt this program? What stakeholders do they need to consult? What levels of approval do they need?" For example, in a school setting, a teacher team leader may hear about a program at a professional meeting and discuss it with other teachers and staff. The team leader may then request the curriculum coordinator or superintendent (depending on the school district's size and personnel structure) to adopt the program. The decision maker may then share the decision with parent groups or other stakeholders. In a clinic setting, a clinic director may need to seek the approval of board members and garner support from clinic managers before adopting a program. He or she may also need to consult with consumer stakeholders.

In clinical practice settings, adoption and implementation of new practices, programs, or policies are often referred to as "practice change." Examples of clinical practice changes are implementation of new guidelines for a procedure and implementation of a program to increase patient uptake of a preventive service, such as colorectal cancer screening (CRCS). The implementation of the FLU-FIT program, designed to help clinical teams increase CRCS by offering home tests to patients at the time of their annual flu shots, is an example of such a program (Potter et al., 2011). The FLU-FIT program has demonstrated effectiveness in increasing colorectal cancer screenings (Potter et al., 2013). The existence of a successful program, such as FLU-FIT, however, does not guarantee its use. For adoption to occur, clinic leaders and managers must become aware of the program, obtain buy-in from clinic board members, select a program champion to coordinate efforts, and involve team members in the planning process (FLU-FIT, 2013). A planner designing an intervention to increase adoption of FLU-FIT must clearly state the adoption performance objectives, which will then lead to decisions about messages, materials, and other resources to increase program adoption. The developers of FLU-FIT have provided these types of resources on a website for prospective adopters and implementers: http://fluFIT.org.

Program adoption outcomes can be specified in this way: [someone/group] adopts the [innovative program] as indicated by [the evidence or document to indicate adoption]. For example, following the implementation of the adapted EBI described in Chapter 10, Highfield (2014) planned a wider dissemination and wrote performance objectives for clinic directors, nurse managers, and patient navigators or schedulers. Adoption outcomes for the mammography-screening program could be stated as follows: the management team at [each] clinic decides to adopt the Peace of Mind Program (PMP) as indicated by the clinic director signing a memorandum of understanding. The answer to the question, "What do the potential program adopters need to do to constitute adoption of the program?" specifies the performance objectives for adoption for the PMP example:

The management team members will do the following:

- Review the description of PMP and evaluation results
- Compare the intended outcomes with current mammography services and completion rates
- Agree to participate in the PMP
- Agree to expand mammography services
- Agree to participate in evaluation
- Provide a program champion for the PMP
- Review the PMP program manual including phone-counseling scripts
- Agree to plan and execute communications
- Work with partners to draft, edit, and sign the Memorandum of Understanding (MOU)
- Gain support from stakeholders' reaction to the program (care providers, decision makers, navigators/schedulers, patients)

Planners might also include objectives to change contextual factors necessary for program adoption. For example, a study of the dissemination of physical activity programs by state health departments found four contextual factors associated with adoption of interventions by communities: available funding, physical activity being a high priority, adequate staffing at the state level, and a supportive legislature at the policy level (Brownson et al., 2007a). If program planners decide that these factors are critical in their local settings and can be addressed as part of their planning for program use, they could state performance objectives, such as the following:

- The state legislature will pass legislation that will provide funding for physical activity programs in local communities.

- The director of the state health department will allocate staff to support communities in adopting and implementing physical activity programs.

- The executive committee for the health department will make physical activity programs a high priority.

## Stating Outcomes and Performance Objectives for Implementation

*Implementation* is the use of a program. Whether implementing a program for the first time or using a selected EBI, planners will need to articulate what is required to implement their program and specify objectives required for program use. Planning interventions to increase program use of existing EBIs is often necessary because many EBIs lack implementation protocols or plans. They do not describe the tasks that should be completed to implement a program nor provide sufficient training or preparation to enable implementers to do so (Bradley, et al., 2004; Scheirer, 1981, 1994). This failure of programs to include implementation plans greatly diminishes the probability that programs will be implemented as planned, with either high fidelity or guided adaptation, to ensure delivery of the program's essential elements to produce change (Lee, Altschul, & Mowbray, 2008).

**Dimensions of Implementation**    At this stage, planners will want to clearly describe the implementation outcomes considering dimensions of implementation, such as fidelity, completeness, and dose, as they define performance objectives for program delivery (Baranowski & Stables, 2000; Linnan & Steckler, 2002; Rossi, Lipsey, & Freeman, 2004; Scheirer, 1981). Fidelity is the degree to which the program is implemented with its change methods and practical applications intact; completeness indicates the proportion of intended program activities and components delivered; and dose is the amount of the program that participants receive. Carroll et al. (2007) present a conceptual framework for implementation fidelity that includes elements of adherence, such as content, coverage, frequency, and duration, and also considers moderators of implementation fidelity, including intervention complexity, facilitation strategies, quality of delivery, and participant responsiveness.

For the initial implementation and testing of a new health promotion program, planners usually place greater emphasis on achieving a high level of fidelity and completeness to ensure that the intervention methods and practical applications are applied as intended. This involves identifying the core or essential elements that are judged necessary to achieve intervention effects. Although this ability to identify the "essential components" of a program is a critical factor that determines the implementation fidelity (Carroll et al., 2007), it is not always an easy task and will require understanding the link between determinants and change methods.

**Implementation Outcomes**    Planners will want to answer the following questions to describe the implementation outcome: What exactly is the program? What would constitute a level of fidelity and a level of completeness consistent with program effectiveness? To a greater extent than for adoption, implementation often includes multiple tasks performed by a variety of individual roles. Program implementation outcomes can be stated in this way: the [organization or individual] will implement [innovative program] including use of [program components]. For example, the clinical manager will implement the PMP program including deployment of phone counselors who use the PMP script to encourage program attendance, use of a mammography tracking system, and participation in follow-up assessment. The statement must answer the question: What do the program implementers need to do to implement the essential program components with acceptable completeness, fidelity, and dose? Once the implementation outcome is clearly stated, the planner can begin to develop the performance objectives for implementation.

To create performance objectives, the health promotion planner will think about the steps necessary to deliver the program and about what structural or organizational infrastructure may be required for implementation of the new program. There may be changes in the implementation environment that are necessary to deliver the program, such as hiring new staff or modifying patient flow in clinic settings. Fixsen et al. (2005) call this changing the environment "installation," making the structural and instrumental changes necessary to implement a program and identifying an implementation team.

To determine the performance objectives, the planners of PMP program asked what clinic managers and staff need to do to implement the program and stated the following:

The clinic decision makers will:

- Respond to e-mail from PMP and schedule appointments with PMP team

- Attend consultation visit—make plan to assess clinic capacity and needs

- Provide program updates to board
- Agree to provide staff and/or allow the Breast Health Collaborative of Texas to provide staff for implementation
- Agree to allow a program champion to dedicate time to PMP
- Agree to share information with staff about the PMP program
- Communicate with staff about practice change/role changes for patients due for mammography
- Identify program champion
- Designate time for EBI training
- Approve and institute systems changes (electronic health records (EHR); work with IT staff to make changes)
- Approve increase in mobile screening/new/expanded relationships with mobile mammography programs
- Review and provide feedback on performance objectives (needed actions for implementation by program champion and navigator)

The program champion will:

- Attend consultation visit—make plan to assess clinic capacity and needs
- Arrange for patient navigator to participate in PMP
- Arrange for new or increased frequency of screening capacity
- Arrange for patient navigator for training
- Arrange for in-house scheduling and reminders
- Arrange for any change to EHR or reporting for PMP
- Arrange for patient referrals for mammograms
- Set screening goals with decision makers
- Arrange/coordinate ongoing participation meetings with staff and research team
- Arrange for gathering/sharing patient stories and manage privacy concerns
- Monitor implementation barriers
- Troubleshoot barriers to implementation
- Recommend or provide retraining
- Recommend adaptation for PMP
- Work with PMP partners to make adaptations to PMP

The patient navigator will:

- Work with the program champion to schedule mammography services
- Pilot test PMP and recommend adaptation for PMP
- Work with PMP partners to make adaptations to PMP
- Recommend adaptation for the PMP when needed
- Search schedule for upcoming appointments
- Conduct telephone barrier counseling
- Identify referred patients for reminder calls and follow-up (outside referrals)
- Make three attempts to reach patient via phone before appointment
- Ask staging question for PMP
- Use active-listening protocol when talking with patient
- Use barrier scripts to respond to patient concerns
- Obtain patient consent for PMP evaluation
- Arrange for gathering/sharing patient stories and manage privacy concern
- Monitor implementation barriers
- Schedule mammography services (will vary by clinic). Communicate/coordinate delivery and implementation progress with program champion
- Enter data related to PMP
- Give patient callback number on every call
- Attend mobile screening days (in some clinics, but not all)
- Record patient barriers in EHR or PMP database
- Track patients for diagnostic referral or treatment (where; time to referral)

**Using Theories and Frameworks**   Consulting organizational theories, such as those described in Chapter 3, and implementation frameworks, such as the ISF (Wandersman et al., 2008) and the CFIR (Damschroder et al., 2009), described above, can help planners identify who the implementers should be and the actions they need to take. For example, both the prevention support system and the prevention delivery system as described by the ISF can help a planner think through which actions and capacity may be required to support the implementation of the program and which resources (including personnel and time) are needed for

actual delivery, including who should deliver the program and what implementation behaviors (performance objectives) are important. The CFIR
describes constructs within the inner setting domain, such as the implementation climate, available resources, readiness for implementation, and
networks for communication, that can provide guidance about who has to
do what for implementation to occur. According to the CFIR, *Readiness
for Implementation* includes involvement of leaders and managers with
implementation, and clear communication about the importance of an
implementation effort. A planner could make sure to include performance
objectives consistent with this construct. For example, "Leaders of the Star
City community health center will publicly express their support for the
implementation of the PMP and will describe their planned involvement in
its implementation."

The CFIR "Process" domain also may stimulate thinking about implementation performance objectives (and possibly maintenance as well). It
includes involving appropriate people in implementation and providing
qualitative and quantitative feedback about the progress and quality of
implementation. A planner could use this information to articulate performance objective, such as, "the clinic manager will monitor phone counseling
and communicate with counselors about their progress in reaching women
in need of mammograms." Other CFIR domains, such as characteristics
of individuals (e.g., self-efficacy, knowledge, and beliefs about the intervention) and characteristics of the innovation, may be more helpful in
identifying the determinants of implementers, discussed below under the
task for developing matrices.

**Using Empirical Literature**    The empirical literature can also help planners address the contextual factors that influence implementation. For
example, a recent study of publicly funded agencies in New Mexico found
that within leadership engagement, availability of resources and access
to information were important contextual factors to prepare providers
for integration of new practices (Bonham et al., 2014). They also found
that transformational leadership, characterized by close supervisory relationships, individual feedback, support, and motivation, influenced EBI
implementation (Bonham et al., 2014). Many studies support the role of
leadership in implementation (Bonham et al., 2014; Damschroder et al.,
2009). For example, Aarons and Sommerfeld (2012) found that supervisor transformational leadership style was associated with positive provider
attitudes toward adoption and use of EBIs and increased positive implementation climate. Panzano and Roth (2006) described key leadership functions
across stages of implementation of evidence-based mental health initiatives
and found that management needed to actively support the practice change
throughout implementation and not just at the beginning of the effort.

They also found that performance monitoring and technical assistance were associated with improved implementation outcomes. Information from studies such as these can help planners identify individuals within an organization (e.g., leaders and quality improvement managers) who play a role in implementation and describe what actions these individuals should take to improve organizational buy-in, readiness, and structural supports that are key to implementation success. For example, performance objectives related to these findings could be as follows: "clinic manager monitors performance of providers and other staff implementing the program and provides feedback," "clinic leader gathers staff in frequent open meetings to discuss implementation and problem solve," "clinic leader schedules one-on-one meetings with staff to review and provide feedback on implementation outcomes," and "leader periodically assesses the need for technical assistance and identifies opportunities to provide additional training and feedback during implementation."

The work of Aarons, Ehrhart, Farahnak, and Sklar (2014) in a recent study to develop an implementation leadership scale can be particularly useful in identifying performance objectives for leaders. Aarons et al. (2014) surveyed 459 mental health clinicians from 93 outpatient mental health programs and defined several subscales including proactive leadership, knowledgeable leadership, supportive leadership, and perseverant leadership. According to this work, performance objectives related to proactive leadership may include that the leader:

- establishes clear standards for implementation,
- develops a plan to facilitate EBI implementation, and
- removes obstacles to implementation of EBI.

Performance objectives related to supportive and perseverant literature may include that the leader:

- supports employee efforts to use EBI by providing needed resources,
- supports employee efforts to learn more about EBI, and
- recognizes and appreciates employee efforts.

**Making Programs Easier to Adapt**    As planners define implementation and describe performance objectives, they may want to find ways to build in implementation options to make the program easier to adapt for new settings. This can improve fit in different settings while maintaining the essential elements or core elements of the program. Although it is essential to describe what constitutes a well-implemented program and to protect its essential elements or "active ingredients," some evidence suggests that program implementation is most successful when it allows for adaptation (Hall & Loucks, 1978; MacDonald & Green, 2001; Ringwalt, Vincus, Ennett,

Johnson, & Rohrbach, 2004; Weiner, Lewis, & Linnan, 2009). Adaptation is so ubiquitous that Rogers (1995) described it as a stage in organizational innovation, calling it reinvention. Actually, quite a bit of reinvention from insignificant changes to major revision usually takes place. From the perspective of the adopting institution, reinvention is a positive process that fosters program ownership and commitment (Chambers, Glasgow, & Stange, 2013). Thus, an awareness of the potential for variations in implementation depending on different contexts is a useful perspective for the health promotion planner to have when designing implementation interventions in Step 5.

## Stating Outcomes and Performance Objectives for Maintenance

Maintenance is the extent to which a program continues over time and is integrated into organizational routines so that it survives beyond the presence of the original program funding, adopters, and program champions (Kegler & McLeroy, 2003; Schell et al., 2013). Many funding agencies require that applicants provide evidence that, once implemented, the program will be maintained over time beyond the funding period of the original project (Schell et al., 2013). We use the term *maintenance* to include institutionalization (the integration of a program into the routines of an organization) and sustainability, sustaining either the program itself of the outcomes of a program that is no longer needed (Shediac-Rizkallah & Bone, 1998).

To think about how a program might be maintained and what the performance objectives should be, planners should consider both threats and facilitators of maintenance. For example, in a systematic assessment of the an evidence-based asthma control program in three school districts, Wilson and Kurz (2008) described a breakdown in the process of dissemination to institutionalization. They found threats in two main areas: low levels of program evaluation and failure of organizations to change in ways to support program institutionalization. The authors proposed a continuous quality improvement (CQI) approach to increase program institutionalization by promoting process changes in the organizations and promoting feedback of program benefit. Without fairly continuous feedback about benefit, a program loses relevance even if it was considered evidence-based and advantageous at the time of adoption and initial implementation.

In a review of the gap between prevention research and practice, Wandersman et al. (2008) described the importance of organizational capacity needed for maintenance. Flaspohler et al. (2008) developed a taxonomy of capacity including skills, structures, and functions to encourage participation, leadership, group process, conflict resolution, leverage of resources, and network maintenance. Over time, programs may need to be adjusted and if this can be anticipated during planning, maintenance performance objectives can include tasks related to the continuous evaluation of program activities and outcomes to allow for planned modifications over time. Kilbourne, Neumann, Pincus, Bauer, and Stall (2007) note that "maintenance and evolution" often can include incorporation into job duties, training, new hires, and that "recustomizing intervention delivery" may be required over time as the circumstances or context evolve. An example of an outcome for maintenance is, "Clinic leadership will maintain the PMP as part of a clinic's standard practice for every appointed mammography patient after initial funding is withdrawn."

Performance objectives for maintenance should include attention to institutionalization (integration into routines). Planners may also want to consider how health effects will be sustained and monitored after a program is no longer needed. In the PMP project, the following are performance objectives for maintenance:

The program champion will:

• Discuss with decision makers the continuation of the PMP after funding

• Work with decision makers to continue contractual arrangements for increased mammography services

• Add PMP tasks to normal clinic reminder calls

• Approve protocols to ensure that that mammography rates continue to be reported (and remain stable or on an upward trend)

• Ensure that no-show rates continue to be reported (and remain stable or on a downward trend)

The decision makers (vary by clinic) will:

• Approve steps to ensure integration of the PMP into normal clinic routines

## Constructing Matrices of Change Objectives for Implementation

This task is similar to Step 2 of IM in that the planner develops a matrix to guide the development of an implementation intervention. The matrix combines performance objectives and determinants in a matrix for adoption, implementation, and maintenance.

*The third task in Step 5 is to construct matrices of change objectives for program adoption, implementation, and maintenance.*

### *Determinants of Adoption, Implementation, and Maintenance*

As with the performance objectives of health-related behaviors and environmental conditions, the performance objectives for program use will have a set of determinants, that is, factors that are likely to influence their performance. These determinants answer the questions: "Why would adopters decide to use the program?" "Why would implementers do what is necessary to implement the program?" and "Why would those responsible do what it takes to make sure the program is continued over time?" The answers to these questions are the determinants of adoption, implementation, and maintenance respectively. Examples of determinants are awareness of the program, perceptions about the program's characteristics, familiarity with the program components, perceived benefits of program use, self-efficacy and skills for implementation, and values supportive of program goals. The accomplishment of performance objectives for program use may also be influenced by social or structural factors that might serve as barriers or facilitators. Examples are time, resources, social support, and reinforcement.

The processes for selecting determinants of program use are the same as those recommended for selecting determinants of health-related behavior and environmental conditions (Chapter 5, Step 2). The team should begin by brainstorming a list of factors that will facilitate or serve as barriers to accomplishing the performance objectives; review the theoretical and empirical literature to refine or add to the list; and collect new data from potential program adopters and implementers.

**An Example of Brainstorming**   Highfield (2014) brainstormed determinants for why clinics (decision makers and staff) for low-income clients would adopt and implement the PMP. The brainstorming was influenced by both Social Cognitive Theory constructs and their use of the CFIR framework (Damschroeder et al., 2009) to conceptualize the overall project. Even though brainstorming is never conducted in a vacuum, that is, team members have read the literature related to their project and are often knowledgeable about D&I theories and frameworks, the rule of brainstorming is that everything proposed by team members goes on the list unedited. Organizing, adding, and deleting come later as the team further reviews the literature and talks to potential adopters and implementers.

On the list of why clinics would *adopt* the PMP were the following factors:

- Belief that providing more mammography services will lower mortality
- Knowledge of what is required; self-efficacy to respond to what is expected (increased screening capacity, implementation of the PMP, providing a program champion, assess and expand clinic resources)
- Expectation of ongoing support from the PMP developers
- Readiness for change

- Clinic staff perception of breast health needs
- Perception that clinic is capable of change
- Expectation that the PMP would result in positive comparison with other clinics
- Expectation that the PMP project is accessible, i.e., is easy to join
- Awareness of availability of staff resources
- Perception that the PMP is an improvement over what is done now
- Belief that the PMP is effective at increasing mammography rates
- Belief that partners (intervention development partners) are here to help
- Belief that PMP fits with organizational goals and needs

As the brainstorming group moved to implementation, the determinants became more related to capacity of the clinic and staff. On the list of why clinics would [be able to] *implement* the PMP included:

- Capacity of the clinic to incorporate new services
- Skills and self-efficacy of decision makers to garner support for new programs from staff
- Skills and self-efficacy of program champion to garner support for the PMP
- Skills and self-efficacy of program champion for program coordination
- Skills of PMP telephone counselor (navigator) to communicate with patients and develop rapport
- Skills of PMP telephone counselor (navigator) to communicate with patients according to protocol
- Expectation (decision makers, champion, navigator) that the interaction with service providers around the program will be positive
- Expectation (decision makers, champion, navigator) that the program will result in satisfied patients
- Expectation (decision makers, champion, navigator) that the program will result in satisfied clinical staff
- Expectation that improvements in mammography may lead to improvements in other services
- Expectations that this program will provide effective/improved outreach to clinic patients
- Expectation that this program will address breast cancer disparities to increase survivorship and improve survival among low-income women

As the brainstorming group moved to *maintenance*, the determinants became more related to perceptions of the benefits and costs from having adopted and implemented the program. The main agent for maintenance shifted to the decision makers for the clinic (as in adoption) with some consideration for determinants of the ability of the program champion to enact systems changes to ensure survival of the program. On the list of why the clinic would [be able to] maintain the PMP were included:

- Perceptions by decision makers that funders and other external constituents support the PMP

- Perceptions by decision makers that the PMP has added benefit to clinic services

- Perceptions by decision makers that the PMP can fit into normal routines of the clinic with little staff burden

- Perceptions by decision makers that the PMP can fit into normal routines of the clinic with little or no additional funding

- Skills and self-efficacy of the program champion to make systems changes

**Reviewing the Literature: Characteristics of Innovations**     A review of the literature begins with studies that report findings regarding determinants of use of similar programs in similar settings. Several authors have identified determinants of adoption and implementation behaviors that focus on perceptions of the intervention itself (as described by Rogers, 1995; Berwick, 2003; Damschroder et al., 2009; Mihalic, Fagan, & Argamaso, 2008; Oldenburg, Hardcastle, & Kok, 1997). They include the relative advantage of the innovation compared to what is being used, compatibility with the intended implementers' current practice, complexity, observability of the results, impact on social relations, reversibility or ease of discontinuation, communicability, required time, risk and uncertainty, required commitment, and ability to be modified. In a study to determine the factors influencing the adoption of the Canadian Heart Health Kit, relative advantage and the observability of the program benefits were associated with intentions to adopt the program (Scott, Plotnikoff, Karunamuni, Bize, & Rodgers, 2008). The planning team must consider characteristics of an innovation as either a facilitator of or a barrier to adoption, both in program design and in the creation of an intervention to influence program adoption. During the development phase, the planner should make decisions about program elements while considering such characteristics of diffusible innovations as required time, complexity, compatibility, and ability to be modified. During dissemination planning, the planner is concerned with the perceptions of the adopters and implementers relative to these characteristics. Determinants related to these constructs then could include attitudes about the intervention's compatibility or value, or perceived benefits of the program in terms of its compatibility; the planner may consider characteristics such as communicability, relative advantage, and required commitment to help identify both performance objectives and determinants. An adoption performance objective related to these characteristics might be as follows: the school principal describes the compatibility of the program with school goals to the parent–teacher organization.

**Reviewing the Literature: Characteristics of Implementers**   Other determinants are characteristics of the implementers, such as perceived needs, values and goals, skills, and perceived social support (Damschroder et al., 2009; Fixsen et al., 2005; Greenhalgh et al., 2004; Nanney et al., 2007; Owen, Glanz, Sallis, & Kelder, 2006; Rogers, 2003; Wejnert, 2002). It is critical to consider theories of personal behavior because adopters, implementers, and maintainers are all individuals who need to do something for full implementation to occur. Therefore, many of the theories presented in Chapter 2, which predict and explain individual behavior, are also highly relevant when identifying determinants of implementation.

As attention shifts from adoption to the implementation, the determinants also shift to an emphasis on behavioral capability, skills, self-efficacy, reinforcement, and organizational factors. An important challenge in planning interventions to promote program implementation is to correctly estimate the level of skills and related self-efficacy. For example, in a program we worked on some years ago (the Cystic Fibrosis Family Education Program) required many different types of skills for putting this complex program into clinical practice (Bartholomew et al., 1991). The planners seriously underestimated the training intensity required to develop skills in communication domains such as mutual goal setting. Skill requirements are also often neglected or taken for granted in community interventions based on activities such as coalitions. Some researchers have suggested that coalition members receive training on how to participate in an effective coalition as a part of the implementation of a coalition-based health promotion program (Holmes, Neville, Donovan, & MacDonald, 2001).

**Reviewing the Literature: Characteristics of Systems**   Because program adoption and implementation often involve organizations and community groups making decisions and changing practices to make use of an innovation, the application of organizational change and community development models is critical to identifying performance objectives and determinants of program adoption and implementation (Hogan et al., 2003). Several reviews and syntheses of implementation theories and frameworks have identified factors that influence implementation outcomes in various settings at multiple levels of influence. Durlak and Dupree (2008), for example, reviewed meta-analyses and qualitative reports from over 500 studies examining factors influencing implementation. They identified 23 factors affecting program implementation organized into five categories: innovation characteristics, provider characteristics, community factors, organizational capacity, and training and technical assistance. In comparing their review to three other reviews, there was agreement on 11 factors that affect implementation: funding, a positive work climate, shared decision making, coordination with other agencies, formulation of tasks, leadership, program champions, administrative support, providers' skills, training, and technical assistance (Fixsen et al., 2005; Greenhalgh et al., 2005; Stith et al., 2006). Chaudoir, Dugan, and Barr (2013) present a framework to guide implementation science research that includes four factors that may be useful for thinking about determinants for implementation. They are as follows:

- Structural level factors (including the political and social climate, public policy, economic climate, and infrastructure).

- Organizational level factors (including leadership effectiveness, culture and climate, organizational values and rewards).

- Implementer level factors including attitudes toward the program and perceived behavioral control (or self-efficacy) for implementation.

- Innovation level factors that include characteristics of the program to be implemented, the perceptions of these characteristics by potential adopters and implementers, and the evidence supporting the program's efficacy.

Implementation frameworks, such as the ISF, can be useful in thinking about necessary skills and capacity needed at both the individual and organizational levels to support the delivery of a program (Wandersman et al., 2008). Additionally, theories of organizational readiness have recently identified concepts, such as change commitment and change efficacy, which even though they are measured at the organizational level, represent individual beliefs related to implementation (Shea, Jacobs, Esserman, Bruce, & Weiner, 2014).

Environmental influences necessary for program adoption, implementation, and continuation are identified as performance objectives that state *who* will need to do *what* to make the changes or create the conditions necessary to accomplish the program use outcomes. These influences can be anticipated when stating performance objects in the previous task, or they can be added as determinants of program use. A useful way to determine whether they should be added as a determinant or as another performance objective is as follows: if the answer to the question "Why would the decision maker adopt the program?" is personal or internal (such as knowledge of the goals of the program, perceived benefits of the program, or perceived compatibility with organization values), these are listed as determinants of adoption. If, however, the answers to the "why?" question are external and are characteristics of the adoption context, such as "the patient advisory board requests the program" or the "state primary care association (PCA) recommends the program," then these should be added as additional adoption performance objectives. In this case, the planner may want to think about what additional determinants may be needed to answer the question of why a patient board would request the program and why would the PCA recommend the program?

**Collecting Data From Adopters and Implementers** Qualitative methods, such as focus groups or interviews, can be helpful in generating new ideas for determinants or in verifying some of the findings from the research literature. Quantitative data collection using questionnaires that measure the determinants and interest or intentions to adopt and implement a program can be especially helpful in judging the strength of the association between determinants and potential adoption and implementation (Mihalic et al., 2008). With both types of data collection, planners can obtain some estimate of the presence or absence of the determinant in the user system.

**Organizing and Prioritizing Determinants** Eventually, the planning team must refine the list of determinants to create a practical list for program development. Planners should rate each determinant in terms of importance (that is, strength of association with program adoption and implementation) and changeability (that is, how likely it is that an implementation intervention influences a change in the determinant). The planners should focus on determinants that have both high importance and high changeability. However, planners may want to retain some determinants with high importance and low changeability because the determinant is likely to be a critical factor in successful program use. For example, the cost of adopting a health promotion program may be a strong determinant, but there may be little that planners can do to lower the cost. Because cost may be a major barrier to adoption, planners should address it in the intervention, for example, by finding sources of compensation or demonstrating that the program costs are worth the benefit.

In the PMP example, the brainstormed list of determinants could be organized into only a few constructs including perceived characteristics of the intervention, outcome expectations for use of the program, beliefs about self-efficacy about program use, skills for program use and feedback, and reinforcement regarding effects of the program (Table 8.1).

### Constructing Matrices for Program Use

This task is completed by linking performance objectives and determinants for adoption, implementation, and sustainability to write change objectives. Planners are now performing the same task as in Step 2, but instead of focusing on change objectives for behavioral and environmental outcomes, they are writing change objectives for adoption, implementation, and maintenance of the health promotion program. To prepare a matrix for program use, planners follow the same process as they did for the matrices developed for planning the intervention. They enter performance objectives in the left column of the table and the determinants in the top row. They then assess cells to decide whether the determinant is likely to be important to the achievement of the performance objective. Next, they write change objectives for the appropriate cells (see Chapter 5). Table 8.1 presents a partial matrix for the PMP.

## Designing Implementation Interventions

### Selecting Change Methods and Practical Applications for Program Use

The final task in Step 5 is to choose change methods and practical applications, design the scope and sequence, and produce materials for an implementation intervention to influence program use.

Much like in Step 3 of IM, where planners select theory-based methods and practical applications, in this task of Step 5, the planners use information from the previous steps to select implementation intervention methods and practical applications. The program planners start with the determinants and list of change objectives from the matrix and brainstorm change methods and practical applications. Next, they review the relevant research and practice literature to confirm, refute, or modify the provisional list of change methods and their practical applications. As we discussed in Chapter 6, the selection of change methods and practical applications may be an iterative process. For example, when they review performance objectives, planners may find that ideas for practical applications occur to them before their ideas for change methods. They then assess practical applications and link them to theoretical methods considering how to address the parameters for effective use of the methods.

For example, in the PMP program, the team talked about delivery channels, how to reach the implementers, and then discussed what change methods could be delivered (Table 8.2). The team had the idea of a webinar to introduce the program to address the determinants of awareness and perceptions of the intervention. Once the idea of webinar was broached, the group had to ask the following: What change methods will we deliver? Information transfer, persuasive communication, and modeling? When thinking about implementation, the PMP group immediately realized that clinics would need program champions to shepherd the program into use,

**Table 8.1**    Examples of Change Objectives from the Peace of Mind Program (Highfield, 2014)

**Personal Determinants**

| Performance Objectives | Awareness and Perceptions of PMP | Outcome Expectations | Skills and Self-Efficacy | Feedback and Reinforcement |
|---|---|---|---|---|
| **Adoption** | | | | |
| The clinic decision makers will:<br>PO1. Agree to participate in the PMP | AP.1a. Perceive that the PMP is easy to join; awareness of availability<br>AP.1.b. Describe PMP as an improvement over what is done now<br>AP.1.c. Perceive that PMP partners are here to help<br>AP.1.d. Describe PMP as fitting with organizational goals and needs | OE.1. Expect that the PMP intervention development partners will provide help with program implementation and resources | SSE.1. Express self-efficacy to respond to what is expected by the PMP (increased screening capacity, implementation of the PMP, providing a program champion, assess and expand clinic resources) | |
| PO2. Agree to expand mammography services | AP.2. Acknowledge the availability of staff | OE.2. Expect that increased and enhanced mammography services will decrease mortality from breast cancer | SSE.2. Express self-efficacy to work with partners to increase screening capacity | |
| PO3. Agree to participate in evaluation | | OE.3a. Expect that evaluation results will add value to clinic reporting<br>OE.3.b. Expect that evaluation results will add value and status compared to other clinics | SSE.3. Express self-efficacy for creating records needed for evaluation | |
| PO4. Provide a program champion for the PMP | | OE.4. Expect that a program champion will enable the PMP to be implemented and maintained | SSE.4. Express self-efficacy to recruit a program champion | |
| PO5. Gain support from stakeholders' reaction to the program (care providers, decision makers, navigators/ schedulers, patients) | | OE.5.a. Expect that care providers, patients, and managers will consider expanded mammography to add value to clinic services.<br>OE.5.b. Expect that stakeholders who are consulted will develop feelings of acceptance and ownership of the program | | |

(continued)

**Table 8.1**    (*Continued*)

| Personal Determinants | | | | |
|---|---|---|---|---|
| **Performance Objectives** | **Awareness and Perceptions of PMP** | **Outcome Expectations** | **Skills and Self-Efficacy** | **Feedback and Reinforcement** |
| **Implementation** | | | | |
| The patient navigator will: PO1. Search schedule for upcoming appointments | AP.1. Describe requirements of the PMP intervention AP.1.a. Describe the data system of the clinic AP.1.b. Describe protections for patient information | | | |
| PO2. Conduct telephone barrier counseling PO2.a. Make three attempts to reach patient via phone before appointment PO2.b. Ask staging question for PMP PO2.c. Use active-listening protocol when talking with patient PO2.d. Use barrier scripts to respond to patient concerns | AP.2. Describe PMP as a protocol-driven intervention AP.2.a. Describe PMP as not too complex and fairly easy to implement AP.2.b. Describe PMP as better than current practice | OE.2. Expect that the PMP will help women keep appointments better than current practice OE.2.a. Expect that mammography can help women detect cancer early when it is more curable OE.2.b. Expect that increasing mammography services and kept appointments will contribute to lowering mortality from breast cancer | SSE.2. Demonstrate skills for initiating conversation SSE.2.a. Demonstrate skills for determining women's intention for keeping appointment SSE.2.b. Demonstrate skills for eliciting barriers and using barrier scripts SSE2.c. Demonstrate skills for supporting conversation with active listening SSE.d. Express self-efficacy for conducting telephone-barrier counseling and specific skills | FB.2. Express satisfaction with women's response to phone calls FB.2a. Express satisfaction with improved no-show rates |
| **Maintenance** | | | | |
| The program champion will: PO1. Discuss with decision makers the continuation of the PMP after funding | AP.1. Describes processes that will help a program survive in an organization (e.g. inclusion in job descriptions, reward structures, budgets) | OE.1. Expects the program to continue to be value added to patients | SSE.1. Demonstrates skills for addressing management issues with decision makers SSE.1.a. Expresses self-efficacy for addressing management issues with decision makers | FR.1. Express continued satisfaction with enhanced services and improved no-show rates |

**Table 8.1**  (*Continued*)

| Personal Determinants | | | | |
|---|---|---|---|---|
| **Performance Objectives** | **Awareness and Perceptions of PMP** | **Outcome Expectations** | **Skills and Self-Efficacy** | **Feedback and Reinforcement** |
| **Maintenance** | | | | |
| PO2. Work with decision makers to continue contractual arrangements for increased mammography services | | | SSE.2.Demonstrates administrative skills to follow-up on contracts and work with clinic administrative structure | |
| PO3. Assure that mammography and no-show rates continue to be reported (and remain stable or on upward trend) | | OE.3. Expect that continued monitoring and evaluation will contribute to likelihood of program continuation | SSE.3. Demonstrates administrative skills to monitor data | FR.3. Express satisfaction with enhanced mammography rates |
| The decision makers will: PO1. Approve steps to assure integration of the PMP into normal clinic routines | | OE.1. Expect that continued monitoring and evaluation will contribute to likelihood of program continuation | | FR.1. Express satisfaction with enhanced mammography rates |

**Table 8.2**  Peace of Mind Program Implementation Intervention Plan

| Stage | Agent | Determinants/Change Objectives | Theoretical Change Methods | Practical Applications |
|---|---|---|---|---|
| Adoption | Decision Maker | Awareness/Perceptions of PMP<br>Outcome Expectations<br>Skills and Self-efficacy | Information<br>Persuasion<br>Role Modeling<br>Organizational Consultation/Planning | E-mail and Webinar<br>Webinar<br>Site visit planning meeting |
| Implementation | Program Champion<br>Navigator | Awareness/Perceptions<br>Outcome Expectations<br>Skills and Self-efficacy<br>Feedback and Reinforcement | Information<br>Persuasion<br>Skill building and guided practice<br>Monitoring and feedback<br>Technical assistance / capacity building<br>Facilitation | Face to face training<br>Instruction manual and computer assisted script<br>Ongoing phone consultations and training booster sessions |
| Maintenance | Program Champion<br>Decision Makers | Outcome Expectations<br>Skills and Self-efficacy<br>Feedback and Reinforcement | Information<br>Persuasion | Face to face meeting |

to help with needed systems changes, and to monitor ongoing quality. A program champion is a special case of a role model who is also capable of providing some instrumental support for implementation. When thinking of this method, the group also had to consider parameters for its use (see Chapter 6). Compared to their colleagues, program champions typically take more risks, are more innovative, and initiate more attempts to influence others (Howell & Higgins, 1990; Peterson et al., 2007). Program champions must be credible to their colleagues, and when an innovation is costly or represents a radical new direction for the organization, the champion must be in a powerful organizational role (see Chapter 3, discussion on organization theory).

The change methods discussed in Chapters 2, 3, and 6 can be applied to interventions to accomplish program use. In other words, change methods and practical applications do not have to be specific for dissemination.

## *Organizing the Intervention: Scope, Sequence, and Materials*

The planning team then can use the selected change methods and practical applications to develop a deliverable intervention. These types of interventions usually comprise at least three major components: one to stimulate awareness and adoption; a second to provide training, capacity development, and ongoing technical support for implementation, and a final component to help implementers and managers to transition an ongoing program to maintenance. The most common materials produced in this task are materials to promote awareness, an implementation manual, and materials to support training for implementers. Box 8.2 describes example materials from the It's Your Game project.

---

### BOX 8.2.  IT'S YOUR GAME . . . KEEP IT REAL

The planning group for It's Your Game . . . Keep It Real used the Intervention Mapping tasks in Step 5 to plan for program implementation during two randomized controlled trials to assess the program's efficacy (see Chapter 6). After the program was demonstrated to be an effective sexual health education program, they used the Step 5 tasks to develop an implementation intervention to enhance the adoption, implementation, and maintenance of It's Your Game (IYG) in other school districts. The planning group reviewed the theoretical and empirical literature on the dissemination of school-based interventions, conducted key informant interviews with school district personnel and principals, observed school board meetings, and conducted surveys with teachers to understand the implementation process.

### Task 1: Identify Program Implementers

Many school districts in the U.S. have a School Health Advisory Council (SHAC) that advises the school board and superintendent on the adoption and implementation of age-appropriate health education programs. In decentralized school districts, school principals may also have the authority to approve or disapprove the adoption of a new health program (Hernandez et al., 2011). Thus, key decision makers for adopting IYG included SHAC and school board members, superintendents, and principals. Implementing IYG required participation from physical or health education teachers to deliver the classroom lessons, computer laboratory or library staff to deliver the computer lessons, and backing from the principal to facilitate teacher training and instructional time. Key decision makers for IYG maintenance included the SHAC, school board members, superintendents, and principals.

### Task 2: State Outcomes and Performance Objectives for Implementation

The planning group developed four outcomes and related performance objectives to facilitate the implementation of IYG (see Table 8.3). For program adoption, they developed two outcomes: one for school district personnel and one for school principals. They used theoretical and empirical evidence to develop specific performance objectives. For example, using DIT (Rogers, 2003), they recognized that it was important for potential adopters to assess the relative advantage of IYG compared with current health education programs, and to assess the program's compatibility with existing teaching practices to identify potential barriers to implementation. For implementation, the planning group asked, what do school personnel need to do to implement IYG with fidelity? Guided by the ISF (Wandersman et al., 2008), they recognized that potential implementers needed training, technical assistance, and support to implement the program with fidelity. For maintenance, the planning group asked, what do school principals and school district personnel need to do to ensure ongoing delivery of IYG? The planning group incorporated specific strategies, such as securing funding, incorporating IYG into existing job duties and the training of new hires (Kilbourne et al., 2007), and maintaining political support (Schell et al, 2013) into their performance objectives to facilitate ongoing program delivery.

### Task 3: Construct Matrices of Change Objectives for Implementation

Based on their literature review and local research, the planning group identified important and changeable determinants for IYG implementation. They found that awareness or knowledge (e.g., awareness of the program's goals and procedural knowledge about how to implement it), outcome expectations or positive attitudes toward program use, and perceived norms were key determinants for program adoption, implementation, and maintenance (Bandura, 1986; Damschroder et al., 2009; Rogers, 2003). Skills and self-efficacy were also critical for program implementation (Bandura, 1986; Brink et al., 1995; Damschroder et al., 2009; Peskin et al., 2011; Steckler, Goodman, McLeroy, Davis, & Koch, 1992). The planning group developed a matrix of change objectives for each of the four implementation outcomes (Table 8.3).

**Table 8.3**    It's Your Game . . . Keep It Real: Matrices of Change Objectives for Implementation

**Adoption**

**Outcome 1: The School Health Advisory Council (SHAC), school board members, and superintendent will approve and adopt It's Your Game . . . Keep It Real (IYG), an effective HIV, STD, and pregnancy prevention program, in their district.**

| Performance Objectives | Personal Determinants | | | |
|---|---|---|---|---|
| | Knowledge | Attitudes | Outcome Expectations | Perceived Norms |
| PO.1. The SHAC evaluates student education needs in HIV, STD, and pregnancy prevention in their district | K.1.a. Summarize sexual behavior, HIV, STD, and pregnancy statistics among students<br>K.1.b. List the Health TEKS objectives for middle school students<br>K.1.c. Describe district policy on sexual health education.<br>K.1.d. Prioritize needs | A.1. Describe review time and effort as necessary and important | OE.1.a. Expect that by evaluating student educational needs in HIV, STD, and pregnancy prevention, the problem can be prioritized and these statistics can be decreased<br>OE.1.b. Expect that reducing teen HIV, STD, and pregnancy rates will result in increased academic achievement and reduced dropout rates | PN.1. Recognize that other school districts see this as a problem that needs to be addressed |
| PO.2. The SHAC reviews IYG and specifically notes program objectives, methods, and relative advantages | K.2.a. Describe IYG objectives and describe applicable TEKS objectives<br>K.2.b. Describe how IYG compares to current HIV, STD, and pregnancy prevention curriculum coverage in district's middle schools<br>K.2.c. List advantages of IYG program | A.2.a.Describe IYG as being worth any modifications needed to school level curricula<br>A.2.b. Review characteristics of IYG in a favorable manner | OE.2.a. Expect that many Health TEKS objectives will be covered by implementing IYG<br>OE.2.b. Expect that IYG will be easy to implement and will easily fit in allotted time for their health curriculum | PN.2.a. Recognize that decision makers in other school districts review program objectives, methods, and relative advantages before adopting a new sexual health education program |
| PO.3. The SHAC obtains information on the experiences of other districts using IYG | K.3. Describe how to obtain information on other districts' experiences with IYG | A.3. Feel positive about obtaining information on other districts' experiences with IYG | OE.3. Expect that by knowing the experiences of other districts that have used the IYG program, they will be able to evaluate the pros and cons of using it | |

**Table 8.3** (Continued)

| Performance Objectives | Personal Determinants | | | |
|---|---|---|---|---|
| | **Knowledge** | **Attitudes** | **Outcome Expectations** | **Perceived Norms** |
| PO.4. The SHAC identifies barriers for implementation as perceived by potential program users | K.4.a. Brainstorm possible barriers for implementation of IYG in middle schools (time, computers, parental attitudes, lack of sexual education training for teachers)<br>K.4.b. List possible ways to overcome barriers | A.4. Feel positive about identifying and overcoming potential barriers | OE.4. Expect that identifying possible barriers and ways to overcome them will facilitate successful IYG implementation | PN.4. Recognize that other districts have overcome these barriers |
| PO.5. The SHAC gains support for IYG adoption from parents, teachers (implementers), and key administrators (principals, director of curriculum, regional superintendents, and school board members). | K.5. List supportive messages from parents, teachers, principals, director of curriculum, and other regional superintendents regarding IYG adoption | A.5. Describe effort to gain support as essential and worthwhile | OE.5. Expect that if key stakeholders endorse IYG then it will be easier to adopt it | PN.5. Recognize that the districts' students, families, teachers, principals, and administrators see HIV, STI, and pregnancy prevention as a problem that needs to be addressed in their schools |
| PO.6. The SHAC prepares a statement of recommendation to the school board for adoption of IYG. | K.6. Describe necessary components of a statement of recommendation | A.6. Feel positive about recommending adoption of IYG | OE.6.a. Believe that if they make the recommendation, the regional superintendents and principals will be more likely to adopt IYG | |
| PO.7. The school board approves the adoption of IYG | K.7. Describe the district's need, relative advantages, and stakeholders' support for IYG | A.7. Feel positive about approving adoption of IYG | OE.7. Expect that adopting IYG will lead to student benefits | PN.7. Recognize that other school boards have approved IYG |
| PO.8. The superintendent completes the adoption forms necessary for IYG | K.8. Describe necessary forms and signatures needed | A.8. Feel positive about adopting IYG | OE.8.Expect that by completing the adoption form, more principals will adopt the beneficial program | PN.8. Recognize that other superintendents are completing the IYG adoption forms |

(continued)

**Table 8.3**    (*Continued*)

**Outcome 2: School principals will adopt IYG, an effective HIV, STD, and pregnancy prevention program, at their middle school.**

| Performance Objectives | Personal Determinants | | | |
| --- | --- | --- | --- | --- |
| | Knowledge | Attitudes | Outcome Expectations | Perceived Norms |
| PO.1. Principals, other school administrators, and/or physical education teachers evaluate student education needs in HIV, STD, and pregnancy prevention at their school | K.1.a. Summarize sexual behavior, HIV, STD, and pregnancy statistics among students<br>K.1.b. Describe the district's policy on sexual health education<br>K.1.c. Prioritize needs | A.1. Describe review time and effort as necessary and important | OE.1. Expect that by evaluating HIV, STD and pregnancy prevalence, the problem can be prioritized and these statistics can be decreased<br>OE.1.b. Expect that reducing teen HIV, STD, and pregnancy rates will result in increased academic achievement and reduced dropout rates | PN.1. Recognize that other principals, school administrators, and physical education teachers see this as a problem that needs to be addressed in their schools |
| PO2. Principals, other school administrators, and physical education teachers review IYG and specifically note program objectives, methods, and relative advantages | K.2.a. Describe IYG objectives and describe applicable TEKS objectives<br>K.2.b. Describe how IYG compares to current HIV, STD, and pregnancy prevalence coverage in their district<br>K.2.c. Describe IYG methods and relative advantages | A.2. Describe IYG as being worth the effort to adopt | OE.2.a. Expect that many Health TEKS objectives will be covered by implementing IYG in schools<br>OE.2.b. Expect that IYG will be modifiable, easy to implement, and will fit in their allotted time for their health curriculum | PN.2. Recognize that other principals, school administrators, and physical education teachers have found IYG has enough relative advantages to be worthwhile to implement |
| PO.3. Principals, other school administrators, and physical education teachers obtain information on the experiences of other schools using IYG | K.3. Describe experiences of schools that have used IYG | A.3. Describe IYG as being congruent with prevalent values and norms of district's students, families, teachers, and principals | OE.3. Expect that by knowing the experiences of other schools that have used IYG, they will be able to better evaluate the pros and cons of using it | |

**Table 8.3** (*Continued*)

| Performance Objectives | Personal Determinants | | | |
|---|---|---|---|---|
| | **Knowledge** | **Attitudes** | **Outcome Expectations** | **Perceived Norms** |
| PO.4. Principals, other school administrators, and physical education teachers identify barriers for implementation, including computer lessons | K.4.a. Assess available resources necessary to adopt the IYG program<br>K.4.b. List barriers to implementing IYG (e.g., computer availability, class size, teacher training times) | A.4. Feel positive about identifying and overcoming potential barriers | OE.4. Expect that identifying possible barriers and ways to overcome them will facilitate successful IYG implementation | PN.4. Recognize that other schools have successfully overcome these barriers |
| PO.5. Principals, other school administrators, and physical education teachers gain input regarding IYG adoption from nonphysical education teachers, computer support staff, and parents | K.5. Describe ways to obtain input from nonphysical education teachers, staff, and parents regarding IYG adoption | A.5. Feel favorable about obtaining input from nonphysical education teachers, computer support staff, and parents | OE.5. Expect that obtaining input from nonphysical education teachers, computer support staff, and parents will facilitate implementation of IYG at their school | PN.5. Recognize that other principals and teachers obtain input from nonphysical education teachers, computer support staff, and parents prior to adopting a sexual health education program |
| PO.6. Principals complete the adoption forms necessary for IYG | K.6.a. Describe necessary forms and signatures needed | A.6. Describe notification as necessary and important to program implementation | OE.6.a. Expect that if they complete the forms then more of their teachers will adopt the beneficial program | PN.6. Recognize that other principals in their district and similar districts have adopted IYG |

**Implementation**

**Outcome 3: Principals, physical education teachers, and necessary nonphysical education teachers/staff will implement IYG, an effective HIV, STD, and pregnancy prevention program, as part of their fulfillment for teaching the state's Health TEKS objectives.**

| Performance Objectives | Personal Determinants | | | |
|---|---|---|---|---|
| | **Knowledge** | **Skills and Self-Efficacy** | **Outcome Expectations** | **Perceived Norms** |
| School | | | | |
| PO.1. All physical education teachers attend IYG training | K.1. Describe where training is and how it will be covered (e.g., substitute coverage for training days) | SSE.1.a. Demonstrate ability to attend the training<br>SSE1.b. Express confidence to attend IYG training | OE.1. Expect that by attending the training they will be able to successfully implement program and students will benefit | PN.1. Recognize that all middle school physical education teachers will attend IYG training |

(continued)

**Table 8.3**    (Continued)

| Performance Objectives | Personal Determinants | | | |
|---|---|---|---|---|
| | **Knowledge** | **Attitudes** | **Outcome Expectations** | **Perceived Norms** |
| PO.2. Physical education teachers plan how and when IYG will be implemented | K.2. Describe when the IYG lessons will be implemented during allotted health class time | SSE.2.a. Demonstrate ability to fit lessons into yearly plan SSE.2.b. Express confidence in ability to fit lessons into yearly plan | OE.2. Expect that IYG lessons are adaptable and easy to include in their curriculum | PN.2. Recognize that other physical education teachers feel this program is important and are including it in their lesson plans |
| PO.3. Physical education teachers obtain program materials from the IYG website | K.3.a. Demonstrate how to locate the IYG website K.3.b. List necessary IYG program materials | SSE.3.a. Demonstrate ability to locate the IYG website and download lesson plans and materials SSE.3.b. Express confidence in ability to locate and download IYG materials | OE.3. Expect that becoming familiar with the IYG website will facilitate successful implementation | PN.3. Recognize that other physical education teachers use the IYG website to download materials |
| PO.4. Physical education teachers secure computer lab/library space and other staff time if necessary | K.5.a. Describe when each student will complete computer lessons, where, and who will be supervising them | | | |
| PO.5. Computer and/or library staff arrange for IYG installation | K.5. Describe computer capabilities and IYG application requirements | SSE.5.a. Demonstrate ability to load IYG onto computers SSE.5.b. Express confidence in ability to load IYG onto computers | OE.5. Expect that by becoming familiar with computer capabilities and IYG application choices, the program will be successfully loaded and able to run | PN.5. Recognize that other computer and/or library staff facilitate installation of IYG |
| PO.6. Physical education teachers teach all IYG lessons as described in the teacher manual (i.e., with fidelity). | K.6.a. Acknowledge personal beliefs regarding sexual health education that may contribute to their level of discomfort K.6.b. Describe effective strategies to create a comfortable environment for student learning | SSE.6.a. Express confidence in ability to acknowledge personal beliefs about sexual health education SSE.6.b. Demonstrate ability to create a safe classroom environment | OE.6.a. Expect that acknowledging personal beliefs will help alleviate discomfort when teaching sensitive material OE.6.b. Expect that creating a comfortable environment will enhance student learning | PN.6. Recognize that other physical education teachers in the district teach all IYG lessons as described in the teacher manual |

**Table 8.3**    *(Continued)*

| Performance Objectives | Personal Determinants | | | |
| --- | --- | --- | --- | --- |
| | **Knowledge** | **Attitudes** | **Outcome Expectations** | **Perceived Norms** |
| | K.6.c. Describe IYG classroom and computer lesson activities<br>K.6.d. Describe acceptable adaptations, if needed | SSE.6.c. Express confidence in ability to create a comfortable classroom environment<br>SSE.6.d. Express confidence in ability to implement all IYG lessons as described in teacher manual | OE.6.c. Expect that teaching all IYG lessons as described in the teacher manual will help students to make responsible decisions about dating and sex | |
| PO.7. Principal ensures teacher training time (including securing substitutes if necessary) and encourages IYG implementation | K.7.a. List dates and times when IYG training will be conducted for physical education teachers<br>K.7.b. List ways to provide classroom coverage during training<br>K.7.c. List ways to support teachers and staff to fully implement the IYG program | SSE.7.a. Demonstrate ability to support teachers and staff to fully implement the IYG program<br>SSE.7.b Express confidence in ability to support teachers and staff to fully implement the IYG program | OE.7. Expect that by supporting teachers and staff to fully implement the IYG program, students will benefit and have lower rates of school dropout, HIV, STD, and pregnancy | |

**Maintenance**

**Outcome 4: The SHAC, superintendent, principals, physical education teachers, and necessary nonphysical education teachers/staff will maintain delivery of IYG, an effective HIV, STD, and pregnancy prevention program, in the district's middle schools.**

| Performance Objectives | Personal Determinants | | | |
| --- | --- | --- | --- | --- |
| | **Knowledge** | **Skills and Self-Efficacy** | **Outcome Expectations** | **Perceived Norms** |
| PO.1. Principals include an annual budget line item for IYG teacher training and materials | K.1. Describe annual cost of IYG teacher training and materials | SSE.1.a. Demonstrate ability to allocate annual funds for IYG teacher training and materials<br>SSE.1.b. Express confidence in ability to maintain IYG teacher training and materials | OE.1. Expect that allocating annual funds for IYG will reduce school dropout related to HIV, STD, and pregnancy, and enhance academic achievement | PN.1. Recognize that other superintendents allocate funds for effective sexual health education programs |

*(continued)*

**Table 8.3**    *(Continued)*

| Performance Objectives | Personal Determinants | | | |
| --- | --- | --- | --- | --- |
| | Knowledge | Skills and Self-Efficacy | Outcome Expectations | Perceived Norms |
| PO.2. Principals include IYG in job descriptions and performance reviews for physical education teachers | K.2. Describe physical education teachers' responsibilities for implementing IYG | SSE.2. Express confidence in ability to include IYG in job descriptions and performance reviews for physical education teachers | OE.2. Expect that including IYG in physical education teachers' job description and performance reviews will ensure ongoing IYG implementation | PN.2. Recognize that other principals require physical education teachers to implement an effective sexual health education program |
| PO.3. Principals support new physical education teachers to attend IYG teacher training (including securing substitutes if necessary) | K.3. List IYG teacher training dates and strategies to provide classroom coverage if necessary | SSE.3.a. Demonstrate ability to provide classroom coverage if needed SSE.3.b. Express confidence in ability to provide classroom coverage if needed | OE.3. Expect that supporting new physical education teachers to attend IYG teacher training will result in continued student benefits from IYG delivery | PN.3. Recognize that other principals support new physical education teachers to attend IYG teacher training |
| PO.4. The SHAC reports IYG program outcomes annually to the superintendent and school board | K.4. List relevant IYG program outcomes (e.g., number of students reached, student and teacher satisfaction data, number of pregnancies) | SSE.4.a. Demonstrate ability to compile and report IYG outcomes SSE.4.b. Express confidence in ability to compile and report IYG outcomes | OE.4. Expect that annual reporting of IYG outcomes will facilitate continued district support for IYG implementation | PN.4. Recognize that other SHACs regularly report program outcomes to their superintendent and school board |

TEKS = Texas Essential Knowledge and Skills. These are state mandated student learning objectives.

### Task 4: Design Implementation Interventions

The planning group identified theoretical methods and practical applications, and developed program materials to promote the implementation of IYG in other school districts across the U.S. (Table 8.4)

To promote the adoption of IYG, the planning group created teen birth rate maps for school districts using GIS. Many of the school districts had areas with teen birth rates in excess of state and national rates, which emphasized the need for effective sexual health education (consciousness raising). The planning group also developed presentation materials to be delivered at SHAC and school board meetings, which included evidence on the consequences of teen pregnancy including decreased academic achievement and increased school dropout

**Table 8.4**   It's Your Game . . . Keep It Real: Methods, Practical Applications, and Program Materials to Enhance Program Implementation

| Responsible Person | Sample Performance Objectives | Determinants | Methods and Practical Application | Program Materials |
|---|---|---|---|---|
| **Adoption** | | | | |
| School district personnel Principals | Identify need Review IYG materials Sign adoption form | Knowledge Attitudes Outcome expectations Perceived norms | Consciousness raising through tailored data Persuasive communication through providing evidence Modeling through testimonials from school district personnel | Teen birth rate maps per school district Presentations at SHAC and school board meetings Promotional video |
| **Implementation** | | | | |
| Teachers Computer or library staff Principals | Attend teacher training Plan for use Teach all lessons as written | Knowledge Skills and self-efficacy Outcome expectations Perceived norms | Modeling by trainers Guided practice with feedback for teachers Facilitation via the Internet Modeling through teacher testimonials | Teacher training IYG website Teacher newsletters |
| **Maintenance** | | | | |
| Principals School district personnel | Budget for IYG Report outcomes | Knowledge Attitudes Outcome expectations Perceived norms | Facilitation through templates | Sample budget Template for outcomes report |

(persuasive communication). A promotional video included testimonials from SHAC and school board members, superintendents, principals, teachers, counselors, parents, and students who reported positive experiences implementing IYG (modeling).

To prepare classroom teachers to implement IYG, the planning group developed a teacher training in which IYG staff provided an overview of the curriculum's content (information transfer) and modeled teaching selected lessons (modeling). Teachers engaged in interactive lesson practice, receiving feedback from the trainers and their peers (guided practice with feedback). Teachers also practiced strategies to create a comfortable classroom environment and to deal with sensitive issues. They reviewed guidelines on acceptable curriculum adaptations and used planning time to prepare for IYG implementation at their school (facilitation).

The IYG, website (www.itsyourgame.org) allowed teachers to access online or download all classroom and computer lessons. It also provided information on the program developers and research findings, technical requirements for computer installation, training videos on how to teach selected lessons, and a list of frequently asked questions (facilitation).

The planning group developed and disseminated teacher newsletters, which included program updates and feedback from teachers on their experience attending the IYG teacher training and implementing the curriculum (modeling). Example quotes included:

"The training will enable me to provide a needed tool to my students. Personally, it has given me an additional tool to use with my own children."

"It's Your Game helped me think more clearly about how a middle school student perceives his/her choices and sexual health."

To support the maintenance of IYG, the program planners provided principals and school district personnel with sample budgets, data collection instruments, and templates for reporting program outcomes to their school board and superintendent (facilitation).

It's Your Game...Keep It Real is nationally recognized as an effective sexual health education program (U.S. Department of Health and Human Services Office of Adolescent Health, 2015). The implementation intervention materials developed in Step 5 have facilitated implementation of IYG in school districts across the U.S., reaching over 33,000 middle school students each year.

## Summary

This chapter presented the development of implementation interventions. There is now a body of literature that planners can use to identify implementers, construct performance objectives for adoption, implementation and maintenance, discover determinants, and identify change methods and practical applications for influencing program use.

There are two distinct situations in which intervention planning can be done to influence program use. One is for the initial use of a program. In some cases, the same agency that is planning the program will also be adopting and implementing the program. This might be referred to as an "in-house" program. In other cases, the planning group is developing a program that will be used by outside agencies or organizations. In both cases, the planning for program use will be one of the six IM steps used to plan the health promotion program. Steps 1 through 4 of IM will be used to plan an intervention to achieve outcomes for changes in behavior and environmental conditions to achieve health and quality-of-life outcome goals. In Step 5, the tasks are used to plan an intervention to achieve program use outcomes for adoption, implantation, and continuation of the health promotion program.

In general practice, it is considered unacceptable to encourage widespread use of a health promotion program unless there is evidence that the program works, in other words, that it is able to accomplish stated objectives and achieve expected outcomes. The initial use of a health promotion program is usually intended to determine whether the program is effective. Once effectiveness of the program is established, the sponsoring agency or planning group may use evaluation findings to improve the program, or use effectiveness findings to justify a broader implementation of the program to reach a greater proportion of the population at risk for the health problem. If a health promotion program is effective and made ready for wider use, then Step 5 of IM is used to plan a dissemination intervention to encourage greater adoption and implementation of the program. The dissemination plan may be different from the plan developed for initial use if the adopters and implementers are different, if the agencies or communities are different, or if there are differences in determinants of program use outcomes for adoption, implementation, and continuation. In this situation, Step 5 of IM becomes the planning tool for designing an intervention for the diffusion of a health promotion program with demonstrated effectiveness.

The second use of Step 5 is to disseminate health promotion programs that have been evaluated and shown to be effective in accomplishing stated objectives and achieving the expected outcomes. There is a strong push in the field to encourage community groups to consider evidence-based programs for adoption and implementation when planning a program to address an identified health problem (Brownson et al., 2007b; Collins, Harshbarger, Sawyer, & Hamdallah, 2006; Glasgow et al., 2004b). The rationale is that programs with evidence of effectiveness may have a better chance of improving the health problem and will save community groups time and resources compared with developing a new program on their own. The advantage for an organization or community group using an evidence-based program is in not having to start from scratch to develop a new program and instead making use of the work that the original program developers had already invested in developing the program and concentrating on the implementation of the already evaluated program using IM Step 5.

## Discussion Questions and Learning Activities

1. Compare and contrast the tasks in Step 5 of IM with Steps 2, 3, and 4. What do they have in common? How are they different?

2. Explain why it is important to plan for program use as part of health promotion program planning.

3. What is meant by a linkage system for program adoption and implementation? Give examples of different ways in which a linkage system can be established.

4. Refer back to Chapter 4, question 4, where you have described your planning group. Do you need to bring any new people to the planning group to begin planning for program adoption and implementation? Who are they and what will they contribute to planning for program adoption and implementation?

5. What theories can be used to identify determinants of program adoption, implementation, and sustainability? Give an example of determinants that have been shown through research and theory to be important determinants of program adoption, implementation, and sustainability.

6. Describe how the matrices created in Step 5 can be used to help guide process evaluation of the health promotion program.

7. Continuing with the health promotion program you are proposing, state adoption, implementation, and sustainability outcomes and write performance objectives for each outcome.

8. Create a matrix for adoption and implementation of the program by linking performance objectives with determinants.

9. Describe methods and practical application you propose to affect the change and performance objectives in the matrices to achieve program adoption and implementation.

## References

Aarons, G. A., Ehrhart, M. G., Farahnak, L. R., & Sklar, M. (2014). Aligning leadership across systems and organizations to develop a strategic climate for evidence-based practice implementation. *Annual Review of Public Health, 35,* 255–274.

Aarons, G. A., Hurlburt, M., & Horwitz, S. M. (2011). Advancing a conceptual model of evidence-based practice implementation in public service sectors. *Administration and Policy in Mental Health and Mental Health Services Research, 38*(1), 4–23.

Aarons, G. A., & Sommerfeld, D. H. (2012). Leadership, innovation climate, and attitudes toward evidence-based practice during a statewide implementation. *Journal of the American Academy of Child & Adolescent Psychiatry, 51*(4), 423–431.

Abbott, P. A., Foster, J., Marin, H. F., & Dykes, P. C. (2014). Complexity and the science of implementation in health IT: Knowledge gaps and future visions. *International Journal of Medical Informatics, 83*(7), e12–e22.

Akers, J. D., Estabrooks, P. A., & Davy, B. M. (2010). Translational research: Bridging the gap between long-term weight loss maintenance research and practice. *Journal of the American Dietetic Association, 110*(10), 1511–1522. e3.

Ammerman, A. S., Lindquist, C. H., Lohr, K. N., & Hersey, J. (2002). The efficacy of behavioral interventions to modify dietary fat and fruit and vegetable intake: A review of the evidence. *Preventive Medicine, 35*(1), 25–41.

Bandura, A. (1986). *Social foundations of thought and action: A Social Cognitive Theory.* Englewood Cliffs, NJ: Prentice-Hall.

Bandura, A. (2001). Social Cognitive Theory: An agentic perspective. *Annual Review of Psychology, 52,* 1–26.

Baranowski, T., & Stables, G. (2000). Process evaluations of the 5-a-day projects. *Health Education & Behavior, 27*(2), 157–166.

Bartholomew, L. K., Parcel, G. S., Seilheimer, D. K., Czyzewski, D., Spinelli, S. H., & Congdon, B. (1991). Development of a health education program to promote the self-management of cystic fibrosis. *Health Education & Behavior, 18*(4), 429–443.

Bero, L. A., Grilli, R., Grimshaw, J. M., Harvey, E., Oxman, A. D., & Thomson, M. A. (1998). Closing the gap between research and practice: An overview of systematic reviews of interventions to promote the implementation of research findings. The Cochrane effective practice and organization of care review group. *BMJ (Clinical Research Ed.), 317*(7156), 465–468.

Berwick, D. M. (2003). Disseminating innovations in health care. *Journal of the American Medical Association, 289*(15), 1969–1975.

Bonham, C. A., Sommerfeld, D., Willging, C., & Aarons, G. A. (2014). Organizational factors influencing implementation of evidence-based practices for integrated treatment in behavioral health agencies. *Psychiatry Journal.* Advance online publication. doi:10.1155/2014/802983

Bradley, E. H., Webster, T. R., Baker, D., Schlesinger, M., Inouye, S. K., Barth, M. C., . . . Joren, M. J. (2004). Translating research into practice: Speeding the adoption of innovative health care programs. *The Commonwealth Fund.* Retrieved from http://www.commonwealthfund.org/programs/elders/bradley_translating_research_724.pdf

Brink, S. G., Basen-Engquist, K. M., O'Hara-Tompkins, N. M., Parcel, G. S., Gottlieb, N. H., & Lovato, C. Y. (1995). Diffusion of an effective tobacco prevention program. Part I: Evaluation of the dissemination phase. *Health Education Research, 10*(3), 283–295.

Brownson, R. C., Ballew, P., Dieffenderfer, B., Haire-Joshu, D., Heath, G. W., Kreuter, M. W., & Myers, B. A. (2007a). Evidence-based interventions to promote physical activity: What contributes to dissemination by state health departments? *American Journal of Preventive Medicine, 33*(1), S66–S78.

Brownson, R. C., Ballew, P., Brown, K. L., Elliott, M. B., Haire-Joshu, D., Heath, G. W., & Kreuter, M. W. (2007b). The effect of disseminating evidence-based interventions that promote physical activity to health departments. *American Journal of Public Health, 97*(10), 1900–1907.

Brownson, R. C., Jacobs, J. A., Tabak, R. G., Hoehner, C. M., & Stamatakis, K. A. (2013). Designing for dissemination among public health researchers: Findings from a national survey in the United States. *American Journal of Public Health, 103*(9), 1693–1699.

Carroll, C., Patterson, M., Wood, S., Booth, A., Rick, J., & Balain, S. (2007). A conceptual framework for implementation fidelity. *Implementation Science, 2*(40), 1–9.

Chambers, D. A., Glasgow, R. E., & Stange, K. C. (2013). The dynamic sustainability framework: Addressing the paradox of sustainment amid ongoing change. *Implementation Science, 8*, 117.

Chaudoir, S. R., Dugan, A. G., & Barr, C. H. (2013). Measuring factors affecting implementation of health innovations: A systematic review of structural, organizational, provider, patient, and innovation level measures. *Implementation Science, 8*(1), 22.

Chin, M. H., Goddu, A. P., Ferguson, M. J., & Peek, M. E. (2014). Expanding and sustaining integrated health care-community efforts to reduce diabetes disparities. *Health Promotion Practice, 15*( Suppl 2), 29S–39S.

Clavier, C., Sénéchal, Y., Vibert, S., & Potvin, L. (2012). A theory-based model of translation practices in public health participatory research. *Sociology of Health & Illness, 34*(5), 791–805.

Cohen, W. M., & Levinthal, D. A. (1990). Absorptive capacity: A new perspective on learning and innovation. *Administrative Science Quarterly, 35*(1), 128–152.

Colditz, G. A. (2012). The promise and challenges of dissemination and implementation research. In R. C. Brownson, G. A. Colditz, & E. K. Proctor (Eds.), *Dissemination and implementation research in health: Translating science to practice* (pp. 3–22). Oxford, United Kingdom: Oxford University Press.

Collins, C., Harshbarger, C., Sawyer, R., & Hamdallah, M. (2006). The diffusion of effective behavioral interventions project: Development, implementation, and lessons learned. *AIDS Education & Prevention, 18*(Suppl), 5–20.

Compernolle, S., De Cocker, K., Lakerveld, J., Mackenbach, J. D., Nijpels, G., Oppert, J. M., ... De Bourdeaudhuij, I. (2014). A RE-AIM evaluation of evidence-based multi-level interventions to improve obesity-related behaviours in adults: A systematic review (the SPOTLIGHT project). *International Journal of Behavioral Nutrition and Physical Activity, 11*(1), 147.

Damschroder, L. J., Aron, D. C., Keith, R. E., Kirsh, S. R., Alexander, J. A., & Lowery, J. C. (2009). Fostering implementation of health services research findings into practice: A consolidated framework for advancing implementation science. *Implementation Science, 4*(1), 50.

Damschroder, L. J., & Hagedorn, H. J. (2011). A guiding framework and approach for implementation research in substance use disorders treatment. *Psychology of Addictive Behaviors, 25*(2), 194.

Damschroder, L. J., & Lowery, J. C. (2013). Evaluation of a large-scale weight management program using the consolidated framework for implementation research (CFIR). *Implementation Science, 8*, 51.

Davies, P., Walker, A. E., & Grimshaw, J. M. (2010). A systematic review of the use of theory in the design of guideline dissemination and implementation strategies and interpretation of the results of rigorous evaluations. *Implementation Science, 5*, 14.

Dearing, J. W. (2009). Applying Diffusion of Innovation Theory to intervention development. *Research on Social Work Practice, 19*(5), 503–518.

Ditty, M. S., Landes, S. J., Doyle, A., & Beidas, R. S. (2014). It takes a village: A mixed method analysis of inner setting variables and dialectical behavior therapy implementation. *Administration and Policy in Mental Health and Mental Health Services Research*, doi:10.1007/s10488-014-0602-0

Donaldson, A., & Poulos, R. G. (2014). Planning the diffusion of a neck-injury prevention programme among community rugby union coaches. *British Journal of Sports Medicine, 48*(2), 151–158.

Dunton, G. F., Lagloire, R., & Robertson, T. (2009). Using the RE-AIM framework to evaluate the statewide dissemination of a school-based physical activity and nutrition curriculum: "Exercise Your Options." *American Journal of Health Promotion, 23*(4), 229–232.

Durlak, J. A., & DuPre, E. P. (2008). Implementation matters: A review of research on the influence of implementation on program outcomes and the factors affecting implementation. *American Journal of Community Psychology, 41*(3–4), 327–350.

Fernández, M. E., Melvin, C. L., Leeman, J., Ribisl, K. M., Allen, J. D., Kegler, M. C.,...Hebert, J. R. (2014). The cancer prevention and control research network: An interactive systems approach to advancing cancer control implementation research and practice. *Cancer Epidemiology, Biomarkers & Prevention, 23*(11), 2512–2521.

Finch, C. F., Gabbe, B. J., Lloyd, D. G., Cook, J., Young, W., Nicholson, M.,... Doyle, T. L. (2011). Towards a national sports safety strategy: Addressing facilitators and barriers towards safety guideline uptake. *Injury Prevention, 17*(3), e4.

Fixsen, D. L., Naoom, S. F., Blase, K. A., & Friedman, R. M. (2005). *Implementation research: A synthesis of the literature.* Tampa, FL: Louis de la Parte Florida Mental Health Institute.

Flaspohler, P., Duffy, J., Wandersman, A., Stillman, L., & Maras, M. A. (2008). Unpacking prevention capacity: An intersection of research-to-practice models and community-centered models. *American Journal of Community Psychology, 41*(3–4), 182–196.

FLU-FIT. (2013). How to do it. 5 simple steps. Retrieved from http://flufit.org/assets/doc/HowToDoIt.pdf

Gaglio, B., Shoup, J. A., & Glasgow, R. E. (2013). The RE-AIM framework: A systematic review of use over time. *American Journal of Public Health, 103*(6), e38–e46.

Glanz, K., Steffen, A., Elliott, T., & O'Riordan, D. (2005). Diffusion of an effective skin cancer prevention program: Design, theoretical foundations, and first-year implementation. *Health Psychology, 24*(5), 477.

Glasgow, R. E., Klesges, L. M., Dzewaltowski, D. A., Bull, S. S., & Estabrooks, P. (2004a). The future of health behavior change research: What is needed to improve translation of research into health promotion practice? *Annals of Behavioral Medicine, 27*(1), 3–12.

Glasgow, R. E., Klesges, L. M., Dzewaltowski, D. A., Estabrooks, P. A., & Vogt, T. M. (2006). Evaluating the impact of health promotion programs: Using the RE-AIM framework to form summary measures for decision making involving complex issues. *Health Education Research, 21*(5), 688–694.

Glasgow, R. E., Marcus, A. C., Bull, S. S., & Wilson, K. M. (2004b). Disseminating effective cancer screening interventions. *Cancer, 101*(S5), 1239–1250.

Glasgow, R. E., McKay, H. G., Piette, J. D., & Reynolds, K. D. (2001). The RE-AIM framework for evaluating interventions: What can it tell us about approaches to chronic illness management? *Patient Education and Counseling, 44*(2), 119–127.

Glasgow, R. E., & Riley, W. T. (2013). Pragmatic measures: What they are and why we need them. *American Journal of Preventive Medicine, 45*(2), 237–243.

Glasgow, R. E., Vogt, T. M., & Boles, S. M. (1999). Evaluating the public health impact of health promotion interventions: The RE-AIM framework. *American Journal of Public Health, 89*(9), 1322–1327.

Green, L. W., & Glasgow, R. E. (2006). Evaluating the relevance, generalization, and applicability of research: Issues in external validation and translation methodology. *Evaluation & the Health Professions, 29*(1), 126–153.

Greenhalgh, T., Robert, G., Macfarlane, F., Bate, P., & Kyriakidou, O. (2004). Diffusion of innovations in service organizations: Systematic review and recommendations. *Milbank Quarterly, 82*(4), 581–629.

Greenhalgh, T., Robert, G., MacFarlane, F., Bate, P., & Kyriakidou, O. (Eds.). (2005). *Diffusion of innovations in health service organizations: A systematic literature review*. Oxford, United Kingdom: Blackwell.

Grimshaw, J. M., Shirran, L., Thomas, R., Mowatt, G., Fraser, C., Bero, L., . . . O'Brien, M. A. (2001). Changing provider behavior: An overview of systematic reviews of interventions. *Medical Care, 8*(Suppl 2), II2–II45.

Hall, G. E., & Loucks, S. F. (1978). *Innovation configurations: Analyzing the adaptations of innovations*. Austin, TX: University of Texas, Research and Development Center for Teacher Education.

Harris, J. R., Cheadle, A., Hannon, P. A., Forehand, M., Lichiello, P., Mahoney, E., . . . Yarrow, J. (2012). A framework for disseminating evidence-based health promotion practices. *Preventing Chronic Disease, 9*, E22.

Havelock, R. G. (1971). The utilisation of educational research and development. *British Journal of Educational Technology, 2*(2), 84–98.

Hernandez, B. F., Peskin, M., Shegog, R., Markham, C., Johnson, K., Ratliff, E. A., . . . Tortolero, S. R. (2011). Choosing and maintaining programs for sex education in schools: The CHAMPSS model. *Journal of Applied Research on Children: Informing Policy for Children at Risk, 2*(2), 7.

Highfield, L. (2014). *Evidence-based dissemination for mammography adherence in safety net communities.* Unpublished manuscript.

Hogan, J. A., Baca, I., Daley, C., Garcia, T., Jaker, J., Lowther, M., & Klitzner, M. (2003). Disseminating science-based prevention: Lessons learned from CSAP's CAPTs. *Journal of Drug Education, 33*(3), 233–243.

Holmes, P., Neville, D., Donovan, C., & MacDonald, C. A. (2001). The Newfoundland and Labrador heart health program dissemination story: The formation and functioning of effective coalitions. *Promotion & Education, Suppl 1,* 8–12.

Howell, J. M., & Higgins, C. A. (1990). Champions of change: Identifying, understanding, and supporting champions of technological innovations. *Organizational Dynamics, 19*(1), 40–55.

Ilott, I., Gerrish, K., Booth, A., & Field, B. (2013). Testing the consolidated framework for implementation research on health care innovations from South Yorkshire. *Journal of Evaluation in Clinical Practice, 19*(5), 915–924.

Jacobs, J. A., Dodson, E. A., Baker, E. A., Deshpande, A. D., & Brownson, R. C. (2010). Barriers to evidence-based decision making in public health: A national survey of chronic disease practitioners. *Public Health Reports, 125*(5), 736–742.

Johnson, K., Hays, C., Center, H., & Daley, C. (2004). Building capacity and sustainable prevention innovations: A sustainability planning model. *Evaluation and Program Planning, 27*(2), 135–149.

Kahwati, L. C., Lance, T. X., Jones, K. R., & Kinsinger, L. S. (2011). RE-AIM evaluation of the veterans health Administration's MOVE! weight management program. *Translational Behavioral Medicine, 1*(4), 551–560.

Kegler, M., & McLeroy, K. R. (2003). Commentary on conceptualizing dissemination research and activity: The case of the Canadian heart health initiative. *Health Education and Behavior, 30*(3), 283–286.

Kessler, R. S., Purcell, E. P., Glasgow, R. E., Klesges, L. M., Benkeser, R. M., & Peek, C. J. (2013). What does it mean to "employ" the RE-AIM model? *Evaluation & the Health Professions, 36*(1), 44–66.

Kilbourne, A. M., Neumann, M. S., Pincus, H. A., Bauer, M. S., & Stall, R. (2007). Implementing evidence-based interventions in health care: Application of the replicating effective programs framework. *Implementation Science, 2*(1), 1–10.

Klabunde, C. N., Riley, G. F., Mandelson, M. T., Frame, P. S., & Brown, M. L. (2004). Health plan policies and programs for colorectal cancer screening: A national profile. *The American Journal of Managed Care, 10*(4), 273–279.

Klesges, L. M., Estabrooks, P. A., Dzewaltowski, D. A., Bull, S. S., & Glasgow, R. E. (2005). Beginning with the application in mind: Designing and planning health behavior change interventions to enhance dissemination. *Annals of Behavioral Medicine, 29*(Suppl), 66–75.

Kocken, P., Voorham, T., Brandsma, J., & Swart, W. (2001). Effects of peer-led AIDS education aimed at Turkish and Moroccan male immigrants in the Netherlands. A randomised controlled evaluation study. *European Journal of Public Health, 11*(2), 153–159.

Kolbe, L. J., & Iverson, D. C. (1981). Implementing comprehensive health education: Educational innovations and social change. *Health Education Quarterly, 8*(1), 57–80.

Kreuter, M. W., Eddens, K. S., Alcaraz, K. I., Rath, S., Lai, C., Caito, N., . . . Wells, A. (2012). Use of cancer control referrals by 2-1-1 callers: A randomized trial. *American Journal of Preventive Medicine, 43*(6), S425–S434.

Lee, S. J., Altschul, I., & Mowbray, C. T. (2008). Using planned adaptation to implement evidence-based programs with new populations. *American Journal of Community Psychology, 41*(3–4), 290–303.

Linnan, L., & Steckler, A. (2002). Process evaluation for public health interventions and research: An overview. In A. Steckler, & L. Linnan (Eds.), *Process evaluation for public health interventions and research* (pp. 1–23). San Francisco, CA: Jossey-Bass.

MacDonald, M. A., & Green, L. W. (2001). Reconciling concept and context: The dilemma of implementation in school-based health promotion. *Health Education & Behavior, 28*(6), 749–768.

Mendel, P., Meredith, L. S., Schoenbaum, M., Sherbourne, C. D., & Wells, K. B. (2008). Interventions in organizational and community context: A framework for building evidence on dissemination and implementation in health services research. *Administration and Policy in Mental Health and Mental Health Services Research, 35*(1–2), 21–37.

Michaels, C. N., & Greene, A. M. (2013). Worksite wellness: Increasing adoption of workplace health promotion programs. *Health Promotion Practice, 14*(4), 473–479.

Michie, S., Johnston, M., Abraham, C., Lawton, R., Parker, D., Walker, A., & "Psychological Theory" Group. (2005). Making psychological theory useful for implementing evidence based practice: A consensus approach. *Quality & Safety in Health Care, 14*(1), 26–33.

Michie, S., Johnston, M., Francis, J., Hardeman, W., & Eccles, M. (2008). From theory to intervention: Mapping theoretically derived behavioural determinants to behaviour change techniques. *Applied Psychology, 57*(4), 660–680.

Mihalic, S. F., Fagan, A. A., & Argamaso, S. (2008). Implementing the LifeSkills training drug prevention program: Factors related to implementation fidelity. *Implementation Science, 3*(5), 1–16.

Miller, R. L., & Shinn, M. (2005). Learning from communities: Overcoming difficulties in dissemination of prevention and promotion efforts. *American Journal of Community Psychology, 35*(3–4), 169–183.

Moullin, J. C., Sabater-Hernández, D., Fernandez-Llimos, F., & Benrimoj, S. I. (2015). A systematic review of implementation frameworks of innovations in healthcare and resulting generic implementation framework. *Health Research Policy and Systems, 13*(1), 16.

Nanney, M. S., Haire-Joshu, D., Brownson, R. C., Kostelc, J., Stephen, M., & Elliott, M. (2007). Awareness and adoption of a nationally disseminated dietary curriculum. *American Journal of Health Behavior, 31*(1), 64–73.

National Cancer Institute, Center for the Advancement of Health, & Robert Wood Johnson Foundation. (2002). *Designing for dissemination.* (Conference Summary Report). Retrieved from http://cancercontrol.cancer.gov/IS/pdfs/d4d_conf_sum_report.pdf

Neta, G., Glasgow, R. E., Carpenter, C. R., Grimshaw, J. M., Rabin, B. A., Fernandez, M. E., & Brownson, R. C. (2015). A framework for enhancing the value of research for dissemination and implementation. *American Journal of Public Health, 105*(1), 49–57.

Noonan, R. K., Wilson, K. M., & Mercer, S. L. (2012). Navigating the road ahead: Public health challenges and the Interactive Systems Framework for dissemination and implementation. *American Journal of Community Psychology, 50*(3–4), 572–580.

Oldenburg, B., & Glanz, K. (2008). Diffusion of innovations. In K. Glanz, B. K. Rimer, & K. Viswanath (Eds.), *Health behavior and health education: Theory, research, and practice* (4th ed., pp. 313–333). San Francisco, CA: Jossey-Bass.

Oldenburg, B., Hardcastle, D. M., & Kok, G. (1997). Diffusion of innovations. In K. Glanz, B. K. Rimer, & F. M. Lewis (Eds.), *Health behavior and health education: Theory, research, and practice* (2nd ed., pp. 270–286). San Francisco, CA: Jossey-Bass.

Orlandi, M. A. (1986). The diffusion and adoption of worksite health promotion innovations: An analysis of barriers. *Preventive Medicine, 15*(5), 522–536.

Orlandi, M. A., Landers, C., Weston, R., & Haley, N. (1990). Diffusion of health promotion innovations. In K. Glanz, F. M. Lewis, & B. K. Rimer (Eds.), *Health behavior and health education: Theory, research, and practice* (1st ed., pp. 288–313). San Francisco, CA: Jossey-Bass.

Owen, N., Glanz, K., Sallis, J. F., & Kelder, S. H. (2006). Evidence-based approaches to dissemination and diffusion of physical activity interventions. *American Journal of Preventive Medicine, 31*(4), 35–44.

Panzano, P. C., & Roth, D. (2006). The decision to adopt evidence-based and other innovative mental health practices: Risky business? *Psychiatric Services, 57*(8), 1153–1161.

Peskin, M. F., Hernandez, B. F., Markham, C., Johnson, K., Tyrrell, S., Addy, R. C., . . . Tortolero, S. R. (2011). Sexual health education from the perspective of school staff: Implications for adoption and implementation of effective programs in middle school. *Journal of Applied Research on Children, 2*(2), 9.

Peterson, J. C., Rogers, E. M., Cunningham-Sabo, L., & Davis, S. M. (2007). A framework for research utilization applied to seven case studies. *American Journal of Preventive Medicine, 33*(1), S21–S34.

Potter, M. B., Ackerson, L. M., Gomez, V., Walsh, J. M., Green, L. W., Levin, T. R., & Somkin, C. P. (2013). Effectiveness and reach of the FLU-FIT program in an integrated health care system: A multisite randomized trial. *American Journal of Public Health, 103*(6), 1128–1133.

Potter, M. B., Somkin, C. P., Ackerson, L. M., Gomez, V., Dao, T., Horberg, M. A., & Walsh, J. M. E. (2011). The FLU-FIT program: An effective colorectal cancer screening program for high volume flu shot clinics. *The American Journal of Managed Care, 17*(8), 577–583.

Proctor, E. K., Landsverk, J., Aarons, G., Chambers, D., Glisson, C., & Mittman, B. (2009). Implementation research in mental health services: An emerging science with conceptual, methodological, and training challenges. *Administration and Policy in Mental Health and Mental Health Services Research, 36*(1), 24–34.

Proctor, E. K., Powell, B. J., & McMillen, J. C. (2013). Implementation strategies: Recommendations for specifying and reporting. *Implementation Science, 8,* 139.

Proctor, E., Silmere, H., Raghavan, R., Hovmand, P., Aarons, G., Bunger, A., . . . Hensley, M. (2011). Outcomes for implementation research: Conceptual distinctions, measurement challenges, and research agenda. *Administration and Policy in Mental Health and Mental Health Services Research, 38*(2), 65–76.

Purnell, J. Q., Kreuter, M. W., Eddens, K. A., Ribisl, K., Hannon, P., Williams, R. S., . . . Fagin, D. (2012). Cancer control needs of 2-1-1 callers in Missouri, North Carolina, Texas, and Washington. *Journal of Health Care for the Poor and Underserved, 23,* 752–767.

Rimer, B. K., Glanz, K., & Rasband, G. (2001). Searching for evidence about health education and health behavior interventions. *Health Education & Behavior, 28*(2), 231–248.

Ringwalt, C., Hanley, S., Ennett, S. T., Vincus, A. A., Bowling, J. M., Haws, S. W., & Rohrbach, L. A. (2011). The effects of No Child Left Behind on the prevalence of evidence-based drug prevention curricula in the nation's middle schools. *Journal of School Health, 81*(5), 265–272.

Ringwalt, C. L., Vincus, A., Ennett, S., Johnson, R., & Rohrbach, L. A. (2004). Reasons for teachers' adaptation of substance use prevention curricula in schools with non-white student populations. *Prevention Science, 5*(1), 61–67.

Robinson, K., Elliott, S. J., Driedger, S. M., Eyles, J., O'Loughlin, J., & Riley, B. (2005). Using linking systems to build capacity and enhance dissemination in heart health promotion: A Canadian multiple-case study. *Health Education Research, 20,* 499–513.

Rogers, E. M. (1983). *Diffusion of innovations* (3rd ed.). New York, NY: Free Press.

Rogers, E. M. (1995). *Diffusion of innovations* (4th ed.). New York, NY: Free Press.

Rogers, E. M. (2003). *Diffusion of innovations* (5th ed.). New York, NY: Free Press.

Rossi, P. H., Lipsey, M. W., & Freeman, H. E. (2004). *Evaluation: A systematic approach* (7th ed.). Thousand Oaks, CA: Sage.

Rubenstein, L. V., & Pugh, J. (2006). Strategies for promoting organizational and practice change by advancing implementation research. *Journal of General Internal Medicine, 21*(S2), S58–S64.

Sanchez, S. H., Sethi, S. S., Santos, S. L., & Boockvar, K. (2014). Implementing medication reconciliation from the planner's perspective: A qualitative study. *BMC Health Services Research, 14*(1), 290.

Saunders, R. P., Evans, M. H., & Joshi, P. (2005). Developing a process-evaluation plan for assessing health promotion program implementation: A how-to guide. *Health Promotion Practice, 6*(2), 134–147.

Scheirer, M. A. (1981). *Program implementation: The organizational context.* Beverly Hills, CA: Sage.

Scheirer, M. A. (1994). Designing and using process evaluation. In J. S. Whole, H. P. Hatry, & K. E. Newcomer (Eds.), *Handbook of practical program evaluation* (pp. 40–68). San Francisco, CA: Jossey-Bass.

Scheirer, M. A., Shediac, M. C., & Cassady, C. E. (1995). Measuring the implementation of health promotion programs: The case of the breast and cervical cancer program in Maryland. *Health Education Research, 10*(1), 11–25.

Schell, S. F., Luke, D. A., Schooley, M. W., Elliott, M. B., Herbers, S. H., Mueller, N. B., & Bunger, A. C. (2013). Public health program capacity for sustainability: A new framework. *Implement Science, 8*(1), 15.

Scott, S. D., Plotnikoff, R. C., Karunamuni, N., Bize, R., & Rodgers, W. (2008). Factors influencing the adoption of an innovation: An examination of the uptake of the Canadian heart health kit (HHK). *Implementation Science, 3*, 41.

Shea, C. M., Jacobs, S. R., Esserman, D. A., Bruce, K., & Weiner, B. J. (2014). Organizational readiness for implementing change: A psychometric assessment of a new measure. *Implementation Science, 9*(7), 1–15.

Shediac-Rizkallah, M. C., & Bone, L. R. (1998). Planning for the sustainability of community-based health programs: Conceptual frameworks and future directions for research, practice and policy. *Health Education Research, 13*(1), 87–108.

Slater, J. S., Finnegan J. R., Jr., & Madigan, S. D. (2005). Incorporation of a successful community-based mammography intervention: Dissemination beyond a community trial. *Health Psychology, 24*(5), 463.

Spoth, R., Rohrbach, L. A., Greenberg, M., Leaf, P., Brown, C. H., Fagan, A., . . . Hawkins, J. D. (2013). Addressing core challenges for the next generation of type 2 translation research and systems: The translation science to population impact (TSci impact) framework. *Prevention Science, 14*(4), 319–351.

Steckler, A., Goodman, R. M., & Kegler, M. (2002). Mobilizing organizations for health enhancement: Theories of organizational change. In K. Glanz, B. K. Rimer, & F. M. Lewis (Eds.), *Health behavior and health education: Theory, research, and practice* (3rd ed., pp. 335–360). San Francisco, CA: Jossey-Bass.

Steckler, A., Goodman, R. M., McLeroy, K. R., Davis, S., & Koch, G. (1992). Measuring the diffusion of innovative health promotion programs. *American Journal of Health Promotion, 6*(3), 214–224.

Stith, S., Pruitt, I., Dees, J., Fronce, M., Green, N., Som, A., & Linkh, D. (2006). Implementing community-based prevention programming: A review of the literature. *Journal of Primary Prevention, 27*(6), 599–617.

Sweet, S. N., Ginis, K. A., Estabrooks, P. A., & Latimer-Cheung, A. E. (2014). Operationalizing the RE-AIM framework to evaluate the impact of multi-sector partnerships. *Implementation Science 9*, 74. doi:10.1186/1748-5908-9-74

Tabak, R. G., Khoong, E. C., Chambers, D. A., & Brownson, R. C. (2012). Bridging research and practice: Models for dissemination and implementation research. *American Journal of Preventive Medicine, 43*(3), 337–350.

Tapp, H., & Dulin, M. (2010). The science of primary health-care improvement: Potential and use of community-based participatory research by practice-based research networks for translation of research into practice. *Experimental Biology and Medicine, 235*(3), 290–299.

Thorpe, K. E., Zwarenstein, M., Oxman, A. D., Treweek, S., Furberg, C. D., Altman, D. G., . . . Magid, D. J. (2009). A pragmatic–explanatory continuum indicator summary (PRECIS): A tool to help trial designers. *Journal of Clinical Epidemiology, 62*(5), 464–475.

Trickett, E. J. (2011). Community-based participatory research as worldview or instrumental strategy: Is it lost in translation(al) research? *American Journal of Public Health, 101*(8), 1353–1355.

U.S. Department of Health and Human Services Office of Adolescent Health. (2015). Teen pregnancy prevention resource center: Evidence-based programs. Retrieved from http://www.hhs.gov/ash/oah/oah-initiatives/teen_pregnancy/db/index.html

Vick, L., Duffy, S. A., Ewing, L. A., Rugen, K., & Zak, C. (2013). Implementation of an inpatient smoking cessation programme in a veterans affairs facility. *Journal of Clinical Nursing, 22*(5–6), 866–880.

Viswanathan, M., Ammerman, A., Eng, E., Garlehner, G., Lohr, K. N., Griffith, D., . . . Lux, L. (2004). AHRQ evidence report summaries 2004. Community-based participatory research: Assessing the evidence: Summary. Retrieved from http://www.ncbi.nlm.nih.gov/books/NBK11852/

Wandersman, A., Duffy, J., Flaspohler, P., Noonan, R., Lubell, K., Stillman, L., . . . Saul, J. (2008). Bridging the gap between prevention research and practice: The Interactive Systems Framework for dissemination and implementation. *American Journal of Community Psychology, 41*(3–4), 171–181.

Weiner, B. J., Amick, H., & Lee, S. Y. (2008). Conceptualization and measurement of organizational readiness for change: A review of the literature in health services research and other fields. *Medical Care Research and Review, 65*(4), 379–436.

Weiner, B. J., Lewis, M. A., & Linnan, L. A. (2009). Using organization theory to understand the determinants of effective implementation of worksite health promotion programs. *Health Education Research, 24*(2), 292–305.

Wejnert, B. (2002). Integrating models of diffusion of innovations: A conceptual framework. *Annual Review of Sociology, 28*, 297–326.

Wilson, K. D., & Kurz, R. S. (2008). Bridging implementation and institutionalization within organizations: Proposed employment of continuous quality improvement to further dissemination. *Journal of Public Health Management and Practice, 14*(2), 109–116.

Zahra, S. A., & George, G. (2002). Absorptive capacity: A review, reconceptualization, and extension. *Academy of Management Review, 27*(2), 185–203.

Zulman, D. M., Damschroder, L. J., Smith, R. G., Resnick, P. J., Sen, A., Krupka, E. L., & Richardson, C. R. (2013). Implementation and evaluation of an incentivized internet-mediated walking program for obese adults. *Translational Behavioral Medicine, 3*(4), 357–369.

Zwarenstein, M., & Treweek, S. (2009). What kind of randomized trials do we need? *Canadian Medical Association Journal, 180*(10), 998–1000.

# CHAPTER 9

# INTERVENTION MAPPING STEP 6

*Evaluation Plan*

**with Patricia Dolan Mullen**

## Competency

* Develop an evaluation plan based on previous steps of Intervention Mapping.

The product of Intervention Mapping Step 6 is a plan to guide evaluation. Excellent textbooks and online resources provide detailed guidance (Centers for Disease Control and Prevention, Program Performance and Evaluation Office, 2015; Fetterman, Kaftarian, & Wandersman, 2014; Patton, 2008; Rossi, Lipsey, & Freeman, 2004; Shadish, Cook, & Campbell, 2002; Windsor, Clark, Boyd, & Goodman, 2003). The purpose of this chapter is to help planners (also called evaluators in this chapter) use the previous steps of Intervention Mapping to facilitate program evaluation.

## Perspectives

Evaluation based on Intervention Mapping (IM) products begins with understanding the program to be evaluated—an easy starting place for those who have systematically developed or adapted a program. Basic perspectives also include the importance of evaluating programs and the critical roles played by stakeholders.

### Understanding the Program

Intervention Mapping as well as most evaluation texts (Fetterman et al., 2014; Rossi et al., 2004; Wholey, Hatry, & Newcomer, 2004; Windsor et al., 2003) promote understanding the program to be evaluated as the first part of

**LEARNING OBJECTIVES AND TASKS**

* Write effect and process evaluation questions
* Develop indicators and measures for assessment
* Specify the evaluation design
* Complete the evaluation plan

evaluation. Questions about the program's conceptualization and design include the following: Is there is need for the program? Have the right priority groups been identified? Do stakeholders agree on the program objectives? Is the logic model of the problem or the logic model of change (sometimes called program theory by evaluators) flawed? Have appropriate delivery channels been selected for the intervention? Answering such questions can help an evaluator avoid wasting resources on evaluating programs with inadequate planning. Programs that have been developed using Steps 1–5 of IM are likely to stand up well to this scrutiny; at the very least, their logic will be transparent. However, evaluators are sometimes asked to evaluate a program after it has been developed. In this case, the evaluator must backtrack and reconstruct the steps in the planning process. The idea that conceptualizing and testing the theory of a program should be a first step in evaluating a program emerged in the 1970s as part of "evaluability assessment" (Wholey, 1994). This refers to a systematic process for describing the program model, assessing how well defined the model is, and identifying stakeholders' ability to use the evaluation results. An important first finding of an evaluation might be that the needs assessment, formulation of objectives, choice of change methods, and translation of methods and practical applications into a coherent and feasible program were not appropriately executed.

Rossi et al. (2004) use a logic model to portray the theory of the program and refer to the logic of the pathways for accomplishing program outcomes. Other evaluation experts refer to a theory of action (Patton, 2008) and to causal models (Scheirer, 1994). Program pathways comprise two parts: the impact pathway, how the program is expected to cause change, and the process pathway, how the program is implemented. In addition, the description of the program pathways includes careful specification of the intended participants.

## Reasons for Program Evaluation

Research evaluation to determine efficacy (does the program work under controlled conditions?) and effectiveness (does the program work in the "real world") adds to the body of science that defines an evidence-based intervention. However, it is equally important to conduct evaluation as a part of program management to provide feedback to improve programs and enable the greatest benefit from scarce program resources (Fetterman et al., 2014; Patton, 2008). Keys to establishing accountability and improving the health promotion programs are to assess whether the program has achieved behavioral, environmental, and implementation outcomes and why or why not. Successful health promotion practitioners monitor the implementation and outcomes of their programs to improve them as they are being conducted, to ensure their ongoing quality, and to justify continued allocation of resources.

Perhaps the most exciting reason to perform program evaluation is to generate knowledge. Knowledge about effective programs, complete implementation, and useful evaluation methods enriches the field of health education and promotion. A program planner who has used a systematic planning framework, such as IM, should be able to express in the scientific literature the theory of the intervention, its operationalization, and its implementation. If so, a contribution to knowledge will be possible and will depend on the quality of the evaluation, because a poorly conceptualized or inadequately described intervention (the downfall of some evaluations) should not be an issue.

## Involving Evaluation Stakeholders

An important goal of an evaluation is that someone uses the results (Fetterman et al., 2014; Patton, 2008; Torres, Preskill, & Pointek, 2004). To ensure that evaluation results are used and are trustworthy, the evaluator must engage the attention of the evaluation stakeholders, including the intended beneficiaries, program participants, funders, planners, and implementers. Many of the stakeholders selected in Step 1 of IM (see Chapter 4, Table 4.1) will be stakeholders for the evaluation. Table 9.1 describes possible evaluation stakeholders. Getting an evaluation used requires identifying stakeholders and gaining their participation. Not all types of stakeholders will be relevant for every evaluation, but most programs have multiple stakeholders (Preskill & Jones, 2009). The first step in thinking about stakeholder participation is identifying stakeholders and deciding the degree and kind of involvement each will have.

Generally, endorsed steps in ensuring stakeholder involvement are the following:

- Identify stakeholders and involve them early
- Plan structures for involving stakeholders in the ongoing evaluation process
- Help stakeholders plan how to use evaluation data
- Present evaluation results in multiple forms

Possibly the most important stakeholders from an ethical point of view are those who stand to be most affected by both formative and summative evaluations: a program's intended beneficiaries. Even when program planners have sought the opinions of potential participants during program development, they often leave this group out of the evaluation process.

**Table 9.1**   Evaluation Stakeholders

| | |
|---|---|
| Policymakers and decision makers | Persons responsible for deciding whether the program is to be started, continued, discontinued, expanded, restructured, or curtailed |
| Program sponsors | Organizations that initiate and fund the program (can overlap with policymakers and decision makers) |
| Evaluation sponsors | Organizations that initiate and fund the evaluation (sometimes program sponsors and evaluation sponsors are the same) |
| Target participants | Persons, households, or other units that receive the intervention or services being evaluated |
| Program managers | Personnel responsible for overseeing and administering the intervention program |
| Program staff | Personnel responsible for delivering the program services or in supporting roles |
| Program competitors | Organizations or groups that compete with the programs for available resources |
| Contextual stakeholders | Organizations, groups, and individuals in the immediate environment of a program with interests in what the program is doing or what happens to it |
| Evaluation and research community | Evaluation professionals who read evaluations and pass judgment on their technical quality and credibility and researchers who work in areas related to the program |

Adapted with permission from Rossi, P. H., Lipsey, M. W., & Freeman, H. E. (2004). *Evaluation: A systematic approach* (7th ed., pp. 48–49). Thousand Oaks, CA: Sage.

When the focus is on evaluation use, intended beneficiaries tend to be considered a low-power group. Many evaluators now strive to use an empowerment approach that aims to enhance the capacity of program stakeholders, especially the at-risk group and program implementers, to perform and use evaluations (Fetterman et al., 2014; Torres et al., 2004). Empowerment goals are similar to community-based participatory research (Israel et al., 2008; Minkler & Wallerstein, 2008).

Although all stakeholders are interested in program efficacy or effectiveness, some have specific interest in cost-benefit or cost-effectiveness and some in process evaluation results. For example, policy and decision makers, including funders, will want to know the cost-benefit of the program. How much does the program cost for each unit of benefit? How does this compare to other programs addressing the problem? Planners may evaluate a program's efficiency in terms of its costs and effects. A cost-benefit analysis monetizes both the inputs and the outputs of a program, whereas cost-effectiveness describes only program inputs in terms of money. Cost-effectiveness avoids controversy that may arise from computing a monetary value for a program's health or social effect by describing the program outputs in programmatic units rather than money.

For example, a cost-effectiveness evaluation of a health program that seeks to prevent cases of measles might report the cost of a case of measles averted rather than determining the monetary value (possibly by determining the productivity loss averted). The concept of opportunity cost is also relevant here, because resources spent on one problem are not available to spend on another problem. The program plan includes a budget and a description of all other program inputs that should provide a basis for an efficiency analysis. This chapter does not present the methods for efficiency analyses; for these, we refer the reader to other works (Drummond, Sculpher, Torrance, O'Brien, & Stoddard, 2005; Green & Kreuter, 2005; Haddix, Teutsch, & Corso, 2003; Rossi et al., 2004; Windsor et al., 2003).

Among other things, program managers will be especially interested in the proportion of the intended audience who participate, how much of the program the participants receive, whether staff members have the skills and credentials needed for implementation, whether the program is implemented as intended, and the satisfaction of participants. Intended beneficiaries are likely to be interested in the barriers and facilitators to participation, opinions of participants and nonparticipants about the program, and assurance that data will be fed back to improve program quality. Reports to the various stakeholders should be tailored to their group's interests.

Stakeholders can help evaluators keep the larger context of the program in mind. Interventions are systems within wider systems with structure and function that evolve, and can thus be a challenge to evaluators. Systems thinking, interdisciplinary approaches, interaction with stakeholders, and qualitative inquiry allow the evaluator to understand how the program and its parts are embedded in a larger, interactive whole (Hawe, Shiell, & Riley, 2009; Patton, 2008; Potvin, Haddad, & Frohlich, 2001; Schorr, 2006).

A final and important consideration for stakeholders is the problem of conflict of interest; usually the interest of finding a positive program effect at all costs. It might be summed up as "human nature" to form attachments, in this case to programs, and not want the object of the attachment to "go away," for example, after an evaluation that finds it inadequate. An alternative to looking at efficacy and effectiveness results as a "yes" or "no" is to look at the size of the effect and consider whether adaptations could be made to improve it. Currently, there is too much temptation to find any effect and to grab on to it—program designers afraid to lose their funding, academics making their careers, funders with their own needs—it is not trivial. The concepts of program improvement and comparative effectiveness studies are important counterbalances to evaluations that result in all or none findings.

## Tasks for Step 6

## Writing Evaluation Questions

### *Effect Questions From Program Logic Models*

The first task in Step 6 is to write process and effectiveness questions. These questions will come from a review of the program logic models, goals, and objectives and the IM matrices.

Effect evaluation (sometimes referred to as outcome or impact) describes the differences in outcomes with and without the program. Possible outcomes of interest include quality of life, health indicators, behaviors, environmental conditions, and program objectives (determinants, performance objectives, and change objectives). Effect evaluation involves determining whether these factors change as a result of the intervention, which usually means comparing the group that had the opportunity to participate in the program to one that did not. An evaluator does not usually propose to measure all intended program outcomes in an evaluation plan. Proposed measures will depend on the logic model for the intervention, as well as on evaluation resources, stakeholders' interests, and evaluation purposes. Evaluation in health promotion often concerns multiple outcomes and evaluators have to decide which is their primary outcome.

Effect evaluation can be described as either efficacy or effectiveness two poles between a continuum. Efficacy refers to a program evaluated under optimal conditions, for instance, with motivated volunteers who will take part in the program no matter how much time and effort is required. Effectiveness means a program evaluated under real-world circumstances, for instance with representatives of the at-risk group some of whom will not take part or will drop out (Gartlehner, Hansen, Nissman, Lohr, & Carey, 2006; Singal, Higgins, & Waljee, 2014). The difference between effectiveness and efficacy is the result of, for example, noncompliance, imperfect implementation, or drop-out. Sometimes artificial incentives, e.g., cash or other rewards for participating in the program or highly selected samples, e.g., only those who have demonstrated compliance, are used to test the efficacy of the program.

Throughout the IM process, a planning group will have developed logic models in order to understand first the causes of the health problem (Chapter 4, Step 1) and then how a program is supposed to work to produce change (Chapter 5, Step 2). Here we reintroduce the logic model of change with types of evaluation added (Figure 9.1). Reviewing the program logic model will enable evaluators to develop evaluation questions.

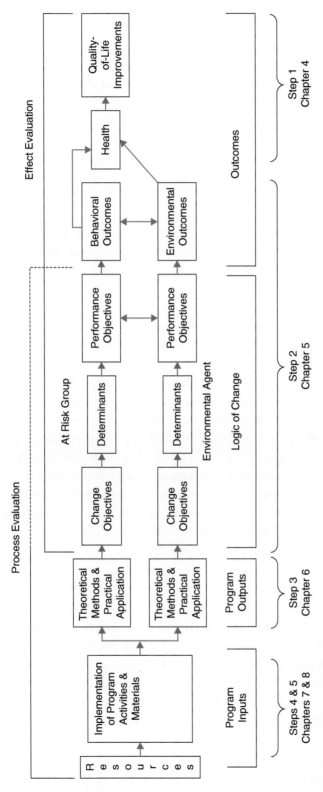

**Figure 9.1** Intervention Logic Model

## BOX 9.1. MAYOR'S PROJECT

Our health educator is hard at work finishing the program plan to present to the city council the next week. She has spread matrices and audiovisuals all across the floor of her office. Just the finishing touches have to be put on the chart that explains the scope and sequence of program activities and the graphic that outlines all of the program partners. Then she can tackle the evaluation plan.

    The department head drops in to make sure that everything is progressing for the next week's meeting.

| | |
|---|---|
| *Department head:* | How is everything coming? |
| *Health educator:* | Oh, just great. Sixteen members of the task force will be at the meeting. Here's the agenda for the flow of the presentation. You can see that you are giving the introduction. Then later on, I have you slated to hand out certificates of appreciation. |
| *Department head:* | Sounds good. Looks like you are just finishing up here. |
| *Health educator:* | Yes, I just have to write the evaluation plan. |
| *Department head:* | (barely under control) What do you mean, write the evaluation plan? Why did you wait until the last moment? |
| *Health educator:* | (pointing out the folder for the evaluation part of her presentation to the mayor) Look, here's the evaluation model. Of course, I didn't wait until the last minute! You know me better than that! The whole intervention planning process is, in a way, developing the evaluation plan as you go along. See, here are our health and quality-of-life objectives, behavior and environment changes, change objectives, methods and practical applications, program, and resources. Here are the pages that show how we are going to measure each outcome, and here is our plan to monitor the process. I just have to wrap some words around it. We have been formulating the plan all along the way. |

**Effect on Health, Quality of Life, Behavior, and Environment**    Working from the right side of the model (Figure 9.1), the evaluator looks at the intended impact of the program on health, quality of life, and on the behavioral and environmental causes of the health problem. In the needs assessment, the planning team will have written program goals about expected changes in these factors. These goals form the basis for evaluation questions:

- How much did the quality-of-life problem change in the designated time frame?

+ How much did the health problem change in the designated time frame?

+ What changes in behavior and environmental conditions occurred?

Some evaluators take a page from pharmaceutical trials and recommend looking for side effects, which may not be a part of the logic model (Scriven, 1991). In practice, this has been a more conceptual idea with not very much practical guidance (House, 2010), but one very feasible strategy is to poll experts to consider potential positive and negative effects of the program. Rossi et al. (2004, p. 213) suggest studying prior research on the topic and keeping in touch with program personnel at all levels, including participants and drop outs. Hawe et al. (2009) suggest four ways to capture system-level change: (a) uncovering how the intervention couples with the context, (b) tracking changes in relationships, (c) focusing on the distribution and transformation of resources, and (d) assessing the activities that are displaced. An evaluator could also consider subgroup analyses to check differential effects of the intervention. For example, interventions to encourage moving out of high-poverty neighborhoods have been associated with *reduced* rates of depression and conduct disorder among girls and *increased* rates of depression, PTSD, and conduct disorder among boys (Kessler et al., 2014). A source of what some stakeholders would consider a negative side effect is the worsening of disparities, which can occur even when the behavior or health status of a disadvantaged group is improved (Mechanic, 2002; Partin & Burgess, 2012). Increased disparity is more likely to occur with interventions that depend on voluntary involvement (because more advantaged individuals have the resources and may be more likely to participate) and with interventions that address prevalent problems when the required behavior is not easy to execute (Mechanic, 2002).

**Effect on Change Objectives**    Next, moving to the left in Figure 9.1, the planner specifies expected changes in objectives from the matrices, that is, performance objectives and change objectives (see Chapter 5). The first questions concern behavior and are derived from the performance objectives.

Change objectives combine hypothesized determinants with expected performance, and both should be well specified and documented from IM Step 2. Planners can write evaluation questions looking at the change objectives by determinants (the columns of the matrices). In the It's Your Game evaluation, the following evaluation questions were derived from the IM work on change objectives: Did the teens who participated in the program increase their knowledge of condom use compared to teens who did not receive the program? Did teens who participated in the program increase their skills and self-efficacy compared to teens who did not participate?

The importance of the exploration of mediator and moderator variables to explain intervention effects is being widely discussed and demonstrated in the literature (Baranowski, Cerin, & Baranowski, 2009; Holmbeck, 1997; Mackinnon, Lockwood, Hoffman, West, & Sheets, 2002). Intervention Mapping guides planners to make an explicit model of these variables throughout planning so that evaluators can analyze their relations to the outcomes in the presence of and without the intervention.

**Determining an Evaluation Time Frame**   Writing evaluation questions, especially about outcomes, requires thinking about the time frame for expected effects. First, intervention outcomes require time to develop. Second, health education is often directed at people's future behavior at a time when a risk behavior has not yet emerged. Third, the intervention itself needs time, especially when the intervention is targeted for long-term change, such as empowerment and community development.

Health and quality-of-life outcomes cannot be evaluated in the short-term for programs that seek to change behavior to prevent late occurring health effects. For example, prevention or reversal of obesity in school children to prevent chronic illnesses that occur primarily in adults would call for very long time frames or focus on intermediate outcomes, such as behavior or environmental change. Because some HIV prevention programs are designed to reach students before they begin having sexual intercourse, even changes in behavior may be outside the time frame for an initial program evaluation (Hofstetter et al., 2014; Table 9.2). At times behavior change is not an appropriate short-term evaluation goal, even though it certainly belongs in the program logic model. In this circumstance, the short-term impacts that program developers expect and seek to measure are changes in determinants such as knowledge, self-efficacy, and skills.

Evaluators may struggle with deciding the optimal way to demonstrate whether a program has reached its goals. On the one hand, the planner wants to show outcomes that are meaningful in relation to the health problem. On the other hand, the planner may not reasonably expect certain changes in health outcomes or risk factors to occur shortly after an intervention. An essential part of the evaluation plan is to decide in advance on the level of effects that can be expected within a given time frame. When health changes are not expected or measured in the evaluation plan, the planner must have strong evidence and logical arguments to justify any assumption of causation that is beyond the evaluation's scope. For instance, the planner must document the relation between skills improvement now and the use

**Table 9.2**    Evaluation of a School HIV Prevention Program

| Intervention Mapping Step | Question Focus | Process Evaluation Variable | Effect Evaluation Variable |
|---|---|---|---|
| Step 1 Needs Assessment | *Quality of Life | NA | Quality of life related to worry about AIDS<br>Quality of life related to AIDS |
| Step 1 Needs Assessment | *Health | NA | HIV infections<br>AIDS cases<br>Mortality |
| Step 1 Needs Assessment | Behavior | NA | Condom use |
| Step 1 Needs Assessment | Environment | NA | Condom availability |
| Step 2 Matrices | Components of behavior | Correctness of objective specification | Condom use performance objectives |
| Step 2 Matrices of Change Objectives | Components of environmental change | Correctness of objective specification | Environmental agent objectives |
| Step 2, Matrices of Change Objectives | Determinants | That chosen determinants are the correct ones<br>That all important behavioral domains are covered | Knowledge<br>Skills<br>Self-Efficacy |
| Steps 3 and 4, Methods and Strategies | Choice of methods<br>Use of methods according to parameters<br>Acceptability of program and materials | Evidence that methods can effect expected change (e.g., modeling is effective in stimulating steps of condom use; skill training results in students able to make counterarguments against taking risk; students can demonstrate refusal and condom use)<br>That strategies convey methods appropriately (e.g., students attend to and remember modeled material)<br>That materials and program are culturally relevant; students and teachers find the program salient<br>That materials and program are acceptable to intended users and implementers (e.g., students and teachers like the program) | NA |
| Step 5 Program Adoption, Implementation, and Sustainability | Interaction of intended intervention group with intervention | Program is delivered to intended recipients<br>Program is adopted<br>Program is implemented with fidelity and completeness; teachers do all lessons as designed; students read magazine and do homework;<br>Program is sustained, e.g., routinized, institutionalized | NA |

*Not included in the final evaluation model because of time frame.

**NOTE. This program has recently been updated.** See Hofstetter, H., Peters, L. W. H., Meijer, S., Van Keulen, H. M., Schutte, L., & van Empelen, P. (2014). Evaluation of the Effectiveness and Implementation of the Sexual Health Program Long Live Love IV. *European Health Psychologist, 16*(S), 489.

of condoms, and a reduction in HIV infections later. The epidemiologic or experimental evidence and arguments could include:

- The relation between behavior or environment change and change in the health problem

- The relation between change in determinants and change in behavior or environment

- The relation between methods and change in determinants

### Program Process Questions

Measuring and attributing outcomes to a program, without insight into how that program was delivered, or whether the program was delivered at all, is sometimes called a "black box evaluation" (Harachi, Abbott, Catalano, Haggerty, & Fleming, 1999; Patton, 2008; Stame, 2004). A black box evaluation contributes little to any field because the evaluator does not know why a program succeeded or failed. If a program was not effective, the cause could be in the program's impact pathways (that is, the program's targeted determinants, change methods, and practical applications) cannot cause the intended effects. On the other hand, ineffectiveness can be because of the process. Patton (2008) offers one example in which the effect of a parenting program was measured before and after the program and compared with a group that was designated not to receive the program. When the results were presented to policy makers, they ended the program because of its ineffectiveness. Several years later, the evaluators found that the program had never been implemented at all because of political sensitivities. This situation is an extreme, but not impossible, example of a black box evaluation.

Process evaluation seeks to describe program implementation (Patton, 2008; Rossi et al., 2004; Scheirer, 1994; Steckler & Linnan, 2002). Implementers use feedback from process measures to correct problems and assure effective delivery. Process evaluation findings also enable interpretation of outcome data and reflection on program design and future implementation (Grimshaw et al., 2007). Program implementation questions include the following: To what extent is the program being delivered to the persons for whom it was intended? How well does the delivery maintain fidelity to the program's original design? How do aspects of implementation explain results of an effect evaluation? Further, process evaluation should ask whether theory- and evidence-based change methods have been appropriately operationalized in the program applications. A program can be poorly implemented because program developers have not adhered to assumptions about how the methods should be used (see Chapter 6). Process evaluation also describes program, organizational, and implementation factors related to why an intervention is being implemented in a certain way. For example, an intervention can be well designed but not well implemented because the planners misjudged the preferences of the at-risk group, because the implementers lack skills, or because there is no one to champion the program in an organization.

In contrast to outcome evaluation, which often makes comparisons between groups, process evaluation is primarily concerned with the group that is designated to receive an intervention. Some process indicators, for example, judgments by the participants about the intervention, can be elicited only from the intervention group. Researchers may also collect process data in a comparison group, but they do this primarily to find out whether an unplanned intervention may have contaminated the evaluation.

Looking at the process components of the program logic model in this way, first the planner needs a correctly implemented intervention (as stated in the adoption and implementation objectives in Chapter 8), in which all the assumptions that were made in the methods and applications steps are realized (Chapters 6 and 7). Next, the planner may expect changes first in the determinants and change objectives, and then in behavior and environmental conditions. Finally, changes are expected in health outcomes and quality of life (as stated in the measurable objectives related to the health problem and the quality-of-life indicators in Chapter 5).

Linnan and Steckler (2002) describe the following key process evaluation components:

- Context: aspects of the larger social environment that may affect implementation
- Reach: the proportion of the intended audience to whom the program is actually delivered
- Dose delivered: the amount of intended units of each program component that is delivered
- Dose received: the extent to which participants engage with the program
- Fidelity: the extent to which the intervention was delivered as intended
- Implementation: the extent to which the program was implemented and received
- Recruitment: a description of the approach used to attract program participants

Table 9.3 shows the plan for a process evaluation based on these dimensions. This is the initial plan for evaluating the process of a program intended to deliver a computerized telephone intervention to increase uptake of colorectal cancer screening in veterans.

**Table 9.3**    Process Evaluation Questions for a Program to Increase Colorectal Cancer Screening (CRCS) Among U.S. Veterans

| Components | Questions | Indicators | Method |
|---|---|---|---|
| Context | During program implementation, has the context changed for CRCS?<br>What changes have been made in screening guidelines, if any?<br>What changes, if any have been made in organizational capacity for CRCS?<br>What CRCS programs or messages have patients been exposed to? | VA CRCS guidelines<br>VA eligibility for and access to CRCS and follow-up<br>VA CRCS capacity<br>VA capacity to integrate new programs<br>Participant exposure to non-VA CRCS health promotion efforts | Tracking CRCS guidelines and access policies<br>Interviews with patients<br>Communication with VA staff |
| Reach | To what extent is the program reaching intended participants?<br>Are any subgroups being missed?<br>Are unintended groups taking part? | Percentage of the intended participants who used the program; distribution by subgroup<br>Percentage of users not part of the intended group | Project records during the delivery period |
| Dose delivered | How much of the program is being delivered?<br>What, if anything, is being omitted/delivered inconsistently? Why? | Tailored phone number and length of completed calls and booster sessions | Project records, including phone counselor checklists and reports generated by the telephone counseling system |
| Dose received | What is the average dose received by program participants?<br>What parts of the intervention, if any, are not received consistently? Why? | Percentage of intended group calling to request educational materials<br>Attention, recall, understanding, and credibility of messages | Toll-free phone records<br>Participant recall and reaction to intervention<br>Interviews with random sample of those getting CRCS and those not getting CRCS |
| Fidelity | | Degree to which the message is linked to theoretical methods and practical applications and to determinants<br>Match of message to stage of change | Narrative analysis of message concept booklets against Intervention Mapping matrices, intervention scripts, and flow charts, checklists, and transcripts of conversations |

VA = Veterans Affairs

**Fidelity and Implementation Performance**    To formulate process questions, the planner must first fully describe the program that should be delivered. What is each program component? What are the program support materials for acceptable delivery of the program? Were the program change methods translated into practical applications with adherence to their parameters? Was the required dose of the program delivered? For example, a program to teach management of Type 1 diabetes might include four meetings with individual families whose children were experiencing frequent high blood sugar. The implementation manual would include

**Table 9.4**    Diabetes Program Performance Standards

| The counselor: | Present | Absent |
|---|:---:|:---:|
| 1. Asks how the family has been since last session or from intake | ☐ | ☐ |
| 2. Establishes or reviews goal statement | ☐ | ☐ |
| 3. Reviews progress on each step of the problem-solving framework, or if first session, teaches the framework | ☐ | ☐ |
| 4. Reviews data collected or presents forms for self-monitoring | ☐ | ☐ |
| 5. Reinforces approximations of the problem-solving steps | ☐ | ☐ |
| 6. Shows video sequence with role-model story | ☐ | ☐ |
| 7. Has the family practice appraisal | ☐ | ☐ |
| 8. Has the family practice generation of alternative solution strategies | ☐ | ☐ |
| 9. Has the family practice evaluation of alternative strategies | ☐ | ☐ |
| 10. Elicits the family's thoughts and feelings about the process | ☐ | ☐ |

Percent of protocol followed is equal to the number from the "Present" column divided by 10.

instructions to guide each 1 hour biweekly meeting (dose). Each of the meetings would follow a protocol in which the interventionist and the family members collaborate to delineate a self-management problem and use specified problem-solving steps to address it (fidelity to change methods and practical applications; Table 9.4).

Inherent in any process evaluation are performance standards: the level of implementer behaviors expected. In the diabetes example, the program manager could express performance standards or acceptable levels of adherence to both the visit schedules and the protocol elements within the visits. Windsor et al. (2003) suggest creating an implementation index that combines the reach of the program with the performance standard. Using a process evaluation example from Windsor et al. (2003), we added fidelity measures and program maintenance measures and created Table 9.5. In the hypothetical diabetes program, staff selected 75 children with poor blood glucose control for the program. Their parents were notified of the new program and encouraged to enroll. Those who enrolled were invited to counseling sessions every 2 weeks for 2 months. The performance standards were that 80 percent of those invited enrolled and that the proportion completing each session showed no more than a 5-percentage-point loss from the session before. The implementation index for program reach was calculated by dividing the proportion reached by the performance standard. In addition, the manager set the standard that 80 percent of the program's intended characteristics should be met in each counseling session. Table 9.5 shows the observation sheet for implementation characteristics that the

**Table 9.5** Hypothetical Process Evaluation of Diabetes Counseling Program

| Procedures Initial Implementation | Number Eligible (A) | Number Exposed (B) | Percent Reached (B/A)=C | Performance Standard for Reach (%) D | Implement. Reach Index C/D=E | Percentage of Protocol Followed* $C^f$ | Performance Standard for Fidelity (%) $D^f$ | Implement. Fidelity Index $C^f/D^f=E^f$ |
|---|---|---|---|---|---|---|---|---|
| Screening for poor control | 200 | 200 | 100 | 80 | 1.20 | NA | NA | NA |
| Enrollment contact | 75 | 75 | 100 | 100 | 1.00 | 63 | 80 | .79 |
| Counseling Session 1 | 75 | 70 | 93 | 95 | .98 | 72 | 80 | .90 |
| Counseling Session 2 | 75 | 67 | 89 | 90 | .99 | 80 | 80 | 1.00 |
| Counseling Session 3 | 75 | 60 | 80 | 85 | .94 | 62 | 80 | .78 |
| Counseling Session 4 | 75 | 59 | 79 | 80 | .99 | 64 | 80 | .80 |
| Counseling Session 5 | 75 | 58 | 77 | 75 | 1.03 | 70 | 80 | .88 |
| Counseling Session 6 | 75 | 55 | 73 | 70 | 1.04 | 62 | 80 | .78 |

| Procedures Program Maintenance | Number Eligible (A) | Exposed (B) | Percent Reached (B/A)=C | Performance Standard for Reach (D) | Implement. Reach Index Maintenance C/D=E | Percentage of* Protocol Followed $C^f$ | Performance Standard for Fidelity (%) $D^f$ | Implement. Fidelity Index Maintenance $C^f/D^f=E^f$ |
|---|---|---|---|---|---|---|---|---|
| Screening for poor control | 125 | 125 | 100 | 100 | 1.00 | NA | NA | NA |
| Enrollment contact | 25 | 25 | 100 | 100 | 1.00 | 72 | 80 | .90 |
| Counseling Session 1 | 25 | 18 | 72 | 95 | .76 | 72 | 80 | .90 |
| Counseling Session 2 | 25 | 16 | 64 | 90 | .71 | 80 | 80 | 1.00 |
| Counseling Session 3 | 25 | 15 | 60 | 85 | .71 | 79 | 80 | .99 |
| Counseling Session 4 | 25 | 14 | 56 | 85 | .66 | 70 | 80 | .88 |
| Counseling Session 5 | 25 | 14 | 56 | 85 | .66 | 70 | 80 | .88 |
| Counseling Session 6 | 25 | 14 | 56 | 85 | .66 | 71 | 80 | .89 |

*Average percentage across all family sessions initial implementation.

manager used to judge the implementation. The implementation index for fidelity was calculated by dividing the proportion of implementation guidelines adhered to by the performance standard.

Further, the manager, concerned that program implementation might change over time, extended the process evaluation table to include implementation beyond the first 75 children (Table 9.5, bottom half). In the continuing implementation, not as many children were eligible because most of the children who had less than adequate control had been recruited and participated initially. However, there were some newly eligible children and also some children whose parents had dropped out of the program in the first phase. As shown in Table 9.5, that group was smaller but 100 percent were screened. They were somewhat more difficult to engage and a much smaller percentage was enrolled (20 percent versus 100 percent in the initial group). On the other hand, the manager had tightened the training requirements for the staff who implemented the protocol, and the fidelity index improved. The performance standard column of Table 9.5 is the average across all families of the proportion of implementation criteria met in each session. Table 9.5 indicates clearly that the checklist was devised from the IM steps because it represents both implementation guidelines and attention to the detail of how the health educator planned that methods, such as role modeling, would be operationalized.

In the HIV prevention program evaluation, interventionists asked teachers about program adoption and use (Table 9.2; Hofstetter et al., 2014; Paulussen, Kok, Schaalma, & Parcel, 1995). For instance, they asked about familiarity with the program and whether the teachers used the program in the previous year. Fidelity was assessed with the question, How did you use the program? Teachers could answer with the following choices: "took some ideas," "took many ideas," "as a guiding principle," "followed most of the instructions," or "followed the instructions completely." The teachers were also asked, "Have you used other materials along with the program materials?"

**Reasons for Implementation Performance**    In the next part of the process evaluation, the evaluator will want explanatory data for the extent and fidelity of implementation. What barriers were there for implementation? For example, in the Cystic Fibrosis Family Education Project evaluation of program diffusion and implementation, the evaluators found that the program was implemented with only moderate fidelity. A major reason for lower fidelity was the lack of skills of program implementers to engage in the goal-setting process (Bartholomew, Cyzewski, Swank, McCormich, & Parcel, 2000). In the HIV prevention program evaluation (Schaalma, Kok, Poelman, & Reinders, 1994; Schaalma et al., 1996), teachers were also asked questions or presented with statements that could explain implementation failure, such as this: "Is AIDS prevention a structural part of your curriculum?" "The program is sufficiently flexible to be used in classes with substantially different subgroups (ethnicity, sexual experience)." Schaalma et al. (1994, 1996) interviewed teachers a second time, based on their responses on the questionnaire, to better understand implementation barriers.

**Reach**    Process evaluation questions about program reach would include the following (Glasgow, Vogt, & Boles, 1999; Rossi et al., 2004):

- What proportions of the intended groups are participating in the program? Which groups are underrepresented?

- Are any persons who are not members of the intended groups participating in the program? How many? Do any of them suggest new groups that should be included?

- How much of the program are intended participants receiving? What are the patterns of incomplete doses? What are the main causes?

**Methods and Practical Applications**    Questions related to the decisions made in program planning, that is, questions about change methods and practical applications and their operationalization, have been addressed to some extent in the pretesting and formative evaluation of the program (see Chapters 6 and 7). The difference is that now the planner can test the intervention in its final form and its final setting instead of in a provisional form and in a simulated setting. Again, evaluators do not deal with effects here but with judgments, such as satisfaction, positive emotional reaction to the materials, an understanding of the message, a determination of whether the program was of help, or conversations with peers about the program.

## Selecting and Developing Measures

The second task in Step 6 is to develop indicators and measures to assess the selected effect and process evaluation questions.

A *measure* is a device for quantifying or categorizing an indicator. Moving from right to left in the evaluation logic model (Figure 9.1), indicators and their measures will be needed for all of the selected evaluation questions. These could include quality of life, health, behavior, environment, determinants, and process. A measure usually entails applying numbers to indicators. For example, an evaluator interested in grades achieved could measure this construct in many different ways. A measure could be a year-end achievement test, an average of numeric grades achieved in all subjects, an average of numerical grades achieved in math and language arts (core subjects), and so forth. Likewise, the other indicators of functional status can be measured in numerous ways. Using the asthma program objective from the previous paragraph, the indicator of participation in physical education could include the number of days the child attended school, the number of days without a doctor- or parent-excused absence, time spent in moderate to vigorous movement, and so forth.

This section presents some guidelines for defining constructs from IM and for developing the measures. However, advice on measurement theory and on the ways that other evaluators have measured similar constructs must come from the measurement literature (DeVellis, 2012; Di Lorio, 2005) and from the literature on a specific construct.

### *Measures of Health and Quality of Life*

Health promotion planners are rarely responsible for developing health and quality-of-life measures and indicators. These measures are generally readily available from national, state, and local data or from data maintained by health facilities and payers as described in Chapter 4. Careful attention should be paid regarding indicators of health status of life before measures are sought. Choosing measurable evaluation indicators that are related to the health problem, as was done in the needs assessment, can be simple or difficult, depending, in part, on the time frame. In an example of fireworks injuries on New Year's Eve, a reasonable health outcome indicator is injuries caused by fireworks. In an example of patient education for chronic diseases, a health outcome indicator could be a reduction in emergency visits to the hospital, which also can be accomplished in a fairly short time frame. However, in cancer prevention, establishing a health outcome indicator can be more difficult. A reduction in cancer morbidity and mortality could only be described over an extended time period (10–25 years or more). Therefore, the best short-term indicators for cancer morbidity and mortality are probably to be found in behavior changes, such as smoking and vaccination, and not in health outcomes.

Sometimes evaluators can identify indicators for the health problem that are measurable at an earlier stage. For cardiovascular diseases, indicators could be serum cholesterol levels, blood pressure, weight, and blood glucose levels. However, the consensus on these indicators is not always strong. Moreover, many health education programs are directed at younger people, anticipating effects on future behavior, which means that the health outcome evaluation objectives are all long-term objectives. Once the indicators are selected, the evaluator develops a protocol for measurement.

For example, a typical protocol for the measurement of lung function would include the daily calibration of the spirometer, the performance of three measures, and the use of the best score.

The selection of indicators for the measurement of quality of life is also based on the needs assessment. In the needs assessment, program planners identified specific outcomes that they considered to be the consequences of the health problem or the behavioral factors and environmental conditions (see Chapter 4; Green & Kreuter, 2005). The indicators may be stated at the individual level, such as days lost from work, happiness, self-esteem, and alienation; or at a societal level, such as crime, crowding, discrimination, and unemployment. Thus, measurement can be made by collecting data from the population to evaluate the program outcomes for individuals, as well as by collecting data from organizations or governmental agencies that track potential social indicators of quality of life. The field of quality of life measurement is developing at a fast pace, concurrent with the incorporation of this type of measurement into many clinical trials. Recently, extensive efforts have been directed at developing measures of quality of life that are especially relevant to and sensitive to health-related factors. The CDC has developed indices for health-related quality of life (HRQOL) based on a series of survey questions that are used in the Behavioral Risk Factor Surveillance System (Jiang & Hesser, 2008; National Center for Chronic Disease Prevention and Health Promotion, Division of Population Health, 2011). The advantage of using a standard measure of quality of life, such as the HRQOL measure, is that results from one study or program evaluation can be compared with data from the Behavioral Risk Factor Surveillance System or with findings from other studies. Such a comparison allows the program evaluators to know how quality-of-life indices for their population compare to those of other populations and allows evaluators to determine whether quality of life improves as a result of the program. The disadvantage of a standardized measure of quality of life is that it may not be specific to the health problem that the program addresses and therefore not sensitive to change even if the health outcomes do improve.

The measurement of quality of life has important time-related factors that need to be considered when developing a program evaluation model. The time needed to detect an improvement in quality-of-life outcomes, as in health outcomes, may be long after the health promotion program takes place, especially for broad societal measures that may require decades of intervention to make a difference. Some of the individual-level indicators, such as pain level or days lost from work, may be more sensitive and therefore measurable within the time frame for evaluating the health promotion program. The point is to select those measures of quality of life that are sensitive to change within the time period allocated to evaluate the program's effectiveness.

For example, a program objective may be to increase the functional status (health and quality of life) of elementary school children with asthma by 25 percent in 2 years. An evaluation question may be, How much did the functional status of elementary school children with asthma change? Now the problem is, What is an indicator of functional status in children that can be measured in a program evaluation? The construct of functional status can be defined as the ability to conduct normal activities of daily living unlimited by disease. Children are usually not limited by disease if they can attend school, can have achievement congruent with aptitude, and can engage in playtime and physical activity with other children. So indicators of functional status in children with asthma could be number of school days attended, grades, achievement, participation in physical education, and time spent playing after school. Following the discussion of the construct, evaluators would look for reliable measures in the published literature.

### *Measures of Behavior and Environment*

Most health problems have a combination of behavioral and environmental causes. Sometimes it is easy to choose a behavioral evaluation objective, for instance, the consistent use of a child restraint device to prevent serious damage to the child in case of an accident. Often the decision is more complex; for example, there are many components to a healthy diet to prevent cardiovascular diseases. One behavior evaluation objective could be a reduction of fat intake by consumers; an environmental condition evaluation objective could be the industry's reduction of the percentage of fat in some popular foods. The best indicator for behavior is the list of performance objectives for behavior changes in IM Step 2, and the best indicator for environmental conditions is the list of performance objectives for environmental changes, also in Step 2. Measurement of these behaviors might best be conducted by observation. However, they could also be measured by self-report of behavior or intentions guided by the performance objectives. When evaluators use self-report measures they should, when feasible, validate them against observation.

For some behaviors, the measurement issues and methods are very complex and will require the program evaluator to become knowledgeable about the scientific basis for their measurement. For example, some behaviors, such as home smoke exposure (Centers for Disease Control and Prevention, 2010), nutrition (Burrows, Martin, & Collins, 2010; Liese et al., 2015; Thompson & Subar, 2011), and physical activity (Chinapaw, Mokkink, van Poppel, van Mechelen, & Terwee, 2010; De Vera, Ratzlaff,

Doerfling, & Kopec, 2010; Janz, Lutuchy, Wenthe, & Levy, 2008), already have established and tested standardized instruments or methods for measurement. Many government agencies and institutes have developed compendia of measures on their health and behavior issues. The National Institute on Alcohol Abuse and Alcoholism and the Division of Cancer Control and Population Science at the National Cancer Institute both have good examples (Division of Cancer Control and Population Sciences, National Cancer Institute, 2011; National Institute on Alcohol Abuse and Alcoholism, n.d.). For each of these behaviors, there is extensive scientific literature on measurement. The program evaluators will need to review this literature and decide whether existing measurement tools match well with the stated performance objectives. If several options are available, then the decision will be to choose the one that best fits the performance objectives and program participants. If there is not a good fit with the performance objectives, then the evaluators may find it necessary to develop new questions or instruments to measure the behaviors. The design of reliable and valid instruments to measure the evaluation objectives is beyond the scope of this chapter; however, readers can use several measurement texts (DeVellis, 2012) and evaluation texts (Patton, 2008; Rossi et al., 2004; Windsor et al., 2003) to guide them.

### *Measures of Determinants*

Like measures of behavior of the at-risk group and behaviors of environmental agents, measures of determinants are more difficult to find in the published literature or online databases. When measures of the specific items found on the IM matrices (Chapter 5) cannot be found, evaluators may need to develop them. The first task in determining an indicator, and then its measure, is to use the matrices developed in Step 2 to define the constructs that require measurement to answer an evaluation question. The matrices are the planner's record of what behaviors and determinants are the immediate targets for change by the intervention. Certainly, considerable effort goes into the development and pilot testing of measures, but even a highly reliable measure will not do an evaluator any good if it is not valid for the intended measurement purpose. In a hypothetical example, an evaluation team wanted to assess whether a program has met its goal of increasing asthma knowledge among school-age children; it must decide whether to use an existing measure or to create one. The team looked at a recently published report of a measure of asthma knowledge for children. The report showed that the measure has good *reliability*–internal consistency (the items measure roughly the same thing) and test-retest reliability (test scores for the same individual are similar over a few weeks' time in the absence of an intervention or disruptive event). It also was

**Table 9.6**   Comparison of Domains of Asthma Knowledge

| Published Measure Domains | Domains Underlying the Program to Be Evaluated |
|---|---|
| Anatomy of the respiratory system | Monitoring asthma symptoms |
| Physiology of asthma | Figuring out personal triggers |
| Causes of asthma exacerbations | Using an asthma action plan |
| Rescue and control medicines for asthma | Managing an episode |
| | Staying in control |

found to be sensitive to pretest and posttest program change. Should the team use that measure? Well, that depends. What does it measure? It is possible that an instrument could measure a very broad construct, asthma knowledge, without the specification of the construct matching what the asthma team needed. What were the items on the measurement blueprint from which the items for the measure were sampled? What domains of asthma knowledge do they represent? How well do the domains and items match the knowledge that was taught in the program the team is assigned to evaluate? Table 9.6 represents the domains of asthma knowledge in which the evaluators were interested compared with the domains reported in the published article. There is not a good match (poor *validity*); therefore, the published measure is not appropriate for the new purpose.

Change objectives from IM matrices are the most specific objectives for program development and for effect evaluation. The evaluator can organize the change objectives by determinant to create a blueprint for each measure related to evaluation questions concerning change in determinants. For example, if there is an evaluation question about change in knowledge, then the change objectives for knowledge (the knowledge column in a matrix) can be used as a blueprint for measuring knowledge. Looking at the columns of a matrix as blueprints for measuring a construct in the specific way it was used for program development is a good way to begin developing construct validity for the specific evaluation purpose. Thus, the indicators for program evaluation are the determinants specified in Step 2, and the change objectives linked to each of the determinants serve as the basis for items in a scale to measure the determinants. The program evaluator then constructs scales for each of the determinants following the measurement methodologies typically applied to the specific type of determinant. For example, if change objectives for adolescents in a program to prevent sexually transmitted infections (STIs) included self-efficacy for performance objectives related to condom acquisition, use, negotiation, disposal, refusal, and so on, then the blueprint includes self-efficacy change objectives for all these behaviors. However, the evaluator must go to the literature on self-efficacy to determine how the construct is typically measured and use this literature as a guide for developing the actual instrument (Bandura, 1986; Dennis, 2003; Hsu & Chiu, 2004; Maurer & Andrews, 2000; Resnick & Jenkins, 2000).

### *Validity and Reliability*

Validity in measurement means that the evaluators are measuring the construct that they think they are measuring. Rossi and colleagues (2004) describe demonstrations of validity as depending on a comparison that shows that the measure "yields the results that would be expected if it were, indeed, valid" (p. 220). Examples of these comparisons are the following:

- When the measure is used with other measures of the same variable, results should be the same

- When the measure is applied in situations thought to be different from the variable, the results should be different

- Results for the measure are correlated with other characteristics expected to be related to the outcome

If planners have used IM carefully, they have clearly specified the health, quality of life, behavioral, environmental, and determinant constructs that will eventually be measured and have provided a good basis for beginning to establish validity. IM Steps 3, 4, and 5 also provide the basis for clarity about what the program is and how it is to be implemented, constructs that will be important in process evaluation.

Reliability, on the other hand, is stability in measurement. If evaluators measure the same construct at two points in time, or if two different observers record the same event, will they get the same answer? Reliability concepts include consideration of sources of error. For example, a child may understand questions about asthma symptoms or self-efficacy, or any other construct differently at two points in time based on the question's complexity, a distraction in the environment, or help received. Reliability can also be diminished through procedural problems, such as asking the question in different ways or transcribing data inaccurately.

IM contributes much less to the consideration of reliability of measurement than to validity questions, and again we refer the reader to the evaluation and measurement literature.

## Specifying Designs for Process and Effect Evaluations

### *Planning Designs for Process Evaluation*

The third task in Step 6 is to specify designs for conducting process and effect evaluations.

We have already stressed the essential role of process evaluation. It is the key to opening the "black box" between the program that the planners envisioned implementing and the outcomes that are measured. Thoughtful selection of the process evaluation questions and measures should be followed by design considerations. It should already be obvious that both quantitative and qualitative methods are fundamental tools of process evaluation. Because the Selecting and Developing Measures section above emphasized the quantitative tools, here we will focus on qualitative tools. We will also discuss Web and "app" analytics because of their importance to the many e-programs that are now being used. (Use of quantitative and qualitative approaches, known as "mixed methods," for both process and effect evaluation will be described in a separate section below.)

**Qualitative Methods**    Qualitative methods often used for process evaluation include focus groups, interviews, observations, document review, and open-ended questions on surveys. We strongly advise against seeing these methods as "quick and dirty" alteratives to quantitative methods. To use these methods, evaluators *must* be concerned with choosing a basic approach to collecting and understanding their data, and with the traditional pillars of rigor in any research—reliability and validity.

The term *qualitative methods* is a broad umbrella covering many research genres that have in common the intense or prolonged contact with participants to gain a holistic overview of the context under study. Users of qualitative methods analyze most data with words and the findings are emergent ("inductive") rather than having been structured in advance ("deductive") (Miles, Huberman, & Saldaña, 2013, p. 9). Miles et al. (2013, p. 10) describe several common approaches in analyzing data: Assigning codes to field notes, interview transcripts, or documents; sorting coded materials to identify relations, patterns, and processes; isolating the patterns and processes and their commonalities and differences to inform the next wave of data collection; writing analytic notes and memos; focusing on a small set of themes and propositions; and comparing the generalizations with a formalized body of constructs and theories.

The basic approaches to qualitative research differ from one another in their philosophy of knowledge, aims, units of analysis, data collection strategies, and methods of analysis, but any may be useful in process and effect evaluation (Creswell, 2013; Merriam, 2009; Miles et al., 2013). Usually evaluation researchers pick one paradigm, but mixed approaches are possible with the caveat that any qualitative method should be consciously planned, with a good understanding of the requirements of data collection and analysis. Creswell (2013) describes five genres, and provides tables comparing them, with useful resources for further study and an example study from each genre. Some genres aim for "thick" description, such as those seen in narrative analysis; they involve collecting stories from individuals through various sources (such as stories about program implementers during startup; Creswell, 2013). Ethnography also aims for description, but of a larger group's shared culture, that is, the social organization of federally qualified health centers and their views of people in their catchment area (Creswell, 2013; Fetterman, 2010). Phenomenology describes what all participants have in common as they experience a phenomenon or concept; both what they experienced and how they experienced it (e.g., being told about "active surveillance" as an alternative to immediate treatment for early stage prostate cancer; Creswell, 2013). The goal of grounded theory (Charmaz, 2011; Corbin & Strauss, 2014; Glaser, 1992) is to discover theory grounded in the data (e.g., how people with chronic illnesses manage their medical regimens, their symptoms, and the illness trajectories). The fifth genre, the case study, applies to a real-life contemporary bounded system (a case) or multiple systems (cases) over time with multiple sources of information (Stake, 2006; Yin, 2013; Merriam, 2009). Cases are often chosen to illustrate typical responses, with in-depth investigation (e.g., how federally qualified health centers implemented a program).

The traditional pillars of rigor in quantitative research, reliability and validity, also apply to qualitative research, although the means for addressing them differ somewhat and come from other scientific perspectives (Long & Johnson, 2000; Malterud, 2001; Mays & Pope, 2000; Tobin & Begley, 2004). For example, reliability has been defined as the extent to which the same observational procedure in the same context yields the same answer however and whenever it is carried out (Kirk & Miller, 1986). Thus, many qualitative researchers emphasize dependability or auditability, meaning that other researchers can follow the decision trail of the original investigator (Miles et al., 2013). Strategies to achieve this type of reliability include:

- Manuals of procedures
- Coding manuals
- Software for managing data
- Multiple coders who work independently

Validity, viewed as the truth value or credibility of findings, is always a research goal. In qualitative research, evaluators can work toward credibility through a combination of procedures including:

- Systematic attention to the impact of the researcher's background and position on choices, such as the object of investigation, the perspective and methods used, and the framing and communication of the conclusions (reflexivity)
- Prolonged engagement with informants

- Repeated engagement with informants

- Attention to negative cases

- Investment of sufficient time to understand the phenomenon being studied

- Persistent observation to understand what aspects of the situation are most relevant (sampling)

- Respondent validation

- Triangulation of sources, methods, investigators, and theories

- Quality of the relation between the evidence collected in the field and the concepts derived or selected

Evaluators conducted a qualitative process evaluation using observation and interviews in five elder care homes in England (Bamford, Heaven, May, & Moynihan, 2012). This work illustrates the use of a conceptual model (theory) to organize the data they collected, that is, pattern matching. The evaluators' aim was to explore the views of managers and staff, including catering staff, regarding the acceptability and feasibility of implementing dietary guidelines for saturated fat, salt, and added sugars (Bamford et al., 2012). They organized their findings to key concepts of an administrative theory (normalization process theory) and found the perception that the guidelines were irrelevant to older people (*coherence*), and as a result, there was little investment in the guidelines (*cognitive participation*). Even among staff who supported the guidelines, minimal technical expertise and institutional support hampered implementation (*collective action*). In addition, lack of observable benefits to clients because of limited reappraisal following implementation confirmed negative preconceptions (*reflexive monitoring*). Importantly, the qualitative findings enabled recommendations for more effective implementation (e.g., the need for specialist support to equip staff with the technical knowledge and skills required for menu development and analysis), and the need for expert consultation to find ways to evaluate the impact of modified menus.

**Web Analytics**   Web-based and mobile health interventions, also called Internet interventions or "eHealth" or "mHealth," are increasingly important tools for public health, and they present specific challenges for process evaluation (Korda & Itani, 2013; Webb, Joseph, Yardley, & Michie, 2010). The editor of the *Journal of Medical Internet Research* and a working group that developed a reporting guideline for Internet, m/eHealth interventions identified "defining and measuring use," "engagement," and "attrition" (non-use and loss to follow-up) as especially important issues for these interventions (Eysenbach & CONSORT–EHEALTH Group, 2011).

Evaluators should track attrition carefully, using analyses similar to a survival curve or other figures or tables that document use/dose/engagement to assess the proportion of users that are still logging in over time. Other advice includes the importance of reporting demographics associated with digital divide issues, such as age, education, gender, social-economic status, and computer/Internet literacy. Also, as related to dose, the average session time (a standard Google analytic) should be accompanied by a description of the timeout policy (e.g., automatic logout after 15 minutes). Additional discussion of human support to enhance adherence to eHealth interventions in the clinical context provides evaluators with a model for evaluating program reach and use (Mohr, Cuijpers, & Lehman, 2011). These authors introduce concepts, such as expectations (e.g., by health care providers), social presence (e.g., e-mail reminders), and bond (e.g., building a therapeutic alliance with the patient). An example of an evaluation of the reach of a Web-assisted tobacco intervention tested the effect of personal referrals by medical and dental providers over and above typical Google advertisements (Sadasivam et al., 2013). They found that recruitment from clinical practices complimented Google recruitment by attracting smokers who are less motivated to quit and less experienced with this type of delivery channel.

## Planning an Evaluation Design for Effect Evaluation

In an effect evaluation, the purpose of the design is to enable the evaluator to answer two questions:

- How do indicators of desired program effects compare with what happened before and after the program?

- Can any changes observed be attributed to the intervention being evaluated?

The first question requires a design in which the evaluators measure program outcomes before the program implementation (usually referred to as baseline or pretest measures), as well as after the program has been conducted (follow-up or posttest measures). Sometimes multiple follow-up measures are made to monitor how long it takes for change to take place or how long change is sustained once it does occur.

However, change in the outcome measures over time may result from influences other than the health promotion program being evaluated; these pertain to the second question and the need for designs that include a comparison group. For example, if a smoking-cessation program is implemented and evaluated during the same period as a national trend in reduced rates of smoking, the possibility exists that the observed evaluation outcomes are the results of secular trends rather than the program interventions.

Therefore, the evaluator also needs to know whether there is a difference between people participating in the program and those not participating.

## *Traditional Designs Including Alternatives to Randomized Controlled Trials*

Traditional designs that address the question of whether the relation between the program and the outcomes observed are valid focus on random assignment and designs with comparison groups measured at the same time. These added features lead to a design containing preprogram and postprogram measures in exposed and nonexposed groups. An important principle in program effect evaluation is ensuring comparability between treatment and control groups on as many factors as possible that may influence the outcomes of interest. This principle is most easily adhered to by using an experimental design with random assignment of participants to the intervention group and a control group. However, it can also be accomplished with "quasi-experimental" designs in which the treatment group is compared to itself at more than two time points or is compared with another group that is not formed by random assignment (Shadish et al., 2002).

In health education practice, randomly assigning individuals is often impossible. For instance, students from secondary schools cannot randomly be assigned to a school program or a control program because the program is school-wide or at least class-wide. In that case, it is possible to randomly assign units to the program condition or the control condition. When randomization of individuals or units (that is, schools, clinics, work sites, communities) is not possible, quasi-experimental designs allow the evaluator to compare two or more groups that are as similar as possible. Evaluators have to expect that the groups are not completely equivalent; meaning not completely comparable on a number of relevant characteristics, and evaluators cannot even assume that they know all of the relevant characteristics. Statistically, evaluators can control for most of these differences, but only when the differences are measured before the program starts (e.g., Schaalma et al., 1996; Shadish et al., 2002). We encourage the reader to consult texts on program evaluation (Moerbeek, van Breukelen, & Berger, 2003; Rossi et al., 2004; Senn, 2007; Shadish et al., 2002; van Breukelen, 2006; Windsor et al., 2003; Winkens, Schouten, van Breukelen, & Berger, 2006) for more specific guidance on selecting a design for program evaluation.

Recognition of the contribution of nonrandomized designs was signaled by publication in 1979 of *Quasi-experimentation: Design and Analysis Issues for Field Settings* (Cook & Campbell, 1979). Acceptance of these designs has grown slowly, however, among funders and review groups, such as the influential Cochrane Collaboration that has only recently accepted non-randomized controlled trials (non-RCT) in their reviews, with adequate justification (Reeves, Deeks, Higgins, & Wells, 2011). In the past decade, federal agencies have sponsored major meetings to look at alternatives to the RCT, culminating in articles about the strengths and weaknesses of the RCT and of various alternatives (Mercer, DeVinney, Fine, Green, & Dougherty, 2007; Sanson-Fisher, Bonevski, Green, & D'Este, 2007; West et al., 2008). Generally speaking, when individual random assignment and experimental control are feasible, the RCT remains the gold standard for assuring that conclusions about causal relations between program and outcome are valid ("internal validity"). At the same time, there is now stronger recognition that RCTs for program evaluation are not always possible in the real world and of the importance of being able to generalize to populations and contexts-of-interest ("external validity"). A third conclusion is that several types of studies are best for determining causality, given that no single study can establish causality (Mercer et al., 2007).

We have highlighted two quasi-experimental designs here because of their applicability to the evaluation of health promotion programs—observational studies with propensity scores and time-series designs (West et al., 2008). We also mention designs with multiple baseline measures (Hawkins, Sanson-Fisher, Shakeshaft, D'Este, & Green, 2007) in conjunction with time-series designs. Interestingly, the basic ideas for these designs were included in the original Cook and Campbell (1979) textbook on quasi-experimental designs and in the update by Shadish et al. (2002). We note that these designs require statistical expertise to assure the appropriate choice of analysis and correct interpretation.

**Observational Studies With Propensity Score Matching**    As we noted above, participants in preexisting or constructed groups may receive programs, often through voluntary selection, with the result that the "treated" and "untreated" groups may be quite different from one another. Propensity score matching is a well-developed statistical strategy, for reducing "selection bias" (i.e., between-group differences that random assignment usually protects against; Haviland, Nagin, & Rosenbaum, 2007; Luellen, Shaddish, & Clark, 2005; McCaffrey, Ridgeway, & Morral, 2004; Rosenbaum, 2002). Propensity scores are based on baseline measures that must be able to represent participants in the experimental and control conditions on all characteristics believed to be potentially related to the treatment election or outcome, or ideally both (West et al., 2008, p. 9). On the other hand, because the propensity score is a function of covariates and not outcomes, repeated analyses attempting to balance covariate distributions across treatment groups do not bias estimates of the treatment effect on outcomes and enable evaluators to design an observational study, including the analysis in advance, before the outcomes are known (Rubin, 2001). For example, Evans Cuellar, McReynolds, and Wasserman (2006) used propensity score matching to evaluate a mental health treatment diversion program (Special Needs Diversionary Program) to reduce crime among youth in Texas. They selected the first six counties funded and used administrative data (all juvenile offenses, demographic and education information, and participation in special education programs) together with mental health diagnoses measured at baseline before a decision was made to detain the youth or send him/her home without further processing. Wait-listed youth were an obvious source of a comparison group, but because of the possibility of differences between the two groups (e.g., youth with certain diagnoses or histories are more likely to be assigned to treatment immediately), the evaluators used propensity scores based on the administrative data and mental health diagnoses to equate the two groups. Their findings indicated that the diversion program delayed or prevented youth recidivism.

**Time Series Designs**    These designs involve a large series of observations on the same variable, consecutively, over time. The *interrupted time-series design* is of particular interest here, where a program or policy is introduced at a specific time. The repeated measures allow the evaluator to examine trends before, during, and after the intervention (Shadish et al., 2002, Chapter 6, pp. 171–206). This design is suited to a situation in which data are part of an ongoing monitoring plan for the population potentially affected by the intervention (e.g., motor vehicle accidents in a particular geographic area) or data can be collected from reasonably unbiased sources on an ongoing basis. Many examples come from evaluations of motor vehicle laws (e.g., A. Muller, 2004; Zwerling & Jones, 1999), but other examples are evaluations of alcohol tax increases on alcohol-related disease mortality (Wagenaar, Salois, & Komro, 2009), the national Cleanyourhands campaign on infections in hospitals in England and Wales (Stone et al., 2012), the National Institute for Clinical Excellence (NICE) and guidance on prescribing (Sheldon et al., 2004). The *multiple baseline design* is essentially a variant of the interrupted time-series design, although the methods of analysis are different. Hawkins et al. (2007) provide an overview and rationale for this design, together with suggestions for strengthening its internal and external validity.

## Designs that Promote External Validity

Two design variations on traditional designs emphasize external validity (Cook & Campbell, 1979; Shadish et al., 2002), and they have captured the attention of program evaluators in the past few years. One is *pragmatic designs* (e.g., Glasgow & Riley, 2013; Green & Glasgow, 2006) and the other is *comparative effectiveness designs* (e.g., Slutsky & Clancy, 2010). (Mixed methods and hybrid designs are presented separately, because they address both process and effect evaluation.) For a guide to propensity score analyses, see Guo and Fraser (2014).

**Pragmatic Designs**    The recent return of emphasis on effectiveness evaluations, that is, "real-world" trials over efficacy trials for medical and public health programs, has been driven by the need to provide more relevant evidence to practice (Glasgow, Klesges, Dzewaltowski, Estabrooks, & Vogt, 2006; Schwartz & Lellouch, 1967; Tunis, Stryer, & Clancy, 2003). The term *pragmatic* was coined by Schwartz and Lellouch (1967) to describe an attitude in trial design, which recognizes that the difference between effectiveness and efficacy studies is a continuum, as we noted above, not simply an either/or. Thorpe et al. (2009) identified 10 dimensions on which trials could be pragmatic, under the acronym PRECIS (PRagmatic-Explanatory Continuum Indicator Summary). These include design dimensions, such as participant eligibility criteria, level of practitioner expertise, follow-up intensity, outcomes, and practitioner adherence (see Figure 9.2). In the figure, each spoke represents a design dimension. The "web" lines connect the dots on each spoke, with dots farther from the center representing

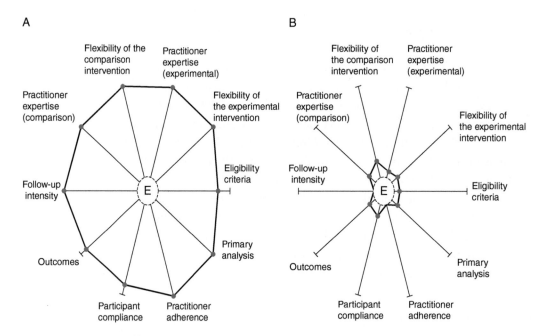

**Figure 9.2**    Illustration of the PRECIS Criteria to Characterize Research Studies
Reprinted with permission from Glasgow, R. E. (2013).

a more pragmatic approach. Thus, Figure 9.2A is very pragmatic on all dimensions, in contrast with Figure 9.2B, a typical efficacy trial. Examples of pragmatic approaches can be found in Thorpe et al. (2009) and Glasgow et al. (2012). According to Zwarenstein et al. (2008), trial results are likely to be more widely applicable if the participants, communities, practitioners, or institutions resemble the at-risk population, and are not narrowly selected; if the intervention is implemented without strenuous efforts to standardize it; if the comparison group receives care or other interventions widely used; and if outcomes studied are important to relevant decision makers (p. 7). Lorig's studies of self-management education for chronic illness serve as examples of pragmatic trials from the health-promotion literature (e.g., Bodenheimer, Lorig, Holman, & Grumbach, 2002; Lorig & Holman, 2003; Lorig, Ritter, Laurent, & Plant, 2006): The participants typically have several chronic conditions, with relatively unlimited comorbidities; the interventions are provided in the community, over the Internet, or through some other "open" setting led by trained volunteer lay leaders; and the outcomes include pain, functional status, and depression—all important to decision makers.

Establishment of a reporting guideline created for pragmatic trials in 2008 (Zwarenstein et al., 2008) and specific calls for pragmatic trials by federal funding agencies have legitimized these designs and provided guidance for designing the evaluation a proposal for funding and reporting the methods and findings.

The randomized encouragement design is a type of pragmatic trial that allows trial participants assigned to an opportunity or an encouragement to receive a specific treatment to choose whether to receive the treatment (Barnard, Frangakis, Hill, & Rubin, 2003; Holland, 1988). This contrasts with the traditional RCT in which strong incentives outside usual practice are applied to increase uptake of the intervention. In addition, this design can reveal participants' decision-making process. A limitation is that the size of the effects that are measured are likely to be smaller than the traditional RCT, and thus, the sample size required is likely to be larger, making the evaluation more expensive (Mercer et al., 2007, p. 143).

**Comparative Effectiveness Designs**    Whether evaluators use a random assignment or a quasi-experimental design, they sometimes want to determine whether their intervention is more successful than the standard program or practice. In this situation, the control or usual care comparison is not a condition without a program but a condition with the usual program. The evaluators here are estimating program effects for the new program or new drug compared to usual care or practice. This is the main idea behind "comparative effectiveness" studies in medicine (Piaggio et al., 2012; Slutsky & Clancy, 2010). This is especially relevant for medical treatments where, for example, the gap between a generic drug widely in use and a new drug is artificially enlarged in trials comparing the new drug to a control group *with placebo drug only*. Comparative effectiveness designs can be helpful in health promotion evaluations when, for example, a more resource-intensive program or difficult-to-implement program should be compared with a less intensive, more readily scalable program.

## Emerging Designs and Analyses for Process and Effect Evaluation

### *Mixed Methods*

Although evaluators have traditionally advocated either qualitative (e.g., Patton, 2005) or quantitative (Shadish et al., 2002) approaches, there is increasing recognition of the value of a strategic mix of the two sets of methods (Bamberger, 2012; Creswell & Clark, 2011; Work Group for Community Health and Development, University of Kansas, 2014). We have already suggested that qualitative methods are often used for process evaluation. Newer applications in conjunction with quantitative methods also include outcome evaluation, as for example when qualitative data, such as key informant interviews, help fill in characteristics of program beneficiaries and nonbeneficiaries at the time the program began; a response to the special problem that arises when an evaluation is initiated after the program begins. A way in which quantitative methods can strengthen qualitative is by linking to the quantitative sampling frame, thereby making it easier to compare findings of the survey data (Bamberger, 2012).

The strengths of quantitative methods include being less time consuming; having lower cost per unit collected; permitting researcher control; and being regarded as unbiased, with standard parameters for reliability and validity, and easily analyzed (Chapel, n.d.). Qualitative methods usually require more time for analysis, and they can be more costly, per unit collected, although fewer units are collected. Reliability and validity are increasingly subject to standard explanations, aided by standards for reporting (O'Brien et al., 2014; Tong et al., 2007, 2012) and software such as Atlas.ti (http://atlasti.com/) and NVivo (http://www.qsrinternational.com/products_nvivo.aspx) for data management. The main idea of mixed methods is to balance concerns about reliability and validity of a single method with a combination of methods that have complementary strengths and nonoverlapping weaknesses (Chapel, n.d.). Mixed methods provide corroboration, that is, better understanding, more credibility, and "triangulation" through multiple perspectives on the same event or phenomenon. Mixed methods help the evaluator see patterns and explore new insights (Chapel, n.d.).

Three general models of mixed methods display the purposes, sequences, and degrees of integration of qualitative and quantitative approaches (Creswell & Clark, 2011; Klasser, Creswell, Clark, Smith, & Meissner, 2012): (a) *Convergent* (parallel or concurrent) mixed methods in which both methods of data collection are used with the goal of both sets of data and comparing their results; (b) *sequential* (explanatory sequential or exploratory sequential) designs in which one method builds on the other, for example, qualitative data may be collected to explain in greater depth the mechanisms underlying quantitative results or qualitative findings from initial exploratory data collection is used to design, for example, a quantitative survey; and (c) *embedded* (nested) designs that use both methods in tandem and embed one in the other, for example, in-depth interviews to produce case studies that may be used to understand how participants experience the program. Consultation with recent textbooks (Bamberger, 2012; Creswell & Clark, 2011) will provide extended examples of each type that will help the evaluator select the optimum combination of methods to address evaluation questions.

A process evaluation (*sequential explanatory*) that used mixed methods found that recruitment for an exercise program through ethnically specific channels and ethnically matched recruiters contributed to its reach and receptivity in ethnic minority mothers in the Netherlands (Hartman, Nierkens, Cremer, Stronks, & Verhoeff, 2013). The evaluators used reply cards and the attendance records to measure reach and participation. Observations of the recruitment process, interviews with 14 key figures, and 32 mothers who responded to the recruitment channel. The qualitative component found that the recruiters were familiar and trusted and could serve as a translator and motivator. Enthusiasm and targeting (the ethnic group) and tailoring to the individual appeared to enhance receptivity to the program.

### Hybrid Designs

"Hybrid designs" blend effectiveness and implementation research and simultaneously evaluate the impact of interventions in real-world settings (effectiveness evaluation) *and* implementation strategies (Bernet, Wilens, & Bauer, 2013). Looking at effectiveness and implementation together enables the evaluator to identify important interactions, with the idea of scaling up interventions more rapidly (see Chapter 10). The quality-improvement initiative of the largest health care system in the U.S., the Department of Veterans' Affairs, has been an important driver of the hybrid concept (Curran, Bauer, Mittman, Pyne, & Stetler, 2012). The interventions most suitable for a hybrid approach are those with at least indirect evidence of effectiveness and strong face validity to support their fit in the new setting or population or to a new delivery method (Bernet et al., 2013). There should also be a solid foundation for the implementation strategy (Curran et al., 2012). The degree of certainty for each will dictate how much emphasis to place on implementation versus effectiveness (Curran et al., 2012). Several examples of clinical applications of hybrid designs with varying emphases can be found in the paper by Curran et al. (2012). One example was a four-site trial in which the chronic care clinical intervention was experimentally assigned with and without a theory-based set of implementation strategies and tools (Brown, Cohen, Chinman, Kessler, & Young, 2008). Their measures included not only patient outcomes but also clinicians' attitudes toward patients and families, view of workload, indicators of implementation, and maintenance of the clinical intervention, as well as qualitative methods to assess implementation barriers and facilitators. We note that hybrid designs are a type of pragmatic design (discussed under Designs that Promote External Validity above).

### *Mediation and Moderation Analyses*

Mediation and moderation analysis is becoming an expected part of the information provided in a program evaluation. For process evaluation, mediation analysis is one way to determine whether the observed effect of the program compared with a control or comparison treatment is mediated by participants' compliance with the intervention. Hayes (2012) points out that as a research area matures, focus eventually shifts away from whether there is an effect toward understanding the mechanism(s) by which the effect operates ("how") and establishing the populations and contexts in which it occurs ("when"). The "how" questions have typically been approached through *mediation analysis*, and the "when" questions, through moderation analysis. For example, in an evaluation of the Incredible Years BASIC Parent Program, a parenting program for preschoolers at risk for conduct problems, mediation analysis found that change in a positive parenting skill (but not a negative parenting skill) predicted change in conduct problems (Gardner, Hutchings, Bywater, Whitaker, 2010). Moderation analysis in the same evaluation found that boys and younger children and those with more depressed mothers showed more improvement in conduct problems on posttest. More recent thinking about mediator and moderator analyses is that answering only one or the other question is not a complete analysis. Terms, such as moderated mediation, mediated moderation, and conditional process modeling, have come into the literature suggesting a blending of the two analyses (Edwards & Lambert, 2007; Fairchild & MacKinnon, 2009; Morgan-Lopez & MacKinnon, 2006;

D. Muller, Judd, & Yzerbyt, 2005; Preacher, Rucker, & Hayes, 2007). Hayes (2012, 2013) provides a primer on these new approaches and he also introduces PROCESS, a freely available computational tool for Statistical Analysis System (SAS) and Statistical Package for the Social Sciences (SPSS) software packages that covers many of the functions of popular procedures for analyses and that avoids the use of specialized software that may not be familiar to evaluators.

## Completing the Evaluation Plan

An evaluation plan includes the effect and process evaluation questions, primary outcome, indicators and measures, the design with the timing of the measures, and details about how the evaluation will be carried out. These details include the sample size that is needed, what data will be collected, who will collect it, what resources will be needed, how the data will be analyzed, and how it will be reported to the stakeholders (Senn, 2007). See Table 9.7 for an example evaluation plan summary from the Dutch School AIDS prevention program.

*The final task in Step 6 is to specify and complete the evaluation plan.*

Reporting guidelines for many types of designs now provide templates for writing evaluation plans (Popham et al., 2012). Although reporting guidelines are designed to increase the transparency of reporting, i.e., writing the evaluation report or journal article, consulting the appropriate guideline in advance will keep the evaluator from being surprised by the expectation of reporting an aspect of design that he or she had not anticipated. Guidelines differ in the degree of research and expertise on which they are founded. Literally, scores now are posted on the EQUATOR (Enhancing the QUAlity and Transparency Of health Research) website at http://www.equator-network.org/. The most helpful (with the strongest foundation) contain checklists of what to report (and plan for), and they are prominently listed, e.g., CONSORT (CONsolidated Standards of Reporting Trials, for randomized trials, CARE (Consensus-based Clinical Case Reporting Guideline) for case reports; SRQR (Standards for reporting qualitative research) and COREQ (COnsolidated criteria for REporting Qualitative research), and SQUIRE (Standards for QUality Improvement in Reporting Excellence) for quality improvement studies. Look for "explanation and elaboration" documents that contain examples of each item on the checklist from published reports together with a rationale for including each item. These guidelines also are primers on the particular type of design, including the best practices (and mistakes often made) in analyses. For example, we cited the CONSORT extensions for pragmatic designs, e-interventions, and comparative effectiveness trials in the section on emerging designs for outcome evaluation as key resources for these designs.

**Table 9.7** Evaluation Plan Summary: School AIDS Prevention Program

| Evaluation Questions, Variables, and Proposed Design | Measures | Sources | Data Collection Timing and Resources | Data Analysis | Reporting |
|---|---|---|---|---|---|
| **Process Evaluation Plan** | | | | | |
| *Adoption* | | | | | |
| Awareness | Survey | Teachers | Prior to program, project research assistant (RA) | Frequencies | Report to the linkage system |
| Agreement to conduct program | Record review | Project records | Prior to program, RA | Frequencies | Report to the linkage system |
| Participation in teacher training | Observation | Teacher training | Prior to program, RA | Summary memos on observations | Report to the linkage system |
| *Implementation* | | | | | |
| Lessons completed | Teacher records | Teachers | During program, RA | Frequencies | To the development team, scientific literature, schools, funder (each implementation indicator) |
| Activities executed | Observation | Research staff | During program, RA | Frequencies | |
| Time/lesson | Surveys | Students | During program, RA | Means | |
| Scheduling of lessons | Interviews | Teachers | During program, RA | Means and summary memos | |
| Use of video | Surveys | Students | After program, RA | Means and summary memos | |
| *Intervention Assumptions* | | | | | |
| User evaluation | Surveys | Teachers | 1 week following program, RA | Frequencies | To the research team, scientific literature, schools, funders, and participants (all intervention assumption indicators) |
| User evaluation | Interviews | Students | 1 week following program, RA | Comment summaries | |
| Participant exposure | Surveys | Students | 1 week following program, RA | Means | |
| Method & strategy assumptions | Content analysis | Materials and lesson review | Before program, project team leaders | Table of content analysis | |

**Effect Evaluation Plan**

***Quality-of-Life and Health***

| | | | | | |
|---|---|---|---|---|---|
| QOL | | | | | |
| Health | Not measured | n/a | n/a | n/a | n/a |
| HIV infection | Not measured | n/a | n/a | n/a | n/a |
| AIDS cases | Not measured | n/a | n/a | n/a | n/a |
| STI cases | Health Department Registry of STIs | Health Department Surveillance | Baseline and years 3, 4, 5 | Change in pre- and postintervention incidence rates compared between groups | To research team, schools, funders, scientific literature, and participants |

***Behavior***

| | | | | | |
|---|---|---|---|---|---|
| Condom use | Survey questions | Intervention and control groups | Baseline, 6 month, and 1 year follow-ups | Pre- and postintervention change scores compared between groups | To research team, schools, funders, and scientific literature (behavior and environmental condition) |

***Environmental Condition***

| | | | | | |
|---|---|---|---|---|---|
| Availability of condoms (condom machines) | Observations | Businesses | Baseline and 1 year follow-ups | Pre- and postintervention change scores compared between groups | |

***Determinants***

| | | | | | |
|---|---|---|---|---|---|
| Knowledge and self-efficacy | Knowledge and self-efficacy scales | Intervention & control groups | Baseline, 6 month, and 1 year follow-ups | Pre- and postintervention change scores compared between groups | To research team, schools, funders, scientific literature, and participants |
| Cues | Observation | Schools | Baseline, 6 month, and 1 year follow-ups | Pre- and postintervention change scores compared between groups | |
| Skills | Not measured | n/a | n/a | n/a | |

## BOX 9.2.  IT'S YOUR GAME . . . KEEP IT REAL

Figure 9.3 is the final logic model for the It's Your Game (IYG) project. It enabled the planning group to review all of the possibilities for asking evaluation questions.

### Evaluation Questions

#### Task 1: Write effect and process evaluation questions

The primary outcome examined the effect of IYG on delayed sexual initiation at the ninth grade follow-up for those students who reported no lifetime sexual activity at baseline. The primary hypothesis tested whether the intervention would decrease the number of students who initiated sexual activity by the 9th grade relative to those in the comparison schools. Sexual activity was defined as participation in vaginal, oral, or anal sex (Tortolero et al., 2010). Secondary outcomes included examining the effect of IYG to reduce the frequency of sex, to reduce the frequency of sex without a condom, to reduce the number of sexual partners, to reduce dating violence victimization and perpetration, and to enhance the targeted determinants related to these behaviors (Peskin et al., 2014; Tortolero et al., 2010). Process evaluation questions examined the reach, dose, and fidelity of implementation. See an abbreviated evaluation plan in Table 9.8.

#### Task 2: Develop indicators and measures for assessment

The planning group developed indicators and measures for each evaluation question, where possible using measures that had been previously validated with urban minority youth (Ball, Pelton, Forehand, Long, & Wallace, 2004; Basen-Engquist, Coyle, et al., 2001; Basen-Engquist, Masse, et al., 1999; Coyle et al., 2001; Coyle, Kirby, Marin, Gomez, & Gregorich, 2004; Miller et al., 1997; Prinstein, Boergers, Spirito, Little, & Grapentine, 2000; Prinstein, Boergers & Vernberg, 2001; Vernberg, Jacobs, & Hershberger, 1999).

### Evaluation Design and Plan

#### Task 3: Specify the evaluation design

The program planners used a randomized controlled trial design to assess the efficacy of IYG to delay sexual initiation, and to reduce dating violence and other risky sexual behaviors. The study design included baseline surveys in 7th grade and follow-up surveys in 8th and 9th grade. This study design also allowed them to examine the program's effect on the determinants of knowledge, self-efficacy, outcome expectations, normative beliefs, and gender role norms.

#### Task 4: Complete the evaluation plan

The planners created an evaluation plan that included the effect and process evaluation questions, the primary outcome, indicators and measures, the timing of measures, and details about how the evaluation would be carried out. Data collectors were hired and trained

**Individual Level**

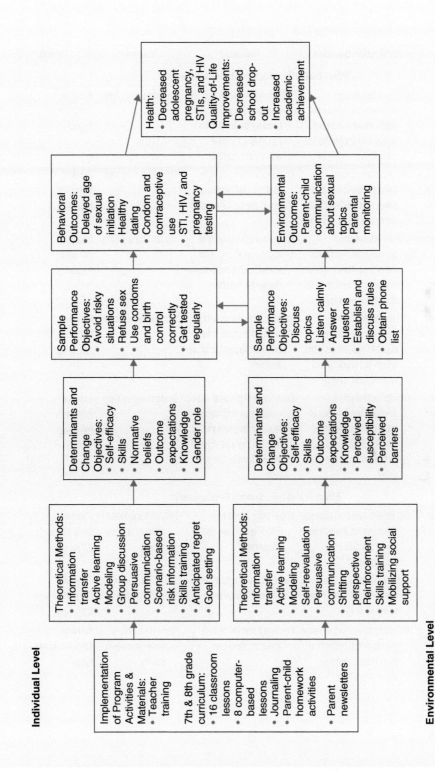

**Environmental Level**

**Figure 9.3** IYG Intervention Logic Model for Evaluation

**Table 9.8**    Partial Evaluation Plan for It's Your Game . . . Keep It Real (IYG)

| Variable | Evaluation Question | Indicator | Measure | Timing |
|---|---|---|---|---|
| **Effect Evaluation: Sample Student Behaviors** | | | | |
| Delayed sexual initiation | Did the intervention decrease the number of students who initiated sexual activity by the 9th grade? | Initiation of vaginal, oral, or anal sex by the 9th grade (among students who reported no sexual activity at baseline) | Student survey item | Baseline 9th grade follow-up |
| Decreased frequency of sex in the past 3 months | Did the intervention decrease the number of times that students had sex in the past 3 months? | Frequency of engaging in vaginal, oral, and anal sex in the past 3 months | Student survey item | Baseline 9th grade follow-up |
| Decreased frequency of sex without a condom in the past 3 months | Did the intervention decrease the number of times that students had sex without a condom in the past 3 months? | Frequency of engaging in vaginal, oral, and anal sex without a condom in the past 3 months | Student survey item | Baseline 9th grade follow-up |
| Decreased number of lifetime sexual partners | Did the intervention decrease the lifetime number of partners with whom the student had vaginal, oral, or anal sex? | Number of partners with whom the student had ever had vaginal, oral, or anal sex | Student survey item | Baseline 9th grade follow-up |
| Decreased physical dating violence victimization | Did the intervention decrease the number of students who reported physical dating violence victimization in the past year? | Experience of physical dating violence victimization (e.g., hitting, kicking, or pushing) by a boyfriend or girlfriend in the past year | Student survey item | Baseline 9th grade follow-up |
| **Effect Evaluation: Sample Determinants** | | | | |
| Knowledge about HIV/STI transmission | Did the intervention increase the students' knowledge about HIV/STI transmission? | Knowledge about how HIV/STIs are / are not transmitted | HIV/STI knowledge scale on student survey | Baseline 8th & 9th grade follow-ups |
| Self-efficacy to refuse sex | Did the intervention increase the students' self-efficacy to refuse sex? | Self-efficacy to refuse sex in different scenarios | Self-efficacy scale on student survey | Baseline 8th & 9th grade follow-ups |
| Normative beliefs about condom use | Did the intervention increase the students' belief that their friends endorse condom use? | Perceived friends' beliefs about condom use | Normative beliefs scale on student survey | Baseline 8th & 9th grade follow-ups |

**Table 9.8**    *(Continued)*

| Variable | Evaluation Question | Indicator | Measure | Timing |
|---|---|---|---|---|
| | | **Process Evaluation** | | |
| Reach | How many 7th and 8th grade students received IYG? | Students receiving IYG | Class roster | 7th & 8th grade |
| Dose | How many IYG lessons did each student receive? | Students attending IYG lessons | Class roster | 7th & 8th grade |
| Fidelity | How many facilitators attended IYG training? | Persons counted in trainings | Sign-in sheet | 7th & 8th grade |
| | Did classroom facilitators implement IYG lessons as written? | Number of activities completed as written | Implementation log Classroom observation | 7th & 8th grade |

to conduct student surveys on laptop computers using an audio-computer-assisted self-interview (ACASI). ACASI systems are reliable for obtaining sensitive information on sexual risk-taking (Booth-Kewley, Larson, & Miyoshi, 2007; Morrison-Beedy, Carey, & Tu, 2006). Surveys were conducted in a quiet location (e.g., school library). To protect student confidentiality, headphones were provided and laptops were positioned so screens were not visible to others. The planners calculated the sample size needed ($n = 750$) to see a statistically significant difference in the primary outcome, given expected attrition over the 2 year evaluation. They also developed an a priori data analysis plan and dissemination plan to ensure that results would be communicated to key stakeholders, including school district and school-level administrators, parents and community members, state personnel, and the scientific community.

### Findings

IYG was evaluated in two randomized controlled trials conducted in a large south-central U.S. school district. In each trial, middle schools serving a low-income, urban population were randomly assigned to the intervention or control condition using a multiattribute randomization protocol (Markham et al., 2012; Tortolero et al., 2010). Each trial comprised a cohort of predominantly African American and Hispanic students followed from 7th grade into 9th grade. In the first trial ($n = 907$), control group students experienced more statistically significant negative outcomes compared to students in the intervention group. They were 1.29 times more likely to initiate sex by 9th grade and students who were sexually active had a higher frequency of vaginal sex in the past three months (adjusted relative risk = 1.30) compared to students who received IYG. Control group students were also more likely to report physical dating violence victimization (adjusted odds ratio [AOR] = 1.52), emotional dating violence victimization (AOR = 1.74), and emotional dating violence perpetration (AOR = 1.58) compared to students who received IYG (Peskin et al, 2014). No other statistically significant outcomes were reported amongst the much smaller number of sexually active youth. Students who received IYG had more positive changes in determinants of behavior. These included greater self-efficacy to refuse sex, greater self-efficacy to use condoms, greater condom and HIV/STI knowledge, more positive norms about waiting to have sex, and more positive norms about condom use. They also reported less exposure to risky situations (Tortolero et al., 2010). The second trial ($n = 627$) reported similar effects on behavior and its determinants, as well as positive reductions in unprotected sex. Students who received IYG were significantly less likely to engage in unprotected sex at last vaginal intercourse, compared to students in the control group. They reported more positive changes in determinants, similar to the original trial; however, they also reported increased parent–child communication about sexual topics and more supportive perceived parental beliefs about waiting to have sex compared to students in the control group (Markham et al., 2012).

It's Your Game . . . Keep It Real is nationally recognized as an effective sexual health education program (U.S. Department of Health and Human Services Office of Adolescent Health, 2015) and has been adopted by school districts across the U.S., reaching more than 33,000 middle school students. Much of the program's success may be attributed to the use of IM to systematically guide program development and dissemination.

## Summary

Chapter 9 describes how to develop a plan of evaluation of a health promotion program based on the previous five IM steps. Evaluation flows from the selection of quality of life, health, behavior, and environmental outcomes following the needs assessment (Step 1), the matrices of performance objectives and change objectives (Step 2), and the description of change methods, applications, and implementation (Steps 3, 4, and 5). The effect evaluation focuses on the differences in outcomes with and without the program, whereas process evaluation addresses program implementation and why the intervention was delivered in a certain way.

The development of indicators—the constructs being measured—and measures—the devices for quantifying or categorizing the indicators—is a major task in the development of an evaluation plan. Clear specification of program outcome objectives in the logic model and change objectives from the matrices allow development of measures that can test the effect of the program and characteristics of its implementation.

The choice of an evaluation design underlies the assurance with which the evaluator can say that indicators have changed from before to after the program and whether these changes can be attributed to the program. Although an experimental design with random assignment of participants or units to the intervention and comparison groups yields the strongest evidence, there are many useful quasi-experimental designs, emerging approaches, and analytic methods that can contribute to credible evaluation findings.

The final product of Step 6 is an evaluation plan, which includes the evaluation questions, design, indicators and measures, timing of the measures, study protocol, resources required, and plan for reporting to stakeholders.

## Discussion Questions and Learning Activities

1. Explain how the products from Steps 1 through 5 of IM can be used to help plan for program evaluation.

2. Explain the difference between outcome and process evaluation and between formative and summative evaluation.

3. Continuing with the health promotion program you proposed from the proceeding chapters, create an intervention logic model and show where effect evaluation and process evaluation relate to the model for your program.

4. State your effect evaluation questions and briefly describe the measures you will use to evaluate program outcomes.

5. State your process evaluation questions and briefly describe the measures you will use to conduct a process evaluation.

6. Briefly describe the evaluation study design you would propose to evaluate your health promotion program.

## References

Ball, J., Pelton, J., Forehand, R., Long, N., & Wallace, S. A. (2004). Methodological overview of the Parents Matter! program. *Journal of Child and Family Studies, 13*(1), 21–34.

Bamberger, M. (2012). *Introduction to mixed methods in impact evaluation. Impact evaluation guidance notes No. 3*. Washington, DC: InterAction and The Rockefeller Foundation.

Bamford, C., Heaven, B., May, C., & Moynihan, P. (2012). Implementing nutrition guidelines for older people in residential care homes: A qualitative study using Normalization Process Theory. *Implementation Science, 7*, 106.

Bandura, A. (1986). *Social foundations of thought and action: A Social Cognitive Theory*. Englewood Cliffs, NJ: Prentice-Hall.

Baranowski, T., Cerin, E., & Baranowski, J. (2009). Steps in the design, development and formative evaluation of obesity prevention-related behavior change trials. *International Journal of Behavioral Nutrition & Physical Activity, 6*, 6.

Barnard, J., Frangakis, C. E., Hill, J. L., & Rubin, D. B. (2003). Principal stratification approach to broken randomized experiments: A case study of school choice vouchers in New York City. *Journal of the American Statistical Association, 98*(462), 299–323.

Bartholomew, K. L., Czyzewski, D. I., Swank, P. R., McCormick, L., & Parcel, G. S. (2000). Maximizing the impact of the cystic fibrosis family education program: Factors related to program diffusion. *Family & Community Health, 22*(4), 27–47.

Basen-Engquist, K., Coyle, K. K., Parcel, G. S., Kirby, D., Banspach, S. W., Carvajal, S. C., & Baumler, E. (2001). Schoolwide effects of a multicomponent HIV, STD, and pregnancy prevention program for high school students. *Health Education & Behavior, 28*(2), 166–185.

Basen-Engquist, K., Masse, L. C., Coyle, K., Kirby, D., Parcel, G. S., Banspach, S., & Nodora, J. (1999). Validity of scales measuring the psychosocial determinants of HIV/STD-related risk behavior in adolescents. *Health Education Research, 14*(1), 25–38.

Bernet, A. C., Willens, D. E., & Bauer, M. S. (2013). Effectiveness-implementation hybrid designs: Implications for quality improvement science. *Implementation Science, 8*(Suppl 1), S2.

Bodenheimer, T., Lorig, K., Holman, H., & Grumbach, K. (2002). Patient self-management of chronic disease in primary care. *JAMA, 288*(19), 2469–2475.

Booth-Kewley, S., Larson, G. E., & Miyoshi, D. K. (2007). Social desirability effects on computerized and paper-and-pencil questionnaires. *Computers in Human Behavior, 23*(1), 463–477.

Brown, A. H., Cohen, A. N., Chinman, M. J., Kessler, C., & Young, A. S. (2008). EQUIP: Implementing chronic care principles and applying formative evaluation methods to improve care for schizophrenia: QUERI series. *Implementation Science, 3*, 9.

Burrows, T. L., Martin, R. J., & Collins, C. E. (2010). A systematic review of the validity of dietary assessment methods in children when compared with the method of doubly labeled water. *Journal of the American Dietetic Association, 110*(10), 1501–1510.

Centers for Disease Control and Prevention (CDC). (2010). Vital signs: Nonsmokers' exposure to secondhand smoke: United States, 1999–2008. *MMWR. Morbidity and Mortality Weekly Report, 59*(35), 1141–1146.

Centers for Disease Control and Prevention, Program Performance and Evaluation Office. (2015). Program evaluation. Retrieved from http://www.cdc.gov/eval/index.htm

Chapel, T. (n.d.). Mixed methods in program evaluation. Retrieved from www.cdc.gov/asthma/program_eval/webinar4B/4B_with_notes.pptx

Charmaz, K. (2011). Grounded theory methods in social justice research. In N. Denzin & Y. Lincoln (Eds.), *The SAGE handbook of qualitative research* (4th ed., pp. 359–380). Thousand Oaks, CA: Sage.

Chinapaw, M. J., Mokkink, L. B., van Poppel, M. N., van Mechelen, W., & Terwee, C. B. (2010). Physical activity questionnaires for youth. *Sports Medicine, 40*(7), 539–563.

Cook, T. D., & Campbell, D. T. (1979). *Quasi-experimentation: Design and analysis issues for field settings.* Boston, MA: Houghton Mifflin.

Corbin, J., & Strauss, A. (2014). *Basics of qualitative research: Techniques and procedures for developing grounded theory* (4th ed.). Thousand Oaks, CA: Sage.

Coyle, K., Basen-Engquist, K., Kirby, D., Parcel, G., Banspach, S., Collins, J., ... Harrist, R. (2001). Safer Choices: Reducing teen pregnancy, HIV, and STDs. *Public Health Reports (Washington, DC: 1974), 116*(Suppl 1), 82–93.

Coyle, K. K., Kirby, D. B., Marin, B. V., Gomez, C. A., & Gregorich, S. E. (2004). Draw the line/respect the line: A randomized trial of a middle school intervention to reduce sexual risk behaviors. *American Journal of Public Health, 94*(5), 843–851.

Creswell, J. W. (2013). *Research design: Qualitative, quantitative, and mixed methods approaches.* Thousand Oaks, CA: Sage.

Creswell, J. W., & Clark, V. L. P. (2011). *Designing and conducting mixed methods research* (2nd ed.). Los Angeles, CA: Sage.

Curran, G. M., Bauer, M., Mittman, B., Pyne, J. M., & Stetler, C. (2012). Effectiveness-implementation hybrid designs: Combining elements of clinical effectiveness and implementation research to enhance public health impact. *Medical Care, 50*(3), 217–226.

Dennis, C. (2003). The breastfeeding self-efficacy scale: Psychometric assessment of the short form. *Journal of Obstetric, Gynecologic, & Neonatal Nursing, 32*(6), 734–744.

DeVellis, R. F. (2012). *Scale development: Theory and applications* (3rd ed.). Thousand Oaks, CA: Sage.

De Vera, M. A., Ratzlaff, C., Doerfling, P., & Kopec, J. (2010). Reliability and validity of an internet-based questionnaire measuring lifetime physical activity. *American Journal of Epidemiology, 172*(10), 1190–1198.

Di Lorio, C. K. (2005). *Measurement in health behavior: Methods for research and education.* San Francisco, CA: Jossey-Bass.

Division of Cancer Control and Population Sciences, National Cancer Institute. (2011). Behavioral measures. Retrieved from http://cancercontrol.cancer.gov/brp/sci-res/behavior.html

Drummond, M. F., Sculpher, M., Torrance, G., O'Brien, B., & Stoddart, G. (2005). *Methods for the economic evaluation of health care programmes.* New York, NY: Oxford University Press.

Edwards, J. R., & Lambert, L. S. (2007). Methods for integrating moderation and mediation: A general analytical framework using moderated path analysis. *Psychological Methods, 12*(1), 1.

Evans Cuellar, A., McReynolds, L. S., & Wasserman, G. A. (2006). A cure for crime: Can mental health treatment diversion reduce crime among youth? *Journal of Policy Analysis and Management, 25*(1), 197–214.

Eysenbach, G., & CONSORT-EHEALTH Group. (2011). CONSORT-EHEALTH: Improving and standardizing evaluation reports of web-based and mobile health interventions. *Journal of Medical Internet Research, 13*(4), e126.

Fairchild, A. J., & MacKinnon, D. P. (2009). A general model for testing mediation and moderation effects. *Prevention Science, 10*(2), 87–99.

Fetterman, D. M. (Ed.). (2010). *Ethnography: Step-by-step* (Vol. 17). Thousand Oaks, CA: Sage.

Fetterman, D. M., Kaftarian, S. J., & Wandersman, A. (2014). *Empowerment evaluation: Knowledge and tools for self-assessment, evaluation capacity building, and accountability.* Thousand Oaks, CA: Sage.

Gardner, F., Hutchings, J., Bywater, T., & Whitaker, C. (2010). Who benefits and how does it work? Moderators and mediators of outcome in an effectiveness trial of a parenting intervention. *Journal of Clinical Child & Adolescent Psychology, 39*(4), 568–580.

Gartlehner, G., Hansen, R. A., Nissman, D., Lohr, K. N., & Carey, T. S. (2006). *Criteria for distinguishing effectiveness from efficacy trials in systematic reviews. Technical review 12* (Prepared by the RTI-International University of North Carolina Evidence-Based Practice Center under contract No. 290-02-0016.) AHRQ publication No. 06-0046. Rockville, MD: Agency for Healthcare Research and Quality.

Glaser, B. G. (1992). *Emergence vs. forcing: Basics of grounded theory analysis.* Mill Valley, CA: Sociology Press.

Glasgow, R.E., (2013). What does it mean to be pragmatic? Pragmatic methods, measures, and models to facilitate research translation. *Health Education & Behavior, 40*(3), 257–265.

Glasgow, R. E., Gaglio, B., Bennett, G., Jerome, G. J., Yeh, H., Sarwer, D. B., . . . Wells, B. (2012). Applying the PRECIS criteria to describe three effectiveness trials of weight loss in obese patients with comorbid conditions. *Health Services Research, 47*(3, Pt. 1), 1051–1067.

Glasgow, R. E., Klesges, L. M., Dzewaltowski, D. A., Estabrooks, P. A., & Vogt, T. M. (2006). Evaluating the impact of health promotion programs: Using the RE-AIM framework to form summary measures for decision making involving complex issues. *Health Education Research, 21*(5), 688–694.

Glasgow, R. E., & Riley, W. T. (2013). Pragmatic measures: What they are and why we need them. *American Journal of Preventive Medicine, 45*(2), 237–243.

Glasgow, R. E., Vogt, T. M., & Boles, S. M. (1999). Evaluating the public health impact of health promotion interventions: The RE-AIM framework. *American Journal of Public Health, 89*(9), 1322–1327.

Green, L. W., & Glasgow, R. E. (2006). Evaluating the relevance, generalization, and applicability of research: Issues in external validation and translation methodology. *Evaluation & the Health Professions, 29*(1), 126–153.

Green, L. W., & Kreuter, M. W. (2005). *Health program planning: An educational and ecological approach* (4th ed.). New York, NY: McGraw Hill Professional.

Grimshaw, J. M., Zwarenstein, M., Tetroe, J. M., Godin, G., Graham, I. D., Lemyre, L., . . . Hux, J. (2007). Looking inside the black box: A theory-based process evaluation alongside a randomised controlled trial of printed educational materials (the Ontario printed educational message, OPEM) to improve referral and prescribing practices in primary care in Ontario, Canada. *Implementation Science, 2*(1), 38.

Guo, S., & Fraser, M. W. (2014). *Propensity score analysis: Statistical methods and applications.* Thousand Oaks, CA: Sage.

Haddix, A. C., Teutsch, S. M., & Corso, P. S. (2003). *Prevention effectiveness: A guide to decision analysis and economic evaluation.* Oxford, United Kingdom: Oxford University Press.

Harachi, T. W., Abbott, R. D., Catalano, R. F., Haggerty, K. P., & Fleming, C. B. (1999). Opening the black box: Using process evaluation measures to assess implementation and theory building. *American Journal of Community Psychology, 27*(5), 711–731.

Hartman, M. A., Nierkens, V., Cremer, S. W., Stronks, K., & Verhoeff, A. P. (2013). A process evaluation: Does recruitment for an exercise program through ethnically specific channels and key figures contribute to its reach and receptivity in ethnic minority mothers? *BMC Public Health, 13*, 768.

Haviland, A., Nagin, D. S., & Rosenbaum, P. R. (2007). Combining propensity score matching and group-based trajectory analysis in an observational study. *Psychological Methods, 12*(3), 247.

Hawe, P., Shiell, A., & Riley, T. (2009). Theorising interventions as events in systems. *American Journal of Community Psychology, 43*(3–4), 267–276.

Hawkins, N. G., Sanson-Fisher, R. W., Shakeshaft, A., D'Este, C., & Green, L. W. (2007). The multiple baseline design for evaluating population-based research. *American Journal of Preventive Medicine, 33*(2), 162–168.

Hayes, A. F. (2012). PROCESS: A versatile computational tool for observed variable mediation, moderation, and conditional process modeling [white paper]. Retrieved from http://www.afhayes.com/ public/process2012.pdf

Hayes, A. F. (2013). *Introduction to mediation, moderation, and conditional process analysis: A regression-based approach.* New York, NY: Guilford Press.

Hofstetter, H., Peters, L., Meijer, S., Van Keulen, H., Schutte, L., & van Empelen, P. (2014). Evaluation of the effectiveness and implementation of the sexual health program Long Live Love IV. *European Health Psychologist, 16*(S), 489.

Holland, P. W. (1988). Causal inference, path analysis and recursive structural equations models. *ETS Research Report Series, 1988*(1), i–50.

Holmbeck, G. N. (1997). Toward terminological, conceptual, and statistical clarity in the study of mediators and moderators: Examples from the child-clinical and pediatric psychology literatures. *Journal of Consulting and Clinical Psychology, 65*(4), 599.

House, E. R. (2010). *Evaluating with validity.* Charlotte, NC: Information Age Publisher.

Hsu, M., & Chiu, C. (2004). Internet self-efficacy and electronic service acceptance. *Decision Support Systems, 38*(3), 369–381.

Israel, B. A., Schultz, A. J., Parker, E. A., Becker, A. B., Allen, A. J., III, & Guzman, J. R. (2008). Critical issues in developing and following community based participatory research principles. In M. Minkler & N. Wallerstein (Eds.),

*Community-based participatory research for health: From process to outcomes* (pp. 47–66). San Francisco, CA: Jossey-Bass.

Janz, K. F., Lutuchy, E. M., Wenthe, P., & Levy, S. M. (2008). Measuring activity in children and adolescents using self-report: PAQ-C and PAQ-A. *Medicine and Science in Sports and Exercise, 40*(4), 767.

Jiang, Y., & Hesser, J. E. (2008). Patterns of health-related quality of life and patterns associated with health risks among Rhode Island adults. *Health and Quality of Life Outcomes, 6,* 49.

Kessler, R. C., Duncan, G. J., Gennetian, L. A., Katz, L. F., Kling, J. R., Sampson, N. A., . . . Ludwig, J. (2014). Associations of housing mobility interventions for children in high-poverty neighborhoods with subsequent mental disorders during adolescence. *JAMA, 311*(9), 937–948.

Kirk, J., & Miller, M. L. (1986). *Reliability and validity in qualitative research.* Thousand Oaks, CA: Sage.

Klassen, A. C., Creswell, J., Clark, V. L. P., Smith, K. C., & Meissner, H. I. (2012). Best practices in mixed methods for quality of life research. *Quality of Life Research, 21*(3), 377–380.

Korda, H., & Itani, Z. (2013). Harnessing social media for health promotion and behavior change. *Health Promotion Practice, 14*(1), 15–23.

Liese, A. D., Crandell, J. L., Tooze, J. A., Fangman, M. T., Couch, S. C., Merchant, A. T., . . . Mayer-Davis, E. J. (2015). Relative validity and reliability of an FFQ in youth with type 1 diabetes. *Public Health Nutrition, 18*(3), 428–437.

Linnan, L., & Steckler, A. (2002). Process evaluation for public health interventions and research: An overview. In A. Steckler & L. Linnan (Eds.), *Process evaluation for public health interventions and research* (pp. 1–23). San Francisco, CA: Jossey-Bass.

Long, T., & Johnson, M. (2000). Rigour, reliability and validity in qualitative research. *Clinical Effectiveness in Nursing, 4*(1), 30–37.

Lorig, K. R., & Holman, H. R. (2003). Self-management education: History, definition, outcomes, and mechanisms. *Annals of Behavioral Medicine, 26*(1), 1–7.

Lorig, K. R., Ritter, P. L., Laurent, D. D., & Plant, K. (2006). Internet-based chronic disease self-management: A randomized trial. *Medical Care, 44*(11), 964–971.

Luellen, J. K., Shadish, W. R., & Clark, M. H. (2005). Propensity scores: An introduction and experimental test. *Evaluation Review, 29*(6), 530–558.

MacKinnon, D. P., Lockwood, C. M., Hoffman, J. M., West, S. G., & Sheets, V. (2002). A comparison of methods to test mediation and other intervening variable effects. *Psychological Methods, 7*(1), 83.

Malterud, K. (2001). Qualitative research: Standards, challenges, and guidelines. *The Lancet, 358*(9280), 483–488.

Markham, C. M., Tortolero, S. R., Peskin, M. F., Shegog, R., Thiel, M., Baumler, E. R., . . . Robin, L. (2012). Sexual risk avoidance and sexual risk reduction interventions for middle school youth: A randomized controlled trial. *Journal of Adolescent Health, 50*(3), 279–288

Maurer, T. J., & Andrews, K. D. (2000). Traditional, Likert, and simplified measures of self-efficacy. *Educational and Psychological Measurement, 60*(6), 965–973.

Mays, N., & Pope, C. (2000). Qualitative research in health care. Assessing quality in qualitative research. *BMJ (Clinical Research Ed.), 320*(7226), 50–52.

McCaffrey, D. F., Ridgeway, G., & Morral, A. R. (2004). Propensity score estimation with boosted regression for evaluating causal effects in observational studies. *Psychological Methods, 9*(4), 403.

Mechanic, D. (2002). Disadvantage, inequality, and social policy. *Health Affairs, 21*(2), 48–59.

Mercer, S. L., DeVinney, B. J., Fine, L. J., Green, L. W., & Dougherty, D. (2007). Study designs for effectiveness and translation research: Identifying trade-offs. *American Journal of Preventive Medicine, 33*(2), 139–154. e2.

Merriam, S. (2009). *Qualitative research. A guide to design and implementation (revised and expanded from qualitative research and case study applications in education).* San Francisco, CA: Jossey-Bass.

Miles, M. B., Huberman, A. M., & Saldaña, J. (2013). *Qualitative data analysis: A methods sourcebook.* Thousand Oaks, CA: Sage.

Miller, K. S., Clark, L. F., Wendell, D. A., Levin, M. L., Gray-Ray, P., Velez, C. N., & Webber, M. P. (1997). Adolescent heterosexual experience: A new typology. *Journal of Adolescent Health, 20*(3), 179–186.

Minkler, M., & Wallerstein, N. (Eds.). (2008). *Community-based participatory research for health: From process to outcomes* (2nd ed.). San Francisco, CA: Jossey-Bass.

Moerbeek, M., van Breukelen, G. J., & Berger, M. P. (2003). A comparison between traditional methods and multilevel regression for the analysis of multicenter intervention studies. *Journal of Clinical Epidemiology, 56*(4), 341–350.

Mohr, D. C., Cuijpers, P., & Lehman, K. (2011). Supportive accountability: A model for providing human support to enhance adherence to eHealth interventions. *Journal of Medical Internet Research, 13*(1), e30.

Morgan-Lopez, A. A., & MacKinnon, D. P. (2006). Demonstration and evaluation of a method for assessing mediated moderation. *Behavior Research Methods, 38*(1), 77–87.

Morrison-Beedy, D., Carey, M., & Tu, X. (2006). Accuracy of audio computer-assisted self-interviewing (ACASI) and self-administered questionnaires for the assessment of sexual behavior. *AIDS and Behavior, 10*(5), 541–552.

Muller, A. (2004). Florida's motorcycle helmet law repeal and fatality rates. *American Journal of Public Health, 94*(4), 556–558.

Muller, D., Judd, C. M., & Yzerbyt, V. Y. (2005). When moderation is mediated and mediation is moderated. *Journal of Personality and Social Psychology, 89*(6), 852.

National Center for Chronic Disease Prevention and Health Promotion, Division of Population Health. (2011). Health related quality of life (HRQOL). Methods and measures. Retrieved from http://www.cdc.gov/hrqol/methods.htm

National Institute on Alcohol Abuse and Alcoholism. (n.d.). National Institute on Alcohol Abuse and Alcoholism of the National Institutes of Health. Retrieved from http://www.niaaa.nih.gov

O'Brien, B. C., Harris, I. B., Beckman, T. J., Reed, D. A., & Cook, D. A. (2014). Standards for reporting qualitative research: A synthesis of recommendations. *Academic Medicine, 89*(9), 1245–1251.

Partin, M. R., & Burgess, D. J. (2012). Reducing health disparities or improving minority health? The end determines the means. *Journal of General Internal Medicine, 27*(8), 887–889.

Patton, M. Q. (2005). Qualitative research. In B. S. Everitt & D. Howell (Eds.), *Encyclopedia of statistics in behavioral science.* Hoboken, NJ: Wiley.

Patton, M. Q. (2008). *Utilization-focused evaluation.* Los Angeles, CA: Sage.

Paulussen, T., Kok, G., Schaalma, H., & Parcel, G. S. (1995). Diffusion of AIDS curricula among Dutch secondary school teachers. *Health Education & Behavior, 22*(2), 227–243.

Peskin, M. F., Markham, C. M., Shegog, R., Baumler, E. R., Addy, R. C., & Tortolero, S. R. (2014). Effects of the It's Your Game . . . Keep It Real program on dating violence in ethnic-minority middle school youths: A group randomized trial. *American Journal of Public Health, 104*(8), 1471–1477.

Piaggio, G., Elbourne, D. R., Pocock, S. J., Evans, S. J., Altman, D. G., & CONSORT Group. (2012). Reporting of noninferiority and equivalence randomized trials: Extension of the CONSORT 2010 statement. *JAMA, 308*(24), 2594–2604.

Popham, K., Calo, W. A., Carpentier, M. Y., Chen, N. E., Kamrudin, S. A., Le, Y. L., . . . Mullen, P. D. (2012). Reporting guidelines: Optimal use in preventive medicine and public health. *American Journal of Preventive Medicine, 43*(4), e31–e42.

Potvin, L., Haddad, S., & Frohlich, K. L. (2001). Beyond process and outcome evaluation: A comprehensive approach for evaluating health promotion programmes. *WHO Regional Publications European Series, 92,* 45–62.

Preacher, K. J., Rucker, D. D., & Hayes, A. F. (2007). Addressing moderated mediation hypotheses: Theory, methods, and prescriptions. *Multivariate Behavioral Research, 42*(1), 185–227.

Preskill, H., & Jones, N. (2009). *A practical guide for engaging stakeholders in developing evaluation questions.* Princeton, NJ: Robert Wood Johnson Foundation.

Prinstein, M. J., Boergers, J., Spirito, A., Little, T. D., & Grapentine, W. (2000). Peer functioning, family dysfunction, and psychological symptoms in a risk factor model for adolescent inpatients' suicidal ideation severity. *Journal of Clinical Child Psychology, 29*(3), 392–405.

Prinstein, M. J., Boergers, J., & Vernberg, E. M. (2001). Overt and relational aggression in adolescents: Social-psychological adjustment of aggressors and victims. *Journal of Clinical Child Psychology, 30*(4), 479–491.

Reeves, B. C., Deeks, J. J., Higgins, J. P. T. & Wells, G. A. (2011). Including non-randomized studies. In J. P. T. Higgins & S. Green (Eds.), *Cochrane handbook for systematic reviews of interventions* (Version 5.1.0 [updated March

2011]). The Cochrane Collaboration, 2011. Retrieved from www.cochrane-handbook.org

Resnick, B., & Jenkins, L. S. (2000). Testing the reliability and validity of the self-efficacy for exercise scale. *Nursing Research, 49*(3), 154–159.

Rosenbaum, P. R. (2002). *Observational studies* (2nd ed.). New York, NY: Springer.

Rossi, P. H., Lipsey, M. W., & Freeman, H. E. (2004). *Evaluation: A systematic approach* (7th ed.). Thousand Oaks, CA: Sage.

Rubin, D. B. (2001). Using propensity scores to help design observational studies: Application to the tobacco litigation. *Health Services and Outcomes Research Methodology, 2*(3–4), 169–188.

Sadasivam, R. S., Kinney, R. L., Delaughter, K., Rao, S. R., Williams, J. H., Coley, H. L., ... QUIT-PRIMO Collaborative Group. (2013). Who participates in web-assisted tobacco interventions? The QUIT-PRIMO and national dental practice-based research network hi-quit studies. *Journal of Medical Internet Research, 15*(5), e77.

Sanson-Fisher, R. W., Bonevski, B., Green, L. W., & D'Este, C. (2007). Limitations of the randomized controlled trial in evaluating population-based health interventions. *American Journal of Preventive Medicine, 33*(2), 155–161.

Schaalma, H. P., Kok, G., Bosker, R. J., Parcel, G. S., Peters, L., Poelman, J., & Reinders, J. (1996). Planned development and evaluation of AIDS/STD education for secondary school students in the Netherlands: Short-term effects. *Health Education & Behavior, 23*(4), 469–487.

Schaalma, H., Kok, G., Poelman, J., & Reinders, J. (1994). The development of AIDS education for Dutch secondary schools: A systematic approach. In D. R. Rutter (Ed.), *The social psychology of health and safety: European perspectives* (pp. 175–194). Aldershot, United Kingdom: Avebury.

Scheirer, M. A. (1994). Designing and using process evaluation. In J. S. Whole, H. P. Hatry, & K. E. Newcomer (Eds.), *Handbook of practical program evaluation* (pp. 40–68). San Francisco, CA: Jossey-Bass.

Schorr, L. B. (2006). *Common purpose: Sharing responsibility for child and family outcomes.* New York, NY: National Center for Children in Poverty.

Schwartz, D., & Lellouch, J. (1967). Explanatory and pragmatic attitudes in therapeutical trials. *Journal of Chronic Diseases, 20*(8), 637–648.

Scriven, M. (1991). Prose and cons about goal-free evaluation. *American Journal of Evaluation, 12*(1), 55–62.

Senn, S. (2007). *Statistical issues in drug development* (2nd ed.). Chichester, United Kingdom: Wiley.

Shadish, W., Cook, T., & Campbell, D. (2002). *Experimental and quasi-experimental designs for generalized causal inference.* Boston, MA: Houghton Mifflin.

Sheldon, T. A., Cullum, N., Dawson, D., Lankshear, A., Lowson, K., Watt, I., ... Wright, J. (2004). What's the evidence that NICE guidance has been implemented? Results from a national evaluation using time series analysis, audit of patients' notes, and interviews. *BMJ (Clinical Research Ed.), 329*(7473), 999.

Singal, A. G., Higgins, P. D. R., & Waljee, A. K. (2014). A primer on effectiveness and efficacy trials. *Clinical and Translational Gastroenterology, 5*(1), e45.

Slutsky, J. R., & Clancy, C. M. (2010). Patient-centered comparative effectiveness research: Essential for high-quality care. *Archives of Internal Medicine, 170*(5), 403–404.

Stake, R. E. (2006). *Multiple case study analysis.* New York, NY: Guilford Press.

Stame, N. (2004). Theory-based evaluation and types of complexity. *Evaluation, 10*(1), 58–76.

Steckler, A., & Linnan, L. A. (2002). *Process evaluation for public health interventions and research.* San Francisco, CA: Jossey-Bass.

Stone, S. P., Fuller, C., Savage, J., Cookson, B., Hayward, A., Cooper, B., . . . Charlett, A. (2012). Evaluation of the national Cleanyourhands campaign to reduce *Staphylococcus aureus* bacteraemia and *Clostridium difficile* infection in hospitals in England and Wales by improved hand hygiene: Four year, prospective, ecological, interrupted time series study. *BMJ (Clinical Research Ed.), 344,* e3005.

Thompson, F. E., & Subar, A. F. (2011). Dietary assessment methodology. In A. Coulton, M. Ferruzzi, & C. J. Boushey (Eds.), *Nutrition in the prevention and treatment of disease* (3rd ed., pp. 5–47). San Diego, CA: Academic Press.

Thorpe, K. E., Zwarenstein, M., Oxman, A. D., Treweek, S., Furberg, C. D., Altman, D. G., . . . Magid, D. J. (2009). A pragmatic–explanatory continuum indicator summary (PRECIS): A tool to help trial designers. *Journal of Clinical Epidemiology, 62*(5), 464–475.

Tobin, G. A., & Begley, C. M. (2004). Methodological rigour within a qualitative framework. *Journal of Advanced Nursing, 48*(4), 388–396.

Tong, A., Flemming, K., McInnes, E., Oliver, S., & Craig, J. (2012). Enhancing transparency in reporting the synthesis of qualitative research: ENTREQ. *BMC Medical Research Methodology, 12,* 181.

Tong, A., Sainsbury, P., & Craig, J. (2007). Consolidated criteria for reporting qualitative research (COREQ): A 32-item checklist for interviews and focus groups. *International Journal for Quality in Health Care, 19*(6), 349–357.

Torres, R. T., Preskill, H., & Piontek, M. E. (2004). *Evaluation strategies for communicating and reporting: Enhancing learning in organizations* (2nd ed.). Thousand Oaks, CA: Sage.

Tortolero, S. R., Markham, C. M., Peskin, M. F., Shegog, R., Addy, R. C., Escobar-Chaves, S. L., & Baumler, E. R. (2010). It's Your Game . . . Keep It Real: Delaying sexual behavior with an effective middle school program. *Journal of Adolescent Health, 46*(2), 169–179.

Tunis, S. R., Stryer, D. B., & Clancy, C. M. (2003). Practical clinical trials: Increasing the value of clinical research for decision making in clinical and health policy. *JAMA, 290*(12), 1624–1632.

U.S. Department of Health and Human Services Office of Adolescent Health. (2015). Teen pregnancy prevention resource center: Evidence-based programs. Retrieved from http://www.hhs.gov/ash/oah/oah-initiatives/teen_pregnancy/db/index.html

van Breukelen, G. (2006). ANCOVA versus change from baseline: More power in randomized studies, more bias in nonrandomized studies. *Journal of Clinical Epidemiology, 59*(9), 920–925.

Vernberg, E. M., Jacobs, A. K., & Hershberger, S. L. (1999). Peer victimization and attitudes about violence during early adolescence. *Journal of Clinical Child Psychology, 28*(3), 386–395.

Wagenaar, A. C., Salois, M. J., & Komro, K. A. (2009). Effects of beverage alcohol price and tax levels on drinking: A meta-analysis of 1003 estimates from 112 studies. *Addiction, 104*(2), 179–190.

Webb, T., Joseph, J., Yardley, L., & Michie, S. (2010). Using the internet to promote health behavior change: A systematic review and meta-analysis of the impact of theoretical basis, use of behavior change techniques, and mode of delivery on efficacy. *Journal of Medical Internet Research, 12*(1), e4.

West, S. G., Duan, N., Pequegnat, W., Gaist, P., Des Jarlais, D. C., Holtgrave, D., . . . Clatts, M. (2008). Alternatives to the randomized controlled trial. *American Journal of Public Health, 98*(8), 1359–1366.

Wholey, J. S. (1994). Assessing the feasibility and likely usefulness of evaluation. In J. S. Wholey, H. P. Hatry, & K. E. Newcomer (Eds.), *Handbook of practical program evaluation* (pp. 15–39). San Francisco, CA: Jossey-Bass.

Wholey, J. S., Hatry, H. P., & Newcomer, K. E. (2004). *Handbook of practical program evaluation* (2nd ed.). San Francisco, CA: Jossey-Bass.

Windsor, R., Clark, N., Boyd, N. R., & Goodman, R. M. (2003). *Evaluation of health promotion, health education and disease prevention programs* (3rd ed.). New York, NY: McGraw-Hill.

Winkens, B., Schouten, H. J., van Breukelen, G. J., & Berger, M. P. (2006). Optimal number of repeated measures and group sizes in clinical trials with linearly divergent treatment effects. *Contemporary Clinical Trials, 27*(1), 57–69.

Work Group for Community Health and Development, University of Kansas. (2014). Community Tool Box. Retrieved from http://ctb.ku.edu/en

Yin, R. K. (2013). *Case study research: Design and methods.* Thousand Oaks, CA: Sage.

Zwarenstein, M., Treweek, S., Gagnier, J. J., Altman, D. G., Tunis, S., Haynes, B., . . . Pragmatic Trials in Healthcare (Practihc) group. (2008). Improving the reporting of pragmatic trials: An extension of the CONSORT statement. *BMJ (Clinical Research Ed.), 337*, a2390.

Zwerling, C., & Jones, M. P. (1999). Evaluation of the effectiveness of low blood alcohol concentration laws for younger drivers. *American Journal of Preventive Medicine, 16*(1), 76–80.

# CHAPTER 10

# USING INTERVENTION MAPPING TO ADAPT EVIDENCE-BASED INTERVENTIONS

### with Linda Highfield, Marieke A. Hartman, Patricia Dolan Mullen, and Joanne N. Leerlooijer

## Competency

• Make decisions about whether and how to adapt an evidence-based intervention (EBI).

In this chapter, we describe how to use Intervention Mapping (IM) to adapt evidence-based interventions (EBIs) for new populations and settings. EBIs are interventions (including programs, policies, or practices) that have shown effectiveness in decreasing a health problem or its causes. Because of the importance of a balance between fidelity to original program design and adaptation to help an intervention better suit a new setting, changes to EBIs should be undertaken systematically with an eye to retention of the critical elements that made the program effective in the first place (Card, Solomon, & Cunningham, 2011; Elliot & Mihalic, 2004; Lee, Altschul, & Mowbray, 2008; Shen, Yang, Cao, & Warfield, 2008; Van Deale, van Audenhove, Hermans, van den Bergh, & van den Broucke, 2014). Despite these cautions, practically speaking, "adaptation happens." The problem is that it sometimes happens poorly and leads to incomplete interventions that have little chance of maintaining effectiveness. For example, planners may choose pieces of interventions that are the most appealing to them or that seem the most feasible, often without soliciting input from the original developers or the new community and without systematically determining what in an EBI needs to change and what must stay the same.

### LEARNING OBJECTIVES AND TASKS

• Conduct a needs assessment to describe the health/behavior problems and develop logic models for the problem and for change

• Search for evidence-based interventions (EBIs)

• Assess fit and plan adaptation

• Make adaptations by modifying materials and activities

• Plan for implementation

• Plan for evaluation with a focus on adaptations

Some adaptation guides are general conceptual models that do not provide a step-by-step approach to adaptation decisions and execution (Lee et al., 2008; Wandersman et al., 2008). Others are specific to HIV prevention (Card et al., 2011; McKleroy et al., 2006; Wingood & DiClemente, 2008) or substance abuse interventions (Backer, 2002; Kumpfer, Pinyuchon, Teixeira de Melo, & Whiteside, 2008; Smith & Caldwell, 2007). More recent guides emphasize adaptation through community engagement (Chen, Reid, Parker, & Pillemer, 2013). Van Deale and colleagues (2014) present the concept of "empowerment evaluation" as a framework for implementing the core elements of a program with fidelity while still allowing for adaptation of the program to fit the needs of the new population or setting. The authors suggest a high level of community participation and collaboration in making decisions about improving program fit. They also advise planners to use IM as a way of identifying and articulating the core components of a program that should be maintained and implemented with fidelity.

Intervention Mapping can provide a systematic approach to adapting EBIs on any health problem that can help program planners identify and retain essential elements in translation to new communities and settings. We present a case study in which a planning team used IM to adapt an EBI to improve appointment keeping for mammography (Highfield, Bartholomew, Hartman, Ford, & Bahile, 2014a).

## Perspectives

Using health promotion programs beyond the settings in which they are originally developed presents unique challenges. These include understanding what constitutes evidence, identifying acceptable programs, policies, and practices, and deciding whether and when it is appropriate to adapt them.

## Challenges in Choosing Evidence Based Interventions

The first challenge in decisions about adaptation is finding an EBI that may fit the new context.

### *Defining Evidence-Based*

Following from a focus on "evidence-based medicine" over the last 30 years, the ideal of "evidence-based" is pursued in many other fields, including public health, social and behavioral interventions, and health promotion (Brownson, Fielding, & Maylahn, 2009). In public health, two levels of evidence are required. The first is evidence that the behavioral or environmental goal is sound, for example, the evidence that colorectal cancer screening for all normal-risk adults 50 years and older reduces mortality

(Brownson, et al., 2009). The second level of evidence, which is the focus here, is evidence that a particular intervention or type of intervention is sufficiently effective (Brownson et al., 2009). Authors have described EBIs as having been systematically and scientifically developed and tested. Both best practices in program development and in research evaluation are important in defining "what is evidence?" (Brownson et al., 2009; Drake et al., 2001; Glasgow, Klesges, Dzelwaltowski, Estabrooks, & Vogt, 2006). An EBI is one that has been shown to be effective through the application of sound scientific testing. Just how rigorous this testing must be, how generalizable the results should be, and how many studies are needed will vary, depending on the source. Further, the descriptions of EBIs grouped together in a systematic review is often very general, such as "mass media," and the effectiveness of the individual EBIs in the review may vary, making decisions about evidence difficult for practitioners and researchers alike. Nevertheless, the first criterion for selecting a program to adopt and replicate, or to adapt, is to show credible evidence that the program is effective. In general, an effective intervention is one that achieves practically important changes in behavior or environmental conditions. If evidence of effectiveness is insufficient for an intervention, researchers may have rationale to adapt and reevaluate an intervention (Shen et al., 2008); however, we do not cover this topic further in this chapter.

## *Finding Evidence-Based Interventions*

Planners need more than evidence and narrative portrayals of EBIs. They need the specific materials and description of activities (here, called the "full EBIs"). Systematic reviews of programs, policies, and processes have made laudable strides toward establishing evidence and are available on the Internet through government and other sponsored sites, such as the Centers for Disease Control and Prevention's Community Guide (http://www.thecommunityguide.org), the Agency for Health Care Research and Quality's Evidence-Based Practice Center reports (http://www.ahrq.gov/research/findings/evidence-based-reports/index.html), Canada's Health Evidence (http://www.healthevidence.org), and the Cochrane Collaboration Library (http://www.cochranelibrary.com). These resources and even individual publications presenting the trials of specific EBIs, however, typically do not facilitate access to full EBIs.

Resources that make full EBIs accessible are available in a growing number of specific health problem areas. Examples include the U.S. National Cancer Institute's Research-Tested Intervention Programs, "RTIPs" (http://rtips.cancer.gov/), the U.S. Centers for Disease Control and Prevention's Effective Interventions: HIV Prevention that Works (https://effectiveinterventions.cdc.gov/en/home.aspx), and the U.S. Substance Abuse and Mental Health Services Administration's National

Registry of Evidence-Based Programs and Practices (http://www.nrepp
.samhsa.gov). The full EBIs on these sites have been evaluated usually in
well-funded trials, which may be difficult to implement in new settings with
limited resources. Even EBIs that are potentially feasible may fail to include
important details about the program (including theoretical underpinnings,
performance objectives, determinants, and intervention methods). These
missing elements are critical for implementation (as is) and for adaptation
to improve fit in communities beyond the test site. Increased attention to
dissemination of EBIs should improve the number and quality of resources
for full EBIs, as well as stimulating authors to provide needed elements in
their publications about specific EBIs.

## Challenges in Adapting EBIs

### *Protecting Essential Elements*

The core of the challenge in adapting EBIs is to identify the elements of an
EBI that are crucial to effectiveness and to retain them. When programs are
adapted in ways that modify their program theory of change, the programs
are no longer evidence-based and may no longer be effective either in the
old population or in the new one, and require new effectiveness trials (Lee
et al., 2008). Therefore, the decision to adapt an EBI is a serious one.

Adaptation must be undertaken with balance between program fidelity
and the needs of the adopting site (Backer, 2001; van Deale et al., 2014).
Barrera, Castro, Strycker, and Toobert (2013) found that behavioral interventions were more effective when adapted for a new cultural group and
that most planners agreed that adaptation begins with data collection and
ends with testing in the new setting. Card and colleagues (2011) point out
that there are often mismatches between the new context and the original
EBI, such as outdated language, images, and examples; in the HIV context,
the mismatch may be particular objectives or activities that are too controversial for the new community or simply not relevant. On the other hand,
in a review of more than 500 studies, Durlak and DuPree (2008) point out
that although higher levels of implementation fidelity were closely tied to
improved program outcomes, levels of fidelity were well below 100 percent
across interventions. Therefore some adaptation occurred and may have
also contributed to programmatic success. The questions surrounding the
need for adaptation versus the importance of maintaining program fidelity
during implementation clearly warrant further investigation. In the mean-
time, however, planners must make careful decisions about whether or not
to adapt a program, and if so, what should be maintained as is and what
can change. We recommend the use of IM to guide these decisions.

In changing an EBI to fit a new setting, we may be inadvertently assuming that program settings are unchangeable — that the program must be adapted to fit the setting rather than the reverse (Elliot and Mihalic, 2004). However, planners should also ask, how does the setting need to change in order to implement this program? In other words, planners might aim to change capacity to deliver the program before changing the program itself. Although it may be easier to change the program, changing local capacity to deliver it as it was designed may be a safer choice (Goddard & Harding, 2003). This concept of necessary capacity building for implementation is consistent with Wandersman and colleagues'(2008) Interactive Systems Framework (ISF) in which both intervention-specific capacity and general organizational capacity building efforts are essential for effective program implementation.

When adaptation is necessary to improve program fit, planners must determine which program elements were essential in making the program successful. Unfortunately, program evaluations rarely report on which features of a program constitute these "core elements" (also called essential elements and active ingredients) and which can be adapted without compromising program impact. A major hazard of program adaptation is that it inadvertently changes core elements of EBIs; but we often do not know what constitutes these (Botvin, 2004). Because separate program aspects are not usually tested independently, new program users may not be able to identify and protect essential elements (Botvin, 2004). We suggest that these "active ingredients" are related to an intervention's logic model of change. The logic model or theory of change is most likely to include the following types of elements: (a) theoretical change methods that are intended to influence determinants of behavior of the at-risk group and the environmental agents, and (b) the practical applications of the change methods. However, any program element can be important to participants to the extent that it adds to credibility, contributes to reach, or embeds a change method. Therefore, intervention delivery channels (especially sensitivity to reaching the intended at-risk group with culturally accessible and credible channels); dose and intensity, or how much of the program the participant are getting; and an ecological approach (taking into consideration changing environmental as well as individual determinants) may also be active ingredients. Lee et al. (2008) encourage program developers to provide guidance both by describing their theory of change, including mediators and moderators of effects, and by suggesting which parts of the EBI are essential and cannot be changed without modifying the theory of change. They also suggest that program developers can proactively suggest the ways in which their EBI can be modified for new populations.

## Formative Research and Summative Evaluation

When a decision is made to adapt an EBI, planners should also be committing to base adaptation on formative evidence that the change will make the program more acceptable to and effective in the new population (Lau, 2006). Lau (2006) suggests strong formative research to create evidence-based adaptation. She also points out that inclusion of diverse populations in initial evaluation studies increases external validity so that adaptation may not be needed.

Program adaptors should also be committing to evaluation research on the effect of adaptation on intervention effectiveness. Users of EBIs and the health promotion community need to know whether program adaptations are successful in increasing reach and for highly adapted programs whether an intervention continues to be effective in its new form.

In a review of published descriptions of program adaptation, Krivitsky and associates (2012) found that one-half (51 percent) obtained direct feedback about the original program from stakeholder groups (Krivitsky et al., 2012). The 2011 review also found that 73 percent reported at least a pilot test of the adapted intervention; only 36 percent evaluated the impact of the adapted program with a comparison group. In another review, Stirman, Miller, Toder, and Calloway (2013) coded 258 adaptations identified in 32 published articles describing interventions implemented in health care or community settings. They identified five types of modifications that included changes to the format, setting, or patient population that did not influence change in the content of the intervention. They also identified 12 different types of content modifications and a smaller number of adaptations of the training or evaluations of EBIs. The review also noted that although many of the changes to existing programs were made prospectively and proactively by identifying differences between the original program and the new implementation setting, some were made after implementation was underway. These changes, in particular, may give rise to concerns about maintaining program impact. The authors propose using fidelity measure along with a framework for making adaptations to guide decisions about whether a particular change may alter the core elements of a program, thus diminishing intervention impact (Stirman et al., 2013).

## Program Adaptation

Several authors have described the processes of dissemination of evidence-based programs including suggested adaptation (Backer, 2001; Centers for Disease Control & Prevention, n.d.; Lee et al., 2008; McKleroy et al. 2006; Wandersman et al. 2008). Most of the frameworks describe the tasks involved, such as: (a) assessing the new priority population, the candidate EBI, and the agency's capacity for implementation; (b) determining whether to adopt a program with or without adaptation; (c) adapting (when necessary) and pretesting the materials; (d) developing an implementation protocol and pilot testing the adapted intervention; and (e) implementing the entire intervention (McKleroy et al., 2006). Other frameworks, such as the ISF, suggest processes that must take place in each adoption, adaptation, and implementation step (Wandersman et al., 2008). Lee and colleagues (2008) recommend that EBI adopters, optimally, in collaboration with or with technical assistance from program developers, first explore the EBI theory of change in the original program and identify elements that cannot be changed. Like the other stepwise guidelines, Lee and colleagues (2008) assess differences between the new population and the original population, execute content adaptation and pretesting, and plan an evaluation of the adapted EBI. Chen and colleagues' (2013) Method for Program Adaptation through Community Engagement (M-PACE) emphasizes obtaining high-quality participant feedback adjudicating recommendations for program changes.

Intervention Mapping provides a systematic approach that adds a detailed "how to" to existing frameworks. In this chapter, we illustrate the use of IM for adapting EBIs. Our main perspective in this chapter is conducting program adaptation using a systematic evidence- and theory-informed approach. Doing so, planners can maintain fidelity while still allowing for program adaptation to improve fit (van Deale et al., 2014), whereas Backer (2001) notes that the question is not whether things will change, but instead, how change can be managed in a way that retains core program components (Backer, 2001). From an IM perspective, systematic adaptation includes: (a) understanding the needs of the community by identifying the correct behavioral and environmental targets for change, and understanding the determinants of these; (b) choosing a program that is the best match to the targets for change; (c) making adaptation decisions by comparing the logic of the EBI with the needs of your community; and (d) only making changes that correspond with mismatches between the EBI and the community needs while avoiding modification of the theory of change of the original program.

## Intervention Mapping for Adaptation

In this chapter, we describe applying IM steps and tasks for adapting and implementing evidence-based programs (Bartholomew & Mullen, 2011; Leerlooijer et al., 2011; Tortolero et al., 2005). We include the questions to be addressed at each step and the products that come from the step.

Planners can apply intervention mapping for adaptation (IM Adapt) to either revising an intervention they have built from the six steps of IM (therefore being able to skip searching for an appropriate new EBI) or to find and make adaptations to an EBI that they have not developed themselves.

IM Adapt is not full-fledged Intervention Mapping. We described IM used for program adaptation in the third edition of this book (Bartholomew & Mullen, 2011) and other authors had applied it for adaptation (Leerlooijer et al., 2011; Tortolero et al., 2005). However, in this edition, we have simplified the application (see Figure 10.1).

We used the IM Adapt framework to conduct the project that provided the case study presented in this chapter. In the project we found, adapted, implemented, and evaluated an EBI to help underserved African American women in Houston, Texas, keep appointments for mammography screening.

A common scenario for an organization considering EBIs is that it has a mission to address certain health problems and would like to avoid developing an intervention from the beginning. This may be because there are insufficient resources for developing an intervention from scratch, or because a funder has required the use of an existing EBI. So, the organization must find a program that has been evaluated, was found to be effective, and is available for use. If a planning group is able to find an EBI that addresses the priority health problem, it will face several questions: Does it fit? Can it be adapted? What changes will make it a better fit while maintaining effectiveness? IM Adapt is a guide for answering these questions and performing a systematic adaptation.

For choosing and adapting an EBI, the IM Adapt framework suggests the following steps: (a) conduct a needs assessment and assess organizational capacity, (b) search for EBIs, (c) assess fit and plan adaptations, (d) modify materials and activities, (e) plan for implementation, and (f) plan for evaluation with a focus on changes to the EBI (see Figure 10.1).

## Step 1. Conduct a Needs Assessment, Assess Organizational Capacity, and Create Logic Models

In Step 1, the planning group will complete four tasks: (a) conduct a needs assessment and developing a logic model of the problem, (b) develop a logic model of change, (c) assess organizational capacity, and (c) write program goals for expected outcomes from implementing the EBI at the new site.

### Developing a Logic Model of the Problem

The first step of adapting an EBI is to fully understand the health problem in the new site. Understanding the problem means confirming its importance

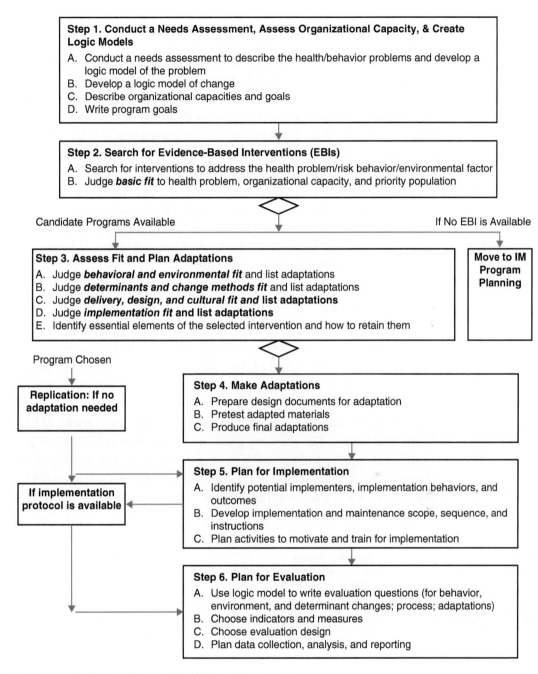

**Step 1. Conduct a Needs Assessment, Assess Organizational Capacity, & Create Logic Models**
A. Conduct a needs assessment to describe the health/behavior problems and develop a logic model of the problem
B. Develop a logic model of change
C. Describe organizational capacities and goals
D. Write program goals

**Step 2. Search for Evidence-Based Interventions (EBIs)**
A. Search for interventions to address the health problem/risk behavior/environmental factor
B. Judge *basic fit* to health problem, organizational capacity, and priority population

Candidate Programs Available                                          If No EBI is Available

**Step 3. Assess Fit and Plan Adaptations**
A. Judge *behavioral and environmental fit* and list adaptations
B. Judge *determinants and change methods fit* and list adaptations
C. Judge *delivery, design, and cultural fit and* list adaptations
D. Judge *implementation fit and list adaptations*
E. Identify essential elements of the selected intervention and how to retain them

Move to IM Program Planning

Program Chosen

**Replication: If no adaptation needed**

**Step 4. Make Adaptations**
A. Prepare design documents for adaptation
B. Pretest adapted materials
C. Produce final adaptations

**If implementation protocol is available**

**Step 5. Plan for Implementation**
A. Identify potential implementers, implementation behaviors, and outcomes
B. Develop implementation and maintenance scope, sequence, and instructions
C. Plan activities to motivate and train for implementation

**Step 6. Plan for Evaluation**
A. Use logic model to write evaluation questions (for behavior, environment, and determinant changes; process; adaptations)
B. Choose indicators and measures
C. Choose evaluation design
D. Plan data collection, analysis, and reporting

**Figure 10.1**   Adapting an Evidence-based Health Promotion Intervention

(prevalence, incidence, impact) in the new community among the risk groups there. If the problem of interest to the community is a behavior, then the group will want to confirm the epidemiological evidence that links the behavior to one or more health problems. We suggest organizing the information about the health problem into a modified PRECEDE model that that will set the stage for comparing EBIs to community needs (Green & Kreuter, 2005). This first logic model is based on a needs assessment, the same as in IM Step 1 (see Chapter 4). However, sometimes for adaptation, if planners already have an EBI in mind. In that case, planners can find the needs assessments performed by the original program developers and then supplement the available information about the health problem with information from the new community. The assessment should help the group narrow its problem focus, as well as describe its particular priority population based on the importance of the health problem and how it compares to other problems in the community. Another important consideration is whether a particular population group carries excess burden including quality-of-life issues. The logic model of the problem depicts the relations between the health problem and its causal behaviors and environmental factors. See Figure 10.2.

## Developing a Logic Model of Change

As in Step 2 of IM for the development of a new program, after understanding the problem, the planners' transition from their logic model of the problem to a logic model of the solution. The logic model of change depicts how theory-based change methods are proposed to influence first the determinants of behavior and environment, then the behavior and environmental factors, and finally the health problem and quality of life (Kirby et al., 2004). The planning group in the new site will create a logic model of change by looking at the needs assessment and suggesting what changes should be the targets of their program. The group will ask, "What needs to change as a result of the program?" The group will look at needed change in the behaviors of the at-risk groups as well as needed change

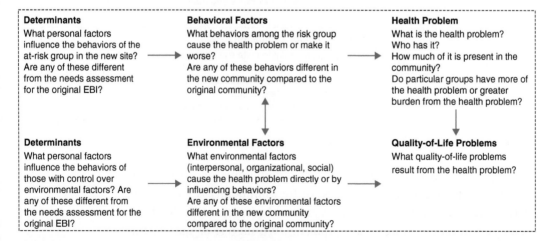

**Figure 10.2** Logic Model of the Problem With Guiding Questions

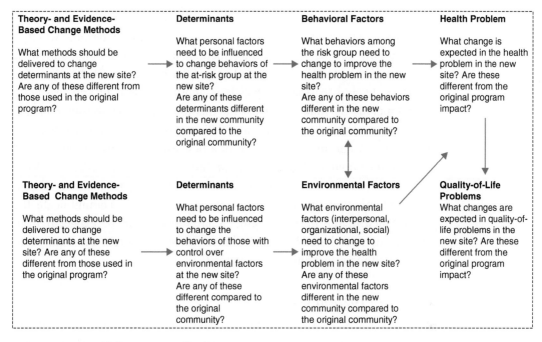

**Figure 10.3** Logic Model of Change With Guiding Questions

in the environment. They may want to break down these behaviors into sub-behaviors (performance objectives). They will then assess the probable determinants of that change and consider theory-based change methods. See Figure 10.3.

## *Assessing Organizational Capacity*

Whether or not a new setting can feasibly use an existing EBI setting depends largely on the capacity and goals of an organization that will implement it. Brownson and colleagues (2012) consider organizational capacity in five domains: workforce, leadership, relationships and partnerships, financial processes, and organizational climate and culture. These categories can help guide planners through thinking about the capacity of the organization to implement an EBI. Frameworks such as the Consolidated Framework for Implementation Research (CFIR, see Chapter 8; Damschroder et al., 2009) and the ISF can also provide information about what specific features of the implementing organization or setting may influence the ability of that organization to implement a program. For example, CFIR includes organizational leadership, communication, and readiness as constructs that all influence implementation. Scaccia and colleagues (2014) describe organizational readiness containing three elements: the motivation to implement an innovation, the general capacities of an organization, and the innovation-specific capacities needed for a particular innovation. A planner may choose to measure these constructs to determine whether certain EBIs can be feasibly implemented in certain settings and what changes (either to the setting or to the EBI) may be needed to increase program fit and feasibility. Questions about potential fit and feasibility might include the following: Does the mission of the organization coincide with the goals of the intervention? What staff are available to work on the adaption and implementation of a new evidence-based intervention? What is the implementation culture of the organization (from CFIR)? What budget is available for this project? What is the organization's readiness for implementing this program? How will the leader communicate the importance of the new program? What support can be expected from management and staff? What technical assistance might be required to complete the project and its evaluation?

### *Writing Program Goals*

Working from the logic model of change, the planning group will set goals for the impact of the implementation of an adapted EBI. What will change regarding health, behavior, and environmental outcomes? How much change is reasonable to expect? Over what period of time will it occur? See Chapter 4, the last task for Step 1 of IM for guidance on writing program goals. At this point in planning for implementation of an EBI, these goals are preliminary. After the planner chooses an EBI, the reports of the evaluation findings for the program should suggest how much change they could expect, and then the program goals can be revised.

## Step 2. Search for Evidence-Based Interventions

This step will help planners identify EBIs that fit their local health problem (or behavioral or environmental risk), organizational capacity, and population. They will most often begin their searches with sites of EBIs such as Effective Interventions: HIV Prevention that Works (https://effectiveinterventions.cdc.gov/en/home.aspx) and RTIPS (http://rtips.cancer.gov/) that offer full intervention descriptions and program materials. As a second option, planners can search sites that describe general intervention strategies with evidence of effectiveness from systematic reviews such as those available in the Guide to Community Preventive Services (http://www.thecommunityguide.org). However, ultimately in order to adapt an intervention, the planning group will identify one or more specific interventions with available materials, that is, "full interventions."

In Step 2, the planning team will complete two tasks: (a) search for an EBI, and (b) judge basic fit to create a "short list" of interventions to carry forward to Step 3. Basic fit is an initial assessment of how well an intervention tested in one setting might fit the needs and resources in another setting. To judge basic fit, the planner considers whether the intervention is a match to the health problem, behaviors, environmental conditions, organizational resources, and characteristics of the population in the new setting or community.

## *Searching for Evidence*

There are several ways in which a team may identify an evidence-based program. It could have been identified and required by a funder or a supervisor, it may have been recommended by a colleague, the planner may have seen it presented at a conference or meeting, or the planner may identify the EBI from an online search. As described above, there are several resources available that can help a planner find EBIs on line. When doing such, a search the team will select the search topics that fit the health problem or the behavioral or environmental risk—at the new site. For example, if the health problem is breast cancer, the search topics might be "Cancer," "Breast Cancer Screening," or "Mammography Screening," and search terms may be added for the setting, such as "Clinic" or "Community," and priority population such as "African American" or "Asian." Then the team will choose whether to look first at website presentations of full interventions (sites that may give access to full programs with a number of different specific strategies) or at systematic reviews of general intervention strategies (that typically do not have direct reviews of or links to full programs).

Depending on what is available from the search, the team will bring a short list with several interventions to Step 3 for judging specific fit and for planning adaptation if needed. To move to Step 3, the team must have detailed descriptions of the program and at least one copy of the materials required to implement the EBI. After the planners have one or more interventions that seem to have at least a basic fit with their site and organizational capacity, they will compare the program with the Logic Model of Change from Step 1. Table 10.1 presents terms and definitions to help planners make sense of search options and what they fill find.

**Levels of Evidence**   All evidence of effectiveness is not created equal. Ratings of the strength or quality of evidence are often presented as a pyramid, typically with systematic reviews and meta-analyses at the top, and "word of mouth" at the bottom (Brownson et al., 2009). Researchers who work on synthesis may sometimes disagree on these hierarchies because the validity of a particular study (and not just a general study type) depends on the study's quality of execution, the likelihood that

**Table 10.1**    Terms for Thinking About Evidence

| Concept | |
| --- | --- |
| Systematic Review | A literature review focused on the question of the effectiveness of a type of program or policy that tries to identify, appraise, select, and synthesize all high-quality evidence relevant to determining evidence for effectiveness. May or may not include a meta-analysis. Also called "evidence review" at the Community Guide website. |
| Evidence Table (or Summary of Finding Table) | A table that presents key information about each study included in a review. In many reviews, descriptions of the interventions tested in each study are included in evidence tables. (The Cochrane Collaboration calls this a "summary of findings table.") When intervention descriptions are *not* included in evidence tables, a reader has to depend on the description of the general category under review and scan the titles of individual studies to decide whether the intervention in a particular study might be of interest. |
| Effect Magnitude or Effect Size (sometimes called Impact) | The size of the intervention's impact on a particular outcome. An odds ratio or standardized mean difference both reflect the effect magnitude. Called "impact" in RTIPs. |
| Meta-analysis | A special type of systematic review that converts the outcomes of the evaluation research studies included in the review to a common statistic that represents the effect size or magnitude of the effect of the intervention on an outcome. The individual intervention effects are then weighted according to their precision or width of their confidence intervals and combined as an overall effect size estimate, with a confidence interval to tell how much certainty there is about the estimate. |
| Evaluation Research Study (Evaluation) | A study conducted to test the effectiveness of an intervention on a particular sample of people (e.g., low income, Latino older adults) or clusters of individuals within an organization (e.g., patients of Migrant Farmworker clinics) in a particular setting (e.g., churches, schools, community clinics). Sometimes called a "primary study" when summarized as a part of a systematic review. Although, an evaluation study is not required to be a randomized controlled trial, it does require attention to threats to validity. |
| Evidence-based intervention | A particular set of activities that has been tested in one or more evaluation/ research studies and found to increase the health promoting behavior, change the environment, and/ or improve the health outcome. |
| Full Intervention | An arrangement that allows a user to download or otherwise have easy access to the intervention materials that were used in the study or studies that evaluated the effectiveness of an intervention. Usually free, but there may be a charge. |
| Intervention Materials | Resources needed to carry out a specific intervention (e.g., implementation protocols, educational materials, training manuals, and tracking logs). The materials should be all that a project team needs to understand and implement the intervention components. |
| General Intervention Strategy | A category of interventions reviewed and labeled in a systematic review. Some categories are relatively simple and specific, e.g., client reminders to get a screening test or provider reminders to recommend and discuss a screening test or vaccination. Others, e.g., "small media" or "group education" do not provide enough detail about an intervention to envision specific programs. |
| Levels of Evidence | Various hierarchies of evidence credibility. |
| Practice-tested interventions | These interventions have been evaluated in practice but have not been tested using more formal research methods; the evaluation reports are not required to be published in peer-reviewed journals. The Canadian Best Practices Portal uses a similar definition, but it does emphasize multiple implementations. This category of evidence would not be called "evidence based" by all funders or public health researchers. Some websites, such as Center TRT, use this label to refer to practitioner-developed interventions that show promise based on their underlying theory, approach, and potential for public health impact *based on findings from an evaluation suggesting they improved one or more behavior or health outcomes.* |
| Emerging or Promising Interventions | Emerging or promising interventions are not evidence based. Defined as interventions that show promise based on their theory, practical applications, and potential for public health impact; they lack data demonstrating effects on relevant behavioral or health outcomes. |

it will deliver the same results in the user's real-world circumstances, and the magnitude and certainty of the impact found in the study. Resources for further discussions of evidence quality are the GRADE Working Group (Grading of Recommendations Assessment, Development, and Evaluation, at http://www.gradeworkinggroup.org/) Partners in Information Access for the Public Health Workforce (http://phpartners.org) and RE-AIM (Reach Effectiveness Adoption Implementation Maintenance at http://www.reaim.org/).

Standards for literature reviews have decreased bias through new reporting standards (Liberati et al., 2009) and quality assessment tools (e.g., Chandler, Churchill, Higgins, Lasserson, & Tovey, 2013) for systematic reviews and meta-analyses. Yet, challenges in understanding evidence summaries remain. Inconsistencies in how intervention strategies are defined and what exactly is being recommended in many other systematic reviews make applying these recommendations in practice challenging. Several researchers have approached addressing some of these inconsistencies by offering more explicit descriptions and standardized classifications of intervention methods (de Bruin, Crutzen, Bishop, & Evers, 2014; de Bruin, Crutzen, & Peters, 2015; Michie & Johnston, 2012; Michie, et al, 2011; Michie, Johnson , & Johnston, 2014; Peters, de Bruin, & Crutzen, 2015).

In general, planners would first be looking for a program described in a Web-based compilation of interventions, such as Research-Tested Intervention Programs (RTIPs) with strong impact score and favorable RE-AIM ratings. Still considered evidence based (but perhaps with somewhat less confidence) is a program with at least one peer-reviewed evaluation research study showing a meaningful impact (effect size) on a behavior or health outcome that is unlikely to be the result of chance alone (moderate to small confidence interval). Examples are EBIs found on RTIPs or the Center for Training and Research Translation (Center TRT) that are labeled "research tested," or all interventions listed on the Canadian Best Practices Portal that are based on a single study.

**Websites for Full EBIs**  We recommend first searching websites that provide descriptions of full programs with explicit availability of the materials needed to judge them for fit and to implement them. For example, planners could begin with the RTIPs website, which describes programs and makes many materials available by download or accessible by contacting the developers. Depending on the health problem, other sites with full intervention descriptions and materials are also available. See Table 10.2.

**Websites for General Intervention Strategies**  Although going to websites with systematic reviews can require more effort to get to specific

**Table 10.2**    Websites for Full EBIs and General Intervention Strategies

| Site | Description |
|---|---|
| *Full EBIs (may include general strategies as well)* ||
| **Effective Interventions: HIV Prevention That Works** (formerly Diffusion of Effective Behavioral Interventions [DEBI]) U.S. Centers for Disease Control & Prevention (CDC) | Descriptions of interventions to prevent HIV and treat HIV infection with links to materials and specific lists of core elements. https://effectiveinterventions.cdc.gov/en/Home.aspx |
| **Healthy People 2020** U.S. Department of Health & Human Services | Descriptions of interventions, strategies, and resources including clinical and consumer guidelines, searchable by health topic. Includes ratings of each resource on publication status, publication type, and number of studies. Resources come from many databases, including gray literature that may vary in rigor. Not all materials are evidence based. www.healthypeople.gov |
| **National Registry of Evidence-Based Programs and Practices** U.S. Substance Abuse & Mental Health Services Administration (SAMHSA) | Descriptions of mental health and substance abuse interventions meeting minimum requirements for review that have been independently assessed and rated for Quality of Research and Readiness for Dissemination. (Users are directed to make their own assessments of an intervention's effectiveness, based on findings.) Includes the research outcomes reviewed, a list of studies and materials reviewed, and contact information for more information about implementation or research. http://www.nrepp.samhsa.gov/ |
| **Smoking & Tobacco Use** U.S. Centers for Disease Control & Prevention (CDC) | Descriptions of interventions and strategies that are evidence-based for states and communities. Includes sample videos, documents, planning tools, and data on tobacco use. http://www.cdc.gov/tobacco/stateandcommunity/best_practices/ |
| **Center for Training & Research Translation** Funded by the U.S. Centers for Disease Control & Prevention (CDC) | Descriptions of interventions and strategies for obesity prevention that are "research-based," "practice-based," or "emerging." Includes Web-based training on implementation of specific programs, evaluation, and techniques for adapting specific programs. Interventions are grouped by level: individual, organizational, or environmental policy. http://www.centertrt.org/ |
| **RTIPs (Research-Tested Intervention Programs)** U.S. National Cancer Institute (NCI) & the U.S. Substance Abuse & Mental Health Services Administration (SAMHSA) | A website within Cancer Control Planet that includes descriptions of programs published within the last 10 years with guaranteed access to materials (most are free). RTIPs rate each program on quality of evaluation, impact, dissemination capability, and readability. For recent postings, it includes the RE-AIM score (reach, effectiveness, adoption, implementation). http://rtips.cancer.gov/rtips/index.do See also a similar website hosted in the Netherlands: http://www.loketgezondleven.nl/algemeen/english/ |
| *General Strategies* ||
| The Community Guide U.S. Centers for Disease Control & Prevention (CDC) | Full-text reviews by topic with evidence tables and logic models. Includes quality ratings for each strategy (i.e., "recommended," "insufficient evidence," and "not recommended"); it also links to other websites, such as RTIPS, when an EBI that is readily available is included in a Guide review. CDC w/contributions from other U.S. Federal health agencies. http://thecommunityguide.org/index.html |
| Health Evidence Canadian National Health Agencies/ McMaster University, Montreal | Over 3,000 quality-rated systematic reviews and meta-analyses of public health strategies with tools and tutorials on developing a search and using evidence-based decision making. The website has and many search filters (e.g., full text available, intervention strategy, intervention delivery method, population) to help guide users to request materials more efficiently. http://www.healthevidence.org/ |

**Table 10.2** *(Continued)*

| Site | Description |
|---|---|
| Canadian Best Practices Portal<br>Canadian National Health Agencies | General strategies on many topics searchable by intervention setting type; some reviews can be downloaded. This website contains tools on evidence-informed decision making and planning public health programs. Not all quality rated and not all are evidence based; full text available for some reviews.<br>http://cbpp-pcpe.phac-aspc.gc.ca/ |
| Trip (formerly, Turning Research Into Practice)<br>Public and Private Sources | Contains quality-rated abstracts of reviews and primary research on health promotion and public program and combines other review databases so you can search all simultaneously. Includes reviews from U.S. Agency for Healthcare Research & Quality, Cochrane Database of Systematic Reviews, and U.K. National Institute for Health & Clinical Excellence (NICE). A new feature is Rapid Review, analyses and syntheses of multiple research articles of single intervention studies on topics where there are no meta-analyses or reviews. Notes: Extensive database; some false-positives; not all materials are evidence based.<br>www.tripdatabase.com |
| National Association of County & City Health Officials Model Practices (NACCHO)<br>Public and Private Sources | Public health programs and toolkits (i.e., templates, training guides, case example, some prepackaged programs) developed and used by the public health community. Includes "promising" as well as "model programs." Search filters guide users. For model practices: state, year, type (i.e., promising, model), category (topic). For toolboxes: can browse toolboxes by keyword, name, toolkit, new tools. Most would be considered practice based. Nonmembers can search for programs; login is required to download materials.<br>http://www.naccho.org/ |

interventions and to their materials, these sites provide a broader view of potential interventions. When planners do not find a good basic fit with a fully described and accessible intervention, they should certainly search these systematic review sites. Conversely, planners may want to review these websites first, to gain an overview of the types or categories of interventions that have been effective in influencing their health problem. Systematic reviews evaluate and summarize the findings across many studies to give an idea whether the intervention strategy will produce the same results in multiple contexts. If the review is a meta-analysis, it will also report the effect size or impact of *each* individual research study and how they compare.

One weakness of the systematic review websites is that they often group together interventions that are superficially similar. For example, a group of programs called "mass media" could be interventions using radio, billboards, or television with various formats, sources, and content. Perhaps more important, these deliveries could be presenting many different theory- and evidence-based change methods. In the case of groups that are too broad or badly defined, conclusions about that particular type of strategy may not be very informative. The websites listed in Table 10.2 also include some strategies with a clear indication of whether there is sufficient evidence to recommend the strategy. Once a strategy looks like it might fit with the problem in the new community, planners will need to look for intervention materials by finding original articles describing the individual programs that were reviewed to come up with the recommended strategies. Planners may then need to contact the program developers to obtain program materials (see Table 10.2).

## Judging Basic Fit

The outcome for this task is a "short list" of programs that planners want to review further for possible use in their sites. We suggest three criteria for judging basic fit: (a) an EBI addresses the target health problem (or risk behavior or environment) and their determinants; (b) organizational capacity is sufficient or can be developed to conduct the program or the EBI can be modestly adapted in light of the resources, and (c) the priority population for the EBI is similar to the population in the new site or the EBI can be adapted for the new population.

**Health Problem and Health Promoting Behavior Fit**   This is the first criterion because it assesses whether a program or strategy is likely to work in a new site at the most basic level. The question for this criterion is: Is there a match of the focus of the original program with the health problem and its causes including behavior or environmental conditions in the new site? To consider whether to adopt a particular program, the planning group will compare the logic model of the problem for the original program with the logic model of the problem in the new setting. The planning group will look for discrepancies between the ways the initial developers described the health problem and how the potential adopters of the program in the new setting understand the problem. In other words, what were the characteristics of the health problem and the priority population in the site where the program was evaluated and how does the original situation compare to the new one? What is the logic model of the problem for the new site? How does it compare to the original needs assessment and logic model? What is the health problem? The behavioral and environmental causes? The determinants of the behavior of the risk group and the determinants of the behavior of the environmental agents? What is different about the problem in the new community? The adopting site? What is the priority population in the new site? How does it compare to the original evaluation site? What are the demographics, context, burden of disease, causes of the health problem?

The answer to whether there is a "health problem fit" is usually a simple "Yes" or "No." In the case of an answer of "No," planners may want to continue searching for programs that match the health problem, behaviors, or environmental conditions or seek programs in closely related areas. For example, a group that found few programs that fit with their topic of being vaccinated against HPV later searched for interventions that addressed other vaccines with the idea to adapt one of these EBIs to HPV.

**Priority Population/At-Risk Group Fit**    The second criterion is fit with the at-risk group at the new site. At first, the question for this criterion seems obvious: Is the group for which the original program was developed the same as the group at the new site? However, a judgment of fit in this criterion may not be so simple. We suggest not rejecting an intervention outright if the population for the original program is not the same as that in the new site. The at-risk group with whom an intervention was tested may have determinants or preferred delivery channels in common with the new population. Therefore, interventions evaluated in a "general" or a slightly different population might still be useful and rated as "maybe" and looked at more closely for the fit of determinants in the next step.

**Organizational Capacity Fit**    This third criterion addresses the match of a program with the adopting organization's ability to successfully implement a specific program. The question for this criterion is: Does the program fit with the organizational mission, strategic goals, and resources? When a planning group recognizes a mismatch due to lack of capacity, it might consider whether training or technical support can help with capacity development. We strongly recommend capacity development rather than cutting a program component because it does not match your organizational capacity. If, however, the program does seem to match on several other criteria but there are changes that may be necessary to make it more feasible based on the existing resources and capacity, planners may choose to proceed carefully with modifications to make delivery more feasible, keeping in mind that these sorts of changes may affect program impact.

## Step 3. Assess Fit and Plan Adaptations

In the previous step, the team created a short list of potential interventions (or it already had a candidate EBI in mind). In this step, the planners can make a final decision about which program to implement by making a more detailed judgement of fit and listing adaptations that would be needed for each program on the short list. With the materials for each candidate intervention as a focus, the team will do the following tasks before making a final program selection: (a) judge behavioral and environmental fit (how well the candidate program fits with the behavioral and environmental conditions in the logic model of the health problem and how well it matches to the desired changes in the logic model of change); (b) judge change methods and determinants fit; (c) judge delivery fit, design features, and cultural fit; (d) judge implementation fit, and (e) consider essential program elements and how to retain them. As the team considers fit and makes a list of needed adaptations, they should remember that less adaptation is the safer choice. Choosing an intervention that requires little adaptation saves resources and protects an evidence-based intervention from changes that may make it less effective.

A recommended starting point for this step is to organize the intervention materials into smaller parts that will be easy to analyze for aspects of fit. Parts of a program might be described as components, such as materials, activities, or sets of materials and activities. See Figure 10.4. For example, an intervention might have a community media campaign, patient support activities, and physician trainings; some planners might think of these as components. Others might be more comfortable describing a program by its activities and materials individually. For example, in Figure 10.4, we analyzed an intervention that was designed to increase physical activity among breast cancer survivors. This intervention seems to have three major components: one for health care providers, one directed toward patients in clinical settings (at-risk group/priority population), and another directed toward community social support for physical activity at worksites. Nested under each of these major components, we encountered both materials and activities. For example, to stimulate patient-provider discussion, the healthcare provider component included the following three materials: guidelines for physical activity in cancer survivors, a prompt in the electronic medical record to stimulate a discussion about the importance of physical activity for survivors, and a patient handout to support the discussion. In the patient component, there was the patient handout (also listed in the provider component), a goal-setting form, and an

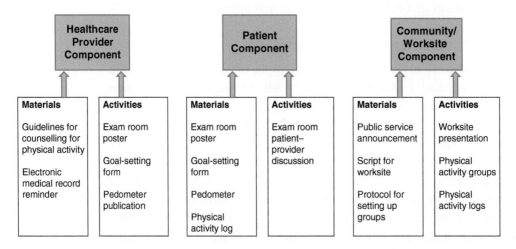

**Figure 10.4**  Parts of a Program

exam-room poster. Again, the materials were in support of one activity, the patient–provider discussion. This program also had a worksite component with activities to form physical activity groups (supported by printed protocols) and a motivational session with a coach (supported by goal setting forms).

Imagine a planning group either sitting at a table with hard copies of program materials for two interventions on their short list of possibilities for EBIs; or, perhaps the group found program materials on a website and can project descriptions and examples on a screen for review. The group also should have one or more descriptions of the evaluation(s) performed on the programs.

## Judging Behavioral and Environmental Fit

For judging behavioral and environmental fit (this task) and change methods and determinants (next task), the planners will then compare the change model in the original program and the proposed logic model of change in the new site. Sometimes, the original developers and evaluators of a program will not have described their original logic model of change in the published literature (or at all). In this case, the planning group for the program adoption will have to work backward from available program materials to try to figure out what behaviors, environmental factors, and determinants the original program developers were trying to influence and what change methods they used. Planners may want to contact the original program developers to obtain more information about the logic of the original program, particularly when this information is not available in published articles or reports.

First, the group members will figure out if the programs have targeted the same risk group behavior and the environmental change they want to target. They will look at the materials, implementation manual, and research articles and/or website description to find descriptions of the behavior of the risk group and of the environmental change agents. They will compare these descriptions to their logic model of change. The questions they will ask are: Does this intervention address the behavioral and environmental changes in the Logic Model of Change and in the project goals for the new population, community, and setting? Where in the program is each behavior addressed? Does the content of the intervention break the behaviors into the steps that it would take to achieve performance? Are these steps those that are necessary to carry out the behavior or make changes in the environment? See Chapter 5 to learn more about creating performance objectives. According to the evaluation results, which health behaviors and environmental factors were changed due to the intervention? Which behaviors are addressed by the content of the intervention? To be a better fit with the planning group's logic model of change and program goals, what adaptations would need to be made? Does the group need to add behaviors or remove behaviors (e.g., behaviors in the original intervention that are not supported by current evidence guidelines)? Does the group need to break behaviors into more detailed, smaller steps? How feasible are the changes the group is recommending? Do proposed changes create the risk of damaging or eliminating the intervention's core elements? Table 10.3 (in the case study below) is an example of a template for capturing ideas about fit and possible adaptations.

## Judging Determinants and Change Methods

After judging whether an intervention targets the correct behaviors for the new community, the next step is to consider determinants and change methods. The following questions can be useful: Does the intervention contain theory-based change methods that will have impact on the determinants from the group's logic model of change? Where in the intervention are these theory-based change methods found? To be a better fit, what modifications in determinants or change methods would need to be made? Does the planning group need to add determinants or add theory-based change methods to a set that may be too weak to influence change in certain determinants? What components of the program might deliver these new change methods? How feasible are these changes? Do they create the risk of damaging or eliminating the intervention's core elements?

Intervention materials and scientific articles describing the intervention may not specifically list the determinants that the developers meant to address. However, by looking at the intervention materials, reviewers can often make an educated guess about whether an intervention addresses a determinant by looking for mentions of the determinant (e.g., messages about risk) and by looking for change methods that can influence the determinant (e.g., role-model stories that help personalize risk). In Chapter 6, the tables of change methods organized by determinants can be very helpful for this task.

Significant adaptations of change methods and determinants may involve altering essential elements of the interventions and should be done only with caution. In general, planners should avoid deletion of change methods and should remember that the EBIs under consideration have been evaluated and judged to be effective. An EBI may also show effectiveness in a new community even with some weaknesses, some lack of fit. When a group chooses to add change methods to strengthen an intervention, it should make sure that the determinants are important in the new community, and that the addition of methods to address them does not create excess burden for either participants or implementers.

**Table 10.3**   Adaptation "To-Do List" for Telephone-Counseling Program

**Intervention 1 Name __Telephone Counseling for Mammography_____**
**Program Resources Available:** ✖ **Materials** ✖ **Description of Program Targets – Behavior** ✖ **Target Population**
   ✖ **Implementation Instructions** ✖ **Results of Research Evaluation**
**Description of Program Targets:** ✖ **Behavior Not Clear-Determinants Not Clear-Change Methods**

| Fit Category | Fit | Location in EBA | Adaptation Ideas |
|---|---|---|---|
| **List Health-Promoting Behaviors From Logic Model** <br> Adherence to mammography | ☐ **Good** <br> ✖ **Adequate** <br> ☐ **Poor** | Manual | Change behavior to "appointment keeping" rather than general mammogram |
| **List Health-Promoting Environmental Conditions From Logic Model** <br> Not Applicable | ☐ **Good** <br> ☐ **Adequate** <br> ☐ **Poor** <br> Not Applicable | Not applicable | No change |
| **List Change Methods (With Determinant) for At-Risk Group** <br> Information dissemination (barriers) <br> Staging (but does not seem closely related to change methods beyond information) | ☐ **Good** <br> ☐ **Adequate** <br> ✖ **Poor** <br> Note: Revise to include local barriers and stronger change methods | Manual: Scripts for each barrier | **Role Modeling:** Quotations from women in the community regarding barriers <br> **Problem Solving:** Regarding logistical barriers <br> **Information Dissemination:** Correcting misinformation <br> **Persuasion:** By culturally congruent navigator <br> **Message Matching to Stage of Change:** Initial message to either preparation/action OR precontemplation/contemplation |
| **List Change Methods (With Determinants) for Environmental Agents** <br> Not applicable | ☐ **Good** <br> ☐ **Adequate** <br> ☐ **Poor** | Not applicable | Not applicable |
| **List Delivery for Components: At-Risk Group** <br> Telephone counseling call | ☐ **Good** <br> ✖ **Adequate** <br> ☐ **Poor** <br> Note: Does not seem to be a conversational structure that would be comfortable for navigators | Manual: Stage of change staging <br> Manual: Barrier scripts | Change staging question and scripts to be less research oriented and more "real-world" navigator approach <br> Develop an active-listening framework for barrier scripts <br> Retain staging but with only two classifications |
| **List Delivery for Components: Environmental Agents** <br> Not applicable | ☐ **Good** <br> ☐ **Adequate** <br> ☐ **Poor** | Not applicable | Not applicable |
| **List Design Features and Cultural Relevance** <br> Barriers are general and information based | ☐ **Good** <br> ✖ **Adequate** <br> ☐ **Poor** <br> Note: Add local barriers and culturally congruent role models | Manual: Barrier scripts | Add barriers described by local women: Perceived likelihood that no cancer <br> Expectation that God will protect against cancer <br> No money for treatment |

(continued)

**Table 10.3**    *(Continued)*

| Fit Category | Fit | Location in EBA | Adaptation Ideas |
|---|---|---|---|
| | | | Becoming less than a woman with the loss of a breast — fear of losing one's partner |
| | | | Cancer is a death sentence |
| | | | Time only for caring for others |
| | | | Logistics: No time off work; no transportation; responsibilities caring for a child or others; money/lack of awareness of programs that can pay for breast cancer treatment |
| **Describe Implementation Plan** Implementation is research-based rather than clinic based. Much of the interview is to ascertain stage of change. It is unclear how the interviewers transition between one barrier and the next and how they move from staging to barriers | ☐ **Good** ☐ **Adequate** ✖ **Poor** Note: Add script with conversational transitions | Manual: staging and barrier scripts | |

## Judging Delivery Fit, Design Features, and Cultural Relevance

Throughout choosing and deciding whether to adapt an intervention, planners have considered cultural issues because both behaviors and determinants are culturally influenced (Nierkens et al., 2013). In this task, the planning group continues to consider culture, particularly whether the EBI will be acceptable to the new population; whether the original delivery will reach the new population; how the design of program materials will resonate with the new participants; and how culturally congruent the entire program will feel to users. At this point, delivery fit focuses on reach to intended users, whereas the next task examines delivery from the point of view of the match of implementation requirement (e.g., personnel and resources) and protocol (exactly who did what, when) with the capacity of the planning organization.

By design fit and cultural relevance, we mean the extent to which the design features of materials used in the original intervention (e.g., credibility, readability, graphics, the aspects of the materials that capture attention and encourage comprehension) match the needs of the new population and setting. These elements are also related to cultural fit, in which, for example, language, people, activities, communities, and values depicted are congruent with an intended population and community.

Here, the planning group continues to judge fit by considering these questions: Will the delivery strategies reach the at-risk group and the environmental change agents? How will participants relate to the format and design of materials in the intervention? How do language, length, specific messages, readability, understandability, pictures, graphics, and layout fit with expectations of the new group of participants? Are materials up to date? Do these features fit with the new population?

A planning group will want the opinions of potential participants about the program, especially views regarding cultural issues, such as language, depictions of family, rules of communication, role of family, spirituality and religiosity, myths, time orientation, ethnic identity, level of acculturation, resilience, medical mistrust, depictions of clothing, music, colors, homes, neighborhoods, and ways of coping. If these perspectives were not garnered in the needs assessment (Step 1), they should be explored here.

When generating ideas for adaptation, planners will need to continue to use caution. For example, when adapting delivery, caution is required because some delivery channels (e.g., community health workers going door to door) are intertwined with change methods, such as role modeling and the cultural credibility of a message. Having a program delivered by a peer to participants or a community health worker may create greater receptivity to a message than would be engendered by another channel. On the other hand, if health professionals were the deliverers, their expertise might play an important role in the credibility of the message and the desire of the participants to comply. Another caution is in decisions to alter design features such as graphics, pictures, music, and layouts. Planners should take care to maintain the content and change methods so that the intended influence on determinants is not lost. For example, changing photographs used for brochures to better reflect a new population may introduce subtle changes in features, such as facial expressions, attire, body language, and so forth. A new photograph with a frowning doctor instead of a smiling doctor may change the content and message. Table 10.4 will continue to be useful as a guide for planning adaptations.

### Judging Implementation Fit

Judging implementation fit begins early in the process of finding an EBI because the way a program is delivered is closely tied to an organization's capacity to deliver it. Therefore, in both Steps 1 and 2 of IM Adapt, the planning team is probably ruling out programs that far exceed local delivery capacity (see Case Study below).

Thinking first about who has to do what to implement the adapted program, and what materials they would need will help the planner make an appropriate assessment of whether or not existing implementation

**Table 10.4**    Examples From the Design Document Template for the Telephone-Counseling Program

| Change | Where | New Content or Content Edits | Delivery |
|---|---|---|---|
| **Change Behavior from Mammography to Appointment Keeping - At-risk Group** | | | |
| **Add: Appointment Keeping** | Throughout manual | Throughout, change making an appointment to keeping an appointment | Throughout manual |
| **Add Determinants and Change Methods** | | | |
| **Add: Foundational Conversation Script** | From beginning of script | SAMPLE Active listening rephrase *"It sounds like you . . . . . . Does that sound right?"* <br><br> SAMPLE Active listening if woman expresses reluctance but does not volunteer reasons *"It sounds like you are little worried/reluctant . . . "* <br><br> SAMPLE Active listening if woman talks about worries/beliefs *"It sounds like you. . . . . "* OR *"What is making you worried about your mammogram? What is making you worried about keeping the appointment?"* | Use active listening throughout phone conversation |
| **Change: Go to barriers scripts as needed [worry barriers first; logistical barriers after all worry barriers probed]** | From beginning of script | SAMPLE Barrier scripts if woman mentions specific barriers *"I have some information on [whatever woman has mentioned]."* Continue to information on barrier. | Use barrier scripts whenever needed throughout conversation |
| **Add: Role Model Story (Outcome Expectations)** | In all barrier scripts | SAMPLE Role model story women mention barrier of too busy *"When we spoke to women in our community, some of them told us that they are too busy taking care of others to take care of themselves. Others said that they are just too busy making a living or doing all the other work that we women do."* <br><br> *"But some women have told us that it's important to have a mammogram to make sure to stay healthy for all of those who depend on them."* | In all barrier scripts |
| **Add: Persuasion** | | SAMPLE of personal persuasion *"I hope that this information has helped ease your worries. I really want you to keep your mammogram appointment even if you do have a few concerns."* | End phone conversation |
| **Change: Initial Designation of Stage of Change** | | SAMPLE of Assessing the woman's "true" intention/reluctance to get a mammogram <br><br> *"Ok, great. Let's talk about your upcoming appointment."* <br><br> *"How confident are you that you will keep your mammogram appointment?"* <br><br> ** If NO barriers — PROBE: *"There have been women in our community who say they are confident in keeping their appointment, but miss because they are worried about something. Is there ANYTHING that concerns you?"* <br><br> ** If STILL NO BARRIERS, PROBE logistical barriers. | Beginning phone conversation |

**Table 10.4**    *(Continued)*

| Change | Where | New Content or Content Edits | Delivery |
|---|---|---|---|
| **Add: Barriers from Local Needs Assessment** | | SAMPLE Woman is afraid of finding cancer *"When we spoke to some women in our community, they said that they would rather not know if they have breast cancer. Some women said that as long as they feel fine, they don't want to look for trouble. One woman said "if it is not broke, don't fix it."* <br> *Other women say something else, which is true: "If you have cancer, you'll find out eventually. It is better to find it early and treat it."* <br> *"And, we have to remember; 9 out of 10 times a mammogram does not find anything abnormal. Getting a mammogram does NOT mean you have cancer."* | Phone conversation |

protocols and materials are appropriate and how they may need to change. Planners are advised to refer to Step 5 in IM for planning implementation interventions to help in this phase.

## *Identifying and Retaining Essential Elements*

Essential elements, also referred to as core elements and active ingredients, are the characteristics of EBIs that are most likely to contribute to demonstrated effectiveness. Although any characteristic of an intervention might be important to its effectiveness in the original research testing, essential elements are most likely to include content (i.e., messages) and theory-based change methods (e.g., modeling, risk appraisal, reinforcement), directed toward specific determinants. We advise great caution and consultation with original developers when changing these elements.

Some elements can be changed with moderate caution. These include adding the following: target behaviors or detail to behaviors (performance objectives) for the at-risk group, health promoting environmental conditions and behaviors of environmental agents, and important determinants and change methods that are possibly weak or absent in the original EBI. Deleting behaviors or performance objectives that are not relevant for the new population or setting or are not supported by guidelines as important to influence health outcomes is also in the category of "moderate caution." However, there is a caveat to dropping behaviors: most EBIs have not been evaluated in a way that allows decisions about whether a behavior can be deleted without decreasing the effectiveness of the program. For example, a program that targeted mammography screening (guideline recommended) might have been effective because it also encouraged breast self-exam (not guideline recommended) perhaps because BSE might raise awareness and interest in breast health.

More caution is recommended if a planner is deleting behaviors that are recommended but that do not fit the goals of the new community. For example, a team may be interested in mammography but has chosen an intervention that also includes Pap testing. Should it remove Pap, or leave it in because its inclusion may have influenced overall program effectiveness? Note that these issues also pertain to deleting environmental conditions. Other elements can be changed with only slight caution: Changing language and graphics to match a new culture, lowering reading level or increasing comprehensibility in some other way (as long as the message remains the same), and adding detail to behaviors of environmental agents and program components to address the behaviors.

## Step 4. Make Adaptations

From Step 3, the planning team has the intervention it has chosen to use and an "adaptation to-do list" to guide this step. Working from the list, the team will do the following tasks: (a) prepare design documents for the adaptations; (b) pretest adapted materials, and (c) produce final adapted materials.

### *Preparing Design Documents for Adaptation*

Table 10.4 (see Case Study below) provides an example of a simple template for preparing a document to guide adaptations. The template links the planned change and the location of the change in program materials and activities. It also cues the team to write the messages that support the change. For example, if the change is to expand the focus on skill development (determinant) with guided practice (change method) a team would write the instructions for guided practice and note what graphics would be necessary to accompany the text. If proposed changes include the *addition* of determinants and change methods (rather than simply enhancing them), we suggest preparing a "minimatrix" that pairs the new determinants with behaviors to create change objectives (see Chapter 5).

### *Pretesting Adapted Materials*

Once the team has decided where adaptations will go in the program and what the new content will be, the next task is pretesting to make sure that their proposed changes are acceptable to the new priority population.

(see Chapter 7). Planners may also want to pretest unchanged program components to judge their impact on new participants. Having potential program participants and implementers respond to intervention materials is important. Pretesting means having individuals or groups respond to program ideas, materials, and components to identify needed corrections. Planners should be sure to show participants discrete program components that they can know exactly to which characteristics participants are responding. Questions to ask include: What do you understand from this material? Tell me about the people depicted: are they like you? Do you find them believable? What would you be likely to do, after seeing this material? What do you especially like? What do you dislike? If you decide to make changes from the pretesting, make sure that you are not deleting essential elements, especially change methods. If you change messages related to change methods, be sure to replace them (see Chapter 7).

### Producing Final Adaptations

Chapter 7 describes how to produce or oversee the production of program materials. One caveat is to make sure not to make unintended changes when making planned adaptations.

## Step 5. Plan for Implementation

In this step, the tasks are the following: (a) identify implementers, implementation behaviors, and outcomes; (b) develop implementation and maintenance scope, sequence, and instructions; and (c) plan activities to motivate and train implementers.

### Identifying Implementers, Behaviors, and Outcomes

This Step should benefit from the assessment of organizational capacity conducted in Step 1 and from instruction in Chapter 8. In Step 5, program planners consider the implementation protocol for the original program (if they can find it) and compare it to implementation considerations and constraints for the new site to create a revised protocol. Wandersman et al. (2008) and Mihalic, Fagan, and Argamaso (2008) underscore the importance of organizational capacity and readiness for implementation. To the extent that the organizations and other implementers in the new setting require additional or different skills, incentives, or conditions for adoption, implementation, or maintenance, these would be reflected in the new implementation plan.

As described in Chapter 8, the implementation plan should include expected implementation outcomes: delivered to whom? When? How much? It should also list the persons who will implement, and their exact roles and required behaviors. How to write performance objectives for implementers is covered in Chapter 8. As in Step 4, modifications to the original implementation protocol should be pretested and pilot tested prior to implementation.

### Developing Scope, Sequence, and Instructions

Developing scope, sequence, and instructions refers to creating a guide that specifies how much of the EBI will be implemented in what sequence, over what period of time, and then writing the instructions explicitly so that new program implementers can know what to do, and when and how (see Chapter 8).

### Planning Activities to Motivate and Train Implementers

Not only do planners have to know what their implementers will do, they have to consider what will motivate them to do the performance objectives. Just like in Step 2 of IM (Chapters 5 and 8), at this step the program adapter explores determinants of implementation and change methods and practical applications that would influence them. Usually for implementation, these methods are woven into trainings, consultation, and technical support activities.

## Step 6. Plan for Evaluation

The tasks in this step are the following: (a) write evaluation questions (for behavior, environment, and determinant changes; process and adaptations); (b) choose indicators and measures; (c) choose the evaluation design; and (d) plan data collection, analysis, and reporting. For extended instruction and examples for each of these tasks, see Chapter 9. Here we comment only differences for adaptation.

An overriding purpose to evaluating an adapted EBI is to determine whether the intervention achieves the same results in the new setting with the changes that have been made ("effect evaluation"). As with other evaluations, questions about how successfully the program was implemented, including how well it reached the priority population ("process evaluation") are necessary. Program adapters who have used a systematic approach to adaptation, such as IM Adapt, will find that they are well prepared to plan their evaluation, because the logic model and explicit adaptation plan provide the foundation for each step of the evaluation. These evaluation findings should be shared widely, including publication in the peer-reviewed literature to contribute to the field's understanding of both the promises and the pitfalls of program adaptation.

## *Writing Evaluation Questions*

"Effect" evaluation questions focus on the impact of the EBI on quality of life, health indicators, behaviors, environmental conditions, and program objectives (determinants, performance objectives, and change objectives). Evaluators usually do not propose to measure all program outcomes, and select only outcomes that are feasible to measure within the program's time frame and provide adequate evidence of the program effect. This means going only as far to the right on the logic model of change for the adapted EBI as did the evaluation of the original EBI. Thus, the main effect evaluation question typically is about behavior and/or an environmental condition rather than a health outcome or quality of life. In the mammography-screening example, the main question would be about the key behavior targeted in the adaptation, "What changes in appointment keeping for scheduled mammograms occurred as the result of the adapted EBI?" The evaluator's questions also should fill in more questions more proximal to the intervention (farther to the left of the main question on the logic model, such as determinants of behavior and environmental conditions). This guarantees that the causal logic will be available to explain the reasons for the results.

Sometimes "shortcuts" can be taken on the logic model. These decisions depend on the extent of the adaptation and strength of the evidence supporting the original intervention. For example, an adaptation may be minimal, with a strong evidence base that includes an evaluation of the original EBI reporting strong relations between determinants and changes in behavior and/or changes in environmental conditions. In such a case, it might be sufficient to measure determinants only.

Of course, a "process evaluation" is essential to determine whom the program reached, whether the adapted program was delivered with completeness and fidelity, and how the participants reacted to it. For an adapted program, the evaluation should also explicitly consider how well accepted were the new and old program elements to the priority population. Some of the questions about acceptability will have been addressed when the adaptations were planned and during pretesting, but adapters may want to reassess at the effect evaluation. Process evaluation questions are concerned primarily with the group receiving the adapted EBI rather than a comparison or control group. Example questions applicable to the mammography case would likely focus on the success in reaching women for telephone counseling, because the use of telephones and the willingness to take calls has shifted so much generally and may be specific to disadvantaged subgroups, and on adherence to scripts by the telephone navigators. Further, the evaluation would probably focus on women's reactions to the calls, the callers, and the new active-listening component to the barriers.

## Choosing Indicators and Measures

Evaluation questions for adapted EBIs can borrow from the evaluation of the original EBI. If the target behavior or environmental condition has been changed in an adaptation, the indicators and measures must match the new logic mode. Switching from adherence to mammography screening recommendations to appointment keeping, for example, clearly defines the behavioral indicator for the effect evaluation. In the mammography example, with the change from general adherence to screening mammography guidelines to appointment keeping (Table 10.3), the primary behavioral indicator would be taken from the logic model for the adapted program, that is, kept appointments (Figure 10.6). Other outcomes also will have been specified in the adaptation process, so it is likely that the main task here is *how* the indicators are to be measured.

A *measure* is a device for quantifying or categorizing an indicator. For example, even appointment keeping for a scheduled mammogram requires thought about the definition of a "kept appointment" (e.g., can the woman have one or more "no-shows" or last minute rescheduled appointments before keeping an appointment and still be called a successful kept appointment so long as this occurs within a defined time window?) and whether to use the clinic scheduling system or some other record. Typically, the same outcome indicators and measures will be used for the adapted program, with the addition of any behaviors or determinants added during the adaptation process. Key ideas in thinking about measures are *validity* (Are the evaluators are measuring the construct they think they are measuring?) and *reliability* (Are the measures stable—at two different times when no change has occurred? For two different observers of the same event?). Again, the original evaluation may provide assistance in selecting measures, and Chapter 9 provides an overview and resources.

## Choosing the Evaluation Design

Many traditional and emerging designs are now available, and Chapter 9 gives an overview and referrals to textbooks and websites. One way or another, the key questions that drive all designs for effect evaluation are as follows: (a) how do indicators of desired program effects compare with what happened before and after the program, and (b) can any changes observed be attributed to the intervention being evaluated?

### Planning Data Collection, Analysis, and Reporting

An evaluation plan includes the effect and process evaluation questions, indicators and measures, and the design, including timing of follow-up measures, analysis plan, resources needed, a time line, and methods of reporting the findings to stakeholders (see Chapter 9, Table 9.7 for an example plan). Although published reports of program evaluations do not often include the time line and resources, they can provide a model for writing the final report.

---

**CASE STUDY**

In the conduct of the project on which this case study is based, we followed each step of IM Adapt. Here we present a summary of the process and the product or outcome for each step.

---

## Step 1. Conduct a Needs Assessment, Assess Organizational Capacity, and Create Logic Models

### Assessing Organizational Capacity

**Setting and Organizational Characteristics**   The setting of the project was Houston, Texas, a metropolitan area of over 3 million population. The city has well-documented health, social, and economic disparities in African American and Hispanic groups (Begley et al., 2012; Highfield, Ottenweller, Pfanz, & Hanks, 2014b).

A local hospital-based charity organization (the Charities), initiated the planning for the project, secured funding, and put together the planning team of stakeholders (referred to here as the project lead agency). Staff at the lead agency had become aware that not only are mammography rates lower and mortality rates from breast cancer higher among African American women in the Houston community as compared to other racial/ethnic groups, among women with appointments for mammography screening, African Americans miss appointments at a higher rate. This type of problem was within the mission of the Charities, and the staff became interested in working with their clinical partner to see if an evidence-based program could reduce the no-show rate for appointments made at mobile mammography sites with primarily African American women.

The planning team included representatives from the lead agency research arm, breast cancer provider organizations, the local breast health collaborative (an organization to establish linkages between organizations with breast health missions), and the local school of public health. All partners had missions that encompassed improving breast health in the Houston area. The researchers from the school of public health and the lead agency also had a commitment to using and evaluating evidence-based programs. The planning team secured funding from the Avon Foundation to find, adapt, implement, and evaluate an evidence-based program to decrease missed appointments among African American women.

**Organizational Capacity**    The main service provider partner was willing to implement a program that could fit into their existing telephone reminder and patient navigator program. The resources acquired from the funder were enough to hire a part-time person to deliver the intervention and to cover the staff time required for the evaluation.

The planning team conducted a site visit of the clinical partner agency to assess resources for this project and determined that some changes were needed in the agency's data collection so that the project could be adequately evaluated.

**Developing a Logic Model of the Problem**    Before searching for an EBI that could address the problem of missed appointments, the planning group conducted a needs assessment of barriers to mammography screening and appointment keeping among African American women in Houston. Working with the Charities' African American community advisors, the planning group conducted a literature review of mammography in African American women, and interviewed and surveyed African American women in the Houston community. We present a brief summary of the assessment outcomes here, with a detailed description of methods and results previously published (Highfield et al. 2014a).

**Summary of the Problem From the Literature Review**    There exists a well-documented and substantial inequality when comparing African American women with other ethnicities' breast cancer mortality rates (American Cancer Society, 2013; Ries et al., 2006). In the last decade, Caucasian and Hispanic women have experienced declining mortality rates (2.5 and 1.2 percent per year, respectively); however, rates for African American women have remained unaffected (Williams et al., 2008). Research attributes the reduction in mortality in the other groups principally to early detection (mammography) and enhanced cancer treatment (Williams et al., 2008). Recent research has shown that African

American women are less likely to make recommended use of mammography screening (Crump, Mayberry, Taylor, Barefield, & Thomas, 2000; Legler et al., 2002; Menashe, Anderson, Jatoi, & Rosenberg, 2009; Schueler, Chu, & Smith-Bindman, 2008; Smith-Bindman et al., 2006; Williams et al., 2008) and are less likely to attend scheduled appointments (Margolis, Lurie, McGovern, & Slater, 1993; Schueler, et al., 2008) with rates of missed appointments at some sites around 30 percent.

African American women experience significant barriers to mammography screening appointment attendance, including individual, environmental, and sociocultural factors (Alexandraki & Mooradian, 2010; Bernstein, Mutschler, & Bernstein, 2000; Crump et al., 2000; Ko, Sadler, Ryujin, & Dong, 2003; Moy, Park, Feibelmann, Chiang, & Weissman, 2006; Ogedegbe et al., 2005; O'Malley, Forrest, & Mandelblatt, 2002; Paskett et al., 2004; Peek, Sayad, & Markwardt, 2008; Schueler et al., 2008; Tejeda, Thompson, Coronado, & Martin, 2009). Facilitators to mammography adherence include physician recommendation (primary driver), recommendation by another health professional (nurse), patient navigation, and mobile mammography programs (Crump et al., 2000; Legler et al., 2002; Wells et al., 2008).

**Local Data Collection**    The planning team worked with African American community members to conduct four focus groups with 34 women. The women described the following barriers to the behavior of mammography: (a) fear of the outcome (it will be cancer), (b) competing demands (taking care of everyone but myself), (c) logistical barriers, such as insurance, cost, and transportation, (d) fear of partner abandonment (loss of womanhood) if cancer is found and mastectomy performed (more common than breast conserving surgery in this group), (e) lack of education (nobody talks about mammography/breast cancer), (f) fear the mammogram would hurt, and (g) belief that their faith would protect them from cancer and thus no need for a mammogram.

The planning group (which included leaders from the local African American community) discussed barriers to mammography in African American women with particular emphasis on community and health care barriers. Access to primary care is a potential barrier because, in Texas, mammography requires a clinical breast exam and a medical order from a healthcare provider who also receives the test results. In addition, low-income women with breast cancer in Houston have breast-conserving surgery at a lower rate than insured women do because of issues with access to radiation treatment. Furthermore, in our local community, women told us that uninsured women have almost no access to reconstructive surgery, thus reinforcing their perceptions that a breast cancer diagnosis can result

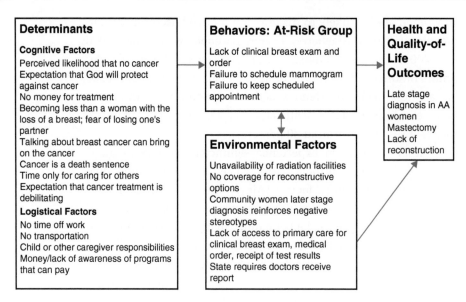

**Figure 10.5**   Case Study Logic Model of the Problem

in permanent loss of a breast leading to rejection by male partners. Furthermore, the higher mortality among women in African American communities may reinforce the sense that the diagnosis of cancer is a "death sentence."

Next, the planning group organized the data from the needs assessment into a logic model of the problem (see Figure 10.5). The planning group focused on both failure to make appointments for mammograms and failure to keep them. They then included all of the information from the community data collection as determinants of the lack of mammograms. These determinants are the community women's perceptions of why they do not get mammograms.

**Developing a Logic Model of Change**   Next, the planning group converted their logic model of the problem to a logic model of change (see Figure 10.6). The logic model of change then served as the foundation for comparing EBIs to the intervention needs in the new site. The team first chose behaviors that needed to change based on the strength of the relation between the behavior and the health outcome, and on whether or not the behavior is changeable. They chose only behaviors of the at-risk group because they did not consider the environmental factors to be changeable in the short run. The group worked from their list of local barriers to determine whether there were categories of barriers

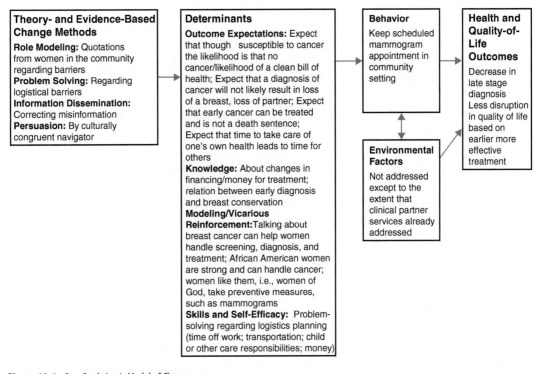

| Theory- and Evidence-Based Change Methods | Determinants | Behavior | Health and Quality-of-Life Outcomes |
|---|---|---|---|
| **Role Modeling:** Quotations from women in the community regarding barriers<br>**Problem Solving:** Regarding logistical barriers<br>**Information Dissemination:** Correcting misinformation<br>**Persuasion:** By culturally congruent navigator | **Outcome Expectations:** Expect that though susceptible to cancer the likelihood is that no cancer/likelihood of a clean bill of health; Expect that a diagnosis of cancer will not likely result in loss of a breast, loss of partner; Expect that early cancer can be treated and is not a death sentence; Expect that time to take care of one's own health leads to time for others<br>**Knowledge:** About changes in financing/money for treatment; relation between early diagnosis and breast conservation<br>**Modeling/Vicarious Reinforcement:** Talking about breast cancer can help women handle screening, diagnosis, and treatment; African American women are strong and can handle cancer; women like them, i.e., women of God, take preventive measures, such as mammograms<br>**Skills and Self-Efficacy:** Problem-solving regarding logistics planning (time off work; transportation; child or other care responsibilities; money) | Keep scheduled mammogram appointment in community setting<br><br>**Environmental Factors**<br>Not addressed except to the extent that clinical partner services already addressed | Decrease in late stage diagnosis Less disruption in quality of life based on earlier more effective treatment |

**Figure 10.6**  Case Study Logic Model of Change

by theoretical constructs that would make the overall list of barriers and counterarguments to barriers more useable in an intervention. The barriers and counterarguments included specific items that fit into the following Social Cognitive Theory (Bandura, 1986) categories of knowledge, outcome expectations, modeling/vicarious reinforcement, skills, and self-efficacy. For example: (a) outcome expectations could constitute a barrier (such as a diagnosis of breast cancer leads to death) and a counter argument (early detection can lead to treatment and cure), and (b) self-efficacy could constitute a barrier (such as logistical problems of caring for others make mammography impossible for me to do) and a counter argument (I can use the problem solving skills I use for other problems). However, it is important to note that these theoretical category labels did not replace the natural language of the women, the way they described barriers. The group completed the logic model of change by adding theory- and evidence-based change methods that are suited to influencing the determinants, such as persuasion, role model stories, culturally congruent role models, and guided practice for problem solving.

### Writing Project Goals

Based on Step 1, the group set the goal to decrease missed appointments of low-income African American women by 20 percent in the first year of program implementation.

## Step 2. Search for Evidence-Based Interventions

### Searching for Evidence

After the group had found definitions of EBIs, they still had to come up with a plan for how to search for one. The planning group was certain that it preferred a program that might be judiciously adapted rather than a general intervention strategy for which they would have to conduct extensive program development. The planning group decided to search broadly for EBIs focused on improving adherence to mammograms in African American women rather than more narrowly on appointment keeping to increase the number of possibly relevant interventions found. They devised the following plan: (a) first look at the Community Guide to review the recommendations for mammography and to see what types of strategies are recommended (prior to searching); (b) search for a program using RTIPS, something that has all the materials available and that can be reviewed, adopted, adapted to fit their community, and implemented without too much redevelopment; (c) if no acceptable program is found in RTIPS, search for evidence that has been synthesized in systematic reviews beginning with the Community Guide and then branching out. If the program was identified from a review, the group members would have to get and review individual primary references. Note: Before the group had this discussion, members had performed a typical academic literature search and came up with hundreds of articles that seemed to be about ways to increase mammography use. They abandoned this first search as being too overwhelming. The group found one promising candidate program (telephone counseling) from RTIPS (Lipkus, Rimer, Halabi, & Strigo, 2000). For the programs found in RTIPS, the team performed a second search with the goal of finding supportive literature (original evaluation research or descriptions of the programs or of program development). While they were searching for these studies, they found articles on three additional programs (one community based, one home visit based, and one church based) that sounded as though they met some of the search criteria (Erwin, Spatz, Stotts, & Hollenberg, 1999; Pasket et al., 1999; Slater et al., 1998).

### Assessing Basic Fit

Before ordering materials or tracking down the original investigators, the team read the peer-reviewed articles, which described the program and its evaluation. The group worked through the main criteria to assess basic fit: Was the health promoting behavior the same as for the new community? Could the organizational capacity support the program? Was the program acceptable for the risk group in the new community?

**Health Problem and Health Promoting Behavior Fit**   The planning group found only programs that encouraged mammography rather than the specific behavior of appointment keeping. Because no programs seemed to be narrowly focused on appointments, the group understood that it would need to adapt the behavioral focus of any of the four candidate programs and continued to keep all four programs on their short list of candidate programs.

**Priority Population/At-Risk Group Fit**   All of the programs targeted either multiple ethnicities or African American women. The planning group realized that any of the programs might be a basic fit for priority population. No matter what program they chose, the group would have to integrate all of the information about local barriers and the way African American women in Houston feel about and talk about mammography and their intentions to get screened or not.

**Organizational Capacity Fit**   The basic fit analysis for organizational capacity led the team to carry only the telephone-counseling program forward for the current project. The main clinical partner did not have the capacity to conduct either community-based, church-based, or home-visiting-based programs. The group thought the telephone-based program fit with the agency resources including funding for a patient navigator to make phone calls. The telephone-counseling program, "Breast Cancer Screening Among Non-Adherent Women," was developed by researchers at Duke University and Kaiser Foundation Health Plan (Lipkus et al., 2000). The intervention is a tailored telephone-counseling reminder based on the Transtheoretical Model of Change (DiClemente and Prochaska, 1998). The program assessed a woman's readiness to attend her appointment through a series of survey questions and counseled her through barriers to attendance. In the original trial, women who were off-schedule with screening were more than twice as likely to get a mammogram if they received the telephone counseling (OR $= 2.10$; 95% confidence interval (1.17, 3.78)).

However, the team continued to be interested in the three remaining programs and may reconsider the community-based, church-based, or home-visiting- based programs for a broader program on mammography among never-screened women in the African American community at a later date.

## Step 3. Assess Fit and Plan Adaptations

In the previous step, the team decided to carry only the telephone counseling program forward to this step to further explore the degree of fit and make a list of proposed adaptations. With the materials for each candidate intervention as a focus, the team judged: (a) behavioral fit; (b) change methods and determinants fit; (c) delivery, design features, and cultural fit; (d) implementation fit; and (e) consideration of essential program elements and how to protect them when making adaptations.

As a starting place for judging fit and planning adaptations, the group obtained the program manual, which included implementation instructions and scripts for telephone counselors to use to discuss barriers. The intervention had only one activity (telephone counseling) and only one program material (manual of instructions and barriers scripts).

### *Judging Behavioral Fit*

Referencing their logic model of change, the group began by assessing how much adaptation would be required to change the behavioral focus from mammogram in general to appointment keeping specifically (see Table 10.3). The template shown in Table 10.3 evolved after this project, but the principles used were the same.

### *Judging Determinants and Change Methods*

After judging whether the interventions targeted the correct behaviors for the new community and suggesting the substitution of "appointment keeping," the group then considered the match of determinants and change methods in the EBI with those on their logic model of change. As Table 10.3 suggests, the planning group thought that the original program was weak in its inclusion of determinants and change methods and suggested the addition of Social Cognitive Theory-based determinants and change methods. In reviewing the manual from the original program, the group could find the script led the telephone counsellor to ascertain the stage of change of the women, possibly for evaluation purposes in the original research, but they did not match specific change methods to stage of change. The group decided to recommend assessing only two stage categories (precontemplation/contemplation and preparation/action) as measured by women's certainty that they would keep their appointments, and then match dialogue to the stage. For example, if the woman seemed unsure (precontemplation/contemplation), the telephone navigator would explore intensively for barriers. The planners then recommended that a conversational script be developed to inquire about barriers in ways that fit with each stage category and that would enable the counsellor to develop rapport with the women. The group thought that change methods such as persuasion, cultural congruence, role modeling, and problem solving would only be effective if conducted in the context of rapport.

The group also found in the manual a comprehensive list of barriers, but barriers were addressed as if most beliefs could be addressed by provision of information. The group noted that most belief change requires change methods beyond information (i.e., role models, persuasion, and guided practice).

## Judging Delivery Fit, Design Features, and Cultural Relevance

In this task, the planning group considered the acceptability of the EBI to the new population, whether the original delivery will reach the new population, how the design of program materials will resonate with the new participants, and how culturally congruent the entire program will feel to users. The planning group understood from the clinical partner that telephone reminders were an effective way to reach the priority population; so the telephone delivery was acceptable. The group also judged that the scripts for barriers were up-to-date, accurate, and understandable, but were not targeted to the exact concerns of local African American women or expressed in the ways that local women talked about their concerns. They also thought that the script would be difficult for clinical navigators to use because it did not have a conversational tone and had no instruction for how to deal with transitions. The group also agreed on an active-listening framework for the scripts to maximize the connection of the navigator with the women through listening to their concerns and acknowledging them.

## Judging Implementation Fit

Implementation fit is closely related to delivery, and the team made several adaptations to delivery as mentioned above. However, implementation also has to do with how the implementing agency will manage the logistics. The planning team worked with the clinical partner to ensure that staff were in place to deliver the telephone counseling, that contact information was available for women with scheduled appointments, and that data from each call and from appointment records could be recorded and accessed for the evaluation.

## Considering Essential Elements of Programs

The planning group considered essential elements of the counseling program. The program was developed over a decade ago, and the developers were not available to answer questions. Therefore, the group independently considered the program to decide the program features that might have been essential to its effectiveness. They listed the following characteristics: (a) barrier-focused counseling (change method), (b) telephone call delivered by a person (rather than a computer [delivery]), and (c) an assessment of stage of change (prerequisite for matching change methods). Looking back at their adaptation "to-do list," they made sure that their suggestions for change did not eliminate seemingly important program elements and sought only to enhance their intensity.

## Step 4. Make Adaptations

From Step 3, the planning team had the manual for the intervention it had chosen to use and an "adaptation to-do list." Working from the list, the team: (a) prepared design documents for the adaptations; (2) pretested adapted materials, and (c) produced the final adapted materials.

### *Preparing Design Documents for Adaptation*

Table 10.4 provides a simple template for preparing a document to guide making adaptations. The template shown here has evolved since this project was conducted, but the principles used prior to the template were the same. The team noted the planned change, described the program materials and activities in which the change should be made, and then wrote or edited messages that supported the change. For example, the team proposed (Table l0.3) to develop a foundation conversational structure based on active listening. Table 10.4 exhibits the change and the script written to support the change. In another example, the team had noted in Table 10.3, the need to insert the specific barriers discussed by local African American women and to reference the fact that the barriers were described by local women who also described strategies for overcoming them (role-model change method). See Table 10.4.

### *Pretesting Adapted Materials*

After the team had adapted the program manual, they pretested the scripts with local African American women. A group of 14 women worked in pairs to role-play the scripts with one woman as a navigator (caller) and the other woman in the pair as a patient. The participants noted needed changes in the scripts to make them as relevant as possible to local women. For example, they recommended taking care not to talk about a cancer diagnosis (and engender fear) in a group that was simply being prepared to undergo screening. The group then thoroughly debriefed the role-plays to the entire project team including the navigator, and the team made the recommended changes to specific language in barrier scripts. The pretesters also strongly urged that the calls be made by a culturally congruent navigator.

### *Producing Final Adaptations*

The team produced the revised manual of barriers and foundational conversation scripts organized in hardcopy form. The hardcopy format was used for the initial implementation and evaluation of the adapted EBI (Highfield, Hartman, Bartholomew, Balihe, & Ausborn, 2015). Following the initial evaluation study, the manual was converted to computer-assisted scripts for use by a live navigator (Highfield, 2014).

## Step 5. Plan for Implementation

In this step, the team identified implementers; defined implementation behaviors and outcomes; developed implementation scope, sequence, and instructions; and trained implementers.

### *Identifying Implementers, Behaviors, and Outcomes*

The team assessed the implementation protocol for the original program and found it to be focused on assessment of stage of change and barriers. The team could find no guidance for the implementer about how to transition from assessment to barriers. In addition, the manual was developed for research staff and not practicing navigators. It was helpful, but not sufficient for this project. The team identified implementers as patient navigators or community health workers familiar with making reminder calls. The implementers would be making standard reminder calls as well as protocol-driven, barrier-focused counselling calls to African American women already scheduled for a mammogram. They also would be documenting the calls. The clinical partners would be providing space and access to appointment records for the navigator. The partner would also provide data on patient appointment attendance for the evaluation study. The desired implementation outcome was the completion of at least 100 EBI calls and 100 standard reminder calls in twelve months.

### *Developing Scope, Sequence, and Instructions*

The scope of the EBI was one completed call per woman. The sequence was seen as the sequence of the call to include: assessment of stage, query regarding barriers, and solutions to barriers based on barrier scripts. The "glue" for moving the conversations forward was based on active listening.

### Planning Activities to Motivate and Train Implementers

The team focused on encouraging self-efficacy, outcome expectations, and skill development of implementers. The adapters developed a training manual that included instructions, scripts for opening, moving, and closing conversations, and barrier scripts. In the training sessions, we explained the theory behind the program, but spent the vast majority of the sessions in informal role-play practice. The role plays were broken into segments and practiced with feedback until the entire team including the navigator could use the scripts in real time.

## Step 6. Plan for Evaluation

The team thought it was important and best practice to evaluate its adapted EBI in the practice setting. The evaluation sought to accomplish two aims: (a) determine the effectiveness of an adapted EBI in improving appointment keeping for mammography in African American women, and (b) describe processes of implementation of an EBI in a practice setting.

### Writing Evaluation Questions

We wrote the following evaluation questions for the effectiveness evaluation: (a) what was the effectiveness in decreasing appointment "no-show" rates in the new setting, and (2) how did the effectiveness of the adapted EBI in improving appointment-keeping compare to the effectiveness of the original EBI in improving mammography rates among nonadherent women? The questions for the process or implementation evaluation included the following: (a) was the adapted EBI delivered to the intended population (i.e., low-income African American women with mobile mammography appointments); (b) did the implementers follow the protocol (i.e., implemented with fidelity); (c) what barriers were discussed in the phone calls; (d) did the women who received the adapted EBI find it helpful and acceptable, and (e) what problems occurred during implementation of the adapted EBI?

### Choosing Indicators and Measures

To measure effectiveness, we obtained kept and missed appointments from the electronic database of the clinical partner's mobile mammography program. We also collected the site of screening; time between phone call and appointment as 0 days, 1 day, 2 days, 3–4 days, and 5 days or more; age in categories of 35–39, 40–49, and 50–64 years old; sponsored status (lack of insurance and ≤200 percent federal poverty level [FPL]); date and time of appointment; and contact information including phone number. We evaluated implementation fidelity by monitoring of intervention phone calls and comparing them to the protocol, making site visits to the clinical partner, and meeting with implementation staff (researchers and practitioners). We coded whether the navigator asked the staging question, used the barrier scripts appropriately, conducted logistical planning, and used active listening: "Is that what you mean?"

In addition, we made postintervention follow-up phone calls to randomly selected patients receiving the intervention to assess their perception of the EBI calls and systems barriers encountered. In these calls, we asked the following questions regarding satisfaction with the phone call: whether anything about the phone call helped with appointment keeping, reasons for keeping the appointment, and recommended improvements to the program.

## Choosing the Evaluation Design

We originally planned a randomized controlled trial but found that the navigator could not readily implement scripts for usual care or the adapted EBI according to a scheme for random assignment. Therefore, we changed to a design in which we assigned contacted women to usual care or adapted intervention in sequential groups of 50 patients.

## Planning Data Collection, Analysis, and Reporting

We sought and obtained funding for the evaluation from the Avon Foundation (project numbers 05-2010-004 & 05-2011-008) and we obtained Institutional Review Board approval from St. Luke's Episcopal Hospital Institutional Review Board.

We enrolled African American females who were age 35–64 years, uninsured, income of ≤200 percent of the federal poverty level and with an upcoming appointment for a mobile screening mammogram. We identified eligible patients from the electronic patient scheduling records at our clinical partner.

We tracked all data for the pilot either in an Access database or paper data collection forms. The database included fields for a unique identifier for each patient, date and time of attempted call(s) with outcome of each (reached, not reached, left message, bad number), barriers, and systems barriers encountered during the session, such as the patient was not aware they needed a doctor's order to receive a mammogram. We included an open text-field for the patient navigator to record notes during the call. Data from both the project database and the clinical partner database were exported to Stata for analysis.

We calculated descriptive statistics and then conducted logistic regression analysis to report attendance in the intervention group compared to the comparison group while controlling for potential confounders (patient age, screening site, number of days from appointment to call, navigator making the reminder call). To determine whether appointment site, time between call and appointment, and age were related to attendance, we fit unadjusted and adjusted logistic regression models. We conducted power analysis using a two-tailed two sample frequencies Fisher Exact test with $\alpha = 0.05$, and adjusted for unequal sample sizes to evaluate our ability to detect a difference between the groups. Following the basic analysis, we further evaluated the effectiveness of the EBI using intent to treat analysis (Gupta, 2011; Heritier, Gebski, & Keech, 2003; LaValley, 2003; Newell, 1992; Wertz, 1995).

## Project Outcomes and Current Status

The evaluation for this project was completed and the results have been used to acquire funding for a larger implementation of the adapted EBI (Highfield, 2014). The project approached women at 41 mammography sites in eight counties. The evaluation results are available elsewhere (Highfield et al., 2015). The effectiveness results were in the range of the results from the original intervention evaluation (Lipkus et al., 2000).

The implementation evaluation allowed us to discover problems in the initial implementation and correct them with a change in evaluation design and eventually in navigator personnel. Other findings from the implementation evaluation were that it is possible to reach women by telephone and engage them in discussion about barriers to screening. Patients reported positive interactions with the navigator saying things such as, "she was warm, friendly, helpful, sweet, supportive, and sincere." When asked if there was something about the phone call from the navigator that helped them to keep their appointment, patients reported that a number of things from the phone call helped them to attend their appointment, including: "the encouragement from her [the navigator] went beyond a reminder call, she cared, put me first, helped me overcome my misconceptions, was nice."

## Summary

This chapter presents an abbreviated version of IM to be used for adaptation of evidence based-interventions (see Figure 10.1). IM Adapt can guide researchers and practitioners in the selection of an EBI, decisions about whether it should be adapted, and plans for and execution of adaptation. The chapter can also help those engaged in adapting an intervention take care to consider parts of the intervention that may be responsible for its effectiveness and should be guarded (rather than adapted).

In this chapter, we present a case study of a community project for which we used the IM Adapt framework to find, adapt, implement, and evaluate an EBI to help underserved African American women in Houston, Texas, keep appointments for mammography screening.

IM Adapt should be useful for planners who are considering EBIs to avoid developing an intervention from the beginning. Not wanting to develop an intervention de novo could be from awareness of insufficient resources for developing an intervention from scratch, or because a funder has required the use of an existing EBI. Therefore, some organizations must find programs that have been evaluated, found to be effective, and are available for use. If a planning group is able to find an EBI that addresses its priority health problem, it will face a core question: Does this program fit with our community and with the characteristics of the health problem in the new setting, and can it be adapted so that it better fits and still works? IM Adapt is a guide for answering these questions and performing a systematic adaptation.

For choosing and adapting an EBI, the IM Adapt framework suggests the following steps: (a) conduct a needs assessment and assess organizational capacity; (b) search for EBIs; (c) assess fit and plan adaptations; (d) modify materials and activities, (e) plan for implementation, and (f) plan for evaluation with a focus on changes to the EBI. See Figure 10.1.

## Discussion Questions and Learning Activities

1. Explain the dilemma in the decision regarding adapting a program for a new setting and retaining fidelity to the original program to assure continuing effectiveness.

2. What is meant by the term *essential elements* in relation to an EBI?

3. Look at Figure 10.1. Describe the sequence of activities in which you would engage to find and adapt an EBI.

4. Describe strengths and weaknesses of the adaption of the mammography program described in the Case Study.

5. Describe strengths and weaknesses of IM Adapt as a systematic process for helping to improve fit of an EBI as it is used in a new site.

## References

Alexandraki, I., & Mooradian, A. D. (2010). Barriers related to mammography use for breast cancer screening among minority women. *Journal of the National Medical Association, 102*(3), 206–218.

American Cancer Society. (2013). Cancer facts & figures 2013. Retrieved from http://www.cancer.org/acs/groups/content/@epidemiologysurveilance/documents/document/acspc-036845.pdf

Backer, T. E. (2001). *Finding the balance: Program fidelity and adaptation in substance abuse prevention: A state of the art review*. Rockville, MD: Department of Health and Human Services, Substance Abuse and Mental Health Services Administration, Center for Substance Abuse Prevention.

Backer, T. E. (2002). *Finding the balance: Program fidelity and adaptation in substance abuse prevention: A state of the art review. 2002 conference edition*. Rockville, MD: Department of Health and Human Services, Substance Abuse and Mental Health Services Administration, Center for Substance Abuse Prevention.

Bandura, A. (1986). *Social foundations of thought and action: A Social Cognitive Theory*. Englewood Cliffs, NJ: Prentice-Hall.

Barrera, M., Jr., Castro, F. G., Strycker, L. A., & Toobert, D. J. (2013). Cultural adaptations of behavioral health interventions: A progress report. *Journal of Consulting and Clinical Psychology, 81*(2), 196–205.

Bartholomew, L. K., & Mullen, P. D. (2011). Five roles for using theory and evidence in the design and testing of behavior change interventions. *Journal of Public Health Dentistry, 71*(S1), S20–S33.

Begley, C., Deshmukh, A., Eschbach, K., Fouladi, N., Liu, Q. J., Reynolds, T., & Deshmukh, A. (2012). Health insurance coverage in the Houston-Galveston area under the Patient Protection and Affordable Care Act. *Texas Medicine, 108*(11), e1.

Bernstein, J., Mutschler, P., & Bernstein, E. (2000). Keeping mammography referral appointments: Motivation, health beliefs, and access barriers experienced by older minority women. *Journal of Midwifery & Women's Health, 45*(4), 308–313.

Botvin, G. J. (2004). Advancing prevention science and practice: Challenges, critical issues, and future directions. *Prevention Science, 5*(1), 69–72.

Brownson, R. C., Allen, P., Duggan, K., Stamatakis, K. A., & Erwin, P. C. (2012). Fostering more-effective public health by identifying administrative evidence-based practices: A review of the literature. *American Journal of Preventive Medicine, 43*(3), 309–319.

Brownson, R. C., Fielding, J. E., & Maylahn, C. M. (2009). Evidence-based public health: A fundamental concept for public health practice. *Annual Review of Public Health, 30*, 175–201.

Card, J. J., Solomon, J., & Cunningham, S. D. (2011). How to adapt effective programs for use in new contexts. *Health Promotion Practice, 12*(1), 25–35.

Centers for Disease Control and Prevention. (n.d.). Effective interventions: HIV prevention that works. Retrieved from https://effectiveinterventions.cdc.gov/

Chandler, J., Churchill, R., Higgins, J., Lasserson, T., & Tovey, D. (2013). Methodological standards for the conduct of new Cochrane intervention reviews. Retrieved from http://editorial-unit.cochrane.org/mecir

Chen, E. K., Reid, M. C., Parker, S. J., & Pillemer, K. (2013). Tailoring evidence-based interventions for new populations: A method for program adaptation through community engagement. *Evaluation & the Health Professions, 36*(1), 73–92.

Crump, S. R., Mayberry, R. M., Taylor, B. D., Barefield, K. P., & Thomas, P. E. (2000). Factors related to noncompliance with screening mammogram appointments among low-income African-American women. *Journal of the National Medical Association, 92*(5), 237–246.

Damschroder, L. J., Aron, D. C., Keith, R. E., Kirsh, S. R., Alexander, J. A., & Lowery, J. C. (2009). Fostering implementation of health services research findings into practice: A consolidated framework for advancing implementation science. *Implementation Science, 4*(1), 50.

de Bruin, M., Crutzen, R., Bishop, F., & Evers, S. (2014). Discussion: Risk of bias in health behaviour change trials: Do we need agenda for research and research practice? *European Health Psychologist,16*(S), 364.

de Bruin, M., Crutzen, R., & Peters, G. Y. (2015). Everything should be as simple as possible, but this will still be complex: A reply to various commentaries on IPEBA. *Health Psychology Review, 9*(1), 38–41.

DiClemente, C. C., & Prochaska, J. O. (1998). Toward a comprehensive Transtheoretical Model of Change. In W. Miller & N. Heather (Eds.), *Treating addictive behaviors* (pp. 3–24). New York, NY: Plenum Press.

Drake, R. E., Goldman, H. H., Leff, H. S., Lehman, A. F., Dixon, L., Mueser, K. T., & Torrey, W. C. (2001). Implementing evidence-based practices in routine mental health service settings. *Psychiatric Services, 52*(2), 179–182.

Durlak, J. A., & DuPre, E. P. (2008). Implementation matters: A review of research on the influence of implementation on program outcomes and the factors affecting implementation. *American Journal of Community Psychology, 41*(3–4), 327–350.

Elliott, D. S., & Mihalic, S. (2004). Issues in disseminating and replicating effective prevention programs. *Prevention Science, 5*(1), 47–53.

Erwin, D. O., Spatz, T. S., Stotts, R. C., & Hollenberg, J. A. (1999). Increasing mammography practice by African American women. *Cancer Practice, 7*(2), 78–85.

Glasgow, R. E., Klesges, L. M., Dzewaltowski, D. A., Estabrooks, P. A., & Vogt, T. M. (2006). Evaluating the impact of health promotion programs: Using the RE-AIM framework to form summary measures for decision making involving complex issues. *Health Education Research, 21*(5), 688–694.

Goddard, C., & Harding, W. (2003). Selecting the program that's right for you: A feasibility assessment tool. Retrieved from http://hhd.org/resources/assessmenttools/selecting-program-s-right-you-feasibility-assessment-tool

Green, L. W., & Kreuter, M. W. (2005). *Health program planning: An educational and ecological approach* (4th ed.). New York, NY: McGraw Hill Professional.

Gupta, S. K. (2011). Intention-to-treat concept: A review. *Perspectives in Clinical Research, 2*(3), 109–112.

Heritier, S. R., Gebski, V. J., & Keech, A. C. (2003). Inclusion of patients in clinical trial analysis: The intention-to-treat principle. *Medical Journal of Australia, 179*(8), 438–440.

Highfield, L. (2014). *Evidence-based dissemination for mammography adherence in safety net communities.* Unpublished manuscript.

Highfield, L., Bartholomew, L. K., Hartman, M. A., Ford, M. M., & Balihe, P. (2014a). Grounding evidence-based approaches to cancer prevention in the community: A case study of mammography barriers in underserved African American women. *Health Promotion Practice, 15*(6), 904–914.

Highfield, L., Hartman, M. A., *Bartholomew,* L. K., Balihe, P., & Ausborn, V. M. (2015). *Evaluation of the effectiveness and implementation of an adapted evidence-based mammography intervention.* Unpublished manuscript.

Highfield, L., Ottenweller, C., Pfanz, A., & Hanks, J. (2014b). Interactive web-based portals to improve patient navigation and connect patients with primary care and specialty services in underserved communities. *Perspectives in Health Information Management, 11*(Spring), 1e.

Kirby, D. B., Baumler, E., Coyle, K. K., Basen-Engquist, K., Parcel, G. S., Harrist, R., & Banspach, S. W. (2004). The "Safer Choices" intervention: Its impact on the sexual behaviors of different subgroups of high school students. *Journal of Adolescent Health, 35*(6), 442–452.

Ko, C. M., Sadler, G. R., Ryujin, L., & Dong, A. (2003). Filipina American women's breast cancer knowledge, attitudes, and screening behaviors. *BMC Public Health, 3,* 27.

Krivitsky, L. N., Parker, S. J., Pal, A., Meckler, L., Shengelia, R., & Reid, M. C. (2012). A systematic review of health promotion and disease prevention program adaptations: How are programs adapted? In E. Wethington & R. E. Dunifon (Eds.), *Research for the public good: Applying the methods of translational research to improve health and well-being* (pp. 73–99). Washington, DC: American Psychological Association.

Kumpfer, K. L., Pinyuchon, M., Teixeira de Melo, A., & Whiteside, H. O. (2008). Cultural adaptation process for international dissemination of the strengthening families program. *Evaluation & the Health Professions, 31*(2), 226–239.

Lau, A. S. (2006). Making the case for selective and directed cultural adaptations of evidence-based treatments: Examples from parent training. *Clinical Psychology: Science and Practice, 13*(4), 295–310.

LaValley, M. P. (2003). *Intent-to-treat analysis of randomized clinical trials.* ACR/ARHP Annual Scientific Meeting, Boston University.

Lee, S. J., Altschul, I., & Mowbray, C. T. (2008). Using planned adaptation to implement evidence-based programs with new populations. *American Journal of Community Psychology, 41*(3–4), 290–303.

Leerlooijer, J. N., Ruiter, R. A. C., Reinders, J., Darwisyah, W., Kok, G., & Bartholomew, L. K. (2011). The world starts with me: Using intervention mapping for the systematic adaptation and transfer of school-based sexuality education from Uganda to Indonesia. *Translational Behavioral Medicine, 1*(2), 331–340.

Legler, J., Meissner, H. I., Coyne, C., Breen, N., Chollette, V., & Rimer, B. K. (2002). The effectiveness of interventions to promote mammography among women with historically lower rates of screening. *Cancer Epidemiology, Biomarkers & Prevention, 11*(1), 59–71.

Liberati, A., Altman, D. G., Tetzlaff, J., Mulrow, C., Gøtzsche, P. C., Ioannidis, J. P.,...Moher, D. (2009). The PRISMA statement for reporting systematic reviews and meta-analyses of studies that evaluate health care interventions: Explanation and elaboration. *Annals of Internal Medicine, 151*(4), W-65–W-94.

Lipkus, I. M., Rimer, B. K., Halabi, S., & Strigo, T. S. (2000). Can tailored interventions increase mammography use among HMO women? *American Journal of Preventive Medicine, 18*(1), 1–10.

Margolis, K. L., Lurie, N., McGovern, P. G., & Slater, J. S. (1993). Predictors of failure to attend scheduled mammography appointments at a public teaching hospital. *Journal of General Internal Medicine, 8*(11), 602–605.

McKleroy, V. S., Galbraith, J. S., Cummings, B., Jones, P., Harshbarger, C., Collins, C., ... ADAPT Team. (2006). Adapting evidence-based behavioral interventions for new settings and target populations. *AIDS Education & Prevention, 18*(Suppl), 59–73.

Menashe, I., Anderson, W. F., Jatoi, I., & Rosenberg, P. S. (2009). Underlying causes of the black-white racial disparity in breast cancer mortality: A population-based analysis. *Journal of the National Cancer Institute, 101*(14), 993–1000.

Michie, S., Ashford, S., Sniehotta, F. F., Dombrowski, S. U., Bishop, A., & French, D. P. (2011). A refined taxonomy of behaviour change techniques to help people change their physical activity and healthy eating behaviours: The CALO-RE taxonomy. *Psychology & Health, 26*(11), 1479–1498.

Michie, S., Johnson, B. T., & Johnston, M. (2014). Advancing cumulative evidence on behaviour change techniques and interventions: A comment on Peters, de Bruin, and Crutzen. *Health Psychology Review, 9*(1), 25–29.

Michie, S., & Johnston, M. (2012). Theories and techniques of behaviour change: Developing a cumulative science of behaviour change. *Health Psychology Review, 6*(1), 1–6.

Mihalic, S. F., Fagan, A. A., & Argamaso, S. (2008). Implementing the LifeSkills training drug prevention program: Factors related to implementation fidelity. *Implementation Science, 3*(5), 1–16.

Moy, B., Park, E. R., Feibelmann, S., Chiang, S., & Weissman, J. S. (2006). Barriers to repeat mammography: Cultural perspectives of African-American, Asian, and Hispanic women. *Psycho-Oncology, 15*(7), 623–634.

Newell, D. J. (1992). Intention-to-treat analysis: Implications for quantitative and qualitative research. *International Journal of Epidemiology, 21*(5), 837–841.

Nierkens, V., Hartman, M. A., Nicolaou, M., Vissenberg, C., Beune, E. J., Hosper, K.,... Stronks, K. (2013). Effectiveness of cultural adaptations of interventions aimed at smoking cessation, diet, and/or physical activity in ethnic minorities. A systematic review. *PloS One, 8*(10), e73373.

Ogedegbe, G., Cassells, A. N., Robinson, C. M., DuHamel, K., Tobin, J. N., Sox, C. H., & Dietrich, A. J. (2005). Perceptions of barriers and facilitators of cancer early detection among low-income minority women in community health centers. *Journal of the National Medical Association, 97*(2), 162–170.

O'Malley, A. S., Forrest, C. B., & Mandelblatt, J. (2002). Adherence of low-income women to cancer screening recommendations. *Journal of General Internal Medicine, 17*(2), 144–154.

Paskett, E. D., Tatum, C. M., D'Agostino, R., Jr., Rushing, J., Velez, R., Michielutte, R., & Dignan, M. (1999). Community-based interventions to improve breast and cervical cancer screening: Results of the Forsyth County cancer screening (FoCaS) project. *Cancer Epidemiology, Biomarkers & Prevention, 8*(5), 453–459.

Paskett, E. D., Tatum, C., Rushing, J., Michielutte, R., Bell, R., Foley, K. L., . . . Dickinson, S. (2004). Racial differences in knowledge, attitudes, and cancer screening practices among a triracial rural population. *Cancer, 101*(11), 2650–2659.

Peek, M. E., Sayad, J. V., & Markwardt, R. (2008). Fear, fatalism and breast cancer screening in low-income African-American women: The role of clinicians and the health care system. *Journal of General Internal Medicine, 23*(11), 1847–1853.

Peters, G. Y., de Bruin, M., & Crutzen, R. (2015). Everything should be as simple as possible, but no simpler: Towards a protocol for accumulating evidence regarding the active content of health behaviour change interventions. *Health Psychology Review, 9*(1), 1–14.

Ries, L. A. G., Harkins, D., Krapcho, M., Mariotto, A., Miller, B. A., Feuer, E. J., . . . (Eds.). (2006). *SEER cancer statistics review, 1975–2003.* Bethesda, MD: National Cancer Institute.

Scaccia, J., Cook, B., Lamont, A., Wandersman, A., Castellow, J., Katz, J., & Beidas, R. (2014). A practical implementation science heuristic for organizational readiness: R= MC2. *Journal of Community Psychology, 43*(4), 484–501.

Schueler, K. M., Chu, P. W., & Smith-Bindman, R. (2008). Factors associated with mammography utilization: A systematic quantitative review of the literature. *Journal of Women's Health, 17*(9), 1477–1498.

Shen, J., Yang, H., Cao, H., & Warfield, C. (2008). The Fidelity–Adaptation relationship in non-evidence-based programs and its implication for program evaluation. *Evaluation, 14*(4), 467–481.

Slater, J. S., Ha, C. N., Malone, M. E., McGovern, P., Madigan, S. D., Finnegan, J. R., . . . Lurie, N. (1998). A randomized community trial to increase mammography utilization among low-income women living in public housing. *Preventive Medicine, 27*(6), 862–870.

Smith, E., & Caldwell, L. (2007). Adapting evidence-based programs to new contexts: What needs to be changed? *Journal of Rural Health, 23*(S1), 37–41.

Smith-Bindman, R., Miglioretti, D. L., Lurie, N., Abraham, L., Barbash, R. B., Strzelczyk, J., . . . Kerlikowske, K. (2006). Does utilization of screening mammography explain racial and ethnic differences in breast cancer? *Annals of Internal Medicine, 144*(8), 541–553.

Stirman, S. W., Miller, C. J., Toder, K., & Calloway, A. (2013). Development of a framework and coding system for modifications and adaptations of evidence-based interventions. *Implementation Science, 8*(1), 65.

Tejeda, S., Thompson, B., Coronado, G. D., & Martin, D. P. (2009). Barriers and facilitators related to mammography use among lower educated Mexican women in the USA. *Social Science & Medicine, 68*(5), 832–839.

Tortolero, S. R., Markham, C. M., Parcel, G. S., Peters, R. J., Jr., Escobar-Chaves, S. L., Basen-Engquist, K., & Lewis, H. L. (2005). Using Intervention Mapping to adapt an effective HIV, sexually transmitted disease, and pregnancy prevention program for high-risk minority youth. *Health Promotion Practice, 6*(3), 286–298.

van Daele, T., van Audenhove, C., Hermans, D., van den Bergh, O., & van den Broucke, S. (2014). Empowerment implementation: Enhancing fidelity and adaptation in a psycho-educational intervention. *Health Promotion International, 29*(2), 212–222.

Wandersman, A., Duffy, J., Flaspohler, P., Noonan, R., Lubell, K., Stillman, L., . . . Saul, J. (2008). Bridging the gap between prevention research and practice: The Interactive Systems Framework for dissemination and implementation. *American Journal of Community Psychology, 41*(3–4), 171–181.

Wells, K. J., Battaglia, T. A., Dudley, D. J., Garcia, R., Greene, A., Calhoun, E., . . . Raich, P. C. (2008). Patient navigation: State of the art or is it science? *Cancer, 113*(8), 1999–2010.

Wertz, R. T. (1995). Intention to treat: Once randomized, always analyzed. *Clinical Aphasiology, 23*, 57–64.

Williams, K. P., Sheppard, V. B., Todem, D., Mabiso, A., Wulu, J. T., Jr., & Hines, R. D. (2008). Family matters in mammography screening among African-American women age >40. *Journal of the National Medical Association, 100*(5), 508–515.

Wingood, G. M., & DiClemente, R. J. (2008). The ADAPT-ITT model: A novel method of adapting evidence-based HIV interventions. *Journal of Acquired Immune Deficiency Syndromes (1999), 47*(Suppl 1), S40–S46.

Page references followed by *fig* indicate an illustrated figure; followed by *t* indicate a table; followed by *b* indicate a box.

active learning
  changing behavior through, 376*t*
  scene from HIV-prevention active learning video, 402
  for translating change methods to application, 401–402
  *See also* learning
Act Knowledge & Aspen Institute Roundtable on Community Change (2003), 14
actual norms, 308
ACT-UP (AIDS Coalition to Unleash Power), 180
adaptation. *See* evidence-based interventions (EBIs) adaptation; IM Adapt framework
adherence and self-management behaviors, 288–289
adolescents
  Dutch HIV/AIDS-Prevention Program for, 371, 400–401, 577, 578*t*–579*t*
  iCHAMPSS Model (Choosing and Maintaining Programs for Sex Education in Schools) for, 367
  identifying determinants when planning an AIDS prevention program for, 306
  matching tobacco use change methods to intervention levels, 353–354
  overestimation of tobacco use by, 308
  participatory approach to implementation planning of TAAG program for girls, 493
  performance objectives for consistent and correct condom use by, 296*t*
  program to increase condom use by sexually active, 22*t*
  U.S. Department of Health and Human Services Office of Adolescent Health, 528*b*
  *See also* children; It's Your Game . . . Keep It Real (IYG) project; school programs
adopters
  characteristics of innovation and, 117–119
  collecting data from, 513
  Diffusion of Innovations Theory (DIT) on innovation and, 61*t*, 116–120
  innovation as an idea, practice, or product new to the, 116
  social norm change process and role of early, 173
  stating outcomes and performance objectives for adoption by, 497–500, 505–506
adoption
  definition of, 497
  determinants of, 507–513
  It's Your Game . . . Keep It Real project stating outcomes and performance objectives for, 520*t*–523*t*
  Peace of Mind Program (PMP) determinants for, 515*t*

performance objective/program outcomes statements for, 497–500, 505–506
advance organizers change method, 381*t*
advocacy
  advocacy and lobbying change method, 392*t*
  description and function of, 180
  health, 180–181
  media, 182–184, 398*t*
  principles underlying effective tactics for, 181*t*
  three stages of, 181–182
advocacy and lobbying change method, 392*t*
Advocacy Coalition Framework
  comparison of Multiple Streams Theory to, 190
  on public policy process, 189–191, 398*t*
  for society and government intervention level, 61*t*
advocacy stages
  direct action or interventions, 181, 182
  research and investigation, 181–182
  strategy, 181, 182
African Americans
  health problems of youth among, 257*b*–258*b*
  HIV-associated risk behaviors of women, 245
  inequality of breast cancer mortality rates of, 630–632
  It's Your Game . . . Keep It Real project focus on, 256*b*–261*b*
  *See also* racial/ethnicity differences
Agency for Health Care Research and Quality's Evidence-based Practice Center, 599
agenda setting change method, 398*t*
AIDS epidemic. *See* HIV/AIDS epidemic
Alzheimer's disease, 235
American Academy of Pediatrics, 237–238
American Association of Public Health, 11
American Cancer Society (ACS), 229, 493–494
*American Journal of Community Psychology,* 8
American Lung Association, 229
answers. *See* working list of answers
anticipated regret
  as behavioral-oriented theory, 80–81
  to change attitudes, beliefs, and outcome expectations, 386*t*
  moving from method to application through use of, 403
APA Publications and Communications Board Working Group on Journal Article Reporting Standards, 355
application examples
  active learning, 401–402
  anticipated regret, 403
  fear arousal, 403–405
  IYG project, 414*t*–416*t*

application examples (*continued*)
    IYG project screen captures, 474*fig*
    modeling, 400–401
    risk perception information, 402–403
applications
    different levels for translating methods into, 406–408*t*
    examples of translating methods to, 400–405
    how to think about, 399
    implementation and selection of change methods and practical, 514, 518, 526*b*–528*b*
    issues to consider for, 398–399
    process evaluation questions on, 558
    stick to the theoretical parameters of change methods for, 400
    theory, 20, 25*t*–26, 485–487*fig*
    *See also* change methods
appreciative inquiry (AI), 243, 249
apps (eHealth technology), 370
archival data
    finding and using, 246
    secondary sources of secondary, 246, 247*t*–248*t*
ART (antiretroviral treatment), 296
ASPIRE (A Smoking Prevention Interactive Experience), 367
asset assessment
    balancing a needs assessment with an, 251–254
    conducting in different types of health promotion programs, 252*t*–253
    description of a, 251–253
    identifying the intervention setting, 254
asset assessment environmental levels
    information environment, 252*t*, 253
    physical environment, 252*t*, 253
    policy/practice environment, 252*t*, 253
    social environment, 252*t*, 253
asthma
    health and quality of life measures for children with, 561
    Partners in School Asthma Management Program, 309
at-risk behaviors
    anticipated regret argument against, 80–81
    ecological model applied to, 61–62*fig*
    epilepsy PRECEDE model on, 234*fig*, 238–239
    It's Your Game . . . Keep It Real project description of adolescent sexual, 258*b*–260*b*
    logic models for, 61–62*fig*
    needs assessment description of determinants and, 236–237, 239–241
    posing question about, 21
    Reflective-Impulsive Model (RIM) on impulsive, 90–91
    sexual, 22*t*, 245, 258*b*–260*b*
    stating behavioral and environmental outcomes by identifying the, 286–289
    tables for selecting change methods for changing, 375–398*t*
    theories of health behavior on using fear to change, 76–77
    unrealistic optimism and, 96–97
    *See also* behaviors; health-promoting behaviors; risk factors
at-risk population
    constructing matrices differentiating the intervention, 309, 312–313

designation of, 229
IM Adapt framework on program fit with the, 615, 635
It's Your Game . . . Keep It Real project task of describing the, 257*b*–258*b*
IYG logic model of change on
needs assessment description of the priority population or, 229–232
PEN-3 model constructs for understanding cultural factors of, 230
*See also* priority population
attitudes
    methods for changing beliefs, outcome expectations, and, 385*t*–386*t*
    modeling to reinforcement objectives and change methods for changing, 372–373*t*
    stereotyping, 90
    theories of automatic behavior and habits on unaware, 89–90
    ToyBox-Study personal determinants of, 310*t*–312*t*
attribution theory and relapse prevention
    attributional retraining and relapse prevention, 100–101
    for individual intervention level, 61*t*
    overview of, 99–100
    summary of, 101
authority power, 152, 153
automatic behavior
    change methods for habits, impulsive, and, 383*t*–384*t*
    habits as special case of, 92–93
    impulsive behavior type of, 90–91
    nudging used to make desired behavior the default, 93–94
    theories of automatic behavior and habits on, 61*t*, 89–95
    training executive function to control, 91–92
autonomy (versus control) need, 108
awareness. *See* raising awareness

BBC World Service Trust (India), 172
behavioral capability
    change methods for overcoming barriers and influencing, 387–390
    description of, 110
    Social Cognitive Theory (SCT) on self-efficacy, outcomes, and, 109–110
    ToyBox-Study personal determinant of, 310*t*–312*t*
behavioral journalism
    as change method, 393*t*
    DIT on appropriate role-model stories used by, 119
    role in changing social norms by, 173
    *See also* health messages
behavioral outcomes
    identifying health-related behaviors of the at-risk group, 286–289
    influence of subjective and actual norms on, 308
    It's Your Game . . . Keep It Real project, 322*b*, 323*t*, 414*t*–415*t*
    specifying performance objectives associated with the, 294–299
    stating the, 286–291
    *See also* performance (or change) objectives; program outcomes
behavior change theory, 356
behavior-oriented theories

attribution theory and relapse prevention, 61*t*,
    99–101
behavior change theory, 356
    common constructs of, 63–64
    competency, 57–58
    cultural sensitivity of, 62–63
    Diffusion of Innovations Theory (DIT), 61*t*, 116–120,
        163–166, 486, 491
    eclectic use of, 59
    ecological interventions, 59–62*fig*
    examples of when to use in intervention planning, 58*t*
    intervention levels and specific theory, 61*t*
    learning theories, 61*t*, 66–70
    Mayor's Project use of, 64*b*–65*b*
    perspectives on, 58
    Social Cognitive Theory, 59, 61*t*, 65, 81, 96, 109–113,
        118, 305, 308, 324*b*, 486
    stage theories, 61*t*, 95–99
    theories of automatic behavior and habits, 61*t*, 89–95
    theories of goal-directed behavior, 84–88
    theories of health behavior, 61*t*, 62–63, 74–78
    Theories of Information Processing, 25*t*, 61*t*, 70–74
    theories of persuasive communication, 101–105
    Theories of Reasoned Action (TRA), 61*t*, 78–84
    theories of self-regulation, 25*t*, 61*t*, 105–109, 308
    theories of stigma and discrimination, 61*t*, 113–116
    *See also specific theory*; theory
behaviors
    adherence (or compliance) and self-management,
        288–289
    challenges of translating method into application of
        modeled, 351–352
    classical conditioning of, 66–67
    Health Belief Model (HBM) on perception-based
        health, 61*t*, 62–63, 74–75, 78
    IM Adapt framework on program fit with judging
        environment and, 617–618
    operant conditioning of, 67–69
    planning team identification of health-promoting,
        16–17
    program evaluation measure for, 561–562
    RAA and TPB on ways to influence the perceived
        norms of, 83–84
    risk-reduction, 287
    Theories of Information Processing for changing, 25*t*,
        61*t*, 70–74
    vicarious (or social) learning of, 69
    writing effect evaluation questions on, 548–549
    *See also* at-risk behaviors; health-promoting behaviors
beliefs
    for changing behavior, 376*t*
    colorectal cancer screening survey (2008) on impact
        of, 245–246
    It's Your Game . . . Keep It Real project determinants
        of normative, 325*t*–327*t*
    methods for changing attitudes, outcome
        expectations, and, 385*t*–386*t*
    RAA distinction between goals, intentions, and, 82
    RAA's approach to intervention for colonoscopy,
        82–83
    *See also* culture; risk perception; social norms
Black Panthers, 178
Bobo doll experiments, 69
brainstorming
    answers, 20–23

idea generation through, 221
    for PMP adoption and implementation,
        508–510
brainstorming answers process
    description of the, 21–23
    provisional list of answers regarding condom use
        among adolescents, 22*t*
    as theory and evidence core process, 20
    *See also* questioning process
breast cancer mortality rate inequality, 630–631
breast cancer screening
    Cultivando La Salud for, 252, 357, 358*fig*
    Friend to Friend program to increase mammography,
        493–494
    Peace of Mind Program (PMP) to increase
        mammography, 499, 501–503, 507, 508–510, 514,
        515*t*–517*t*
    social norms theories on encouraging mammograms
        for, 173
    study on farm-working women 50 years and older
        and, 243, 252
    U.S. programs using Intervention Mapping in, 34*t*
Brown Berets, 178
budgets
    hiring and working with creative consultants to
        develop materials, 453–455
    program structure and organization task of checking
        the, 437–438
    video production, 462–463
Bureau of Epidemiology, 257*b*


Canada's health evidence, 599
Canadian Heart Health Initiative, 493
Canadian Heart Health Kit, 510
Cancer Prevention and Control Research Network,
    491
cancer screening
    Cultivando La Salud intervention for breast- and
        cervical, 252, 357, 358*fig*
    FLU-FIT program to increase CRCS,
        498–499
    focus groups research on impact of beliefs on
        colorectal, 245
    Peace of Mind Program (PMP) to increase
        mammography, 499, 501–503, 507, 508–510, 514,
        515*t*–517*t*
    predicting Ghana women's cervical, 24
    process evaluation questions for a program to
        increase CRCS, 553–554*t*
    social norms theory on encouraging mammograms,
        173
    study on farm-working women 50 years or older and
        colorectal, 243, 252
    survey (2008) on impact of beliefs on colorectal,
        245–246
    U.S. programs using Intervention Mapping in breast,
        34*t*
capability. *See* behavioral capability
capacity
    community, 61*t*, 169–172
    organizational, 607–608, 615, 629–633*fig*, 635,
        636–638
CARE (Consensus-based Clinical Case Reporting
    Guidelines), 577

CATCH (Coordinated Approach To Child Health)
program
program theme of the, 357
teachers as environmental agents and program
implementers of, 318–319
Center for the Advancement of Health & Robert Wood
Johnson Foundation, 465
Centers for Disease Control and Prevention
as archival data source, 246, 247t
Community Guide of, 599
on creating work group timeline, 218
Diffusion of Effective Disease Control Interventions
(DEBI) of the, 599, 608
HRQOL (health-related quality-of-life) measure by,
560
logic models as fundamental framework for program
evaluation used by, 14
on need for meaningful participation by stakeholders,
214
on overestimation of adolescent tobacco use, 308
on youth health problems among African American
and Hispanic youth, 257b
Center TRT (Center for Training and Research
Translation), 611
cervical cancer screening
Cultivando La Salud for, 252, 357, 358fig
predicting Ghana women's, 24
CF FEP (Cystic Fibrosis Family Education Program), 399
CFIR (Consolidated Framework for Implementation
Research), 119, 489, 491–492, 503–504
change agents
differing from stage to stage, 164
Diffusion of Innovations Theory (DIT) on, 116–117
Force Field Analysis on role of, 161
health promotion practitioners working as external
organizational, 160, 162
power theories on using power to create change by,
153
program design that includes practical applications
of, 348–350
change methods
channels and vehicles for health messages and,
359–364t
classical conditioning, 66–67
examples of various levels and objectives and,
372–373t
Force Field Analysis, 160–161
health behavior change techniques (BCTs), 355
IM Adapt framework on program fit with, 618,
636–637
implementation and selection of, 514, 518, 526b–528b
It's Your Game . . . Keep It Real project, 414t–416t,
474fig
often missing in the health education literature,
350–351
operant conditioning, 67–68
posing question about, 21
process evaluation questions on applications and, 558
program design matching different levels of
intervention with different, 352–354
program design with correct usage of, 351–352
taxonomy of, 355
using power to create change at higher environmental
levels, 153
vicarious (or social) learning of behavior, 69

See also applications; evidence-based change
methods; logic model of change; theory-based
change methods
change methods/theories/evidence tables
behavior change, 378t, 380
change attitudes, beliefs, and outcome expectations,
385t–386t
change awareness and risk perception, 380, 382t–383t
change communities, 395–397t
change habitual, automatic, and impulsive behaviors,
380, 383t–384t
change of environmental conditions, 390, 392t–393t
change organizations, 394–395t
change policy, 397–398t
change social norms, 390, 393t
change social support and social networks, 391–394t
changing social influence, 386–387t
how to use the, 379–380
increase knowledge, 380, 381t
influence skills, capability, and self-efficacy and
overcome barriers, 387–390
reduce public stigma, 390, 391t
change objectives. See performance (or change)
objectives
change process
changing organizational change, 161–162
Force Field Analysis and unfreezing, moving, and
refreezing, 160–161
raising awareness as first step in, 98–99, 371t
Social Cognitive Theory (SCT) on behavior, 59
systems theory on changing systems, 151
charismatic power, 152, 153
CHESS (Comprehensive Health Enhancement Support
System), 366
CHEW (Checklist of Health Promotion Environments at
Worksites), 253
children
asthma and health and quality of life, 561
HOPE project focusing on young Cambodian girls
living in the U.S., 159
Mayor's Project on planning program fighting
childhood obesity of, 4b–7b
The ToyBox-Study focus on increasing physical
activity by, 292
TV viewing hours by, 237–238
See also adolescents; school programs
chlamydia infection/fear arousal change method,
404–405
chunking
increasing knowledge through, 381t
memorizing through, 71
circulating print or online channel/vehicle, 362t
classical (or Pavlovian) conditioning, overview of, 66–67
class inequalities change method, 391t
Cleanyourhands campaign, 571
coalitions
Advocacy Coalition Framework on public policy and,
61t, 189–191
definition and purpose of community, 168
formation and key tasks of community, 168–169
formed as a change method, 397t
interpersonal communication channels and vehicles
used by, 360, 361t
coalition theory
communication intervention level using, 61t

Community Coalition Action Theory, 168–169
Cochrane Collaboration, 570, 599
coercion change method, 392t
collaborative participation principles, 214–215
collective efficacy
    community participation for building, 178
    empowerment at higher ecological levels as similar to, 154
    See also self-efficacy
colorectal cancer screening (CRCS)
    FLU-FIT program to increase, 498–499
    focus groups research on impact of beliefs on, 245–246
    as "practice change" or clinical practice change, 498
    process evaluation questions for a program to increase, 553–554t
    study on farm-working women 50 years or older and, 243, 252
commitment change methods
    early commitment, 384t
    public commitment, 384t, 389t
Committee on Health Literacy, 452
communication
    changing behavior through persuasive, 376t
    Communication-Persuasion Matrix (CPM) on, 61t
    group facilitation processes related to, 219t
    See also health messages; risk communication
communication channels
    for change methods and health messages, 359–364t
    description of, 359–360
    display print and circulating print or online, 362t
    interventions that include an interpersonal, 360, 361t
Communication-Persuasion Matrix (CPM)
    for individual intervention level, 61t
    overview of, 101–102
communication vehicles
    for change methods and health messages, 359–364t
    description of, 359–360
    display print and circulating print or online, 362t
    interventions that include an interpersonal, 360, 361t
    issues to consider when choosing, 360
communities
    coalitions formed within, 61t, 168–169
    of evaluation and research community as evaluation stakeholders, 544t
    program design documents created for, 448
    social capital and capacity of, 61t, 169–172
    table on change methods for changing, 395–397t
    understood as networks of networks, 156
    See also opinion leaders
community assessment change method, 396t
community-based participatory research (CBPR), 492
community capacity
    democratic management as essential to development of, 171
    dimensions and functions of, 171
    related to and inclusive of social capital, 170–171
    social capital theory on, 61t, 169–172
Community Coalition Action Theory, 168–169
community development change method, 396t
community empowering level, 154t, 155
community environmental outcomes
    identifying and stating, 293
    to reduce stigma and promote HIV testing, 298–299, 301t

Community Guide (CDC), 599
community intervention level
    community environmental outcomes at the, 293, 298–299, 301t
    program design documents created for the, 448
    table on change methods at the, 395–397t
    theories impacting, 61t, 167–184
community-level theories
    Community Coalition Action Theory, 61t, 168–169
    for community intervention level, 61t
    community organization theories, 61t, 175–184
    conscientization, 61fig, 173–175
    description of, 167
    social capital and community capacity, 61t, 169–172
    social norms theories, 61t, 172–173
community organization theories/models
    advocacy, 180–184
    locality development, 175
    social action, 152, 153, 175, 178
    social movements, 179–180
    social planning, 175
    summary of, 184
community participation
    building collective efficacy through, 178
    community-based participatory research (CBPR) for, 492
    Contra Costa County Health Services Department's Health Neighborhood Project, 177–178
    as core method of community work, 176
    health promotion applications of, 176–178
    Healthy Cities movement, 176
    "wicked problems" issue of, 10
    See also participation
comparative effectiveness designs, 573–574
competence need, 108
complex adaptive systems (CASs), 149–150
compliance (or adherence) behaviors, 288
Comprehensive Health Enhancement Support System (CHESS), 366
computer-based tailored interventions
    description and advantages of, 364–367
    developing tailored feedback, 365, 366fig
conditioned stimulus (CS), 66–67
condom use
    examples of objectives and methods for changing awareness and risk perception of, 371t
    increasing among adolescents to prevent STIs, 22t
    It's Your Game . . . Keep It Real project goals to increase, 260b–261b, 314, 317, 322b–330t
    performance objectives for adolescence consistent and correct, 296t
    performance objectives for among HIV-positive men who have sex with men (MSM), 303t
    qualitative study on HIV/AIDS and, 245
conscientization
    community intervention level using, 61t
    Freirian method of, 173–174, 242
    three stages passing from apathy to social responsibility action process of, 175
consciousness raising change method, 382t
consensus
    description of, 222
    work group processes for creating, 222

Consolidated Framework for Implementation Research (CFIR), 119, 489, 491–492, 503–504
CONSORT (CONsolidated Standards of Reporting Trials), 577
CONSORT Work Group on Pragmatic Trials, 485
CONSORT–EHEALTH Group, 568
constructs
    common behavior-oriented, 63–64
    Health Belief Model (HBM) used of, 62–63
    self-efficacy as, 99, 305
    *See also* theory
contextual stakeholders, 544*t*
contingent rewards change method, 389*t*
continuous quality improvement (CQI), 506
Contra Costa County Health Services Department
    Health Neighborhood Project of, 177–178
    Public and Environmental Health Advisory Board of, 178
cooperative learning change method, 391*t*
Coordinated Approach To Child Health (CATCH) program
    program theme of the, 357
    teachers as environmental agents and program implementers of, 318–319
coping. *See* planning coping responses change method
core elements (essential elements)
    adapting EBIs and challenge of protecting the, 600–601
    description of the, 623
    identifying and retaining, 623–624
    planning group consideration of the, 637–638
COREQ (COnsolidated criteria for REporting Qualitative research), 577
counterconditioning change method, 383*t*
critical consciousness (conscientization), 61*t*, 173–175, 242
critical incident technique, 242
cue altering change methods
    for changing habitual, automatic, and impulsive behaviors, 384*t*
    for changing skills, capability, and self-efficacy and overcome barriers, 389*t*
cues
    how health promoters can provide people with health information, 74
    increasing knowledge by providing, 381*t*
    retrieving information through, 73
    theories of automatic behavior and habits on guiding behavior with environmental, 89
Cultivando La Salud program
    cancer screening intervention focus of, 252
    program theme and message of, 357, 358*fig*
cultural humility
    description of, 28
    Intervention Mapping and role of, 28–30
cultural relevance
    judging delivery fit, design features, and, 620–621, 637
    of program materials, 438–440
cultural relevant program materials
    considering deep and surface culture dimensions for, 439–440
    planning and preparing, 438–440
cultural self-awareness, 222–224
cultural sensitivity
    defining, 438–439

preparing program materials aiming at cultural relevance and, 438–440
    writing program messages with, 458
cultural similarity change method, 386*t*
culture
    behavior-oriented theories and role of cultural sensitivity and, 62–63
    Communication-Persuasion Matrix (CPM) on communication role of, 102
    deep structure and surface structure of, 439–440
    exploring and working in another, 224–225
    as pattern of basic assumptions to cope with problems, 161
    PEN-3 model constructs for understanding "population at risk" factors related to, 224, 230
    work group, 222–225
    writing health messages taking a perspective on participants,' 458
    *See also* beliefs; organizational culture
culture-oriented formative research, 440–441
Cystic Fibrosis Family Education Program (CF FEP), 399

data
    acquiring needs assessment, 241–242
    finding and using archival, 246
    needs assessment combining qualitative and quantitative, 242–246
    pretesting and pilot-testing, 464–468
    primary, 246, 248–249
    secondary, 247*t*–248*t*
data analysis
    IM Adapt framework on planning on evaluation, 629, 641–642
    pretesting and pilot-testing, 467–468
    qualitative methods for, 243–244
    quantitative methods for, 243
data collection
    acquiring needs assessment data, 241–242
    from adopters and implementers, 513
    archival data, 246
    on breast cancer mortality rates inequality, 631–632
    IM Adapt framework on planning, 629, 641–642
    pretesting and pilot-testing for, 464–468
    primary data, 246, 248–249
    qualitative and quantitative, 243–244, 306
    secondary data, 247*t*–248*t*
data needs
    description of the process for identifying, 26–27
    theory and evidence core process of identifying, 21
data sources
    primary, 246, 248–251
    secondary, 247*t*–248*t*
decision makers
    creating consensus among, 222
    as evaluation stakeholder, 544*t*
decision making
    for adoption of outcomes and performance objectives, 497–500
    facilitation of power equity and inclusive, 220
    work group processes for consensus, 222
decision making tools
    CHESS (Comprehensive Health Enhancement Support System), 366

MINDSET (Management Information Decision-Support Epilepsy Tool) as, 106–107, 233–236, 255–256, 307, 367
deconditioning change method, 383t
deep structure of culture, 439–440
Delphi technique, 250–251
design documents
    created for community processes, 448
    determining reading level of, 451–453
    IM Adapt framework on preparing them for EBI adaptation, 624, 638
    It's Your Game . . . Keep It Real project example of, 472fig
    Mayor's Project development of, 455b
    MINDSET (Management Information Decision-Support Epilepsy Tool) examples of, 444fig–447fig
    process of developing the, 441–448
    reviewing available material for use in, 448–453
    SAM (Suitability Assessment of Materials) for determining suitability of, 449, 450t
    telephone-counseling program template for, 621, 622t–623t
    T.L.L. Temple Foundation Stroke Project examples of, 442t–443t
    two different types of, 441
    See also program materials
determinants
    of adoption, implementation, and maintenance, 507–513
    of an agent's power, 151, 153
    caution against placing automaticity or habit in the matrix as a, 318
    conscientization, 61t, 173–175, 242
    ecological model on, 60–62fig
    epilepsy PRECEDE model on, 234fig, 240–241
    examples of objectives and methods at various levels, 372–373t
    examples of objectives and methods for changing awareness and risk perception of condom use, 371t
    IM Adapt framework on program fit with, 618, 636–637
    It's Your Game . . . Keep It Real project, 258b, 314–317, 414t–416t
    logic models for, 61–62fig
    matrices creates at intersection of objectives and at-risk, 283–284
    measuring TPB and RAA, 82
    needs assessment description of behavioral and environmental risks, 236–237, 239–241
    organizing and prioritizing, 513
    PAPM incorporation of Social Cognitive Theory change methods and, 98
    Peace of Mind Program (PMP) personal, 515t–517t
    planning group selection of personal, 304–308
    posing questions about, 21
    program evaluation measures of, 562–564
    rating their importance to performance objectives, 306–308, 307t
    selecting personal, 304–308, 322b, 323b–324b
    of self-efficacy, 99–100, 116
    Social Cognitive Theory (SCT), 65, 113
    social network and social support theories, 159
    The ToyBox-Study matrices of change objectives and personal, 309, 310t–311t

Dietary Guidelines Advisory Committee, 297
Diffusion of Innovations Theory (DIT)
    on characteristics of adopters and innovations, 117–119
    implementation frameworks of, 119, 486, 492
    on interpersonal environment, 61t
    overview of, 116–117
    stage theory of organizational change/diffusion of innovation, 163–166
    summary of the, 120
diffusion phases
    adoption, 117
    dissemination, 117
    implementation, 117, 119
    maintenance, sustainability, and institutionalization, 117
diffusion theories
    Diffusion of Innovations Theory (DIT), 61t, 116–120
    Intervention Mapping step, question, and, 25t
    stage theory of organizational change/diffusion of innovation, 163–166
direct experience change method, 386t
discrimination and stigma theories, 113–116
    See also racism
discussion change method, 381t
display print channel/vehicle, 362t
dissemination
    designing health promotion programs for, 484–485
    Intervention Mapping step, question, model for implementation and, 25t
    theory- and evidence-based approaches to implementation and, 485–487fig
    Veterans Administration (VA) dissemination and implementation (D&I) workgroup on, 485
    See also implementation
dissemination frameworks
    for informing Step 5, 487–490
    Intervention Mapping step, question, model for implementation and, 25t
Division of Cancer Control and Population Science (National Cancer Institute), 562
dramatic relief change method, 382t
dual-systems theory
    on individual intervention level, 61t
    Reflective-Impulsive Model (RIM), 90–91
Dutch HIV/AIDS-Prevention Program
    evaluation plan for the, 577, 578t–579t
    guided practice used in, 371
    modeling used in the, 400–401

early adopters. See adopters
early commitment change method, 384t
EBIs. See evidence-based interventions (EBIs)
ecological models
    applied to different intervention levels, 59–62
    Intervention Mapping and, 8–10
    logic model for methods, determinants, behaviors, environmental conditions, and health, 62fig
    for planning program outcomes, 284–285

effect evaluation
    determining a time frame for the, 550–552
    planning design for, 568–574
    of school HIV-prevention program, 550–551t
    selecting and developing measures for, 558–564
    writing effect questions of, 546–552
    *See also* process evaluation
effect evaluation design
    hybrid designs, 575–576
    mediation and moderation analyses, 576–577
    mixed methods, 574–575
    non-randomized controlled trials (RCT), 570
    observational studies with propensity score matching,
        570–571
    planning an, 568–574
    that promote external validity, 571–574
    time series designs, 571
    traditional types of, 569–570
effect evaluation questions
    on change objectives, 549–550
    on health, quality of life, behavior, and environment,
        548–549
    IYG project, 580b, 582t–583t
    for Mayor's Project, 548b
    written from logic models, 546–552
eHealth interventions
    ASPIRE (A Smoking Prevention Interactive
        Experience), 367
    CHESS (Comprehensive Health Enhancement
        Support System), 366
    computer- and Internet-based tailored, 364–367
    description of, 364
    emerging technology for, 370
    iCHAMPSS Model (Choosing and Maintaining
        Programs for Sex Education in Schools), 367
    serious gaming, 368–369
    social media, 367–368
    telephone and smartphone, 369–370
    Web analytics of, 567–568
    *See also* MINDSET (Management Information
        Decision-Support Epilepsy Tool)
elaboration change method
    to change attitudes, beliefs, and outcome
        expectations, 386t
    to increase knowledge, 381t
Elaboration Likelihood Model (ELM)
    for individual intervention level, 61t
    overview of, 102–104
    on persuasive arguments, 104–105
    promoting skills for information processing issue in,
        73
empathy training change method, 391t
empirical literature. *See* literature review
empowerment theories
    comparison of individual, organizational, and
        community levels of empowerment, 154t, 155
    empowerment defined as "social action process" in,
        153
    as multilevel theory, 61t
enhancing network linkages change method, 394t
entertainment-education (E-E) programs
    as change method, 393t
    description of, 172
environmental agents

creating a logic model of change and role of,
    319–320fig
creating matrices that identify the program
    implementers and, 318–319, 320fig
environmental outcomes and logic of change role of,
    285fig, 286
*See also* program implementers
environmental conditions/factors
    CHEW (Checklist of Health Promotion
        Environments at Worksites) audit of, 253
    epilepsy PRECEDE model on, 234fig, 238–239
    It's Your Game . . . Keep It Real project description of
        adolescent sexual risk behaviors, 258b–260b
    logic models for, 61–62fig
    needs assessment description of determinants of risks
        and, 237–238, 239–241
    program evaluation measure for, 561–562
    program fit with judging behavioral and, 617–618
    roles, determinants, and change methods for,
        372–373t
    Social Cognitive Theory (SCT) on observational
        learning and, 110–111
    tables on change methods for changing, 390,
        392t–393t
    using power to create change at higher levels of, 153
    writing effect evaluation questions on, 548–549
    *See also* risk factors
environmental levels
    information environment asset assessment, 252t, 253
    physical environment asset assessment, 252t, 253
    policy/practice environment asset assessment, 252t,
        253
    program design on the intervention logic model,
        347–348fig
    roles, determinants, and change methods for various,
        372–373t
    schematic representation of shift in program design,
        348fig
    social environmental asset assessment, 252t, 253
environmental-oriented theories
    community-level theories, 61t, 167–184
    competency of, 145
    general environmental-oriented theories, 149–155
    interpersonal-level theories, 155–159
    looking at healthy environments as outcomes, 148
    model for change of environmental conditions,
        146–147
    organizational-level theories, 61t, 160–167
    perspectives on, 146
    societal and governmental theories, 184–192
    *See also* theory
environmental outcomes
    community, 293
    identifying health-related behaviors of the at-risk
        group for, 286–289
    interpersonal, 291–292
    It's Your Game . . . Keep It Real project, 322b,
        323t–324t
    logic of change role of environmental agents and,
        285fig–286
    organizational, 292–293
    selecting personal determinants for, 304–308
    societal, 294
    specifying performance objectives associated with the,
        294, 297–299, 301t
    stating the, 291–294

environmental reevaluation change method, 383*t*
Environmental Systems Research Institute (ESRI), 251
epilepsy
    description and statistics of, 235
    PRECEDE model on, 233–236, 238–239, 240–241
    program goals for patients using MINDSET, 255–256
    *See also* MINDSET (Management Information
        Decision-Support Epilepsy Tool)
epilepsy PRECEDE model
    on at-risk behaviors, 234*fig*, 238–239
    on determinants, 234*fig*, 240–241
    development of the, 233–236
    on environmental conditions/factors, 234*fig*, 238–239
essential elements (core elements)
    adapting EBIs and challenge of protecting the,
        600–601
    description of the, 623
    identifying and retaining, 623–624
    planning group consideration of the, 637–638
ethical health promotion guidelines
    diverse participation in intervention development,
        11–12
    human rights of all people, 12
    interventions should be based on thorough evidence,
        11
    program goals should relate to public health, 11
ethnicity. *See* racial/ethnicity differences
ethnographic data collection methods
    ethnographic interviews as, 242
    overview of, 248–249
EUQATOR (Enhancing the QUAlity and Transparency
    Of health Research) website), 577
European Union *Health in All Policies* strategy, 185
evaluation
    evidence-based interventions (EBIs) and summative
        and formative, 602
    formative, 212, 440–441, 602
    *See also* program evaluation
evaluation and research community, 544*t*
evidence
    ecological models and systems thinking underlying,
        8–10
    IM Adapt framework on searching for, 609–614, 634
    implementation interventions to increase program
        application of theory and, 485–487*fig*
    program design based on change methods based on,
        346–348*fig*
    responding to a paper or presentation of, 221–222
    terms for thinking about, 610*t*
evidence and theory processes
    posing questions, 20, 21
    brainstorming answers, 20, 21–23
    reviewing findings from empirical literature and
        evidence-based answers, 20, 23–24
    accessing and using theory, 20, 25–26
evidence-based change methods
    choosing to address program objectives, 370–398*t*
    description of, 370
    moving to applications from, 398–408*t*
    overview of theory-based and, 346–348*fig*
    *See also* change methods; theory-based change
        methods
evidence-based change method selection
    issues to consider and examples of, 370–371*t*
    It's Your Game . . . Keep It Real project, 410*b*, 416*b*

Mayor's Project example of, 374*b*–375*b*
    roles, determinants, and change methods for
        environmental conditions, 372–373*t*
    tables of methods for changing behavior, 375–398*t*
    using core processes for, 373–374
evidence-based interventions (EBIs)
    essential elements (or core elements) of, 600–601,
        623–624
    IM Adapt framework case study on adaptation of a,
        629–642
    implementation intervention targets and outcomes,
        486–487*fig*
    include potential program implementers in, 492–493
    to inform Step 5, 489
    Peace of Mind Program (PMP) implementation of the
        adapted, 499, 507
    perspectives on, 598–603
    protecting essential elements challenge of adapting,
        600–601
    using empirical literature on implementation of,
        504–505
    *See also* IM Adapt framework; interventions
evidence-based interventions (EBIs) adaptation
    assess fit and plan adaptations, 615–624, 636–638
    evaluation plan with focus on adaptation, 626–629,
        640–642
    modifying materials and programs, 624–625,
        638–639
    needs assessment and assess organizational capacity,
        604–608, 629–634
    plan for implementation, 625–626, 639–640
    search for EBIs, 608–615, 634–635
evidence-based interventions (EBIs) perspectives
    on challenges in adapting EBIs, 600–601
    on challenges in choosing EBIs, 598–600
    on formative research and summative evaluation
        issues, 602
    on program adaptation, 602–603
evidence-based interventions (EBIs) program fit
    adaptation "to-do list" for telephone-counseling
        program, 618, 619*t*–620*t*
    basic, 614–615, 634–635
    behavioral and environmental, 617–618
    design features, cultural relevance, and delivery,
        620–621, 637
    determinant and change methods, 618, 636–637
    health problem and health promoting behavior,
        614–615, 635, 636
    IM Adapt framework on planning adaptations and
        assessing, 615–624, 634–638
    implementation, 621, 623, 637
    organizational capacity, 615, 635
    priority population/at-risk group, 615, 635
evidence-based interventions (EBIs) selection
    defining evidence-based for, 598–599
    finding resources on "full" EBIs for, 599–600, 611
    IM Adapt framework on search and, 608–615
evidence/theories/change methods tables
    behavior change, 378*t*, 380
    change attitudes, beliefs, and outcome expectations,
        385*t*–386*t*
    change awareness and risk perception, 380, 382*t*–383*t*
    change communities, 395–397*t*
    change habitual, automatic, and impulsive behaviors,
        380, 383*t*–384*t*

evidence/theories/change methods tables *(continued)*
  change of environmental conditions, 390, 392*t*–393*t*
  change organizations, 394–395*t*
  change policy, 397–398*t*
  change social norms, 390, 393*t*
  change social support and social networks, 391–394*t*
  changing social influence, 386–387*t*
  how to use the, 379–380
  increase knowledge, 380, 381*t*
  influence skills, capability, and self-efficacy and
    overcome barriers, 387–390
  reduce public stigma, 390, 391*t*
executive function
  improving control with practice, 92
  inhibitory control of the, 91–92
  training executive function change method, 384*t*
experience change method
  changing skills, capability, and self-efficacy and
    overcome barriers with direct, 386*t*
  changing skills, capability, and self-efficacy and
    overcome barriers with effective mastery, 388*t*
explanatory vs. change theories, 66
exposure effect
  to change attitudes, beliefs, and outcome
    expectations, 386*t*
  learning and, 69
Extended Parallel Process Model (EPPM)
  as consciousness raising, 78
  description of, 76
  for individual intervention level, 61*t*
external validity
  comparative effectiveness designs, 573–574
  evaluation designs that promote, 571–574
  of PRECIS criteria for pragmatic designs, 572*fig*–573

Facebook, 368
facilitation
  changing behavior through, 378*t*
  of power equity and inclusive decision making, 220
  work task group need for, 218–220
facilitation processes
  communication, 219*t*
  maintenance and team-building functions, 219*t*
  task functions, 219*t*
fear arousal
  as change method, 383*t*
  moving from change method to application using,
    403–405
fear-based health messages
  on at-risk behaviors, 76–77
  Self-Affirmation Theory to make people less defensive
    of, 77
federally qualified health centers (FAHCs)
  appreciative inquiry (AI) approach to in-depth
    interviewing at, 249
  PPGIS (public participation GIS) to collect data from,
    251
feedback
  changing behavior through, 377*t*
  classical conditioning and, 66–67
  as effective method to create changes, 69–70
  operant conditioning and, 67–68
  organizational diagnosis and feedback change
    method, 395*t*

fit. *See* evidence-based interventions (EBIs) program fit
Flesch-Kincaid grade level, 452
Flickr, 368
FLU-FIT program, 498–499
focus groups, 250
Force Field Analysis, 160–161
formative research
  culture-oriented, 440–441
  evidence-based interventions (EBIs) and, 602
  needs assessment and, 212
  preparing program materials and role of, 440
forming coalitions change method, 397*t*
framing
  changing awareness and risk perception through, 382*t*
  of health messages, 77–78
  media advocacy, 183–184
  to shift perspectives, 397*t*
  of social movements, 179–180
free association, 221
Friend to Friend program, 493–494
Fry Readability Graph, 452
full EBIs (evidence-based interventions)
  description and sources of, 599–600
  website sources for, 611, 612*t*–613*t*


gender
  It's Your Game . . . Keep It Real project gender role
    norms determinant, 325*t*–327*t*
  reducing inequalities of class, race, gender and
    sexuality change method, 391*t*
general environmental-oriented theories
  description of, 149
  empowerment theories, 61*t*, 154*t*, 155
  systems theory, 61*t*, 149–151
  theories of power, 151–153
geographic information systems (GIS), 251
Gestalt school of psychology, 71
goal-setting change method, 389*t*
goal-setting theory
  on characteristics of goals, 86
  on implementation intentions, 86–88
  for individual intervention level, 61*t*
  overview of, 85–86
  on unconscious goal pursuit, 88
  *See also* health promotion goals
Google analytics, 568
governmental theories. *See* societal and governmental
    theories
government intervention level
  Advocacy Coalition Framework for, 61*t*, 189–191,
    398*t*
  Multiple Streams Theory for, 61*fig*, 187–189, 190,
    397–398*t*
  table on methods to change public policy at the,
    397–398*t*
  theories impacting societal and, 61*t*, 184–191
  *See also* public policy
GRADE Working Group, 611
Greenpeace actions, 178
group management processes
  for consensus, 222
  creating a timeline fro, 218
  facilitation, 218, 220
  for idea generation, 220–222
  overview of, 217–218

guided practice
    changing skills, capability, and self-efficacy and
        overcome barriers, 388t
    HIV-prevention program for Dutch adolescents
        using, 371

habits
    caution against placing it in the matrix as a
        determinant, 318
    change methods for behaviors that are automatic,
        impulsive, and, 383t–384t
    difficulty of changing, 92–93
    examples of cells to address a habitual behaviors in a
        matrix, 319t
    possible intervention to change, 93
    process of changing, 318
    as special case of automatic behavior, 92
    See also performance (or change) objectives
health
    logic models for, 61–62fig
    program evaluation measures of, 559–561
    social relationships linked to status of, 156
    writing effect evaluation questions on, 548–549
    See also public health
health advocacy
    description of, 180–181
    media advocacy approach to, 182–184
    principles underlying effective tactics for, 181t
    three stages of, 181–182
health behavior change techniques (BCTs), 355
    See also logic model of change
Health Belief Model (HBM)
    as consciousness raising, 78
    constructs to describe health behavior in various
        cultures in the, 62–63
    four psychological constructs of, 74–75
    on health action based on perceptions, 74–75
    for individual intervention level, 61t
health care costs (epilepsy PRECEDE model), 235
health education
    entertainment-education (E-E) programs change
        method, 172, 393t
    Freirian method for, 173–174
    peer education change method for, 394t
    problem-posing, 396t
    use of lay health workers change method for, 394t
health educators, 3
    See also program implementers
Health in All Policies strategy (European Union), 185
health literacy
    program materials consideration of participant
        literacy and, 451–453
    program messages that include presentation of
        medical terminology to facilitate, 459
    reading level assessments should be focused on
        literacy and not on, 453
    Short-TOFHLA (Test of Functional Health Literacy
        in Adults) assessment of, 452
    TOFHLA (Test of Functional Health Literacy in
        Adults) assessment of, 452
    See also literacy
health messages
    communication channels and vehicles for change
        methods and, 359–364t
    cues used to provide health information and, 73–74

Diffusion of Innovations Theory (DIT) on, 61t,
    116–120
Elaboration Likelihood Model (ELM) on persuasion
    effects of, 61t, 73, 102–104
fear-based, 76–77
framing, 77–78
raising awareness through, 98–99
See also behavioral journalism; communication;
    program messages; risk communication
health problems
    example of epilepsy PRECEDE model, 233–236
    IM Adapt framework on fit with health promoting
        behaviors and, 614–615, 635, 636, 639
    IM Adapt framework on literature review to
        summarize, 630–631
    It's Your Game . . . Keep It Real project task of
        describing the, 257b–258b
    needs assessment description possible causes of,
        236–239
    needs assessment description of quality of life and,
        232–236
    posing question about, 21
    rates and risk concepts and statistics on, 233
health promoters
    definition of, 3
    Mayor's Project case study on planning process of,
        4b–7b
    providing cues as method to help people retrieve
        information, 74
    working as external organizational change agents,
        160, 162
health-promoting behaviors
    IM Adapt framework on it with health problem and,
        614–615, 635, 636, 639
    stating behavioral and environmental outcomes for,
        287–288
    See also at-risk behaviors; behaviors
health promotion
    definition of, 3
    efficacy testing in controlled environments, 151
    racism as explicit consideration in, 225
    See also interventions
health promotion goals
    characteristics of, 86
    examples of, 255–256
    IM Adapt framework on writing, 608, 634
    Intervention Mapping framework definition of, 255
    It's Your Game . . . Keep It Real project task of stating,
        260b–261b
    media advocacy, 184
    mental processes and behaviors of, 85
    RAA distinction between intentions, beliefs, and, 82
    setting needs assessment priorities and stating
        program, 254–256
    should relate to public health, 11
    theories of goal-directed behavior on content of,
        84–85
    unconscious pursuit of, 88
    See also goal-setting theory; logic model of change;
        performance (or change) objectives

health promotion programs
conducting asset assessment in different types of, 252t–253
examples developed using Intervention Mapping, 34t–38t
implementation of, 117, 119, 318–319, 320fig, 436–437, 483–529
production and materials of, 13fig, 18, 435–475
scope of, 355–359t, 409b–410b
sequence of, 355–359t, 409b–410b
setting needs assessment priorities and stating goals of, 254–256
themes of, 355–357, 409b–410b
*See also* Mayor's Project; program outcomes; *specific programs*
health/quality-of-life logic models, 61–62fig
health-related quality-of-life (HRQOL), 560
Healthy Cities movement, 176
Healthy Neighborhoods Project (Contra Costa County Health Services Department), 177–178
The Heart Truth Campaign, 368
Hispanic population
declining breast cancer mortality rates among women, 630–631
health problems of youth among, 257b–258b
It's Your Game . . . Keep It Real project focus on, 256b–261b
study on colorectal and breast cancer screening by farm-working 50 years and older women, 243, 252
*See also* racial/ethnicity differences
HIV/AIDS epidemic
ART (antiretroviral treatment) for patients of the, 296
public policy response to, 190
qualitative study on risk behaviors associated with, 245
reducing stigmatization associated to, 114–115
stigma and discrimination related to the, 113–114
*See also* sexually transmitted infections (STIs); sexual risk behaviors
HIV/AIDS programs
ACT-UP (AIDS Coalition to Unleash Power), 180
Dutch HIV/AIDS-Prevention Program, 371, 400–401, 577, 578t–579t
evaluation of a school HIV-prevention program, 550, 551t
health promotion goals of Austin (Texas), 255
identifying determinants when planning, 306
importance of determinants when planning an Internet, 307
for increasing condom use by adolescents, 22t
Intervention Mapping used for, 35t
It's Your Game . . . Keep It Real project goals to reduce HIV infection, 260b–261b
performance objectives for condom use for HIV-positive men who have sex with men (MSM), 303t
role of culture in intervention planning for, 29
scene from HIV-prevention active learning video, 402
School AIDS Prevention Program evaluation plan, 577, 578t–579t
social norms theories on prevention used in, 173–174
specifying performance objectives to promote HIV testing and reduce stigma, 298t–301t
*See also* Mayor's Project

Houston Department of Health and Human Services, 257b
HRQOL (health-related quality-of-life), 560
human relations and team building training, 395t
human rights, 12
hybrid designs for evaluation, 575–576

iCHAMPSS Model (Choosing and Maintaining Programs for Sex Education in Schools), 367
idea generation processes
brainstorming or free association, 221
nominal group technique, 221
overview of, 220–221
responding to a paper or presentation of evidence, 221–222
IM Adapt framework
alternatives to the, 602–603
competency in, 597–598
illustrated diagram on process of the, 604, 605fig
introduction to the, 603–604
overview of adapting EBIs using the, 603–604
*See also* evidence-based interventions (EBIs); Intervention Mapping (IM)
IM Adapt framework case study
project outcomes and current status of the, 642
Step 1: needs assessment and assess organizational capacity, 629–634
Step 2: search for evidence-based interventions, 634–635
Step 3: assess fit and plan adaptations, 636–638
Step 4: make adaptations, 638–639
Step 5: plan for implementation, 639–640
Step 6: plan for evaluation, 640–642
IM Adapt framework steps
Step 1: needs assessment and assess organizational capacity, 604–608
Step 2: search for evidence-based interventions, 608–615
Step 3: assess fit and plan adaptations, 615–624
Step 4: make adaptations, 624–625
Step 5: plan for implementation, 625–626
Step 6: plan for evaluation, 626–629
imagery change method, 381t
implementation
constructing matrices for change objectives, 507–514, 515t–517t
definition of, 497
designing program production and materials for, 436–437
determinants of, 507–514
dimensions of, 500–501
identifying environmental agents and program implements for, 318–319, 320fig
IM Adapt framework on judging program fit of, 621, 623, 637
IM Adapt framework on planning for, 625–626, 639–640
interventions to increase program use during, 485–487
It's Your Game . . . Keep It Real project stating outcomes and performance objectives for, 523t–525t
It's Your Game . . . Keep It Real project Step 5 tasks for, 518b–528b
outcomes of, 501–503

Peace of Mind Program (PMP), 499, 507, 516t
as phase of diffusion, 117
process evaluation questions on, 554–558
stating outcomes and performance objectives for, 500–506
three frameworks of influence for diffusion, 119
using theories and frameworks for, 503–504
Veterans Administration (VA) dissemination and implementation (D&I) workgroup on, 485
*See also* dissemination; Intervention Mapping tasks (Step 5)
implementation frameworks
Consolidated Framework for Implementation Research (CFIR), 119, 489, 491–492, 503–504
Diffusion of Innovations Theory (DIT), 119, 486, 492
Interactive Systems Framework (ISF), 119, 489, 490–491, 503–504, 601
RE-AIM framework, 119, 489, 490, 611
used for implementation, 503–504
used to inform Step 5, 487–490
*See also* theory
implementation intentions change method, 383t
implementation interventions
organizing the intervention scope, sequence, and materials, 518, 526b–528b
selecting change methods and practical applications, 514, 518, 526b–528b
implementation planning
competency in, 483–484
a participatory approach to, 492–494
Peace of Mind Program (PMP), 517t
perspectives on, 484–494
implementation planning perspectives
designing health promotion programs for dissemination, 484–485
on frameworks for dissemination and implementation, 490–492
implementation interventions to increase program use, 485–487
participatory approach to implementation planning, 492–494
using dissemination and implementation frameworks to inform Step 5, 487–490
improving physical/emotional states, 388t
impulsive behavior
change methods for habits, automatic, and, 383t–384t
inhibitory control of executive function to control, 91–92
Reflective-Impulsive Model (RIM) on, 90–91
increasing stakeholder influence change method, 395t
Incredible Years BASIC Parent Program, 576
individual empowering level, 154t
individual intervention level
individual empowering level, 154t
modeling to reinforcement attitude change at the, 372–373t
table on basic change methods at the, 376t–386t
theories to use at the, 61t
*See also* intervention levels
individualization intervention method
changing behavior through, 377t
description of the, 112
infomercials channel/vehicle, 363t
information environment asset assessment, 252t, 253
Information-Motivation-Behavioral Skills model, 81

innovation
characteristics of adopters and, 117–119
definition of, 116, 497
Diffusion of Innovations Theory (DIT) on, 61t, 116–120
literature review on characteristics of, 510–511
Institute of Medicine, 230, 452
Institutional Review Board (St. Luke's Episcopal Hospital), 641
Integrated Behavioral Model (IBM)
for individual intervention level, 61t
overview of, 81
Interactive Systems Framework (ISF), 119, 489, 490–491, 503–504, 601
interactive voice recognition (IVR), 369–370
Internet-based tailored interventions
description and advantages of, 364–367
developing tailored feedback, 365, 366fig
interpersonal contact change method, 391t
interpersonal environmental outcomes
identifying and stating, 291–292
to reduce stigma and promote HIV testing, 298–299, 301t
The ToyBox-Study, 292, 298, 299t
interpersonal intervention level
communication channels and vehicles, 360, 361t
environmental outcomes, 291–292, 298, 299t, 301t
modeling to reinforcement attitude change at the, 372–373t
table on methods for changing social support and social networks at, 386, 393t
theories that impact the, 59, 61t, 65, 81, 96, 109–120, 156–159
ToyBox-Study matrices of change objectives at the, 309, 311t
*See also* intervention levels
interpersonal-level theories
description of, 155
Diffusion of Innovations Theory, 61t, 116–120
Social Cognitive Theory, 59, 61t, 65, 81, 96, 109–113, 118
social network theory, 61t, 155–156, 159
social support theory, 61t, 156–159
theories of stigma and discrimination, 61t, 113–116
interrupted time-series design, 571
intervention levels
community, 61t, 167–184, 293, 298–299, 301t, 395–396t, 448
constructing matrices of change objectives and selecting the, 309, 310t–312t
multilevel, 61t, 146–147
program design using different change methods at different, 352–354
societal and governmental, 61t, 184–191, 294, 298–299, 301t, 386–387t, 397–398t
tobacco control application to differing, 38
The ToyBox-Study matrices of change objectives and specific, 309, 310t–312t
translating change methods into applications at different, 406–408t
*See also* individual intervention level; interpersonal intervention level; organization intervention level
Intervention Mapping (IM)
adapting evidence-based interventions (EBIs) by using, 603–643

Intervention Mapping (IM) (*continued*)
  competency of, 3
  ecological models and systems thinking in, 8–10
  ethical practice of health promotion and, 11–12
  examples of programs developed using, 34*t*–38*t*
  health promotion planning role of, 3
  introduction to theory and evidence and processes
    applied to, 7–8, 11, 20–28
  mapping steps, 12–20
  participation in health promotion planning and,
    10–11
  perspectives on, 7
  program goals as defined by, 255
  role of culture in, 28–30
  *See also* IM Adapt framework; Mayor's Project
Intervention Mapping steps/questions
  1: logic model of the problem/needs assessment, 13*fig*,
    14, 15*fig*, 25*t*, 213–261*b*
  2: program outcomes and objectives and logic model
    of change, 13*fig*, 15–17, 25*t*, 283–330*t*
  3: program design, 13*fig*, 17–18, 25*t*, 345–408*t*
  4: program production, 11*fig*, 18, 25*t*, 435–476
  5: program implementation plan, 13*fig*, 18–19, 25*t*,
    483–530
  6: evaluation plan, 13*fig*, 19–20, 25*t*, 541–585
Intervention Mapping tasks (Step 1)
  1: establishing and working with a planning group,
    214–226*b*, 256*b*
  2: conducting a needs assessment, 226–251,
    256*b*–260*b*
  3: describing the context for the intervention,
    251–254, 260*b*
  4: stating program goals, 254–256, 260*b*–261*b*
  *See also* intervention planning: work planning groups
Intervention Mapping tasks (Step 2)
  1: stating behavioral and environmental outcomes,
    286–304, 322*t*
  2: selecting personal determinants, 304–308, 322*b*,
    323*b*–324*b*
  3: constructing matrices of change objectives,
    308–309, 310*t*–312*t*, 313–314, 315*t*–317*t*,
    317–319
  4: creating a logic model of change, 319–320*fig*
  5: using matrices of change objectives for program
    evaluation, 321–330*t*
  *See also* performance (or change) objectives
Intervention Mapping tasks (Step 3)
  1: generating program themes, components, scope,
    and sequence, 355–370, 409*b*–410*b*, 411*t*–413*t*
  2: choosing theory- and evidence-based change
    methods to address objectives, 370–398*t*, 410*b*,
    414*t*–416*t*
  3: moving from methods to applications, 398–408*t*
  *See also* program design
Intervention Mapping tasks (Step 4)
  1: refining program structure and organization,
    437–438, 468*b*
  2: preparing plans for program materials, 438–455*b*,
    468*b*–469*b*
  3: drafting messages, materials, and protocols,
    456–464, 469*b*
  4: pretesting, pilot-testing, refining, and producing
    materials, 464–468, 469*b*–475*b*
  *See also* program production
Intervention Mapping tasks (Step 5)

  1: identifying program implementers, 494–496*b*, 519*b*
  2: stating outcomes and performance objectives for
    program use, 497–507, 519*b*, 520*t*–526*t*
  3: constructing matrices of change objectives for
    implementation, 507–514, 515*t*–517*t*, 519*b*
  4: designing implementation interventions, 514,
    517*t*,518, 526*b*–528*b*, 580*b*, 583*b*
  *See also* implementation
Intervention Mapping tasks (Step 6)
  1: writing evaluation questions, 546–558, 580*b*,
    582*t*–583*t*
  2: selecting and developing measures, 558–564, 580*b*
  3: specifying designs for process and effect
    evaluations, 564–568, 580*b*
  4: planning an evaluation design for effect evaluation,
    568–574, 586*b*
  5: emerging designs and analyses for process and
    effect evaluation, 574–577
  6: completing the evaluation plan, 577–579*t*
  *See also* program evaluation planning
intervention planning
  examples of when to use behavior-oriented theories
    in, 58*t*
  for implementation, 484–529
  as an iterative process, 31
  It's Your Game . . . Keep It Real project task of,
    256*b*–261*b*
  with limited resources, 32
  matrices as the foundation of, 31
  needs assessment as part of the, 212–214
  participation in, 10–11
  for program materials, 438–455*b*
  *See also* Intervention Mapping (Step 1); logic model of
    change; logic model of the problem; work planning
    groups
interventions
  based on thorough evidence to increase effectiveness,
    11
  diverse participation of, 11
  eHealth, 364–370, 567–568
  logic model of the, 547*fig*
  role of culture in, 28–30
  social support, 157–159
  tailoring, relevance, and individualization methods in,
    112
  *See also* evidence-based interventions (EBIs); health
    promotion
intervention settings
  asset assessment to identify the, 254
  It's Your Game . . . Keep It Real project task of
    establishing, 260*b*
interviews
  appreciate inquiry (AI) use of in-depth, 249
  as data collection method, 248
  ethnographic, 242
  focus groups, 250
  Motivational Interviewing (MI), 108–109, 378*t*
It's Your Game . . . Keep It Real (IYG) project
  computer lessons of the, 470*fig*–471*fig*
  design document of, 472*fig*
  example of role play activity from, 473*fig*
  final logic model for, 580*b*, 581*fig*
  Intervention Mapping Step 1 tasks, 254, 256*b*–261*b*
  Intervention Mapping Step 2 tasks, 322*b*–330*b*
  Intervention Mapping Step 3 tasks, 409*b*–416*b*

Intervention Mapping Step 4 tasks, 468b–475b
Intervention Mapping Step 5 tasks, 518b–519b, 520t–528t
Intervention Mapping Step 6 tasks, 580b–584b
matrix showing personal determinants and change objectives for, 314–317
program components of, 358
program scope and sequence of, 359
program theme of, 357
refining program materials by the, 467
screen captures depicting change methods and practical applications from, 474fig
See also adolescents; school programs
It's Your Game . . . Keep It Real (IYG) project tasks
conduct needs assessment to create logic model of the problem, 256b–260b
construct matrices of change objectives for implementation, 519b
create the matrices, 324b–330t
describe population, setting, and community context for intervention, 260b
develop indicators and measures for assessment, 580b
establish and work with a planning group, 256b
identify program implementers, 519b
preparing plans for program materials, 468b–469
refine the program structure and organization, 468b
select determinants of health behavior and environmental outcomes, 322b–324t
state outcomes and performance objectives for implementation, 519b, 520t–526t
state program goals, 260b–261b
state what health behaviors and environmental conditions need to change, 322b
subdivide behavioral and environmental outcomes into objectives, 322b
write effect and process evaluation questions, 580b
IVR (interactive voice recognition), 369–370

Jasoos (Detective) Vijay (BBC crime drama show), 172
Journal of Medical Internet Research, 567

knowledge
action words for writing change objectives related to, 317t
change methods for increasing, 380, 381t
It's Your Game . . . Keep It Real project determinants of, 315t–316t, 325t–330t
ToyBox Study personal determinants of, 311t–312t

La Raza Unida, 178
laws and regulations change method, 398t
lay health workers change method, 394t
League of Women Voters, 180
learning
cooperative learning change method, 391t
elaboration to add meaning and enhance memory and, 73
Social Cognitive Theory (SCT) on environment and observational, 110–111
text comprehension and, 71–73
vicarious (or social), 69
See also active learning
learning theories
classical (or Pavlovian) conditioning, 66–67

description of, 66
on exposure effect, 69
for individual intervention level, 61t
operant conditioning, 67–68
summary on changing behavior using, 69–70
legitimacy power, 152, 153
literacy
program materials consideration of participant, 451–453
reading level assessments focused on, 452–453
REALM (Rapid Estimate of Adult Literacy in Medicine) assessment of, 452
See also health literacy; reading level assessments
literature review
on characteristics of implementers, 511
on characteristics of innovations, 510–511
on characteristics of systems, 511–513
IM Adapt framework on summary of the problem from, 630–631
questions to help guide a basic, 23–24
stating outcomes and performance objectives for implementation and use of, 504–505
as theory and evidence core process, 20
lobbying and advocacy change method, 392t
locality development community organization model, 175
loci (Greek oratory method), 73
logic model of change
description of, 13fig
ecological model applied to, 61–62fig
effect evaluation questions written from, 546–552
illustrated diagram of development of the, 16fig
IM Adapt framework on developing a, 606–607fig, 632fig–633fig
It's Your Game . . . Keep It Real project task to create a, 330b
planning step of depicting pathways of program causation, 13fig, 15–17, 285fig–286
program outcomes task of creating pathways to program effects, 319–320fig
tasks involved in completing the, 15–17
See also change methods; health behavior change techniques (BCTs); health promotion goals; intervention planning
logic model of the problem
competency of, 211–212
effect evaluation questions written from, 546–552
IM Adapt framework, 604–606fig, 630
It's Your Game . . . Keep It Real project task of creating, 256b–261b
needs assessment for developing a, 13, 211–214, 226, 227fig
perspectives on, 212
steps in the development of the, 14–15, 15fig
tasks for development of a, 214–261b
theories used for, 25t
working list of answers for, 21, 27–28
See also intervention planning; PRECEDE model
logic models
IYG project intervention logic model for evaluation, 580b, 581fig
for methods, determinants, behaviors, environmental conditions, and health, 61–62fig
process and effect intervention, 547fig
understanding PRCEDE model as a, 227–229

logic models  (*continued*)
  writing effect evaluation questions from the program,
    546–552
long-term memory
  how cues can be used to retrieve information from,
    73–74
  imagery stored in the, 72–73
  knowledge as associative network stored in, 71–72

maintenance
  continuous quality improvement (CQI) approach to,
    506
  definition of, 497, 506
  determinants of, 507–514
  It's Your Game . . . Keep It Real project stating
    outcomes and performance objectives for,
    525t–526t
  Peace of Mind Program (PMP) determinants for,
    516t–517t
  stating outcomes and performance objectives for,
    506–507
mammography programs
  Friend to Friend program, 493–494
  Peace of Mind Program (PMP), 499, 501–503, 507,
    508–510, 514, 515t–517t, 518
  social norms theories on encouraging mammograms,
    173
Management Information Decision-Support Epilepsy
    Tool (MINDSET). *See* MINDSET (Management
    Information Decision-Support Epilepsy Tool)
mass media
  public service announcements (PSAs) messages of,
    358
  social norms theories on influence of, 172–173
  TV viewing hours by children, 237–238
mass media role-modeling change method, 393t
materials. *See* program materials
matrices
  caution against placing automaticy or habit as a
    determinant in the, 318
  constructing change objectives for implementation,
    507–514, 515t–517t
  created at intersection of objectives and at-risk
    determinants, 283–284
  dealing with automaticity in the matrix of change
    objectives, 317–318, 319t
  differentiating the intervention population, 309,
    312–313
  examples of cells to address a habitual behavior, 319t
  identifying environmental agents and program
    implementers, 318–319
  It's Your Game . . . Keep It Real project construction
    of implementation, 519b
  It's Your Game . . . Keep It Real project creation of
    the, 314, 315t–317t, 317–318, 324b–330t
  It's Your Game . . . Keep It Real project task to create
    the, 324b–330b
  program evaluation using change objectives, 321–322
  selecting intervention levels for,
    309, 310t–312t
  writing change objectives and constructing the, 314,
    315t–317t, 317–318
Mayor's Project
  behavior-oriented theories used in, in, 64b–65b

core processes for selecting theory- and
    evidence-based change theories, 374b–375b
  identifying, program implementers, 498b
  Intervention Mapping used in, 4b–7b
  planning program outcomes of, 284b
  program materials and design document planning by,
    455b
  work group of the, 235b–236b
  writing effect evaluation questions for, 548b
  *See also* health promotion programs; Intervention
    Mapping (IM)
media advocacy
  for changing policy, 398t
  framing, 183–184
  three steps of, 183
  Wallack's approach to, 182–184
media advocacy change method, 398t
mediation analysis, 576–577
Memorandum of Understanding (MOU), 499
memorizing through chunking, 71
memory
  elaboration to add meaning and enhance learning
    and, 73
  how cues can be used to retrieve information from,
    73–74
  imagery stored in the long-term, 72–73
  knowledge as associative network stored in
    long-term, 71–72
  memorizing through chunking, 71
  writing program messages to enhance cognitive
    processing and, 457–458
Mental Model Theory, 71
men who have sex with men (MSM)
  importance of determinants when planning an
    Internet HIV-prevention program for, 307
  performance objectives for condom use among
    HIV-positive, 303t
Method for Program Adaptation through Community
    Engagement (M-PACE), 603
Microsoft Word readability protocols, 452
MINDSET (Management Information Decision-Support
    Epilepsy Tool)
  design documents of the, 444fig–447fig
  epilepsy PRECEDE model developed using, 233–236
  program goals for patients with epilepsy using,
    255–256
  providing decision support to patients and health care
    providers, 367
  self-regulation theories used to develop, 106–107
  using findings from empirical studies in the
    development of, 307–308
  *See also* eHealth interventions; epilepsy
mixed methods evaluation design, 574–575
mobilizing social networks change method, 393t
mobilizing social support change method, 387t
modeled behavior
  challenges of translating method into application of,
    351–352
  changing behavior through, 377t, 392t
  mass media role-modeling change method, 393t
  to reinforcement objectives and change methods for
    attitude change, 372–373t
  for translating change methods to application,
    400–401
moderation analysis, 576–577

motivation
  Motivational Interviewing (MI) for change, 108–109,
    378*t*
  Self-Determination Theory on three basic needs at
    core of human, 108
motivational enhancement therapy, 308
Motivational Interviewing (MI)
  effectiveness in changing behavior, 378*t*
  for motivating behavior change, 108–109
M-PACE (Method for Program Adaptation through
    Community Engagement), 603
multilevel interventions
  theories for, 61*t*, 146–184
  for tobacco control, 147
multilevel theories
  community-level theories, 61*t*, 167–184
  empowerment theories, 61*t*, 154*t*–155
  interpersonal-level theories, 61*t*, 155–159
  model for change of environmental conditions,
    146–147
  organizational-level theories, 61*t*, 160–166
  societal and governmental theories, 61*t*, 184–192
  stakeholder theory, 61*t*, 166–167
  systems theory, 61*t*, 149–151
  theories of power, 25*t*, 61*t*, 151–153
multiple baseline design, 571
Multiple Streams Theory
  comparison of Advocacy Coalition Framework to, 190
  on public policy process, 187–189, 397–398*t*
  for society and government intervention level, 61*fig*
MySpace, 368

narrative "print" material production, 460–461*fig*
National Cancer Institute, 102, 149, 151, 465, 562, 599
National Implementation Research Network (NIRN),
    489
National Institute for Clinical Excellence (NICE), 571
National Institute for Mental Health (National Institutes
    of Health), 256*b*
National Institute on Alcohol Abuse and Alcoholism,
    562
National Institutes of Health (NIH), 256*b*, 485
National Registry of Evidence-based Programs and
    Practices (SAMHSA), 599–600
needs assessment
  balancing with an asset assessment, 251–252
  conducting a, 226–251
  description and function of the, 212–213
  IM Adapt framework step of, 604–608, 629–634
  It's Your Game . . . Keep It Real project task of,
    256*b*–260*b*
  partnering with the community during the, 213–214
  as part of the intervention planning, 212–214
needs assessment data
  acquiring, 241–242
  combining qualitative and quantitative, 242–246
  finding and using archival data for, 246
  primary sources used for, 246, 248–249
  secondary sources for, 247*t*–248*t*
needs assessment process
  acquiring needs assessment data, 241–242
  combining qualitative and quantitative data, 242–246
  describing determinants of behavioral and
    environmental risks, 236–238, 239–241

  describing health problems and quality of life,
    232–236
  describing possible causes of health problems,
    236–239
  describing the priority population, 229–232
  logic model of the problem used for, 13, 212–214,
    226, 227*fig*
  PRECEDE model to plan the, 226
nominal group technique, 221, 242
non-behavioral factors (epilepsy PRECEDE model),
    234*fig*
non-randomized controlled trials (RCT), 570
norms. *See* social norms
nudging
  changing behavior through, 378*t*
  how to apply for changing automatic behavior, 93–94
  to make desired behavior as default choice, 93
  Self-Determination Theory on autonomous decision
    making role in, 94

Oak Ridge Institute for Science and Education, 218
objectives. *See* performance objectives
observational learning, 110–111
observational studies with propensity score matching,
    570–571
Office of Cancer Communications, 102
operant conditioning, 67–68
opinion leaders
  demonstrating support of health-promoting behavior,
    173
  identifying community, 495
  *See also* communities; program implementers
organizational capacity
  IM Adapt framework on needs assessment and
    assessment of, 607–608, 629–633, 633*fig*, 636–638
  IM Adapt framework on the program fit with, 615,
    635
organizational change theories
  on changing organizational culture, 161–162
  Force Field Analysis, 160–161
  organization intervention level using, 61*t*
  overview of, 160–161
  summary on, 162
  used in change methods, 394–395*t*
organizational culture
  changing, 161–162
  Communication-Persuasion Matrix (CPM) on
    communication role of, 102
  exploring and working in another, 224–225
  as pattern of basic assumptions to cope with
    problems, 161
  work group, 222–225
  *See also* culture
organizational development theories
  description of, 162
  organization intervention level using, 61*t*
  planned change framework of, 162–163
  stage theory of organizational change/diffusion of
    innovation, 163–166
  T.L.L. Temple Foundation Stroke Project, 298, 300*t*
organizational diagnosis and feedback change method,
    395*t*
organizational empowering level, 154*t*

organizational environmental outcomes
    identifying and stating, 292–293
    to reduce stigma and promote HIV testing, 298–299,
        301t
    T.L.L. Temple Foundation Stroke Project, 298, 300t
    The ToyBox-Study, 292, 298, 299t
    See also environmental levels
organization intervention level
    organizational change theories on the, 61t, 160–162,
        394–395t
    organizational development theories on the, 61t,
        162–166, 293, 298, 300t
    organizational empowering, 154t
    organization environmental outcomes at the,
        292–293, 298–299, 301t
    table on change methods at the, 394–395t
    See also intervention levels
organization-level theories
    description of, 160
    for organization intervention level, 61t
    stakeholder theory, 61t, 166–167
    theories of organizational change, 61t, 160–162
    theories of organizational development, 61t, 162–166
others' approval change method, 387t
outcome expectations. See program outcome
    expectations
outcomes. See program outcomes

participants
    considering literacy and health literacy of the,
        451–453
    ensuring appropriate reading level of materials for,
        451–453
    evaluation stakeholders made up of target, 544t
    program material and suitability for, 449–450t
    program structure and organization that reaches the
        intended, 437
    translation of program materials for non-speaking,
        458–459
    writing program messages to enhance cognitive
        processing and memory of, 457–458
participation
    for changing behavior, 376t
    ensuring program planning, 214–217
    ethical guidelines on having inclusive and diverse,
        11–12
    in health promotion planning and Intervention
        Mapping, 10–11
    implementation planning using an approach of,
        492–494
    importance of stakeholder, 214
    involving evaluation stakeholders, 543–546
    See also community participation
participatory action
    community-based participatory research (CBPR), 492
    in health promotion planning, 10
    principles of, 10–11
    See also community participation
participatory problem solving change method, 392t
Partners in School Asthma Management Program, 309
Pavlovian (or classical) conditioning, 66–67
Peace of Mind Program (PMP)
    brainstorming determinants for adoption and
        implementation of, 508–510

examples of change objectives and determinants
    from, 515t–517t
implementation intervention plan for, 517t
selecting change methods and applications, 514, 517t,
    518
stating outcomes and performance objectives for
    adoption, 499
stating outcomes and performance objectives for
    implementation, 501–503
stating outcomes and performance objectives for
    maintenance, 507
peer education change method, 394t
PEN-3 model, 224, 230
perceived barriers determinants, 328t–330t
perceived susceptibility determinants, 328t–330t
performance objective/program outcomes statements
    for adoption, 497–500
    for implementation, 500–506
    It's Your Game . . . Keep It Real project, 519b
    for maintenance, 506–507
performance objectives writing processes
    overview of, 302–303
    using theory as a basis for, 302–303t
    validating performance objectives, 303–304
performance (or change) objectives
    for adolescence consistent and correct condom use,
        296t
    choosing theory- and evidence-based change
        methods to address, 370–398t
    choosing theory- and evidence-based change
        methods to address performance and, 370–398t
    constructing matrices by selecting interventions levels
        and, 309, 310t–312t
    constructing matrices for implementation of,
        507–514, 515t–517t
    dealing with automaticity in the matrix of, 317–318,
        319t
    examples from the Peace of Mind Program (PMP),
        515t–517t
    It's Your Game . . . Keep It Real project, 314–317,
        414t–416t
    It's Your Game . . . Keep It Real project construction
        of implementation matrices on, 519b
    list of action words for writing, 317t
    logic model of change to achieve, 13fig, 15–17
    matrices creates at intersection of at-risk
        determinants and, 283–284
    media advocacy, 184
    planning team addressing any missing, 408–409
    program evaluation using matrices of, 321–330t
    rating importance of determinants to, 306–308, 307t
    specifying those associated with behavioral outcomes,
        294–296
    specifying those associated with environmental
        outcomes, 294, 297–299, 299t
    stating for program use, 497–507
    The ToyBox-Study matrices on personal
        determinants and, 309, 310t, 311t
    using the core processes to write, 299, 301–304
    various levels of change methods for various,
        372–373t
    writing effect evaluation questions on, 549–550
    See also behavioral outcomes; habits; health
        promotion goals; Intervention Mapping tasks (Step
        2); program outcomes

personal determinants. *See* determinants

personalize risk change method, 382*t*

persuasive communication
changing behavior through, 376*t*
theories on, 25*t*

persuasive-communication theories, 25*t*

phones and smartphones
apps as eHealth technology, 370
as communication channel/vehicles, 363*t*
eHealth interventions using, 369–370

photovoice, 242

physical environment asset assessment, 252*t*, 253

pilot-testing program materials
description and process of, 464–465
making sense of the data gathered from, 467–468
purposes and methods used for, 466*t*
reviewing parameters for change methods during the, 467

planned change framework, 162–163

planning coping responses change method
for changing habitual, automatic, and impulsive behaviors, 384*t*
for changing skills, capability, and self-efficacy to overcome barriers, 389*t*

planning. *See* intervention planning; program evaluation planning; work planning groups

PMOST/KIRSCH document readability formula, 452

policymaker evaluation stakeholders, 544*t*

policy/practice environment asset assessment, 252*t*, 253

"population at risk." *See* risk population

power
distinguishing between *power with* and *power over* concepts of, 153
Max Weber on authority, charisma, and legitimacy determinants of, 152, 153
role in the three types of social change, 152
social movements as challenges to *power over* form of, 179–180
used to create change at higher environmental levels, 153
*See also* theories of power

power equity facilitation, 220

PPGIS (public participation GIS), 251

"practice change," 498

pragmatic designs, 572–573

Precaution-Adoption Process Model (PAPM)
for behavior change, 59
for individual intervention level, 61*t*
overview of, 96–97*t*, 99
on unrealistic optimism condition, 96–97

PRECEDE model
of epilepsy health problem, 233–236, 238–239, 240–241
It's Your Game . . . Keep It Real project intervention planning using the, 256*b*–261*b*
logic model (theory) of the problem created by, 13, 14, 211–214, 226, 227*fig*
planning program goals using the, 255
understood as a logic model, 227–229
*See also* logic model of the problem

PRECIS (Pragmatic Explanatory Continuum Indicator Summary), 485, 572*fig*–573

preference determinants (Toy-Boy Study), 310*t*

prejudice (conscious regulation of impulsive stereotyping and prejudice change method), 391*t*

pretesting program materials
description of process for, 464–465
IM Adapt framework on EMI adapted materials, 625, 638–639
making sense of the data gathered from, 467–468
purposes and methods used for, 466*t*
reviewing parameters for change methods during the, 467

primary data collection
appreciative inquiry (AI), 249
Delphi technique, 250–251
description of sources for, 246
ethnographic methods, 248–249
focus groups, 250
geographic methods, 351
interviews, 246
planning groups, 249–250
surveys, 248

"print" narrative material production, 460–461*fig*

priority population
designation "population at risk" of, 229
needs assessment process of describing the, 229–232
*See also* at-risk population

problem-posing education change method, 396*t*

PROCESS computational tool, 577

process evaluation
planning design for, 564–568
selecting and developing measures for, 558–564
writing questions for, 552–558
*See also* effect evaluation

process evaluation design
hybrid designs, 575–576
mediation and moderation analysis, 576–577
mixed methods, 574–575
planning the, 564–568
qualitative methods used for, 565–567
Web analytics used for, 567–568

process evaluation questions
description and purpose of, 552
on fidelity and implementation, 554–557
IYG project, 580*b*, 582*t*–583*t*
on methods and practical applications, 558
on program reach, 558
for program to increase CRCS among U.S. veterans, 552–554*t*
on reasons for implementation performance, 557–558
*See also* questioning process

program champions, 495

program competitors, 544*t*

program components
description and function of, 357–358
It's Your Game . . . Keep It Real project, 409*b*–410*b*, 411*t*–413*t*
task of generating the, 355–356

program design
communication channels and vehicles, 359–364*t*
competency in, 345
decision how to start the, 345–346
description of, 13*fig*
eHealth intervention applications of, 364–370
IM Adapt framework on judging delivery fit, cultural relevance, and, 620–621, 637
perspectives on, 350–355
practical applications for, 348–350
program aspects included in the, 346

program design (*continued*)
  tasks for completing the, 17–18
  theory- and evidence-based change methods used for intervention logic model and, 346–448*fig*
  *See also* Intervention Mapping tasks (Step 3)
program design perspectives
  on enabling creativity to flourish, 350
  on missing methods in literature, 350–351
  on taxonomy of change methods, 355
  on using different methods at different levels of intervention, 352–354
  on using methods correctly, 351–352
program design tasks
  generating program themes, components, scope, and sequence, 355–370, 409*b*–410*b*, 411*t*–413*t*
  choosing theory- and evidence-based change methods to address objectives, 370–398*t*, 410*b*, 414*t*–416*t*
  moving from methods to applications, 398–409
program evaluation
  action words for writing change objectives related to, 317*t*
  cost-effectiveness issue of, 544–545
  It's Your Game . . . Keep It Real project findings of, 583*b*–584*b*
  PRECIS (Pragmatic Explanatory Continuum Indicator Summary) criteria used in, 485
  reasons for, 542–543
  using matrices of change objectives, 321–322
  *See also* evaluation
program evaluation design
  for effect evaluation, 568–574
  emerging designs and analyses for process and effect, 574–577
  IM Adapt framework on choosing the, 641
  It's Your Game . . . Keep It Real project task of, 580*b*
  for process evaluation, 564–568
program evaluation measures
  of behavior and environment, 561–562
  description and purpose of, 558–559
  of determinants, 562–564
  of health and quality of life, 559–561
  IM Adapt framework on choosing indicators and, 640–641
  IYG project indicators and, 580*b*
  selecting and developing, 558–564
  validity and reliability of, 564
program evaluation planning
  competency of, 541
  completing the, 577
  description of, 13*fig*
  with focus on adaptations, 626–629
  IYG project task of completing the, 383*b*, 580*b*
  logic models as fundamental framework used by CDC for, 14
  overview of evaluation and, 32
  perspectives on, 541–546
  the School AIDS Prevention Program plan, 577, 578*t*–579*t*
  tasks required to complete the, 19–20
  *See also* Intervention Mapping tasks (Step 6)
program evaluation planning perspectives
  involving evaluation stakeholders, 543–546
  on reasons for program evaluation, 542–543
  on understanding the program, 541–542
program evaluation questions

effect evaluation questions written from logic models, 546–552
  IM Adapt framework on writing, 640
  IYG project development of indicators and measures for, 580*b*
  IYG project tasks of writing, 580*b*, 582*t*–583*t*
  program process questions, 552–558
program evaluation stakeholders
  considerations when involving the, 543–546
  potential conflict of issue problem with, 545–546
  types listed, 544*t*
program evaluation time frames
  evaluation of a school HIV-prevention program, 550, 551*t*
  writing effect evaluation questions and determining, 550–552
program fit. *See* evidence-based interventions (EBIs) program fit
program goals. *See* health promotion goals
program implementation plan
  description of, 13*fig*
  tasks required for completing the, 18–19
program implementers
  CATCH program use of teachers as environmental agents and, 318–319
  collecting data from, 513
  creating matrices that identify the, 318–319, 320*fig*
  identifying, 494–498*b*
  IM Adapt framework on identifying and including, 492–493, 639
  IM Adapt framework on training, 626, 640
  It's Your Game . . . Keep It Real project identification of, 519*b*
  literature review on characteristics of, 511
  *See also* environmental agents; health educators; opinion leaders
program instruction adaptation, 626, 639
program managers
  as evaluation stakeholder, 544*t*
  interest in the program evaluation by, 545
program materials
  competency in, 435–436
  determining availability of, 449, 451
  determining reading level of, 451–453
  drafting messages, materials, and protocols, 456–464
  hiring and working with creative consultants on the, 453–455
  including presentation of medical terminology as part of the, 459
  It's Your Game . . . Keep It Real project, 468*b*–475*b*
  making adaptations by modifying, 624–625
  Mayor's Project development of, 455*b*
  multimedia approach to, 464
  perspectives on, 436–437
  preparing plans for program materials, 438–455*b*
  pretesting, pilot-testing, refining, and producing, 464–468
  SAM (Suitability Assessment of Materials) for determining suitability of, 449, 450*t*
  videos included in the, 363*t*, 461–464
  visuals and nontext messages included in the, 459–460
  *See also* design documents
program materials perspectives
  designing for implementation, 436–437

using Steps 1, 2, and 3 to complete the Step 4 tasks for, 436

program materials planning
aiming at cultural relevance, 438–440
conducting formative research for, 440–441
creating design document for community processes, 448
developing design documents, 441–448
hiring and working with creative consultants for, 453–455
It's Your Game . . . Keep It Real project, 468b–469b
Mayor's Project process of, 455b
reviewing available material, 448–453

program messages
including visuals as nontext component of the, 459–460
multimedia approach to creating the, 464
process of producing narrative "print" material to convey the, 460–461fig
producing narrative "print" material for, 460–461fig
videos used as part of the, 363t, 461–464
writing the, 456–459
See also health messages

program message writing
cultural perspective on, 458
to enhance cognitive processing, 457–458
issues to consider for, 456–457
presentation of medical terminology included in, 459
translation consideration of, 458–459

program outcome expectations
It's Your Game . . . Keep It Real project determinants of, 325t–330t
methods for changing attitudes, beliefs, and, 385t–386t
Social Cognitive Theory (SCT), on self-efficacy, behavioral capability, and, 109–110, 112

program outcomes
competency in, 283–384
epilepsy PRECEDE model on quality of life and, 234fig, 235–236
IM Adapt framework on, 639, 642
It's Your Game . . . Keep It Real project determinants of expected, 315t–316t
logic model of change used to plan the, 13fig, 15–17, 285fig, 286
perspectives on, 284–286
planning the Mayor's Project, 284b
Social Cognitive Theory (SCT) on self-efficacy, behavioral capability, and, 109–110
stating for program use, 497–507
tasks for, 286–330t
See also behavioral outcomes; performance (or change) objectives

program outcomes/performance objectives statements
for adoption, 497–500
for implementation, 500–506
It's Your Game . . . Keep It Real project, 519b
for maintenance, 506–507

program outcomes perspectives
on continuing with the ecological framework, 284–294
on the logic model of change, 285fig–286

program outcomes tasks
constructing matrices of change objectives, 309–310t
creating a logic model of change, 319–320fig

It's Your Game . . . Keep It Real project process for all of the, 322b–330b
selecting personal determinants, 304–308
stating behavioral and environmental outcomes, 286–304

program planners
constructing matrices of change objectives for implementation, 507–514, 515t–517t
definition of, 3
designing implementation interventions, 514, 518, 526b–528b
identifying program implementers, 494–496b
stating outcomes and performance objectives for program use, 497–507
See also work planning groups

program production
competency in, 435–436
description of, 13fig
It's Your Game . . . Keep It Real project, 468b–475b
perspectives on, 436–437
tasks required for completing the, 18
See also Intervention Mapping tasks (Step 4)

program production perspectives
designing for implementation, 436–437
using Steps 1, 2, and 3 to complete the Step 4 tasks for, 436

program production tasks
drafting messages, materials, and protocols, 456–464
preparing plans for program materials, 438–455b
pretesting, pilot-testing, refining, and producing materials, 464–468
refining program structure and organization, 437–438

program scope
IM Adapt framework on adapting, 626, 639
It's Your Game . . . Keep It Real project, 409b–410b
task of generating the, 355–357
T.L.L. Temple Foundation Stroke Project, 358–359t

program sequence
IM Adapt framework on adapting, 626, 639
It's Your Game . . . Keep It Real project, 409b–410b
task of generating the, 355–356
T.L.L. Temple Foundation Stroke Project, 358–359t

program sponsors, 544t
program staff, 544t

program structure/organization
checking budget and time constraints, 437–438
reaching the intended program participants with the, 437
school curriculum illustration of desired, 438

program themes
description of a, 356–357
It's Your Game . . . Keep It Real project, 409b–410b
task of generating the, 355–356
types of, 357

project work groups. See work planning groups

Protection Motivation Theory (PMT)
as consciousness raising, 78
description of, 75–76
for individual intervention level, 61t

public commitment change method
for changing habitual, automatic, and impulsive behaviors, 384t
for changing skills, capability, and self-efficacy and overcome barriers, 389t

public health
  Advocacy Coalition Framework on, 61t, 189–191
  empowerment defined as "social action process" in, 154
  health promotion goals should relate to, 11
  importance of political ideology in, 190–191
  Multiple Streams Theory on public policy for, 61t, 187–189, 190
  *See also* health
public participation GIS (PPGIS), 251
public policy
  definition of, 184
  function of, 185
  health policy relationship to, 184
  phases and process of, 185–187
  policy/practice environment asset assessment, 252t, 253
  table on change methods for, 397–398t
  timing to coincide with policy windows for change, 398t
  *See also* government intervention level
public policy phases
  policy formation, 185
  policy implementation, 185
  policy modification, 185
  processes of the, 185–187
public policy theories
  Advocacy Coalition Framework, 61t, 189–191, 398t
  Multiple Streams Theory, 61t, 187–189, 190, 397–398t
  overview of, 184–187
  summary on, 191–192
public service announcements (PSAs), 358
public stigma, 114, 115–116
punishment
  changing behavior through, 378t
  classical and operant conditioning with reinforcement and, 67–68

qualitative methods
  comparing quantitative and, 242–243, 244–246
  data collection, 243
  integrating quantitative and, 244fig
  mixed methods for evaluation design use of, 574–575
  for process evaluation design, 565–567
  to select determinants, 306
quality of life
  epilepsy PRECEDE model on health outcomes and, 234fig, 235–236
  HRQOL (health-related quality-of-life), 560
  It's Your Game . . . Keep It Real project task of describing the issue of, 257b–258b
  logic models for, 61–62fig
  primary data sources on, 246, 248–251
  program evaluation measures of, 559–561
  secondary data sources on, 247t–248t
  writing effect evaluation questions on, 548–549
quantitative methods
  comparing qualitative and, 243–246
  data collection, 243–244
  description and function of, 242–243
  integrating qualitative and, 244fig
  mixed methods for evaluation design use of, 574–575
  to select determinants, 306

*Quasi-experimentation: Design and Analysis Issues for Field Settings* (Cook and Campbell), 569
Quebec's 1998 Tobacco Act, 191
questioning process
  examples of posing, 21
  examples of theories for Intervention Mapping steps and, 25t
  as theory and evidence core process, 20
  working list of answers for, 21, 27–28
  *See also* brainstorming answers process; problem evaluation questions
questions types
  at-risk behaviors, 21
  change methods, 21
  determinants, 21
  health problem, 21

race concepts
  race consciousness, 225
  reducing inequalities of class, race, gender and sexuality change method, 391t
racial/ethnicity differences
  epilepsy ratios of, 235
  HIV-associated risk behaviors of African American women, 245
  inequality of breast cancer mortality rates, 630–632
  PEN-3 model constructs for moving beyond labels of, 224, 230
  *See also* African Americans; Hispanic population
racism, 225
  *See also* discrimination and stigma theories
radio channel/vehicle, 362t
raising awareness
  change methods to change risk perception and, 380, 382t–383t
  examples of objectives and methods for condom use and, 371t
  as first step in the change process, 98–99
rates
  health problems described in terms of risk and, 233
  importance and functions of, 233
readability
  ensuring program material, 451–453
  participant literacy and health literacy that may impact, 451–452
reading level assessments
  Flesch-Kincaid grade level, 452
  Flesch Reading Ease score, 452
  focus on literacy and not health literacy by, 453
  Fry Readability Graph, 452
  Microsoft Word protocols used as, 452
  PMOST/KIRSCH document readability formula, 452
  SMOG formula, 452
  *See also* literacy
RE-AIM framework, 119, 489, 490, 611
REALM (Rapid Estimate of Adult Literacy in Medicine), 452
Reasoned Action Approach (RAA)
  change method application using, 403
  distinction between goals, intentions, and beliefs in, 82–83
  guidelines for measuring determinants, 82
  for identifying determinants of behavior, 59
  for individual intervention level, 61t
  overview of, 81

on three ways to influence the perceived norms in, 83–84

reattribution training change method, 388*t*

regulations and laws change method, 398*t*

reinforcement
   changing behavior through, 377*t*
   classical conditioning using, 66–67
   contingent rewards change method form of, 389*t*
   as effective method to create changes, 69–70
   operant conditioning using, 67–68
   three types of directly applied, 70

relapse prevention
   attributional retraining and, 100–101
   attribution theory and, 61*t*, 99–100, 101

relatedness need, 108

relationships
   health status link to extend and nature of social, 156–157
   social network theory on, 61*t*, 155–156, 159
   social support theory on, 61*t*, 156–159
   *See also* social networks

relevance intervention method, 112

reliability (evaluation measures), 564

Research-tested Intervention Programs (RTIPs)
   [National Cancer Institute], 599, 608, 611, 634

resistance to social pressure change method, 387*t*

reviewing findings. *See* literature review

rewards (contingent) change method, 389*t*

risk communication
   for individual intervention level, 61*t*
   stages theories on effects of, 97–98
   *See also* communication; health messages

risk factors
   describing health problems causes and, 236–239
   health problems described in terms of rates and, 233
   probability sensitive to the period of time of observation, 233
   *See also* at-risk behaviors; environmental conditions/factors

risk perception
   change methods to change awareness and, 380, 382*t*–383*t*
   examples of objectives and methods for condom use and, 371*t*
   framing to shift, 397*t*
   Health Belief Model (HBM) on health behaviors based on, 61*t*, 62–63, 74–75, 78
   moving from method to application by dispensing information on, 402–403
   *See also* beliefs

risk population. *See* at-risk population

risk-reduction behaviors, 287

RTIPs (Research-tested Intervention Programs)
   [National Cancer Institute], 599, 608, 611, 634

St. Luke's Episcopal Hospital Institutional Review Board, 641

SAM (Suitability Assessment of Materials), 449, 450*t*

scenario-based risk information change method, 382*t*

School Health Advisory Council (SHAC), 519*b*

school programs
   Dutch HIV/AIDS-Prevention Program, 371, 400–401, 577, 578*t*–579*t*
   evaluation of a school HIV-prevention program, 550, 551*t*

iCHAMPSS Model (Choosing and Maintaining Programs for Sex Education in Schools), 367

Incredible Years BASIC Parent Program, 576

Partners in School Asthma Management Program, 309

School Health Advisory Council (SHAC) role in, 519*b*

The ToyBox-Study on, 292, 298–299*t*, 309, 310*t*–312*t*

*See also* adolescents; children; It's Your Game . . . Keep It Real (IYG) project

screening tests
   breast cancer, 34*t*, 173, 243, 252
   colorectal cancer, 243, 245–246, 252
   as health-promoting behavior, 288

self-affirmation change method, 383*t*

Self-Affirmation Theory, 77

self-control
   self-management "strength model" for, 106
   theories of self-regulation on, 25*t*, 61*t*, 105–109

Self-Determination Theory (SDT)
   for individual intervention level, 61*t*
   on nudging and role of autonomous decision making, 94
   overview of, 107–108
   on three basic needs at core of human motivation, 108

self-efficacy
   attributional retraining and relapse prevention role of, 100–101
   attribution theory and relapse prevention role of, 99–100
   Communication-Persuasion Matrix (CPM) on receiver's changes in, 101
   competence need as similar to, 108
   as a coping with stigma determinant, 116
   Elaboration Likelihood Model (ELM) on persuasion effects on, 102–104
   It's Your Game . . . Keep It Real project determinants of, 315*t*–316*t*, 325*t*–330*t*
   overcome barriers and influence skills, capability, and, 387–390
   Social Cognitive Theory (SCT) on, 109–110, 112
   ToyBox-Study personal determinants of, 310*t*, 311*t*–312*t*
   *See also* collective efficacy

self-management behaviors
   adherence (compliance) and, 288–289
   self-management "strength model," 106
   *See also* theories of self-regulation

self-management "strength model," 106

self-monitoring change method, 388*t*

self-reevaluation change method, 382*t*

self-regulatory theories. *See* theories of self-regulation

self-stigma, 114

Semantic Network Theory, 71

sense-making change method, 395*t*

serious gaming interventions, 368–369

set graded tasks change method, 389*t*

sexuality
   reducing inequalities of class, race, gender and sexuality change method, 391*t*
   risk behaviors associated with adolescent, 22*t*, 245, 258*b*–260*b*

sexually transmitted infections (STIs)
   among African American and Hispanic youth, 258*b*
   chlamydia infection/fear arousal change method, 404–405

sexually transmitted infections (STIs) (*continued*)
  examples of objectives and methods for changing
    awareness and risk perception of condom use to
    prevent, 371*t*
  iCHAMPSS Model (Choosing and Maintaining
    Programs for Sex Education in Schools) to prevent,
    367
  identifying the population at risk for, 231
  increasing condom use by adolescents to prevent, 22*t*
  It's Your Game . . . Keep It Real project goals to
    reduce, 260*b*–261*b*
  performance objectives for adolescence consistent
    and correct condom use to prevent, 296*t*
  *See also* HIV/AIDS epidemic
sexual risk behaviors
  increasing condom use among adolescents to prevent
    STIs due to, 22*t*
  It's Your Game . . . Keep It Real project description of
    adolescent, 258*b*–260*b*
  qualitative study on HIV/AIDS and lack of condom
    use, 245
  *See also* HIV/AIDS epidemic
shifting focus change method, 387*t*
Short-TOFHLA (Test of Functional Health Literacy in
    Adults), 452
skills
  change methods for overcoming barriers and
    influencing, 387–390
  Elaboration Likelihood Model (ELM) on promoting
    information processing, 73
  It's Your Game . . . Keep It Real project determinants
    of, 315*t*–316*t*, 325*t*–330*t*
smartphones and phones
  apps as eHealth technology, 370
  as communication channel/vehicle, 363*t*
  eHealth interventions using, 369–370
SMOG formula assessment, 452
smoking prevention. *See* tobacco control
social action
  as change method, 396*t*
  community organization model of, 175
  overview and examples of, 178
  public health empowerment defined as "social action
    process," 153
  role of power in three types of, 152
social capital
  age-adjusted mortality association with, 170
  bonding, bridging, and linking types of, 170
  community capacity related to and inclusive of,
    170–171
  definitions and meanings of, 169–170
social capital theory
  community intervention level using, 61*t*
  on social capital and community capacity, 169–172
social change
  public health empowerment defined as "social action
    process" for, 153
  role of power in three types of, 152
Social Cognitive Theory (SCT)
  for behavior change, 59
  on behavior change, 111–112
  description of the, 109
  determinants of, 65, 113
  implementation and dissemination application of, 486

importance of determinants to performance
    objectives in, 308
  Integrated Behavioral Model (IBM) also reflected in,
    81
  on interpersonal environment, 61*t*
  It's Your Game . . . Keep It Real project application of,
    324*b*
  on outcome expectations, self-efficacy, and behavioral
    capability, 109–110, 112
  PAPM incorporation of determinants and methods
    for change from, 96
  on psychological mechanisms by which diffusion
    occurs, 118
  self-efficacy as central construct of, 306
  summary of, 113
  tailoring, relevance, and individualization, 112
social comparison change method, 387*t*
social environmental asset assessment, 252*t*, 253
social influence
  table on methods for changing, 386–387*t*
  ToyBox-Study personal determinants of, 311*t*–312*t*
social media
  for communication channels/vehicles, 364*t*
  eHealth interventions using, 367–368
  The Heart Truth Campaign on, 368
social movements
  as challenging *power over*, 179
  framing of, 179–180
social networks
  community coalitions, 61*t*, 168–169
  enhancing network linkages change method, 394*t*
  influencing social norms by mobilizing, 173
  mobilizing social networks change method, 393*t*
  social capital and community capacity of, 61*t*,
    169–172
  table on methods for changing social support and,
    386, 394*t*
  *See also* relationships
social network theory
  interpersonal environment intervention using, 61*t*
  overview of, 155–156
  summary on, 159
social norms
  behavioral journalism role in changing, 173
  definition of, 172
  influence on behavioral outcomes of subjective and
    actual, 308
  It's Your Game . . . Keep It Real project determinants
    of gender role, 325*t*–327*t*
  It's Your Game . . . Keep It Real project determinants
    of perceived, 315*t*–316*t*
  mass media portrayals of, 172–173
  mobilizing social networks to influence, 173
  RAA and TPB on ways to influence the perceived,
    83–84
  tables on change methods for changing, 390, 393*t*
  *See also* beliefs
social norms theories
  community intervention level using, 61*t*
  description and summary of, 172–173
social (or vicarious) learning, 69
social planning case method, 397*t*
social planning community organization model, 175
social pressure resistance change method, 387*t*
social support interventions

altering the network itself by changing the network type of, 157

description of, 159

method for changing influence by mobilizing social support, 387t

peer-to-peer interaction to create message diffusion type of, 157

segmentation to identify groups of people to change at same time type of, 157

tables on change methods for changing, 391, 394t

used to increase social support, 157–159

using network data to identify champions for change type of, 157

social support theory

interpersonal environment intervention using, 61t

overview of, 156–157

on social support interventions, 157–159

summary on, 159

societal and governmental theories

Advocacy Coalition Framework, 61t, 189–191, 398t

description of, 184

Multiple Streams Theory, 61t, 187–189, 190, 397–398t

public policy theories, 184–192

societal environmental outcomes

identifying and stating, 294

to reduce stigma and promote HIV testing, 298–299, 301t

See also environment levels

societal intervention level

Advocacy Coalition Framework for, 61t, 189–191, 398t

environmental outcomes at the, 294, 298–299, 301t

methods for changing social influence, 386–387t

Multiple Streams Theory for, 61t, 187–189, 190, 397–398t

table on change methods, 397–398t

theories impacting governmental and, 61t, 184–191

See also intervention levels

Society for Public Health Education (SOPHE)

on diverse participation in development of interventions, 11–12

ethical and professional guidelines for public health educations by, 11

socioecological models, 8–10

SQUIRE (Standards for QUality Improvement in Reporting Excellence), 577

stage theories

overview of, 95

Precaution-Adoption Process Model (PAPM), 96–97t, 99

on raising awareness, 98–99

on risk communication, 97–98

stage theory of organizational change/diffusion of innovation, 163–166

summary on, 99

Transtheoretical Model of Behavior Change (TTM), 61t, 81, 95–96, 99

stakeholders

increasing stakeholder influence change method, 395t

involving evaluation, 543–546

meaningful participation by, 214

questions to guide work groups in recruitment of, 215–216t

stakeholder analysis to identify, 166–167

"wicked problems" and, 10

stakeholder theory

organization intervention level using, 61t

overview and summary of, 166–167

Statistical Analysis System (SAS), 577

Statistical Package for the Social Sciences (SPSS), 577

stereotype-inconsistent information change method, 391t

stereotyping

conscious regulation of impulsive stereotyping and prejudice change method, 391t

reducing public stigma using stereotype-inconsistent information change method, 391t

reducing stigmatization by conscious repression of, 115

as unaware attitude, 90

stigma

definition of, 113

how to reduce stigmatization and, 114–116

social-psychological and sociological views on, 113–114

specifying performance objectives to promote HIV testing and reduce, 298–301t, 302

tables on change methods to reduce public, 391t

theories of discrimination and, 113–116

stigma by association, 114

stigma types

AIDS-related stigma, 115

public, 114, 115–116

self-stigma, 114

stigma by association, 114

structural stigma, 114

stimulus control change method, 384t

"strength model" of self-management, 106

structural redesign change method, 395t

structural stigma, 114

Student Nonviolent Coordinating Committee (SNCC), 178

Students for a Democratic Society (SDS), 178

subjective norms, 308

summative evaluation (evidence-based interventions, EBIs), 602

surface structure of culture, 439–440

survey data collection, 248

synthesis action words, 317t

systems

literature review on characteristics of systems, 511–513

systems change method, 392t

systems theory

complex adaptive systems (CASs), 149–150

Intervention Mapping and systems thinking, 8–10

as multilevel theory, 61t, 149–151

on processes for changing systems, 150–151

summary on, 151

TAAG program participatory implementation planning, 493

tailoring intervention method

changing behavior through, 377t

description of, 112

Watch, Discover, Think, and Act asthma computer instruction as, 112

target participants (evaluation stakeholders), 544t

taxonomy of change methods, 355

team building and human relations training, 395*t*
technical assistance change method, 393*t*
telephone
   as communication channel/vehicles, 363*t*
   health interventions using the, 369–370
   TLC (telephone linked communication) system, 369
telephone-counseling program
   adaptation "to-do list" for, 618, 619*t*–620*t*
   examples from design document template for the, 621, 622*t*–623*t*
television channel/vehicle, 363*t*
Texas Department of State Health Services, 257*b*
text comprehension, 71–73
theatre channel/vehicle, 363*t*
theories/evidence/change methods tables
   behavior change, 378*t*, 380
   change attitudes, beliefs, and outcome expectations, 385*t*–386*t*
   change awareness and risk perception, 380, 382*t*–383*t*
   change communities, 395–397*t*
   change habitual, automatic, and impulsive behaviors, 380, 383*t*–384*t*
   change of environmental conditions, 390, 392*t*–393*t*
   change organizations, 394–395*t*
   change policy, 397–398*t*
   change social norms, 390, 393*t*
   change social support and social networks, 391–394*t*
   changing social influence, 386–387*t*
   how to use the, 379–380
   increase knowledge, 380, 381*t*
   influence skills, capability, and self-efficacy and overcome barriers, 387–390
   reduce public stigma, 390, 391*t*
theories of automatic behavior and habits
   dual-systems models, 61*t*, 90–91
   on habits as automatic behavior, 92–93
   for individual intervention level, 61*t*
   nudging used to make desired behavior easier, 93–94
   overview of, 89–90
   summary of, 94–95
   training executive function using, 91–92
theories of goal-directed behavior
   on characteristics of goals, 86
   goal-setting theory, 61*t*, 85–88
   on implementation intentions, 86–88
   for individual intervention level, 61*t*
   overview of, 84–85
   summary on, 88
   on unconscious goal pursuit, 88
theories of health behavior
   Extended Parallel Process Model (EPPM), 61*t*, 76, 78
   on framing health messages, 77–78
   Health Belief Model (HBM), 61*t*, 62–63, 74–75, 78
   Protection Motivation Theory (PMT), 61*t*, 75–76, 78
   on using fear to change risk behavior, 76–77
Theories of Information Processing
   on cues to retrieve information from memory, 73–74
   on elaboration to enhance learning and memory, 73
   examples of Intervention Mapping steps and questions that apply, 25*t*
   for individual intervention level, 61*t*
   on memorizing through chunking, 71
   Mental Model Theory, 71
   overview of, 70–71
   Semantic Network Theory, 71

summary of, 74
   on text comprehension and learning, 71–73
theories of persuasive communication
   Communication-Persuasion Matrix (CPM), 61*t*, 101–102
   on cultural similarity, 102
   Elaboration Likelihood Model (ELM), 61*t*, 73, 102–105
   summary of, 105
theories of power
   Intervention Mapping step, question, and, 25*t*
   as multilevel theory, 61*t*
   overview of, 151–153
   summary on, 153
   on using power to create change at higher environmental levels, 153
   *See also* power
Theories of Reasoned Action (TRA)
   on anticipated regret, 80–81
   for individual intervention level, 61*t*
   Integrated Behavioral Model (IBM), 61*t*, 81
   overview of the, 78–79
   Reasoned Action Approach (RAA), 59, 61*t*, 81–84, 403
   summary on, 84
   Theory of Planned Behavior (TPB), 61*t*, 78, 79–80, 82, 83–84, 324*b*
theories of self-regulation
   importance of determinants to performance objectives in, 308
   for individual intervention level, 61*t*
   Intervention Mapping step, question, and, 25*t*
   interventions based on self-regulation, 106–107
   Motivational Interviewing (MI), 108–109
   overview of, 105–106
   Self-Determination Theory (SDT), 61*t*, 94, 107–108
   summary on, 109
   *See also* self-management behaviors
theories of stigma and discrimination
   description of, 113
   on interpersonal environment, 61*t*
   on reducing stigmatization, 114–116
   social-psychological and sociological views on stigma, 113–114
   summary of, 116
theory
   comparing theories of change and explanatory theories, 66
   ecological models and systems thinking, 8–10
   examples of theories for Intervention Mapping steps and questions, 25*t*
   health promotion intervention effectiveness through, 11
   introduction to Intervention Mapping, 7–8
   program design based on change methods based on, 346–348*fig*
   *See also* behavior-oriented theories; constructs; environmental-oriented theories; implementation frameworks
theory and evidence processes
   posing questions, 20, 21
   brainstorming answers, 20, 21–23
   reviewing findings from empirical literature and evidence-based answers, 20, 23–24
   accessing and using theory, 20, 25–26

theory application
description of the, 25–26
examples of theories for Intervention Mapping steps and questions, 25*t*
implementation interventions to increase program use as, 485–487*fig*
as theory and evidence core process, 20
theory-based change methods
choosing to address program objectives, 370–398*t*
description of, 370
moving to applications from, 398–408*t*
overview of evidence-based and, 346–348*fig*
Precaution-adoption Process Model (PAMA), 96, 97*t*
Self-Determination Theory (SDT), 61*t*, 107–108
social network and social support theories, 159
tables of methods for changing behavior, 375–398*t*
theories of health behavior on using fear to change at-risk behaviors, 76–77
Theories of Information Processing, 25*t*, 61*t*, 70–74
theories of organizational change, 61*t*
*See also* change methods; evidence-based change methods
theory-based change method selection
issues to consider and examples of, 370–371*t*
It's Your Game . . . Keep It Real project, 410*b*, 416*b*
Mayor's Project example of, 374*b*–375*b*
roles, determinants, and change methods for environmental conditions, 372–373*t*
tables of methods for changing behavior, 375–398*t*
using core processes for, 373–374
Theory of Planned Behavior (TPB)
ecological levels linked in, 65–66
guidelines for measuring determinants, 82
for individual intervention level, 61*t*
It's Your Game . . . Keep It Real project application of, 324*b*
on three ways to influence the perceived norms in, 83–84
theory of the problem and theory of change (logic model diagram), 14
time frames
evaluation of a school HIV-prevention program, 550, 551*t*
program structure and organization task of checking any constraints on the, 437–438
writing effect evaluation questions and determining evaluation, 550–552
time series designs, 571
TLC (telephone linked communication) system, 369
T.L.L. Temple Foundation Stroke Project
constructing matrices of change objects for intervention level, 309
design documents from the, 442*t*–443*t*
identifying organizational environment outcomes, 293, 300*t*
specifying performance objectives for environmental outcomes, 298–299
translating change method into application by the, 407–408*t*
Tobacco Act (1998, Quebec), 191
tobacco control
ASPIRE (A Smoking Prevention Interactive Experience), 367
differing intervention levels applied to, 38

Healthy Neighborhoods Project (Contra Costa County Health Services Department) efforts for, 178
ideological arguments to benefit, 191
multilevel interventions for, 147
Multiple Streams Theory applied to, 180
normative influences of tobacco industry on, 80
persuasive arguments on health consequences of tobacco used for, 104
program design matching different intervention levels with change methods for, 353–354
Quebec's 1998 Tobacco Act, 191
tobacco use
matching change methods to intervention levels to address adolescent, 353–354
overestimation of proportion of youth, 308
TOFHLA (Test of Functional Health Literacy in Adults), 452
The ToyBox-Study
constructing matrices of change objectives and intervention levels, 309, 310*t*–312*t*
identifying interpersonal and organizational environment outcomes in the, 292, 299*t*
multiple environmental levels of the, 372
specifying performance objectives for environmental outcomes, 298
training executive function change method, 384*t*
translated program materials, 458–459
Transtheoretical Model of Behavior Change (TTM)
for individual intervention level, 61*t*
Integrated Behavioral Model (IBM) reflected in, 81
overview of, 95–96, 99
TV viewing hours, 237–238
Twitter, 368

unconditioned response (UR), 66–67
unconditioned stimulus (UCS), 66–67
United Farm Workers movement, 178
unrealistic optimism, 96–97
U.S. Department of Agriculture, 287
U.S. Department of Health and Human Services, 102, 286, 287
U.S. Department of Health and Human Services Office of Adolescent Health, 528*b*
U.S. Department of Labor, 9
U.S. Food and Drug Administration, 293
U.S. Preventive Services Task Force, 288
U.S. Substance Abuse and Mental Health Services Administration's National Registry of Evidence-based Programs and Practices, 599–600

validity
evaluation designs that promote external, 571–574
of evaluation measures, 564
value-expectancy theories, 25*t*
verbal persuasion change method, 388*t*
Veterans Administration (VA) dissemination and implementation (D&I) workgroup, 485
vicarious (or social) learning, 69
videos
as a communication channel and vehicle, 363*t*
creating a multimedia program that includes, 464
scripts, script treatments, and storyboards for production of, 463–464

videos (*continued*)
  securing contracts and budget for production of,
    462–463
  tasks for producing a program message, 461–462*fig*
visuals
  characteristics of effective, 460
  included to help convey the program messages,
    459–460
  videos included as part of the program, 363*t*, 461–464

Watch, Discover, Think, and Act asthma computer
  application, 112
Web-based computer-tailored intervention
  description and advantages of, 364–367
  developing tailored feedback, 365, 366*fig*
websites
  for full EBIs (evidence-based interventions), 611,
    612*t*–613*t*
  for general intervention strategies, 611–614
"Where Science Meets Advocacy" (Corrigan and
  Kosyluk), 115
"wicked problems," 10
W.K. Kellogg Foundation, 14
women
  autonomy in sexual contexts and opportunity to
    protect health of, 180
  Cultivando La Salud cancer screening intervention
    for, 252
  HIV-associated risk behaviors of African American,
    245
  HOPE project focusing on young Cambodian girls
    living in the U.S., 159
  participatory approach to implementation planning
    of TAAG program for girls, 493
  predicting cervical cancer screening in Ghana of, 24
  racial/ethnic inequalities of breast cancer mortality
    rates among, 630–631
  reflection-action-reflection cycle in public policy for
    Chinese, 174
  social norms theory on encouraging mammograms
    by, 173
  study on colorectal and breast cancer screening by
    farm-working 50 years and older, 243, 252
  UCS and body satisfaction by, 67
  U.S. programs using Intervention Mapping in breast
    cancer screening for, 34*t*
work group culture
  considering the, 222–225

exploring and working in another culture, 224–225
  exploring personal ethnocentricity, 223–224
work group facilitation processes
  communication, 219*t*
  maintenance and team-building functions, 219*t*
  task functions, 219*t*
work group management processes
  for consensus, 222
  creating a timeline fro, 218
  facilitation, 218, 220
  for idea generation, 220–222
  overview of, 217–218
working list of answers
  description of developing a, 27–28
  as theory and evidence process, 21
work planning groups
  collecting primary data from, 249–250
  composing and maintaining, 215–217
  considering culture in the, 222–225
  ensuring participation in program planning by,
    214–215
  generating program themes, components, scope, and
    sequence, 355–370
  group management processes for productive,
    217–222
  identification of health-promoting behaviors by,
    16–17
  It's Your Game . . . Keep It Real project task with, 256*b*
  Mayor's Project, 235*b*–236*b*
  principles of collaboration used by, 214–215
  questions to guide recruitment of stakeholders,
    215–216*t*
  *See also* Intervention Mapping tasks (Step 1);
    intervention planning; program planners
work planning group tasks
  conducting a needs assessment, 226–251
  describing the context for the intervention, 251–254
  establishing and working with a planning group,
    214–226*b*
  preparing plans for program materials, 438–455*b*
  producing narrative "print" material to convey
    program messages, 460–461*fig*
  producing videos used for program message, 461–464
  stating program goals, 254–261*b*
World Health Organization (WHO), 11, 94, 247*t*

YouTube, 368